Major Complications of Female Pelvic Surgery

Mitchel Hoffman • Tracy L. Hull
Bernard H. Bochner
Editors

Major Complications of Female Pelvic Surgery

A Multidisciplinary Approach

Springer

Editors
Mitchel Hoffman
Moffitt Cancer Center
USF Morsani College of Medicine
Tampa, FL, USA

Tracy L. Hull
Department of Colorectal Surgery
Cleveland Clinic
Cleveland, OH, USA

Bernard H. Bochner
Urology Service, Department of Surgery
Memorial Sloan Kettering Cancer
Center
New York, NY, USA

ISBN 978-3-031-66771-8 ISBN 978-3-031-66772-5 (eBook)
https://doi.org/10.1007/978-3-031-66772-5

This Springer imprint is published by the registered company Springer Nature Switzerland AG
The registered company address is: Gewerbestrasse 11, 6330 Cham, Switzerland

This book is dedicated to all pelvic surgeons: past, present, and future. To the surgeons who came before us, thank you for your mentorship, generosity, and paving the way. To the surgeons who are and will be operating in the female pelvis, we hope the information contained in this book will be of some help. You will inevitably encounter difficulties associated with this challenging and complex anatomic region and the pelvic diseases and disorders that our female patients suffer from.

Foreword

The pelvis is one of the most complex areas in the human body. It involves vascular, nerve, lymphatic as well as urologic, gynecologic, and GI structures. Over the years, medicine has evolved to address each of these organ systems by discipline. However, any of us who has ever ventured surgically into the pelvis recognizes that one discipline can easily spill over into another. The book *Major Complications of Female Pelvic Surgery: A Multi-Disciplinary Approach* is edited by three international experts from different disciplines involving gynecology, urology, and colorectal surgery. They have combined their expertise and years of experience to focus on possible complications that might arise from pelvic surgery. One of the unique features of this book is the emphasis on anatomy and prevention of possible complications. Each chapter is worth careful reading, since prevention is much easier than treatment of any given complication. The co-editors have assembled an adept panel of experts who focus on a multi-disciplinary approach to prevent potential complications, recognition of the complication if it occurs, and then a multi-disciplinary approach to ideal management of the situation. Frequently, different approaches to the management of a complication are presented to broaden the effectiveness of techniques that might be applied in any situation. I would imagine that this book will quickly become a reference guide for any surgeon who performs surgery in the pelvis.

As a Cancer Center Director and Surgical Oncologist, I have been a proponent of a multi-disciplinary approach to oncologic care. The entire premise of this book is to provide expert opinions from different disciplines to provide ideal advice for prevention, recognition, and management of possible complications. This book will become a "must read" for anyone who endeavors to take on the challenge of a complex pelvic surgery. The patient who requires surgical intervention in the pelvis will be the ultimate beneficiary of this publication.

Timothy J. Eberlein

Cancer Programs
Washington University School of Medicine
St. Louis, MO, USA

The Alvin J. Siteman Cancer Center At Barnes-Jewish Hospital
Washington University School of Medicine
St. Louis, MO, USA

Preface

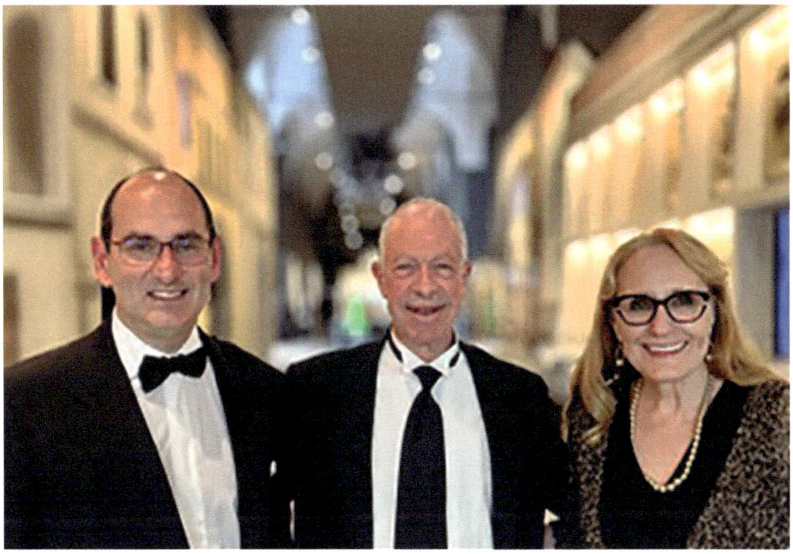

The editors of this book have a long-term friendship that started with our mutual interests in, and shared struggles with, pelvic surgery. Our specialties are different (gynecology, urology, colorectal surgery), but we have consistently encountered many of the same challenges when operating in the female pelvis. An unfortunate but very significant part of these shared experiences are the major complications that occur in association with pelvic surgery. As our careers have progressed, we have noted a transdisciplinary comradery among pelvic surgeons regarding the ever-present, looming potential for the serious morbidity that may occur in association with the operations we perform. Our days in the operating room are generally rewarding, sometimes stressful, and very occasionally unsuccessful.

We try our best and help women, but complications do occur…never intentionally and most often unavoidably. Complications of surgery and the resulting suffering that the patient experiences stay with us. They haunt us during surgery and in the middle of the night.

Being a surgeon carries with it great responsibilities to our patients. They trust that we know what we are doing and will always do our best. They deserve nothing less.

Understanding that despite our skill and best efforts there will be complications, we as surgeons must be committed to life-long learning and constantly seeking to enhance our knowledge, skills, and dedication to prevent or manage these potential adverse outcomes. The three editors of this book have learned much from each other regarding the importance of drawing from the knowledge and experience of each other's disciplines. It is with this in mind that we decided to produce a multidisciplinary book specifically about major complications of female pelvic surgery.

Tampa, FL, USA Mitchel Hoffman
Cleveland, OH, USA Tracy L. Hull
New York, NY, USA Bernard H. Bochner

Acknowledgments

Most surgeons have been the fortunate recipients of career mentorship. Mentors may themselves be surgeons or might have provided some other type of guidance. We often think of such people as those who had a significant positive impact on us during our development as surgeons. However, ongoing mentorship supports professional growth throughout our careers. It is impossible to overstate the importance and profound influence mentors have on our professional growth and development, as well as emotional health. We readily acknowledge a great debt and gratitude to all of our mentors, past and present. These individuals guided the editors and authors to gain the knowledge, experience, and judgement that went into the writing of this book. With this writing, we hope to pay it forward.

Colleagues support the many facets of our daily professional lives. They listen, have our backs, are our clinical sounding board, and understand better than anyone our daily professional struggles. Colleagues are our professional family. We acknowledge them for all of their support and for undoubtedly shaping many of the ideas put forward in this book.

Eugenia Judson, Production Editor for this book, has been outstanding to work with. She has been responsive, patient, and diligent. We very much enjoyed working with Eugene and greatly appreciate all of her efforts that helped bring this book to fruition.

Margaret Moore, Senior Editor for Clinical Medicine at Springer, believed in the concept and importance of this book and was extremely supportive throughout the entire process. Margaret also gave us the leeway needed to adjust to unanticipated challenges with coverage of material, and this ultimately resulted in substantially improved content.

The publishers assigned a team of artists to this book. The outstanding quality of the illustrations done by this team was a very pleasant surprise. We had conceptualized basic black and white line drawings but the artists instead returned our crude examples and instructions with beautiful, meticulous, and accurate color illustrations. We are most appreciative of the artistic talent and dedication of this team. This appreciation also extends to the publishers for providing and supporting their services.

The authors and co-authors of the chapters are the backbone of this book. Their knowledge, experience, and dedication to pelvic surgery are clearly demonstrated in each chapter. It was an honor to work with them. It is with heartfelt acknowledgement that it is these authors who have graciously passed on this wealth of information to the benefit of other pelvic surgeons and the patients they care for.

Most importantly we wish to acknowledge the vital role that our families and loved ones have played in allowing us to focus and spend the time necessary to develop our careers.

We are forever grateful for their patience, understanding, and forgiveness. We know that our lives, career, and indeed this book would not be possible if not for their never-ending support.

Introduction

The pelvis is a confined space where portions of the urinary, genital, and intestinal tract become intimately associated. Surrounding these organ systems is an extensive neural network and the major vascular supply to the pelvic organs and lower extremities. Supporting the pelvic organs with their innervations are the pelvic bones, ligaments, and muscles. The major surgical disciplines that operate within the pelvis are urology, gynecology, and colorectal surgery. A wide range of extirpative and reconstructive procedures are performed by pelvic surgeons. Other disciplines operate within the pelvis as well, including general, oncologic, orthopedic, pediatric, vascular, and plastic surgeons as well as neurosurgeons.

Diseases and other abnormalities within the confines of the pelvis frequently affect more than one organ system as well as the surrounding neurovascular structures. Less commonly, tumor extends to the boney pelvis. The intimate relationships within the pelvis preclude a clear separation of the pelvic surgical disciplines. Complications of pelvic surgery are common to all of these disciplines. All surgeons who perform pelvic operations must have a clear understanding of the complications that may arise and their prevention, recognition, and management. As pelvic diseases and abnormalities cross organ systems and disciplines, so do the complications that arise from their surgical management.

Each pelvic surgical discipline has a range of capabilities for managing operative complications. However, a multidisciplinary approach may at times be required. In some instances, the various surgical disciplines have developed specialty-specific methodology for managing similar complications.

For the reasons described above, pelvic surgery by its very nature is multidisciplinary. The editors of this book are from the three pelvic surgical disciplines mentioned. The contribution of chapters are by experts from these same specialties as well as the extended surgical disciplines who operate on the often challenging conditions in this complex region of female anatomy.

The main objective of this book is to give a multidisciplinary perspective on complications of female pelvic surgery.

Contents

Part I General Perioperative Considerations

1 **Perioperative Venous Thromboembolism** 3
Kristen A. Ban, Stefan D. Holubar, and Daniel L. Clarke-Pearson

2 **Modern-Enhanced Recovery After Surgery (ERAS) for Major Pelvic Surgery** 13
Leilei Xia and Siamak Daneshmand

3 **Frailty** 23
Armin Shahrokni

4 **Nutrition for the Surgical Patient** 31
Richard A. Jacobson, Ankita Mishra, and Sean P. Dineen

Part II Lower Genital Tract

5 **Uterine Surgery for Infertility** 43
Jensen Reckhow and Zaraq Khan

6 **Hysterectomy** 61
Jessica Selle and John Gebhart

7 **Genital Tract Prolapse** 73
Brittany L. Roberts and Rebecca G. Rogers

Part III Lower Urinary Tract

8 **Operations for Stress Urinary Incontinence** 83
Lauren M. Conroy and O. Lenaine Westney

9 **Urethral Diverticulectomy** 93
Richard Lee and Leo Dreyfuss

10 **Segmental or Total Female Urethrectomy** 103
Kirolos N. Meilika and Jaspreet S. Sandhu

11 **Transurethral Bladder Surgery** 117
Joshua J. Meeks

12 Partial Cystectomy 123
Óscar Rodríguez Faba, Alberto Breda, and Joan Palou

13 Complications of Radical Cystectomy 129
Kelly R. Pekala and Bernard H. Bochner

14 Complications in Orthotopic Neobladders 137
Kathrin Meisterhofer, Bastian Amend, and Arnulf Stenzl

15 Continent Cutaneous Urinary Diversion in Women 145
Jakob Klemm, Malte W. Vetterlein, and Margit Fisch

16 Complications of Ileal Conduit Urinary Diversion: A Comprehensive Review 157
Timothy Donahue and Charissa Chu

Part IV Upper Urinary Tract

17 Injury Repair of Pelvic Ureter 167
Kyrollis Attalla and John P. Sfakianos

18 Ureteroscopy 175
Jonathan Modai and Matthew D. Dunn

Part V Anus and Rectum

19 Transanal Local Excisions and Endoluminal Approaches 189
Kamil Erozkan and Emre Gorgun

20 Perianal Abscess and Fistula 207
Valery Vilchez and Amy L. Lightner

21 Fecal Incontinence 221
Anna R. Spivak

22 Operations for Rectal Prolapse 231
Jennifer Shearer, Brooke Gurland, and Caitlin Bungo

Part VI Miscellaneous

23 Complications of Minimally Invasive Surgery 245
Dandi Huang and Kenneth H. Kim

24 Composite Pelvic Resection for Deeply Infiltrating Endometriosis 255
Aparna R. Ramanathan, Rebecca E. Thompson, Elissa Trieu, and Vadim Morozov

25 Inflammatory Bowel Disease 265
Scott A. Strong

26 Complications of Resection of Retroperitoneal Tumors in the Female Pelvis 275
Emmanuel Zervos and Nasreen A. Vohra

Part VII Pregnancy

27 **Cesarean Section** 291
Anthony Kendle and Haywood Brown

28 **Management of Ectopic Pregnancy and Surgical Considerations** 301
Theresa Fisher and Kristin Powell

29 **Surgical Abortion** 309
Christy M. Boraas and Jessika A. Ralph

30 **Cesarean Hysterectomy** 319
Brett D. Einerson and Andrew P. Soisson

Part VIII Cancer

31 **Inguinal Lymphadenectomy, Radical Vulvectomy** 333
Clarissa Lam and Mario M. Leitao

32 **Pelvic and Paraaortic Lymphadenectomy** 351
Mitchel Hoffman, Murray Shames, and Bernard H. Bochner

33 **Radical Hysterectomy** 363
Mitchel Hoffman, Nadim Bou Zgheib, Monica Avila, and Jing-Yi Chern

34 **Composite Pelvic Resection for Ovarian Cancer** 377
Beverly Long and William A. Cliby

35 **Anal Cancer** 387
Anne Macleod and Susan Galandiuk

36 **Rectal and Rectosigmoid Carcinoma** 401
Michelle DeLeon and Luca Stocchi

37 **Pelvic Radiation Therapy** 417
Sudha Amarnath

38 **Pelvic Exenteration for Central Pelvic Cancer** 427
Desmond P. Barton, Owen M. Heath, Rasheed Shahnawaz, Qiu Sheng, Thompson Alan, and Kumar Pardeep

39 **Resection of Recurrent Pelvic Sidewall Tumor** 439
James D. McDonald and Ricardo J. Gonzalez

40 **Resection of Tumors Involving the Pelvic Girdle** 449
Alexander L. Lazarides, Shawna L. Watson, Guston G. Zervoudakis, Nora L. Watson, and David M. Joyce

41 **Pelvic Reconstructive Procedures** 463
Julian Pribaz and Kristen Whalen

Index 473

Contributors

Thompson Alan Department of Uro-oncology, The Royal Marsden Foundation Trust, London, UK

Sudha Amarnath Department of Radiation Oncology, Cleveland Clinic Foundation, Cleveland, OH, USA

Bastian Amend Department of Urology, University Hospital of Tuebingen, Eberhard Karls University, Tuebingen, Germany

Kyrollis Attalla Department of Urology, Icahn School of Medicine at Mount Sinai, New York, NY, USA

Monica Avila Department of Gynecologic Oncology, Moffitt Cancer Center and USF Morsani College of Medicine, Tampa, FL, USA

Kristen A. Ban Department of Colon & Rectal Surgery, Cleveland Clinic, Cleveland, OH, USA

Desmond P. Barton Department of Gynaecological Oncology, The Royal Marsden Foundation Trust, London, UK

Bernard H. Bochner Urology Service, Department of Surgery, Memorial Sloan Kettering Cancer Center, New York, NY, USA

Department of Urology, Weill Cornell Medical College, New York, NY, USA

Christy M. Boraas Department of Obstetrics, Gynecology and Women's Health, University of Minnesota Medical School, Minneapolis, MN, USA

Alberto Breda Urology Department, Universitat Autònoma de Barcelona, Fundació Puigvert, Barcelona, Spain

Haywood Brown Obstetrics and Gynecology, University of South Florida, Tampa, FL, USA

Caitlin Bungo Department of Surgery, Division of Colorectal Surgery, Stanford University, Palo Alto, CA, USA

Jing-Yi Chern Department of Gynecologic Oncology, Moffitt Cancer Center and USF Morsani College of Medicine, Tampa, FL, USA

Charissa Chu Department of Urology, University of California, San Francisco, San Francisco, CA, USA

Daniel L. Clarke-Pearson Department of Obstetrics & Gynecology, University of North Carolina, Chapel Hill, NC, USA

William A. Cliby Division of Gynecologic Oncology, Mayo Clinic, Rochester, MN, USA

Lauren M. Conroy Department of Urology, University of Texas Health Science Center at Houston, Houston, TX, USA

Siamak Daneshmand Department of Urology, USC/Norris Comprehensive Cancer Center, Los Angeles, CA, USA

Michelle DeLeon Division of Colon and Rectal Surgery, Mayo Clinic, Jacksonville, FL, USA

Sean P. Dineen GI Oncology, Moffitt Cancer Center, Tampa, FL, USA

Timothy Donahue Department of Surgery, Memorial Sloan Kettering Cancer Center, New York, NY, USA

Leo Dreyfuss Department of Urology, Weill Cornell Medical College, New York Presbyterian Hospital, New York, NY, USA

Matthew D. Dunn Department of Urology, University of California Los Angeles, Los Angeles, CA, USA

Brett D. Einerson Department of Obstetrics & Gynecology, University of Utah, Salt Lake City, UT, USA

Kamil Erozkan Department of Colorectal Surgery, Digestive Disease and Surgery Institute, Cleveland Clinic, Cleveland, OH, USA

Óscar Rodríguez Faba Urology Department, Universitat Autònoma de Barcelona, Fundació Puigvert, Barcelona, Spain

Margit Fisch Department of Urology, University Medical Center Hamburg-Eppendorf, Hamburg, Germany

Theresa Fisher, MD Obstetrics and Gynecology, Platte Valley Medical Center, Brighton, CO, USA

Susan Galandiuk Division of Colon & Rectal Surgery, Hiram C Polk Jr., MD Department of Surgery, University of Louisville, Louisville, KY, USA

John Gebhart Department of OBGYN, Division Chair Urogynecology, Mayo Clinic, Rochester, MN, USA

Ricardo J. Gonzalez Sarcoma Department, Moffitt Cancer Center, Tampa, FL, USA

Emre Gorgun Department of Colorectal Surgery, Digestive Disease and Surgery Institute, Cleveland Clinic, Cleveland, OH, USA

Brooke Gurland Department of Surgery, Division of Colorectal Surgery, Stanford University, Palo Alto, CA, USA

Owen M. Heath Department of Gynaecological Oncology, The Royal Marsden Foundation Trust, London, UK

Mitchel Hoffman Department of Gynecologic Oncology, Moffitt Cancer Center, USF Morsani College of Medicine, Tampa, FL, USA

Stefan D. Holubar Department of Colon & Rectal Surgery, Cleveland Clinic, Cleveland, OH, USA

Dandi Huang Department of Obstetrics and Gynecology, Division of Gynecologic Oncology, Cedars-Sinai Medical Center, West Hollywood, CA, USA

Richard A. Jacobson GI Oncology, Moffitt Cancer Center, Tampa, FL, USA

David M. Joyce Department of Sarcoma, Moffitt Cancer Center, Tampa, FL, USA

Anthony Kendle Obstetrics and Gynecology, Division of Maternal Fetal Medicine, University of South Florida, Tampa, FL, USA

Zaraq Khan Division Chair for Reproductive Endocrinology and Infertility, Mayo Clinic, Rochester, MN, USA

Kenneth H. Kim Department of Obstetrics and Gynecology, Division of Gynecologic Oncology, Cedars-Sinai Medical Center, West Hollywood, CA, USA

Jakob Klemm Department of Urology, University Medical Center Hamburg-Eppendorf, Hamburg, Germany

Clarissa Lam Gynecology Service, Department of Surgery, Memorial Sloan Kettering Cancer Center, New York, NY, USA

Alexander L. Lazarides Department of Sarcoma, Moffitt Cancer Center, Tampa, FL, USA

Richard Lee Department of Urology, Weill Cornell Medical College, New York Presbyterian Hospital, New York, NY, USA

Mario M. Leitao Gynecology Service, Department of Surgery, Memorial Sloan Kettering Cancer Center, New York, NY, USA

Department of Obstetrics and Gynecology, Weill Cornell Medical College, New York, NY, USA

Amy L. Lightner Department of General Surgery, Scripps Clinic Medical Group, San Diego, CA, USA

Beverly Long Division of Gynecologic Oncology, Sarasota Memorial Healthcare System, Sarasota, FL, USA

Anne Macleod Price Institute of Surgical Research, University of Louisville, Louisville, KY, USA

James D. McDonald Department of Surgery, University Surgixal Oncology, University of Tennessee Graduate School of Medicine, Knoxville, TN, USA

Joshua J. Meeks Departments of Urology and Biochemistry, Feinberg School of Medicine, Northwestern University, Chicago, IL, USA

Kirolos N. Meilika Department of Urology, University of Rochester Medical Center, Rochester, NY, USA

Kathrin Meisterhofer Department of Urology, University Hospital of Tuebingen, Eberhard Karls University, Tuebingen, Germany

Ankita Mishra GI Oncology, Moffitt Cancer Center, Tampa, FL, USA

Jonathan Modai Department of Urology, University of California Los Angeles, Los Angeles, CA, USA

Vadim Morozov Obstetrics and Gynecology, MedStar Washington Hospital Center/Georgetown University School of Medicine, Washington, DC, USA

Joan Palou Urology Department, Universitat Autònoma de Barcelona, Fundació Puigvert, Barcelona, Spain

Kumar Pardeep Department of Uro-oncology, The Royal Marsden Foundation Trust, London, UK

Kelly R. Pekala Urology Service, Department of Surgery, Memorial Sloan Kettering Cancer Center, New York, NY, USA

Kristin Powell, MD, MS Obstetrics and Gynecology, Denver Health, Denver, CO, USA

Julian Pribaz Department of Plastic Surgery, University of South Florida Morsani College of Medicine, Tampa, FL, USA

Jessika A. Ralph Department of Obstetrics, Gynecology and Women's Health, University of Minnesota Medical School, Minneapolis, MN, USA

Aparna R. Ramanathan Obstetrics and Gynecology, Division of Minimally Invasive Gynecologic Surgery, MedStar Washington Hospital Center, Washington, DC, USA

Jensen Reckhow Department of Obstetrics and Gynecology, Mayo Clinic, Rochester, MN, USA

Brittany L. Roberts Department of Obstetrics and Gynecology, Division of Urogynecology and Reconstructive Pelvic Surgery Albany Medical Center, Albany, NY, USA

Rebecca G. Rogers Department of Obstetrics and Gynecology, Division of Urogynecology and Reconstructive Pelvic Surgery Albany Medical Center, Albany, NY, USA

Jaspreet S. Sandhu Department of Surgery, Memorial Sloan Kettering Cancer Center, New York, NY, USA

Jessica Selle Department of OBGYN, Division of Urogynecology, Mayo Clinic, Rochester, MN, USA

John P. Sfakianos Department of Urology, Icahn School of Medicine at Mount Sinai, New York, NY, USA

Rasheed Shahnawaz Department of Colorectal Surgery, The Royal Marsden Foundation Trust, London, UK

Armin Shahrokni Department of Medicine, Jersey Shore University Medical Center, Neptune, NJ, USA

Murray Shames Department of Surgery, Division of Vascular Surgery, USF Morsani College of Medicine, Tampa, FL, USA

Jennifer Shearer Department of Surgery, Division of Colorectal Surgery, Stanford University, Palo Alto, CA, USA

Qiu Sheng Department of Colorectal Surgery, The Royal Marsden Foundation Trust, London, UK

Andrew P. Soisson Division of Gynecologic Oncology, Department of Obstetrics & Gynecology, University of Utah, Salt Lake City, UT, USA

Anna R. Spivak Cleveland Clinic Foundation, Cleveland, OH, USA

Arnulf Stenzl Department of Urology, University Hospital of Tuebingen, Eberhard Karls University, Tuebingen, Germany

Luca Stocchi Division of Colon and Rectal Surgery, Mayo Clinic, Jacksonville, FL, USA

Scott A. Strong Department of Surgery, Feinberg School of Medicine, Northwestern University, Chicago, IL, USA

Rebecca E. Thompson Obstetrics and Gynecology, Division of Minimally Invasive Gynecologic Surgery, MedStar Washington Hospital Center, Washington, DC, USA

Elissa Trieu Obstetrics & Gynecology, Washington Hospital Center, Washington, DC, USA

Malte W. Vetterlein Department of Urology, University Medical Center Hamburg-Eppendorf, Hamburg, Germany

Valery Vilchez Division of Colon and Rectal Surgery, University of California at Irvine, Irvine, CA, USA

Nasreen A. Vohra Surgery, Division of Surgical Oncology, ECU Health Medical Center, East Carolina University, Greenville, NC, USA

Nora L. Watson Department of Sarcoma, Moffitt Cancer Center, Tampa, FL, USA

Shawna L. Watson Department of Orthopaedic Surgery, University of South Florida, Tampa, FL, USA

O. Lenaine Westney Department of Urology, University of Texas—MD Anderson Cancer Center, Houston, TX, USA

Kristen Whalen Department of Plastic Surgery, University of South Florida Morsani College of Medicine, Tampa, FL, USA

Leilei Xia Department of Urology, USC/Norris Comprehensive Cancer Center, Los Angeles, CA, USA

Emmanuel Zervos Surgery, Division of Surgical Oncology, ECU Health Medical Center, East Carolina University, Greenville, NC, USA

Guston G. Zervoudakis Department of Sarcoma, Moffitt Cancer Center, Tampa, FL, USA

Nadim Bou Zgheib Department of Oncology, Edwards Comprehensive Cancer Center and Joan C. Edwards School of Medicine, Huntington, WV, USA

Part I

General Perioperative Considerations

Perioperative Venous Thromboembolism

1

Kristen A. Ban, Stefan D. Holubar, and Daniel L. Clarke-Pearson

Background

Epidemiology

Perioperative venous thromboembolism (VTE), including deep venous thrombosis (DVT) and pulmonary embolism (PE), remains an important source of morbidity and mortality following pelvic surgery [1]. There is also significant cost associated with a VTE event, with each inpatient VTE event associated with an estimated $32,000 in added costs [2]. The Center for Medicare and Medicaid Services (CMS) considers VTE a "never event" and penalizes hospitals for higher-than-expected VTE complications following specific procedures [3].

The incidence of perioperative VTE is estimated between <1% and 29% following pelvic surgery overall, with incidence varying depending on the indication for surgery and procedure performed [4, 5]. Surgery for pelvic organ prolapse carries a low risk of VTE, 0.2% for all approaches, with the highest risk in patients undergoing an abdominal approach with concurrent hysterectomy (0.7%) [6]. Pelvic surgery for malignancy and inflammatory bowel disease carries the highest risk with incidence of 4–12% [7, 8]. The incidence of VTE in cancer patients undergoing surgery without chemoprophylaxis was previously measured at 29% but is lower in the era of routine VTE chemoprophylaxis [5]. VTE rates following surgery for gynecologic malignancy range from 3% for cervical cancer up to 38% for ovarian cancer [9]. The risk of VTE is also elevated in patients undergoing pelvic surgery for inflammatory bowel disease, with ulcerative colitis having the highest incidence [8, 10]. The incidence of VTE following proctectomy is highest for ulcerative colitis (UC) patients at 3.2% followed by Crohn's disease (CD) at 1.5% and lowest for malignancy (1.4%) [11].

VTE events are the most common preventable cause of 30-day mortality in patients undergoing surgery for malignancy [12]. Notably, many postoperative VTE events occur after discharge from the hospital. One third of VTE events following oncologic surgery occur after discharge and an even higher proportion occur following discharge after surgery for pelvic organ prolapse [6, 13].

Risk Factors

General risk factors for VTE in addition to indication for surgery include older age, higher body mass index (BMI), inpatient hospitalization after

K. A. Ban (✉) · S. D. Holubar
Department of Colon & Rectal Surgery, Cleveland Clinic, Cleveland, OH, USA
e-mail: bank4@ccf.org; holubas@ccf.org

D. L. Clarke-Pearson
Department of Obstetrics & Gynecology, University of North Carolina, Chapel Hill, NC, USA
e-mail: daniel_clarkepearson@med.unc.edu

M. Hoffman et al. (eds.), *Major Complications of Female Pelvic Surgery*,
https://doi.org/10.1007/978-3-031-66772-5_1

surgery, American Society of Anesthesiologists (ASA) Classification 3 or 4, prolonged operative time, preoperative renal failure, and chronic steroid use [4, 6, 14]. Important risk factors include prior history of VTE (especially "unprovoked") and known clotting disorders. Preoperative Hematology or Vascular Medicine referral for thrombophilia testing and perioperative management should be considered [15].

Estrogen-based contraception or therapy and tamoxifen treatment are also important modifiable preoperative risk factors in women [16–19]. Oral combined hormonal menopausal therapy was associated with the highest risk of VTE in the nonsurgical population [19].

In the IBD population, surgery-specific risk factors for postoperative VTE include open surgery, emergency surgery, corticosteroids, malnutrition, functional status, ileostomy creation, and others [8, 14]. Patients with anemia, bleeding disorders, and bleeding are a particularly at-risk group as they often have their chemoprophylaxis held. Preoperative hospitalization was also shown to be a risk factor in a dose-dependent manner [20]. VTE risk in the perioperative period can be assessed with a validated measure such as the Caprini score, but this measure is relatively insensitive within sub-populations such as IBD or gynecologic cancer [21–23]. The Caprini score considers age, gender, type of surgery, comorbidities, venous disease, and clotting disorder risk. Most pelvic surgery is considered "Major" according to the Caprini score definition of more than 45 min under anesthesia or any surgery with a laparoscopic approach.

Prevention

A variety of modalities are employed to prevent perioperative VTE [Fig. 1.1]. Early mobilization after surgery, mechanical prophylaxis with compression stockings and/or sequential compression devices (SCDs), and chemoprophylaxis are all thromboprophylaxis interventions [1]. Most, if not all, of these modalities are routinely included in perioperative care pathways like enhanced recovery after surgery (ERAS) protocols [24]. Extended chemoprophylaxis following discharge from the hospital is also selectively employed to decrease VTE events in high-risk populations [13, 25].

Chemoprophylaxis

Chemoprophylaxis refers to the prevention of VTE with administration of medication. Acceptable chemoprophylaxis agents include subcutaneous unfractionated heparin and low-molecular weight heparin (enoxaparin) as well as oral agents like apixaban and rivaroxaban. In the immediate postoperative period, subcutaneous agents are often favored as their shorter half-life (i.e., reversibility) is advantageous in the event of a bleeding complication.

Preoperative Chemoprophylaxis

Preoperative chemoprophylaxis is generally employed for patients undergoing major pelvic

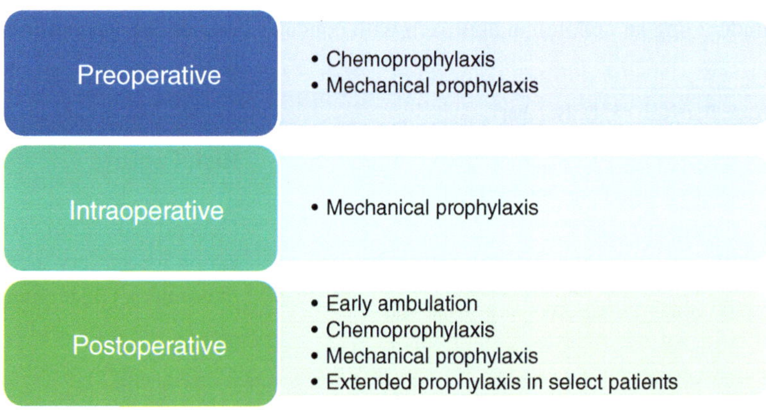

Fig. 1.1 Perioperative VTE prevention measures

surgery under general anesthesia extrapolating from data in the cancer population that this practice reduces perioperative VTE without increasing bleeding risk [26]. The American Society of Clinical Oncology (ASCO) Guidelines recommend chemoprophylaxis prior to major oncologic surgery with subcutaneous unfractionated heparin or enoxaparin unless contraindicated due to active bleeding, high risk of bleeding, or other contraindications [27]. Most enhanced recovery after surgery (ERAS) guidelines recommend preoperative mechanical and chemoprophylaxis prior to induction of general anesthesia for major pelvic operations in the absence of contraindications [9, 28].

Timing of Postoperative Chemoprophylaxis

In the absence of postoperative bleeding concerns, chemoprophylaxis should be re-administered within 24 h of surgery. In patients who receive regional anesthesia with an epidural, consideration must be given to the timing of the most recent dose of chemoprophylaxis prior to epidural removal; a strategy of dosing in the evening so the epidural catheter may be removed the following morning may be helpful.

Mechanical Prophylaxis

Mechanical prophylaxis with compression stockings or SCDs can be employed to prevent perioperative VTE. Mechanical prophylaxis with SCDs is initiated prior to the induction of general anesthesia in the operating room. The CHEST Guidelines support the use of mechanical prophylaxis postoperatively for patients who have undergone inpatient pelvic surgery with intermittent pneumatic compression (e.g., SCDs) preferred over compression stockings [1]. Patients at moderate to high risk of VTE (most patients undergoing inpatient pelvic surgery) should receive both mechanical and chemoprophylaxis, but in patients at high risk for bleeding, mechanical prophylaxis alone is recommended over no prophylaxis [1]. In the cancer population, ASCO Guidelines also recommend mechanical prophylaxis as an adjunct to chemoprophylaxis and do not endorse mechanical prophylaxis as monotherapy unless chemoprophylaxis is contraindicated [27].

Early Mobilization

Early mobilization after surgery is an effective means of decreasing VTE events and is now supported by guidelines and emphasized in most ERAS pathways, regardless of the indication for surgery [1, 24]. Although early ambulation decreases VTE risk during hospital admission following surgery, the use of mechanical prophylaxis with SCDs and chemoprophylaxis is still recommended in patients at moderate to high risk of postoperative VTE.

Extended Postoperative Chemoprophylaxis

Extended chemoprophylaxis in high-risk populations has been evaluated in both randomized controlled trials and observational studies and has been found to be safe and effective [7, 29–31]. A systematic review and meta-analysis confirmed these findings [25]. Multiple guidelines support the use of extended chemoprophylaxis in the oncology population including the American College of Chest Physicians (ACCP), the ASCO, and the National Comprehensive Cancer Network (NCCN) [1, 27, 32]. The ASCO Guidelines recommend extended chemoprophylaxis following major oncologic surgery for a minimum of 7 days and up to 4 weeks in high-risk patients including those with restricted mobility, obesity, history of VTE, and others [27, 33].

Given the elevated risk of postoperative VTE in the IBD population relative to the oncology population, extended chemoprophylaxis is also recommended following major abdominal or pelvic surgery for IBD [34]. A systematic review of extended chemoprophylaxis in patients with IBD undergoing major surgery found that no data exist at present to guide extended chemoprophylaxis recommendations [14]. Within the identified studies, VTE events occurred within varying timeframes up to 30 days from surgery [14]. Based on these findings and the demonstrated safety of extended VTE chemoprophylaxis in the oncology population, extended chemoprophylaxis is also recommended for patients with IBD undergoing major pelvic surgery. The American Society of Colon & Rectal Surgeons has also recently updated their Venous Thromboembolism Clinical Practice Guidelines to include strong consideration of extended prophylaxis for colorectal cancer patients and consideration for IBD patients [33]. The main barriers to postdischarge chemoprophylaxis are adherence and patient cost. Orthopedic literature suggests oral agents were not associated with increased adherence, and cost was recently shown to be a significant barrier for most colorectal surgery patients [35, 36].

Prophylactic IVC Filters

IVC filters are not recommended for prophylaxis prior to or following surgery in the general surgical population. Even among patients undergoing major oncologic surgery with contraindications to chemoprophylaxis, the ASCO Guidelines do not recommend prophylactic placement of IVC filters, noting an absence of randomized trials evaluating this practice and data on the potential long-term harm of IVC filters [27].

Diagnosis

Clinical Assessment and Physical Exam

Clinical symptoms of DVT or PE can prompt further workup to confirm a VTE event. The assessment should begin with a history and physical exam to elicit risk factors for VTE and to evaluate for physical exam findings. Extremity swelling with associated tenderness is consistent with DVT, while acute dyspnea, chest pain, hemoptysis, tachycardia, and increased oxygen requirements are signs concerning for PE. There are often additional diagnoses in the differential for symptoms like lower extremity swelling or dyspnea, so an initial workup should be broad. Of note, portomesenteric vein thrombosis is often detected incidentally during routine cross-sectional imaging for postoperative ileus or high-ileostomy output [37].

Labs and Testing

Useful laboratory testing in the assessment of a possible VTE event includes D-dimer to assess for DVT and/or PE and an arterial blood gas (ABG) and electrocardiogram (ECG) for PE. Because additional diagnoses are initially included in the differential, additional testing is typically warranted. A complete blood count (CBC) and basic metabolic panel (BMP) may be included, and depending on symptoms, a chest X-ray, B-type natriuretic peptide (BNP), or troponin may also be appropriate.

D-dimer is a sensitive marker for VTE in the nonsurgical population but can be elevated in the inflammatory state that follows major pelvic surgery. D-dimer levels greater than 500 mg/mL suggest presence of a PE; however, D-dimer levels normally increase with age. To avoid false-positive results, an age-adjusted D-dimer threshold should be employed, calculated as the patient's age multiplied by 10 ng/mL for patients over 50 years [38]. A normal age-adjusted D-dimer can help avoid unnecessary imaging and rule out PE when the Pulmonary Embolism Rule-Out Criteria pretest probability is low [38]. An elevated D-dimer should prompt additional evaluation with imaging to confirm the diagnosis.

ABG and ECG findings are not sensitive but can increase or decrease index of suspicion for a clinically significant PE. An ABG may demonstrate hypoxemia and hypocapnia (respiratory alkalosis), and an ECG may demonstrate signs of right-heart strain including a new right bundle branch block, rightward shift of the QRS axis, ST segment elevation in V_1, atrial premature contractions, sinus tachycardia, atrial fibrillation/flutter, or T wave inversions in leads V_1–V_4 [39].

In the evaluation of extremity swelling, a CBC, BNP, and assessment of volume status can help evaluate for cellulitis, heart failure exacerbation, and volume overload resulting in bilateral peripheral edema. In the evaluation of PE, a CXR, ECG, and troponin can evaluate for other pathology such as pneumonia, pneumothorax, and acute coronary syndrome.

Imaging

The diagnosis of a VTE event is confirmed with imaging. Compression ultrasonography is employed to confirm the presence of a DVT but may be limited in the morbidly obese, and venous-phase computed tomography (CT) of the pelvic vessels may show large groin clots. Computed tomography pulmonary angiography (CT-PE) is considered the gold-standard for diagnosis of acute PE. In patients with a contraindication to the contrast medium employed in CT-PE (allergy to contrast, acute or chronic renal failure), ventilation/perfusion (V/Q) scintigraphy may be considered. Alternatively, compression ultrasonography of the lower extremities can be obtained, as a proximal DVT in a patient with suspected PE is highly predictive and justifies treatment. Importantly, though, a negative lower extremity ultrasound does not rule out PE.

Treatment

Therapeutic Anticoagulation

In patients without a contraindication, therapeutic anticoagulation is the preferred management of acute VTE [1, 27]. Therapeutic anticoagulation promotes clot resorption while preventing clot extension, hemodynamic collapse, DVT progression to PE, recurrent VTE, and mortality in the acute phase [38]. These benefits must be weighed against the risk of bleeding, particularly in the postoperative setting. A postoperative VTE is considered "provoked," with the risk of recurrence after treatment being low at <1% after 1-year and 3% after 5-years [40]. Anticoagulation is recommended for 3 months because randomized trials have demonstrated that the long-term bleeding risk outweighs the risk of recurrent VTE beyond this timeframe, apart from patients with cancer in whom the annualized risk of VTE is much higher at 15% [27, 38].

Medication Options

Initial therapeutic options include unfractionated heparin as a continuous infusion with dosing guided by activated partial thromboplastin time (aPTT) assessment and therapeutic weight-based subcutaneous enoxaparin, which are appealing as they can be quickly held with a relatively short half-life in the case of bleeding. If the bleeding risk is low, oral anticoagulants are recommended due to ease of administration. Direct oral anticoagulants (DOACs), including direct thrombin inhibitors like dabigatran and factor Xa inhibitors like rivaroxaban, apixaban, and edoxaban, have been evaluated and are recommended by multiple guidelines for the treatment of acute DVT and PE [40–42]. The DOAC agents are favored due to their rapid onset of action and predictable pharmacokinetics, which do not require ongoing laboratory assessment to titrate [38]. Vitamin K antagonists like warfarin remain preferred for patients with severe renal impairment [38]. A summary of recommended therapeutic agents is provided in Table 1.1 along with populations in whom a particular agent might be preferred.

In the oncology population, the ASCO Guidelines support initial therapeutic anticoagulation with agents including unfractionated heparin, enoxaparin, fondaparinux, and rivaroxaban [27]. The NCCN Guidelines endorse monotherapy with unfractionated heparin, enoxaparin, dalteparin, and fondaparinux at doses listed in Table 1.2 [43]. Guidelines endorse additional agents including warfarin or edoxaban with a bridge like enoxaparin or dalteparin until the patient reaches therapeutic drug levels [43].

Table 1.1 Summary of therapeutic anticoagulation medication options per studies considered in CHEST Guidelines [40]

Medication	Dose	Preferred populations
Unfractionated heparin	IV 80 units/kg or 5000 units loading dose then 18 units/kg/hr, target APTT of 2–2.5 x control, then SC 250 units/kg q 12 hrs	
Enoxaparin	1–1.5 mg/kg SC q 12 hrs	Malignancy Liver disease and coagulopathy Pregnancy
Dabigatran	150 mg PO BID	
Rivaroxaban	15–20 mg PO BID	Once daily dosing
Apixaban	2.5 mg PO BID or 5 mg daily	History of GI bleed
Edoxaban	60 mg PO daily	Once daily dosing
Warfarin	Dose varies PO daily Target INR 2.0–3.5	Once daily dosing Renal disease History of GI bleed Poor compliance

Table 1.2 Summary of therapeutic anticoagulation medication options per NCCN guidelines [43]

Medication	Dose
Unfractionated heparin	IV 80 units/kg load then 18 units/kg/hr, target APTT of 2–2.5 x control, then SC 250 units/kg q 12 hrs
Enoxaparin	1 mg/kg SC q 12 hrs
Dalteparin	200 units/kg SC daily for 30 days, then 150 units/kg once daily for 2–6 months
Fondaparinux	5 mg [<50 kg]; 7.5 mg [50–100 kg]; 10 mg [>100 kg] SC daily

Thrombolysis and Suction Thrombectomy

Thrombolysis should be considered in the setting of a DVT where the extremity is at risk or in patients with a PE and hemodynamic instability. Catheter-directed thrombolysis can be considered for DVT, and systemic thrombolysis or suction thrombectomy can be considered for hemodynamically unstable PE [38]. In patients with large central clots who are high risk of bleeding preoperatively, suction thrombectomy may be considered [44]. Many hospitals have implemented PE response teams to facilitate timely interventional treatment for unstable patients. Thrombolysis carries a risk of bleeding, which is even more significant in the setting of recent major pelvic surgery. The risks of interventional procedures must therefore be weighed against the risk of bleeding in the immediate postsurgical period. Patients in whom the bleeding risk is felt to be prohibitive should be evaluated for IVC filter placement.

IVC Filter Placement

IVC filter placement can be considered for patients with acute proximal DVT or PE who are not candidates for systemic anticoagulation or thrombolysis [38]. The use of an IVC filter for 3 months in combination with therapeutic anticoagulation for patients with severe acute PE was recently evaluated in a randomized trial with no reduction in recurrent PE or death at 3- and 6-month follow-up [45]. In the cancer population, the ASCO Guidelines recommend against the insertion of IVC filters as prophylaxis in patients with chronic thrombosis (VTE diagnosis more than 4 weeks prior) but support IVC filter placement consideration in patients with acute VTE (diagnosis within the last 4 weeks) with absolute contraindication to anticoagulant therapy if the thrombus burden is considered life-threatening [27]. There is increased awareness about short- and long-term risks associated with the presence of an IVC filter. When no longer necessary, IVC filters should be removed. Some patients are candidates for therapeutic anticoagulation further out from surgery, at which point surveillance imaging may demonstrate resolution of the thrombus. In these cases, IVC filters can and should be removed to prevent complications like filter migration, fracture, perforation, filter thrombus, and caval and/or iliac thrombosis.

Duration of Anticoagulation

The recommended duration of anticoagulation following a provoked (postsurgical) VTE is 3 months [38, 40], except in the cancer population where treatment should be continued until the cancer has been treated or at the discretion of the patient's medical oncologist.

References

1. Gould MK, Garcia DA, Wren SM, Karanicolas PJ, Arcelus JI, Heit JA, et al. Prevention of VTE in nonorthopedic surgical patients: Antithrombotic Therapy and Prevention of Thrombosis, 9th ed: American College of Chest Physicians Evidence-Based Clinical Practice Guidelines. Chest. 2012;141(2 Suppl):e227S–e77S. https://doi.org/10.1378/chest.11-2297.
2. Lee CHA, Jia X, Lipman JM, Lightner AL, Hull TL, Steele SR, et al. Defining the economic burden of perioperative venous thromboembolism in inflammatory bowel disease in the United States. Dis Colon Rectum. 2021;64(7):871–80. https://doi.org/10.1097/DCR.0000000000001942.
3. Sutedjo JL, Ng RK, Piazza G, Goldhaber SZ. Medicare's new regulations for deep vein thrombosis as a "never event": wise or worrisome? Am J Med. 2009;122(11):975–6. https://doi.org/10.1016/j.amjmed.2009.04.019.
4. Hokenstad ED, Habermann EB, Glasgow AE, Occhino JA. Risk of venous thromboembolism in patients undergoing surgery for pelvic organ prolapse. Int Urogynecol J. 2016;27(10):1525–8. https://doi.org/10.1007/s00192-016-2990-z.
5. Geerts WH, Heit JA, Clagett GP, Pineo GF, Colwell CW, Anderson FA Jr, et al. Prevention of venous thromboembolism. Chest. 2001;119(1 Suppl):132S–75S. https://doi.org/10.1378/chest.119.1_suppl.132s.
6. Chong W, Bui AH, Menhaji K. Incidence and risk factors for venous thromboembolism events after different routes of pelvic organ prolapse repairs. Am J Obstet Gynecol. 2020;223(2):268e1–e26. https://doi.org/10.1016/j.ajog.2020.05.020.
7. Bergqvist D, Agnelli G, Cohen AT, Eldor A, Nilsson PE, Le Moigne-Amrani A, et al. Duration of prophylaxis against venous thromboembolism with enoxaparin after surgery for cancer. N Engl J Med. 2002;346(13):975–80. https://doi.org/10.1056/NEJMoa012385.
8. Wallaert JB, De Martino RR, Marsicovetere PS, Goodney PP, Finlayson SR, Murray JJ, et al. Venous thromboembolism after surgery for inflammatory bowel disease: are there modifiable risk factors? Data from ACS NSQIP. Dis Colon Rectum. 2012;55(11):1138–44. https://doi.org/10.1097/DCR.0b013e3182698f60.
9. Nelson G, Bakkum-Gamez J, Kalogera E, Glaser G, Altman A, Meyer LA, et al. Guidelines for perioperative care in gynecologic/oncology: Enhanced Recovery After Surgery (ERAS) Society recommendations-2019 update. Int J Gynecol Cancer. 2019;29(4):651–68. https://doi.org/10.1136/ijgc-2019-000356.
10. Merrill A, Millham F. Increased risk of postoperative deep vein thrombosis and pulmonary embolism in patients with inflammatory bowel disease: a study of National Surgical Quality Improvement Program patients. Arch Surg. 2012;147(2):120–4. https://doi.org/10.1001/archsurg.2011.297.
11. Clement E, Dang J, Laffin M, Wang H. Incidence of venous thromboembolism following proctectomy is greater in ulcerative colitis than in malignancy or crohn's disease. J Gastrointest Surg. 2020;24(11):2664–6. https://doi.org/10.1007/s11605-020-04738-9.
12. Agnelli G, Bolis G, Capussotti L, Scarpa RM, Tonelli F, Bonizzoni E, et al. A clinical outcome-based prospective study on venous thromboembolism after cancer surgery: the @RISTOS project. Ann Surg. 2006;243(1):89–95. https://doi.org/10.1097/01.sla.0000193959.44677.48.
13. Merkow RP, Bilimoria KY, McCarter MD, Cohen ME, Barnett CC, Raval MV, et al. Post-discharge venous thromboembolism after cancer surgery: extending the case for extended prophylaxis. Ann Surg. 2011;254(1):131–7. https://doi.org/10.1097/SLA.0b013e31821b98da.
14. McKechnie T, Wang J, Springer JE, Gross PL, Forbes S, Eskicioglu C. Extended thromboprophylaxis following colorectal surgery in patients with inflammatory bowel disease: a comprehensive systematic clinical review. Color Dis. 2020;22(6):663–78. https://doi.org/10.1111/codi.14853.
15. Middeldorp S, Nieuwlaat R, Baumann Kreuziger L, Coppens M, Houghton DE, James AH, et al. American Society of Hematology 2023 guidelines for management of venous thromboembolism: thrombophilia testing. Blood Adv. 2023;7(22):7101–38. https://doi.org/10.1182/bloodadvances.2023010177.
16. Kozek-Langenecker S, Fenger-Eriksen C, Thienpont E, Barauskas G, Force EVGT. European guidelines on perioperative venous thromboembolism prophylaxis: surgery in the elderly. Eur J Anaesthesiol. 2018;35(2):116–22. https://doi.org/10.1097/EJA.0000000000000705.

17. Hussain T, Kneeshaw PJ. Stopping tamoxifen perioperatively for VTE risk reduction: a proposed management algorithm. Int J Surg. 2012;10(6):313–6. https://doi.org/10.1016/j.ijsu.2012.05.001.
18. Grandone E, Antonucci E, Colaizzo D, De Laurenzo A, Cosmi B, Cini M, et al. Venous thromboembolism in women of childbearing age: insights from the START registry. Thromb Haemost. 2023;123(11):1060–8. https://doi.org/10.1055/s-0043-1769592.
19. Weller SC, Davis JW, Porterfield L, Chen L, Wilkinson G. Hormone exposure and venous thromboembolism in commercially insured women aged 50 to 64 years. Res Pract Thromb Haemost. 2023;7(3):100135. https://doi.org/10.1016/j.rpth.2023.100135.
20. Greaves SW, Holubar SD. Preoperative hospitalization is independently associated with increased risk for venous thromboembolism in patients undergoing colorectal surgery: a National Surgical Quality Improvement Program Database Study. Dis Colon Rectum. 2015;58(8):782–91. https://doi.org/10.1097/DCR.0000000000000411.
21. Bahl V, Hu HM, Henke PK, Wakefield TW, Campbell DA Jr, Caprini JA. A validation study of a retrospective venous thromboembolism risk scoring method. Ann Surg. 2010;251(2):344–50. https://doi.org/10.1097/SLA.0b013e3181b7fca6.
22. Benlice C, Holubar SD, Gorgun E, Stocchi L, Lipman JM, Kalady MF, et al. Extended venous thromboembolism prophylaxis after elective surgery for IBD patients: nomogram-based risk assessment and prediction from nationwide cohort. Dis Colon Rectum. 2018;61(10):1170–9. https://doi.org/10.1097/DCR.0000000000001189.
23. Cheong JY, Connelly TM, Russell T, Valente M, Bhama A, Lightner A, et al. Venous thromboembolism risk stratification for patients undergoing surgery for IBD using a novel six factor scoring system using NSQIP-IBD registry. ANZ J Surg. 2023;93(6):1620–5. https://doi.org/10.1111/ans.18242.
24. Ban KA, Gibbons MM, Ko CY, Wick EC. Surgical technical evidence review for colorectal surgery conducted for the AHRQ safety program for improving surgical care and recovery. J Am Coll Surg. 2017;225(4):548–57 e3. https://doi.org/10.1016/j.jamcollsurg.2017.06.017.
25. Fagarasanu A, Alotaibi GS, Hrimiuc R, Lee AY, Wu C. Role of extended thromboprophylaxis after abdominal and pelvic surgery in cancer patients: a systematic review and meta-analysis. Ann Surg Oncol. 2016;23(5):1422–30. https://doi.org/10.1245/s10434-016-5127-1.
26. Selby LV, Sovel M, Sjoberg DD, McSweeney M, Douglas D, Jones DR, et al. Preoperative chemoprophylaxis is safe in major oncology operations and effective at preventing venous thromboembolism. J Am Coll Surg. 2016;222(2):129–37. https://doi.org/10.1016/j.jamcollsurg.2015.11.011.
27. Key NS, Khorana AA, Kuderer NM, Bohlke K, Lee AYY, Arcelus JI, et al. Venous thromboembolism prophylaxis and treatment in patients with cancer: ASCO clinical practice guideline update. J Clin Oncol. 2020;38(5):496–520. https://doi.org/10.1200/JCO.19.01461.
28. Ban KA, Gibbons MM, Ko CY, Wick EC, Cannesson M, Scott MJ, et al. Evidence review conducted for the Agency for Healthcare Research and Quality Safety Program for improving surgical care and recovery: focus on anesthesiology for colorectal surgery. Anesth Analg. 2019;128(5):879–89. https://doi.org/10.1213/ANE.0000000000003366.
29. ENOXACAN Study Group. Efficacy and safety of enoxaparin versus unfractionated heparin for prevention of deep vein thrombosis in elective cancer surgery: a double-blind randomized multicentre trial with venographic assessment. Br J Surg. 1997;84(8):1099–103.
30. Kakkar VV, Balibrea JL, Martinez-Gonzalez J, Prandoni P, Group CS. Extended prophylaxis with bemiparin for the prevention of venous thromboembolism after abdominal or pelvic surgery for cancer: the CANBESURE randomized study. J Thromb Haemost. 2010;8(6):1223–9. https://doi.org/10.1111/j.1538-7836.2010.03892.x.
31. Vedovati MC, Becattini C, Rondelli F, Boncompagni M, Camporese G, Balzarotti R, et al. A randomized study on 1-week versus 4-week prophylaxis for venous thromboembolism after laparoscopic surgery for colorectal cancer. Ann Surg. 2014;259(4):665–9. https://doi.org/10.1097/SLA.0000000000000340.
32. Khorana AA. The NCCN clinical practice guidelines on venous thromboembolic disease: strategies for improving VTE prophylaxis in hospitalized cancer patients. Oncologist. 2007;12(11):1361–70. https://doi.org/10.1634/theoncologist.12-11-1361.
33. Fleming F, Gaertner W, Ternent CA, Finlayson E, Herzig D, Paquette IM, et al. The American Society of Colon and Rectal Surgeons clinical practice guideline for the prevention of venous thromboembolic disease in colorectal surgery. Dis Colon Rectum. 2018;61(1):14–20. https://doi.org/10.1097/DCR.0000000000000982.
34. Gross ME, Vogler SA, Mone MC, Sheng X, Sklow B. The importance of extended postoperative venous thromboembolism prophylaxis in IBD: a National Surgical Quality Improvement Program analysis. Dis Colon Rectum. 2014;57(4):482–9. https://doi.org/10.1097/DCR.0000000000000090.
35. Prien C, Ribakow D, Steele SR, Liska D, Kessler H, Hull TL, et al. What about patient cost? Defining copay and out-of-pocket costs of extended venous thromboembolism chemoprophylaxis after colorectal surgery. J Gastrointest Surg. 2023;27(1):152–4. https://doi.org/10.1007/s11605-022-05416-8.
36. Sidhu V, Naylor JM, Adie S, Bastiras D, Buchbinder R, Ackerman I, et al. Post-discharge patient-reported non-adherence to aspirin compared to enoxaparin for venous thromboembolism prophylaxis after hip or knee arthroplasty. ANZ J Surg. 2023;93(4):989–94. https://doi.org/10.1111/ans.18284.

37. McKenna NP, Lightner AL. Importance of considering Portomesenteric vein thrombosis and operation in the risk of venous thromboembolism after colorectal surgery. Dis Colon Rectum. 2018;61(7):e350. https://doi.org/10.1097/DCR.0000000000001115.
38. Tritschler T, Kraaijpoel N, Le Gal G, Wells PS. Venous thromboembolism: advances in diagnosis and treatment. JAMA. 2018;320(15):1583–94. https://doi.org/10.1001/jama.2018.14346.
39. Levis JT. ECG diagnosis: pulmonary embolism. Perm J. 2011;15(4):75. https://doi.org/10.7812/tpp/11-112.
40. Stevens SM, Woller SC, Kreuziger LB, Bounameaux H, Doerschug K, Geersing GJ, et al. Antithrombotic therapy for VTE disease: second update of the CHEST guideline and expert panel report. Chest. 2021;160(6):e545–608. https://doi.org/10.1016/j.chest.2021.07.055.
41. Konstantinides SV, Meyer G, Becattini C, Bueno H, Geersing GJ, Harjola VP, et al. ESC Guidelines for the diagnosis and management of acute pulmonary embolism developed in collaboration with the European Respiratory Society (ERS): the Task Force for the diagnosis and management of acute pulmonary embolism of the European Society of Cardiology (ESC). Eur Respir J. 2019;54(3):1901647. https://doi.org/10.1183/13993003.01647-2019.
42. Mazzolai L, Aboyans V, Ageno W, Agnelli G, Alatri A, Bauersachs R, et al. Diagnosis and management of acute deep vein thrombosis: a joint consensus document from the European Society of Cardiology working groups of aorta and peripheral vascular diseases and pulmonary circulation and right ventricular function. Eur Heart J. 2018;39(47):4208–18. https://doi.org/10.1093/eurheartj/ehx003.
43. Streiff MB, Holmstrom B, Angelini D, Ashrani A, Elshoury A, Fanikos J, et al. Cancer-associated venous thromboembolic disease, version 2.2021, NCCN clinical practice guidelines in oncology. J Natl Compr Cancer Netw. 2021;19(10):1181–201. https://doi.org/10.6004/jnccn.2021.0047.
44. Mubashir M, Carnell C, Haddadin I, Holubar SD. Refractory ulcerative colitis requiring preoperative suction Thrombectomy of submassive bilateral pulmonary emboli before Total abdominal colectomy. Dig Dis Sci. 2023;68(5):1656–7. https://doi.org/10.1007/s10620-023-07843-2.
45. Mismetti P, Laporte S, Pellerin O, Ennezat PV, Couturaud F, Elias A, et al. Effect of a retrievable inferior vena cava filter plus anticoagulation vs anticoagulation alone on risk of recurrent pulmonary embolism: a randomized clinical trial. JAMA. 2015;313(16):1627–35. https://doi.org/10.1001/jama.2015.3780.

2 Modern-Enhanced Recovery After Surgery (ERAS) for Major Pelvic Surgery

Leilei Xia and Siamak Daneshmand

In 1997, Dr. Henrik Kehlet from Denmark asked "why a technically successful operation, whether a colonic resection, hip replacement, or cardiac operation, should result in an unsuccessful outcome" [1]. He then described the multifactorial surgical stress response that can potentially be addressed with interventions. The goal of reducing the stress response from surgery and shortening the time required for full recovery to improve patient outcomes was the foundation of the modern Enhanced Recovery After Surgery (ERAS).

ERAS is a patient-centered, multidisciplinary, and evidence-based approach to surgical care. The original ERAS pathway was developed from colorectal surgery and the first ERAS Study Group evidence-based consensus protocol was published in 2005 for those undergoing colorectal surgery [2]. After that, these multidisciplinary efforts to improve perioperative care across a wide spectrum of patients have been implemented within many surgical disciplines, including urology [3]. A growing body of evidence indicates that structured application of evidence-based principles and standardization of perioperative care significantly improve clinical outcomes [3–7]. In 2010, the ERAS® Society was officially registered as a nonprofit medical society based in Stockholm, Sweden (https://erassociety.org/). There are more than 30 guidelines published by the ERAS® Society and collaborators (https://erassociety.org/guidelines/). In 2013, the ERAS Society published guidelines for perioperative care after radical cystectomy (RC) [8]. In 2016, the ERAS® Society—Urology chapter was formed at the world congress in Lisbon.

RC with pelvic lymph node dissection (PLND) and urinary diversion (UD) is among the most complex urologic operations associated with considerable morbidity and prolonged inpatient stay [9–11]. Hospital stay after RC/PLND/UD is still among the minimally changed in the past decade, and the length of stays (LOS) remains in the 6–7 days range in the United States and 10–17 days range in Europe [5]. RC/PLND/UD has been the target for ERAS pathways because of the complexity of care and the incidence of perioperative complications. A meta-analysis from 2016 included 13 studies (801 ERAS patients versus 692 controls) that showed complication rates favored the ERAS group (39.6% versus 51.5%) in patients undergoing RC [5]. It also showed reduced LOS and faster return of bowel function. Multiple other meta-analyses with updated studies confirmed ERAS for radical cystectomy can achieve better perioperative outcomes [4, 12, 13]. This chapter will be mainly using RC/PLND/UD as an example to further discuss ERAS protocols and we believe

L. Xia · S. Daneshmand (✉)
Department of Urology, USC/Norris Comprehensive Cancer Center, Los Angeles, CA, USA
e-mail: daneshma@med.usc.edu

M. Hoffman et al. (eds.), *Major Complications of Female Pelvic Surgery*,
https://doi.org/10.1007/978-3-031-66772-5_2

that some of the principles or protocols discussed here apply to other major pelvic surgeries, such as colorectal and gynecologic oncologic surgeries.

The University of Southern California ERAS Protocol

The original 22 items published in 2013 RC ERAS guidelines were mainly based on colorectal literature [8]. Since the publication of the guidelines and formation of the Urology chapter, evidence supporting the use of ERAS after RC has grown rapidly, including our University of Southern California (USC) experience [7, 14–23]. Our institutional experience with ERAS for RC has extended from 2012 when we first implemented a multidisciplinary evidence-based ERAS protocol. Table 2.1 lists the modern protocols we use for RC/PLND/UD at USC [14, 17]. Our initial reports showed significantly shortened LOS without increased risks of readmissions after we started to implement the ERAS pathway [14, 17].

Preoperative Considerations

Preoperatively, an educational class for patients and caregivers is completed with an emphasis on expectations for hospitalization and discharge planning. For patients with RC, education about urinary diversions is extremely important since it may affect early discharge [8]. Carbohydrate loading is encouraged as it has been demonstrated to facilitate improved recovery after various surgeries and potentially decrease infection rates [24, 25].

It has been well established that preoperative mechanical bowel preparation (MBP) can be safely omitted in both urologic and colorectal literature [26, 27]. Slim et al. [27] included 14 randomized controlled trials (RCTs) with a total of 4859 patients before colorectal surgery in a meta-analysis: 2452 in the MBP group and 2407 in the no MBP group. The results showed the use of different MBP regimes did not influence primary and secondary outcomes (complications). Deng et al. [26] included two RCT and five cohort studies in a meta-analysis focusing on the role of MBP before ileal UD. The meta-analysis suggested that MBP did not reduce the incidence of perioperative complications in UD.

Table 2.1 The USC ERAS protocol

Preoperative	Precystectomy educational class Carbohydrate loading No bowel preparation Alvimopan 12 mg oral first dose 12 h before operation No epidural
Intraoperative	Opioid sparing anesthesia Minimize intravenous fluid based on stroke volume/central venous pressure
Postoperative	No nasogastric tube Nausea and vomiting prophylaxis Prokinetics (metoclopramide 10 mg intravenously every 6 h as needed) Alvimopan (12 mg twice daily until bowel activity for maximum of 7 days) Neostigmine (0.5 mg subcutaneously twice daily starting on POD 1 until bowel activity for maximum of 72 h) H2 blocker and proton pump inhibitor Early enteral feeding (cystectomy/regular diet—POD 1) Nonnarcotic pain control 24-h perioperative prophylactic antibiotics Prophylactic antibiotics until catheter/stent removal Home intravenous hydration Oral sodium bicarbonate at time of discharge if needed

POD postoperative day

The impact of narcotic pain medications on slowing bowel function is well known. However, adequate pain control following any surgical intervention is essential for appropriate recovery. Regional anesthesia has been advocated for patients undergoing RC. Retrospective studies have shown that epidural anesthesia may be associated with increased postoperative complications [28, 29]. Another alternative is the rectus sheath catheter, and a recent RCT has shown non-inferiority of rectus sheath catheter insertion compared to epidural for opiate usage and satisfaction with pain control [30]. We do not routinely place epidural catheters for RC at USC, but we do use rectus sheath catheter analgesia with an elastomeric pump, along with around the clock acetaminophen and nonsteroidal anti-inflammatory drugs (NSAIDs) for pain control and minimize opioid usage in patients.

Intraoperative Considerations

We emphasize opioid-sparing anesthesia and goal-directed fluid therapy for the surgery [31]. Goal-directed fluid therapy aims to decrease complications associated with fluid excess or hypovolemia. The original 2013 ERAS society guidelines suggested fluid balance should be optimized by targeting cardiac output using the esophageal Doppler system or other systems for this purpose and avoiding overhydration. Judicious use of vasopressors was recommended with arterial hypotension [8]. Fluid monitoring in cystectomy patients can be challenging as urine output is not reliable.

Another consideration worth discussing is robot-assisted RC (RARC). Most of the RCTs showed decreased blood loss but longer operative time with the RARC compared to open RC (ORC) [32–35]. No convincing evidence suggests that RARC enhances recovery in terms of LOS or rates of complications when compared with modern open series applying ERAS care pathways. Current data seem to indicate that clinical outcomes are impacted more by perioperative care patterns (ERAS) than by surgical approaches [20, 36]. Indeed, our series suggested that the surgical approach was not a determinant of readmission or major complications following RC in the context of an ERAS protocol [20]. We believe smaller incisions, less bowel manipulation, efficient/expeditious surgery, minimization of blood loss/transfusion, and consistency play important roles in ERAS for RC.

Postoperative Considerations

Gastrointestinal (GI) complications such as ileus are very common after RC, and they are associated with prolonged LOS, increased morbidity, and increased cost [16]. Therefore, interventions to address GI complications are among the most closely studied [3, 7]. As we can see from Table 2.1, most of the postoperative items are used to target GI complications, especially postoperative ileus.

Nasogastric tubes (or orogastric tubes if used) are removed at the end of surgery and not routinely continued postoperatively. A Cochrane analysis for RCTs comparing groups with and without nasogastric tubes for major abdominal surgeries showed patients without NG tubes had earlier return to bowel function [37]. Bowel preps and prolonged use of NG tubes are no longer recommended.

We tend to be very aggressive in terms of using antiemetics and/or prokinetics. The most notable medication is Alvimopan, a peripheral μ-opioid receptor agonist in the GI tract. Its usage is supported by the highest level of evidence [38–40]. A multicenter double-blinded RCT that included RCs performed in 31 high-volume centers from the United States showed that the perioperative use of Alvimopan was associated with 1.3 days decrease in GI recovery time and almost 2.7 days decrease in LOS compared to placebo [38]. Ileus-related morbidity was only 8.4% in the Alvimopan group compared to 29.1% in the placebo group. The need for postoperative NG tubes and prolonged LOS due to ileus-related morbidity were also significantly lower in the Alvimopan group. FDA approved Alvimopan for perioperative use in patients undergoing RC based on this trial, and Alvimopan has become an essential part of modern ERAS protocols. Of note, there is a difference between the duration of Alvimopan between our institution and the protocol used in the trial. We typically discontinue the medication after the first few bowel movements while it was continued for 7 days or until the time of discharge in the trial. It is unclear whether resuming Alvimopan after the return of regular bowel movements would have any additional benefits. One major disadvantage of Alvimopan is the cost, and our modified administration protocol could potentially relieve some of the concerns regarding the cost of this medication while still ensuring a significant reduction in GI complications.

As part of our USC protocol, we have used neostigmine to further stimulate bowel recovery. All patients who receive low-dose neostigmine postoperatively remain on cardiac monitoring for at least 24–48 h given the potential risk of cardiac arrhythmias reported with this medication. Neostigmine is typically discontinued after the first bowel movement [14]. With previously mentioned protocols to accelerate bowel recovery, early feeding is well tolerated in our RC patients. Early feeding is also well supported in the literature [41, 42]. Patients at USC start a regular diet on the first postoperative day.

In our recent series of 292 patients who underwent RC under ERAS protocol, the GI complication rate was only 15.4% with ileus being the most common one at 11.6% [43]. When compared to non-ERAS perioperative care, the 30-day GI complication rate in the ERAS group was significantly lower (13% versus 27%). The most significant reduction in GI complications was noted for ileus (7% versus 23%). The median time from surgery to first flatus was 2 d (range 1–6) in the ERAS cohort and 5 d (range 2–8) in the control group. The median time to first bowel movement was 2 d (range 1–7) in the ERAS cohort and 5 d (range 2–13) in the control group. Median LOS was significantly shorter in the ERAS cohort (4 d, range 3–16) than in the control group (9 d, range 5–23).

Infectious complications, especially urinary tract infections (UTIs), are also very common after RC and are associated with significant morbidity and risk of readmission [17, 44]. One study reported a UTI rate of approximately 36% and the urosepsis rate of 7.2% within 90 days of surgery in a large cohort of RC patients even with ERAS protocol [44]. UTIs are common in RC because of the nature of urinary diversion (using bowel segments, refluxing ureteroenteric anastomosis, using catheters and ureteral stents). As a standard procedure, all patients undergoing RC receive 24-h perioperative antibiotics. Although there is no high level of evidence to support prolonged prophylactic antibiotic usage, some retrospective data suggested the potential benefits [45, 46]. However, the use of prophylactic antibiotics beyond 24 h after surgery to prevent UTI is still debatable, and its duration is widely variable among different institutions [45]. In our institution, all patients are placed on prophylactic oral antibiotics after the first 24 h until the time of the stent removal which varies based on the type of UD (10 days for ileal conduit and 21 days for orthotopic neobladder). The antibiotic of choice in our institution is currently nitrofurantoin (100 mg daily) based on our internal review of antimicrobial sensitivity analysis of urine culture results and institutional antibiogram.

Finally, all patients are arranged to receive home intravenous hydration following discharge to prevent complications of dehydration and acidosis [10, 47]. For acidosis, oral sodium bicarbonate will also be prescribed if needed. At our institution, a comparatively high volume of continent urinary diversions is performed in eligible patients. It is our experience that these patients are particularly prone to dehydration in the early postoperative period, and the provision of intravenous fluid can limit this complication.

Future Directions

ERAS continues to evolve and improve as comprehensive multidisciplinary approaches to the care of complex surgical patients. Several important issues remain to be answered with more or higher levels of data.

Thromboembolic Events

Patients undergoing pelvic surgery of significant length are at an increased risk for VTE [48–50]. Neoadjuvant chemotherapy, older age, PLND, and malignancy put RC patients at even higher risk. The incidence of symptomatic venous thromboembolism in short-term follow-up after RC is 3%–11.6%, of which more than 50% of cases will occur after hospital discharge [49, 50]. Meta-analyses of clinical trials in patients undergoing major abdominal or pelvic cancer surgeries suggest a decreased risk of venous thromboembolisms for patients receiving extended (4 weeks) venous thromboembolism prophylaxis [51, 52]. Literature on RC also suggested extended prophylaxis (most commonly Enoxaparin) should be considered in all RC cases [49, 53]. Most recent data showed that oral anticoagulants (e.g., apixaban, rivaroxaban) are acceptable alternatives to enoxaparin with similar safety and efficacy profiles [54, 55]. For other pelvic surgeries, one RCT showed oral apixaban is comparable to subcutaneous enoxaparin for thromboembolism prophylaxis after surgery for gynecologic cancer [56].

Prehabilitation

There is emerging evidence supporting multimodal prehabilitation as a strategy to reduce the risk of complications and improve functional recovery after major surgery [57–59]. There are a few studies that investigated the impact of single modal or multimodal prehabilitation programs on functional recovery following RC [60–62]. The program in one study included only 4-week supervised preoperative exercise training [60]. Successful compliance, defined as adherence to >70% of sessions, was achieved by 80% of patients. A multimodal preoperative conditioning intervention in one study included aerobic and resistance exercise, diet therapy, and relaxation techniques [62]. Four weeks postoperatively, the prehabilitation group had significantly improved functional capacity as measured by a 6-min walk test compared to the standard group. Despite these studies, the role of prehabilitation in the ERAS pathway and its benefits in surgical outcomes are not well understood. No adequately powered trial has been performed, but several larger multi-centered RCTs are being conducted, including PREPARE-ABC trial, Prehab4cancer trial, and ENHANCE trial [63–65].

Immunonutrition

It is well known that nutritional status is associated with postoperative outcomes, and ERAS society has incorporated some of the nutritional care into their guidelines [24]. In recent years, studies have shown the use of immunonutrition in patients who have undergone oncological surgery decreases the levels of inflammatory markers and infectious postoperative complications [66, 67]. More studies about the use of immunonutrition in ERAS protocols for different types of surgeries are still needed. SWOG 1600, a randomized phase III double-blind clinical trial, was designed to evaluate the effect of a specialized immunonutritional supplement containing arginine, omega-3 fatty acids, dietary nucleotides, and vitamin A on outcomes after RC [68]. The study is expected to be completed by December 2023 and will answer some of the pending questions in terms of its role in ERAS protocol.

Summary

ERAS has been well studied in various surgical specialties and has been firmly established as an effective care to improve outcomes. ERAS represents a patient-centered and evidence-based approach to providing high-quality care to surgical patients and should be embraced at all levels of care. Most of the major pelvic surgeries such as colorectal and gynecologic oncologic surgeries should benefit from ERAS. Ongoing research and future studies will continue to refine care pathways for each operation and reveal the best methods for improving the care of these patients.

References

1. Kehlet H. Multimodal approach to control postoperative pathophysiology and rehabilitation. Br J Anaesth. 1997;78(5):606–17.
2. Fearon KC, Ljungqvist O, Von Meyenfeldt M, Revhaug A, Dejong CH, Lassen K, Nygren J, Hausel J, Soop M, Andersen J, Kehlet H. Enhanced Recovery After Surgery: a consensus review of clinical care for patients undergoing colonic resection. Clin Nutr. 2005;24(3):466–77.
3. Visioni A, Shah R, Gabriel E, Attwood K, Kukar M, Nurkin S. Enhanced Recovery After Surgery for noncolorectal surgery?: a systematic review and meta-analysis of major abdominal surgery. Ann Surg. 2018;267(1):57–65.
4. Williams SB, Cumberbatch MGK, Kamat AM, Jubber I, Kerr PS, McGrath JS, Djaladat H, Collins JW, Packiam VT, Steinberg GD, Lee E, Kassouf W, Black PC, Cerantola Y, Catto JWF, Daneshmand S. Reporting radical cystectomy outcomes following implementation of Enhanced Recovery After Surgery protocols: a systematic review and individual patient data meta-analysis. Eur Urol. 2020;78(5):719–30.
5. Tyson MD, Chang SS. Enhanced recovery pathways versus standard care after cystectomy: a meta-analysis of the effect on perioperative outcomes. Eur Urol. 2016;70(6):995–1003.
6. Hong T, Bisaillon A, Black P, So A, Mayson K. Implementation of an Enhanced Recovery After Surgery (ERAS) protocol can improve outcomes for patients undergoing radical cystectomy. Clin Nutr ESPEN. 2016;12:e46.
7. Stangl-Kremser J, Lambertini L, Di Maida F, Martinez-Fundichely A, Ferro M, Pradere B, Soria F, Albisinni S, Wu Z, Del Giudice F, Cacciamani GE, Valerio M, Briganti A, Roupret M, Shariat SF, Lee C, Minervini A, Moschini M, Mari A, European Association of Urology-Young Academic Urologists Urothelial Carcinoma Working G. Enhancing recovery after major bladder cancer surgery: comprehensive review and assessment of application of the Enhanced Recovery After Surgery guidelines. Eur Urol Focus. 2022;8(6):1622–6.
8. Cerantola Y, Valerio M, Persson B, Jichlinski P, Ljungqvist O, Hubner M, Kassouf W, Muller S, Baldini G, Carli F, Naesheimh T, Ytrebo L, Revhaug A, Lassen K, Knutsen T, Aarsether E, Wiklund P, Patel HR. Guidelines for perioperative care after radical cystectomy for bladder cancer: Enhanced Recovery After Surgery (ERAS((R))) society recommendations. Clin Nutr. 2013;32(6):879–87.
9. Sobhani S, Ghoreifi A, Douglawi A, Ahmadi H, Miranda G, Cai J, Aron M, Schuckman A, Desai M, Gill I, Daneshmand S, Djaladat H. Perioperative mortality for radical cystectomy in the modern era: experience from a tertiary referral center. Int Braz J Urol. 2023;49(3):351–8.
10. Ahmadi H, Daneshmand S. Association between use of ERAS protocols and complications after radical cystectomy. World J Urol. 2022;40(6):1311–6.
11. Smith A, Anders M, Auffenberg G, Chrouser K, Daneshmand S, Elllimootil C, Fellows J, Gilbert S, Gore JL, Merrill S, Nepple K, Richbourg L, Stoffel JT, Vollmer C. Optimizing outcomes in urological surgery: postoperative care. Urol Pract. 2020;7(6):521–9.
12. Zhou Y, Li R, Liu Z, Qi W, Lv G, Zhong M, Liu X, Zhu M, Jiang Z, Chen S, Shi B, Zhu Y. The effect of the Enhanced Recovery After Surgery program on radical cystectomy: a meta-analysis and systematic review. Front Surg. 2023;10:1101098.
13. Giannarini G, Crestani A, Inferrera A, Rossanese M, Subba E, Novara G, Ficarra V. Impact of Enhanced Recovery After Surgery protocols versus standard of care on perioperative outcomes of radical cystectomy: a systematic review and meta-analysis of comparative studies. Minerva Urol Nefrol. 2019;71(4):309–23.
14. Daneshmand S, Ahmadi H, Schuckman AK, Mitra AP, Cai J, Miranda G, Djaladat H. Enhanced recovery protocol after radical cystectomy for bladder cancer. J Urol. 2014;192(1):50–5.
15. Xu W, Daneshmand S, Bazargani ST, Cai J, Miranda G, Schuckman AK, Djaladat H. Postoperative pain management after radical cystectomy: comparing traditional versus enhanced recovery protocol pathway. J Urol. 2015;194(5):1209–13.
16. Djaladat H, Daneshmand S. Gastrointestinal complications in patients who undergo radical cystectomy with enhanced recovery protocol. Curr Urol Rep. 2016;17(7):50.
17. Djaladat H, Katebian B, Bazargani ST, Miranda G, Cai J, Schuckman AK, Daneshmand S. 90-day complication rate in patients undergoing radical cystectomy with enhanced recovery protocol: a prospective cohort study. World J Urol. 2017;35(6):907–11.
18. Zainfeld D, Chen J, Cai J, Miranda G, Schuckman A, Daneshmand S, Djaladat H. The impact of patient-related nonmodifiable factors on perioperative outcomes following radical cystectomy with enhanced recovery protocol. Ther Adv Urol. 2018;10(12):393–401.
19. Zainfeld D, Shah A, Daneshmand S. Enhanced Recovery After Surgery pathways: role and outcomes in the Management of Muscle Invasive Bladder Cancer. Urol Clin North Am. 2018;45(2):229–39.
20. Chen J, Djaladat H, Schuckman AK, Aron M, Desai M, Gill IS, Clifford TG, Ghodoussipour S, Miranda G, Cai J, Daneshmand S. Surgical approach as a determinant factor of clinical outcome following radical cystectomy: does Enhanced Recovery After Surgery (ERAS) level the playing field? Urol Oncol. 2019;37(10):765–73.
21. Ghodoussipour S, Naser-Tavakolian A, Cameron B, Mitra AP, Miranda G, Cai J, Bhanvadia S, Aron M, Desai M, Gill I, Schuckman A, Daneshmand S, Djaladat H. Internal audit of an Enhanced Recovery After Surgery protocol for radical cystectomy. World J Urol. 2020;38(12):3131–7.

22. Segelman J, Nygren J. Best practice in major elective rectal/pelvic surgery: Enhanced Recovery After Surgery (ERAS). Updat Surg. 2017;69(4):435–9.
23. Pang KH, Groves R, Venugopal S, Noon AP, Catto JWF. Prospective implementation of Enhanced Recovery After Surgery protocols to radical cystectomy. Eur Urol. 2018;73(3):363–71.
24. Cochran A, Cassady BA, Kerr KW, Milas Z, Riggs S, Iannitti DA, Vrochides D. Impact of nutritional compliance within ERAS protocols for hepatopancreatobiliary, radical cystectomy, and head and neck procedures: a case-matched analysis adjusted for major complications. Clin Nutr ESPEN. 2023;55:109–15.
25. Noblett SE, Watson DS, Huong H, Davison B, Hainsworth PJ, Horgan AF. Pre-operative oral carbohydrate loading in colorectal surgery: a randomized controlled trial. Color Dis. 2006;8(7):563–9.
26. Deng S, Dong Q, Wang J, Zhang P. The role of mechanical bowel preparation before ileal urinary diversion: a systematic review and meta-analysis. Urol Int. 2014;92(3):339–48.
27. Slim K, Vicaut E, Launay-Savary MV, Contant C, Chipponi J. Updated systematic review and meta-analysis of randomized clinical trials on the role of mechanical bowel preparation before colorectal surgery. Ann Surg. 2009;249(2):203–9.
28. Mishra K, Fernstrum A, Mahran A, Sidagam V, Adamic B, Shekar A, Calaway A, Nguyen C, Ponsky L, Bukavina L. Epidural anesthesia is associated with increased complications in cystectomy patients: a NSQIP analysis. Urology. 2020;138:77–83.
29. Patel SY, Ackerman RS, Boulware D, Poch MA. Epidural anesthesia may be associated with increased postoperative complications in the elderly population undergoing radical cystectomy: an analysis from the National Surgical Quality Improvement Project (NSQIP) database. World J Urol. 2021;39(2):433–41.
30. Chedgy ECP, Tang R, Struss WJ, Lowe G, Sawka A, Vaghadia H, Froehlich K, Black PC, Gleave ME, So AI. A randomized controlled trial investigating rectus sheath catheters following radical cystectomy. BJU Int. 2023;132(5):554–9.
31. Bazargani ST, Ghodoussipour S, Tse B, Miranda G, Cai J, Schuckman A, Daneshmand S, Djaladat H. The association between intraoperative fluid intake and postoperative complications in patients undergoing radical cystectomy with an enhanced recovery protocol. World J Urol. 2018;36(3):401–7.
32. Catto JWF, Khetrapal P, Ricciardi F, Ambler G, Williams NR, Al-Hammouri T, Khan MS, Thurairaja R, Nair R, Feber A, Dixon S, Nathan S, Briggs T, Sridhar A, Ahmad I, Bhatt J, Charlesworth P, Blick C, Cumberbatch MG, Hussain SA, Kotwal S, Koupparis A, McGrath J, Noon AP, Rowe E, Vasdev N, Hanchanale V, Hagan D, Brew-Graves C, Kelly JD. I ROCST: effect of robot-assisted radical cystectomy with Intracorporeal urinary diversion vs open radical cystectomy on 90-day morbidity and mortality among patients with bladder cancer: a randomized clinical trial. JAMA. 2022;327(21):2092–103.
33. Parekh DJ, Reis IM, Castle EP, Gonzalgo ML, Woods ME, Svatek RS, Weizer AZ, Konety BR, Tollefson M, Krupski TL, Smith ND, Shabsigh A, Barocas DA, Quek ML, Dash A, Kibel AS, Shemanski L, Pruthi RS, Montgomery JS, Weight CJ, Sharp DS, Chang SS, Cookson MS, Gupta GN, Gorbonos A, Uchio EM, Skinner E, Venkatramani V, Soodana-Prakash N, Kendrick K, Smith JA Jr, Thompson IM. Robot-assisted radical cystectomy versus open radical cystectomy in patients with bladder cancer (RAZOR): an open-label, randomised, phase 3, non-inferiority trial. Lancet. 2018;391(10139):2525–36.
34. Bochner BH, Dalbagni G, Marzouk KH, Sjoberg DD, Lee J, Donat SM, Coleman JA, Vickers A, Herr HW, Laudone VP. Randomized trial comparing open radical cystectomy and robot-assisted laparoscopic radical cystectomy: oncologic outcomes. Eur Urol. 2018;74(4):465–71.
35. Bochner BH, Dalbagni G, Sjoberg DD, Silberstein J, Keren Paz GE, Donat SM, Coleman JA, Mathew S, Vickers A, Schnorr GC, Feuerstein MA, Rapkin B, Parra RO, Herr HW, Laudone VP. Comparing open radical cystectomy and robot-assisted laparoscopic radical cystectomy: a randomized clinical trial. Eur Urol. 2015;67(6):1042–50.
36. Tan WS, Tan MY, Lamb BW, Sridhar A, Mohammed A, Baker H, Nathan S, Briggs T, Tan M, Kelly JD. Intracorporeal robot-assisted radical cystectomy, together with an enhanced recovery programme, improves postoperative outcomes by aggregating marginal gains. BJU Int. 2018;121(4):632–9.
37. Nelson R, Edwards S, Tse B. Prophylactic nasogastric decompression after abdominal surgery. Cochrane Database Syst Rev. 2007;2007(3):CD004929.
38. Lee CT, Chang SS, Kamat AM, Amiel G, Beard TL, Fergany A, Karnes RJ, Kurz A, Menon V, Sexton WJ, Slaton JW, Svatek RS, Wilson SS, Techner L, Bihrle R, Steinberg GD, Koch M. Alvimopan accelerates gastrointestinal recovery after radical cystectomy: a multicenter randomized placebo-controlled trial. Eur Urol. 2014;66(2):265–72.
39. Alhashemi M, Hamad R, El-Kefraoui C, Blouin MC, Amar-Zifkin A, Landry T, Lee L, Baldini G, Feldman LS, Fiore JF Jr. The association of alvimopan treatment with postoperative outcomes after abdominal surgery: a systematic review across different surgical procedures and contexts of perioperative care. Surgery. 2021;169(4):934–44.
40. Xu LL, Zhou XQ, Yi PS, Zhang M, Li J, Xu MQ. Alvimopan combined with enhanced recovery strategy for managing postoperative ileus after open abdominal surgery: a systematic review and meta-analysis. J Surg Res. 2016;203(1):211–21.
41. Deibert CM, Silva MV, RoyChoudhury A, McKiernan JM, Scherr DS, Seres D, Benson MC. A prospective randomized trial of the effects of early enteral feeding after radical cystectomy. Urology. 2016;96:69–73.

42. Lewis SJ, Andersen HK, Thomas S. Early enteral nutrition within 24 h of intestinal surgery versus later commencement of feeding: a systematic review and meta-analysis. J Gastrointest Surg. 2009;13(3):569–75.
43. Bazargani ST, Djaladat H, Ahmadi H, Miranda G, Cai J, Schuckman AK, Daneshmand S. Gastrointestinal complications following radical cystectomy using enhanced recovery protocol. Eur Urol Focus. 2018;4(6):889–94.
44. Ghoreifi A, Van Horn CM, Xu W, Cai J, Miranda G, Bhanvadia S, Schuckman AK, Daneshmand S, Djaladat H. Urinary tract infections following radical cystectomy with enhanced recovery protocol: a prospective study. Urol Oncol. 2020;38(3):75 e79–14.
45. Antonelli L, Sebro K, Lahmar A, Black PC, Ghodoussipour S, Hamilton-Reeves JM, Shah J, Bente Thoft J, Lerner SP, Llorente C, Lucca I, Preston MA, Psutka SP, Sfakianos JP, Vahr Lauridsen S, Williams SB, Catto J, Djaladat H, Kassouf W, Loftus K, Daneshmand S, Fankhauser CD. Enhanced Recovery After Surgery ECC: association between antibiotic prophylaxis before cystectomy or stent removal and infection complications: a systematic review. Eur Urol Focus. 2023;9(4):631–6.
46. Werntz RP, Martinez-Acevedo A, Amadi H, Kopp R, La Rochelle J, Koppie T, Amling C, Sajadi KP. Prophylactic antibiotics following radical cystectomy reduces urinary tract infections and readmission for sepsis from a urinary source. Urol Oncol. 2018;36(5):238 e231–5.
47. Zainfeld D, Djaladat H. Enhanced recovery after urologic surgery-current applications and future directions. J Surg Oncol. 2017;116(5):630–7.
48. Garas SN, McAlpine K, Ross J, Carrier M, Bosse D, Yachnin D, Mallick R, Cagiannos I, Morash C, Breau RH, Lavallee LT. Venous thromboembolism risk in patients receiving neoadjuvant chemotherapy for bladder cancer. Urol Oncol. 2022;40(8):381 e381–7.
49. Klaassen Z, Arora K, Goldberg H, Chandrasekar T, Wallis CJD, Sayyid RK, Fleshner NE, Finelli A, Kutikov A, Violette PD, Kulkarni GS. Extended venous thromboembolism prophylaxis after radical cystectomy: a call for adherence to current guidelines. J Urol. 2018;199(4):906–14.
50. Sun AJ, Djaladat H, Schuckman A, Miranda G, Cai J, Daneshmand S. Venous thromboembolism following radical cystectomy: significant predictors, comparison of different anticoagulants and timing of events. J Urol. 2015;193(2):565–9.
51. Fagarasanu A, Alotaibi GS, Hrimiuc R, Lee AY, Wu C. Role of extended thromboprophylaxis after abdominal and pelvic surgery in cancer patients: a systematic review and meta-analysis. Ann Surg Oncol. 2016;23(5):1422–30.
52. Guo Q, Huang B, Zhao J, Ma Y, Yuan D, Yang Y, Du X. Perioperative pharmacological thromboprophylaxis in patients with cancer: a systematic review and meta-analysis. Ann Surg. 2017;265(6):1087–93.
53. Pariser JJ, Pearce SM, Anderson BB, Packiam VT, Prachand VN, Smith ND, Steinberg GD. Extended duration enoxaparin decreases the rate of venous thromboembolic events after radical cystectomy compared to inpatient only subcutaneous heparin. J Urol. 2017;197(2):302–7.
54. Rosen G, Anwar T, Syed J, Weinstein D, Ravichandran S, Bailey J, Hamilton Z, Murray KS. Initial experience with apixaban for extended venous thromboembolism prophylaxis after radical cystectomy. Eur Urol Focus. 2022;8(2):480–2.
55. Faraj KS, Durant A, Mauler D, Choudry M, Singh R, Chang YH, Tyson MD. Extended anticoagulation after radical cystectomy using direct acting oral anticoagulants: a single-institutional experience. Urol Pract. 2022;9(5):451–8.
56. Guntupalli SR, Brennecke A, Behbakht K, Tayebnejad A, Breed CA, Babayan LM, Cheng G, Ramzan AA, Wheeler LJ, Corr BR, Lefkowits C, Sheeder J, Matsuo K, Flink D. Safety and efficacy of apixaban vs enoxaparin for preventing postoperative venous thromboembolism in women undergoing surgery for gynecologic malignant neoplasm: a randomized clinical trial. JAMA Netw Open. 2020;3(6):e207410.
57. Chang MC, Choo YJ, Kim S. Effect of prehabilitation on patients with frailty undergoing colorectal cancer surgery: a systematic review and meta-analysis. Ann Surg Treat Res. 2023;104(6):313–24.
58. Zarate Rodriguez JG, Cos H, Koenen M, Cook J, Lmsw CK, Raper L, Guthrie T, Strasberg SM, Hawkins WG, Hammill CW, Fields RC, Chapman WC, Eberlein TJ, Kozower BD, Sanford DE. Impact of prehabilitation on postoperative mortality and the need for non-home discharge in high-risk surgical patients. J Am Coll Surg. 2023;237(3):558–67.
59. Molenaar CJ, van Rooijen SJ, Fokkenrood HJ, Roumen RM, Janssen L, Slooter GD. Prehabilitation versus no prehabilitation to improve functional capacity, reduce postoperative complications and improve quality of life in colorectal cancer surgery. Cochrane Database Syst Rev. 2023;5(5):CD013259.
60. Kaye DR, Schafer C, Thelen-Perry S, Parker C, Iglay-Reger H, Daignault-Newton S, Qin Y, Morgan TM, Weizer AZ, Kaffenberger SD, Herrel LA, Hafez KS, Lee CT, Skolarus TA, Englesbe MJ, Montgomery JS. The feasibility and impact of a Presurgical exercise intervention program (Prehabilitation) for patients undergoing cystectomy for bladder cancer. Urology. 2020;145:106–12.
61. Banerjee S, Manley K, Shaw B, Lewis L, Cucato G, Mills R, Rochester M, Clark A, Saxton JM. Vigorous intensity aerobic interval exercise in bladder cancer patients prior to radical cystectomy: a feasibility randomised controlled trial. Support Care Cancer. 2018;26(5):1515–23.
62. Minnella EM, Awasthi R, Bousquet-Dion G, Ferreira V, Austin B, Audi C, Tanguay S, Aprikian A, Carli F, Kassouf W. Multimodal Prehabilitation to Enhance functional capacity following radical cystectomy:

a randomized controlled trial. Eur Urol Focus. 2021;7(1):132–8.
63. Collaborative P-AT. SupPoRtive exercise Programmes for Accelerating REcovery after major ABdominal Cancer surgery trial (PREPARE-ABC): pilot phase of a multicentre randomised controlled trial. Color Dis. 2021;23(11):3008–22.
64. Moore J, Merchant Z, Rowlinson K, McEwan K, Evison M, Faulkner G, Sultan J, McPhee JS, Steele J. Implementing a system-wide cancer prehabilitation programme: the journey of Greater Manchester's 'Prehab4cancer'. Eur J Surg Oncol. 2021;47(3 Pt A):524–32.
65. Akdemir E, Sweegers MG, Vrieling A, Rundqvist H, Meijer RP, Leliveld-Kors AM, van der Heijden AG, Rutten VC, Koldewijn EL, Bos SD, Wijburg CJ, Marcelissen TAT, Bongers BC, Retel VP, van Harten WH, May AM, Groen WG, Stuiver MM. EffectiveNess of a multimodal preHAbilitation program in patieNts with bladder canCEr undergoing radical cystectomy: protocol of the ENHANCE multicentre randomised controlled trial. BMJ Open. 2023;13(3):e071304.
66. Garcia-Malpartida K, Aragon-Valera C, Botella-Romero F, Ocon-Breton MJ, Lopez-Gomez JJ. Effects of immunonutrition on cancer patients undergoing surgery: a scoping review. Nutrients. 2023;15(7):1776.
67. Khaleel S, Regmi S, Hannah P, Watarai B, Sathianathen N, Weight C, Konety B. Impact of preoperative immunonutrition on perioperative outcomes following cystectomy. J Urol. 2021;206(5):1132–8.
68. Hamilton-Reeves J, Holzbeierlein JM, Unger JM, Lew DL, Fisch MJ, Henry NL. A randomized phase III double-blind clinical trial (S1600) evaluating the effect of immune-enhancing nutrition on radical cystectomy outcomes. J Clin Oncol. 2018;36(6_suppl):TPS529.

Frailty

3

Armin Shahrokni

Frailty

Frailty is defined as the reduced ability of the body to tolerate stress [1]. It argues that if you apply the same level of distress to the bodies of two persons of the same age through, for example, surgery, the person who is more frail will experience a poorer outcome compared to the person who is more fit. However, as we age, the likelihood and degree of frailty increase [2]. This is the reason that many studies based on real-world datasets which include the typical community dwelling older adults have found that older age is associated with poorer outcomes, while in randomized control trials with restrictive exclusion criteria such as the patient's performance status, kidney or liver function, the relationship between older age and poorer outcomes becomes less pronounced. Frailty is also dynamic rather than static [3]. Patients can experience improvements or worsening of their frailty over time, depending on medical events and/or other stressors. For example, a systematic review showed that among nonfrail patients who survived at least 3 years, about 14% of them became frail during that time period [4]. Hence the need for reassessing frailty, especially after major health-related events.

Biological age is also associated with significant molecular and physiological changes [5]. Some have argued that a combination of nine factors, namely telomere attrition, epigenetic alterations, loss of proteostasis, deregulated nutrient sensing, mitochondrial dysfunction, cellular senescence, stem cell exhaustion, and altered intercellular communication, could lead to the aging process and/or its acceleration [6]. Aging is also associated with significant physiological changes [5]. Aging affects all organs, but its association is different from one patient to another, and in one patient, one organ may be affected more than others. An example of a major physiological change is decreased compliance of large vessels such as the aorta. Stiff arteries can lead to an increase in systolic blood pressure and a decrease in diastolic blood pressure, leading to a widening of pulse pressure. In the same line, the left ventricle compliance decreases, and its relaxation is delayed. These and other changes predispose the heart to the aging process, leading to an increase in blood pressure, aortic stenosis, heart failure, and nerve conduction abnormalities. Decreased lung function remains one of the hallmarks of the aging process. Peak aerobic exercise capacity falls by about 20% for every 10 years after age 70. Respiratory compliance decreases and as a result functional residual capacity decreases. The aging process is also associated with decreased ability of respiratory muscles in response to issues like hypoxia. Aging is also associated with diffuse glo-

A. Shahrokni (✉)
Department of Medicine, Jersey Shore University Medical Center, Neptune, NJ, USA
e-mail: armin.shahrokni@hmhn.org

M. Hoffman et al. (eds.), *Major Complications of Female Pelvic Surgery*,
https://doi.org/10.1007/978-3-031-66772-5_3

merulosclerosis. While serum creatinine may remain constant during aging, the glomerular filtration rate will fall. The immune system, both adaptive and innate, also declines with aging. As we age, our bone marrow is more infiltrated with fat which results in a decrease in bone marrow hematopoietic tissue. Other organs also experience changes with aging. For example, liver mass decreases by about 20–40%. Age-related muscle loss is a result of infiltration of muscles by fat and connective tissues.

Assessing Frailty

The gold standard for assessing frailty is the geriatric assessment, which is usually performed by geriatricians [7]. This is a comprehensive assessment of older adults that typically starts by assessing cognitive function through tools such as the Mini-Cog [8] or Mini-Mental State Exam [9]. It then proceeds to assess patients for the presence and severity of various comorbidities, nutritional status, polypharmacy, gait and balance, history of falls, social support and activity, and emotional well-being. However, a comprehensive geriatric assessment may take up to 60 min to complete, making it unfeasible in fast-paced clinics. Despite this, many argue that the value of the geriatric assessment is so high that healthcare institutions should make every effort to perform it routinely [10]. Alternatively, some have explored other solutions to increase the likelihood of this assessment being performed as routine care. For example, instead of using paper questionnaires and hiring personnel to administer the assessment, some have developed web-based geriatric assessment tools. These tools have been shown to be feasible in patients older than age 75 going for surgery, older patients who are receiving even toxic treatment such as chemotherapy, and minority patients [11–14]. Some have explored innovative approaches such as voice-assisted solutions [15]. These solutions, which some might be familiar with names like Alexa or Siri, automatically read the questions to the patients and then register patients' responses without any involvement from personnel.

There are various frailty assessment tools available for patients and healthcare providers who may not have the time, resources, or necessary skills to perform a full geriatric assessment. These tools can be categorized into two models: the phenotype model and the cumulative aging-impairment model [16].

The Fried Frailty Index [17] is one of the most commonly used frailty assessment tools based on the phenotype model. It assesses five factors, including involuntary loss of 10 pounds or more in the past 6 months, reduced grip strength, difficulty initiating movements, reduced walking speed, and fatigue. Patients with no impairments are considered fit, those with one or two impairments are pre-frail, and those with a higher number of impairments are considered frail. On the other hand, the cumulative aging-impairment model is based on the theory that as we age, we accumulate various aging-related impairments [18]. The more we accumulate these impairments, the more frail we become and, consequently, we become more susceptible to adverse outcomes during and after cancer treatment. In one study, researchers used a web-based geriatric assessment tool called electronic rapid fitness assessment to assess the frailty of cancer patients [19]. The study found that the number of aging-related impairments was associated with a six-month survival rate following cancer surgery. Even after adjusting for factors such as age and American Society of Anesthesiologists-Physical Status classification, each additional aging-related impairment was associated with a 14% increase in six-month mortality following cancer surgery. Other studies have also shown that the accumulation of aging-related impairments is associated with mortality, chemotherapy toxicity, and the risk of institutionalization [20–24].

In addition to instruments based on frailty phenotype or cumulative deficits, there are also many frailty screening tools that are shorter and take much less time to complete. An umbrella review of frailty screening tools reviewed 26 questionnaires aimed at detecting frailty and eight frailty indicators [25]. Huisingh-Scheetz and colleague described some of these frailty screening tools and provided guidance on how to approach frailty (assessment) in older patients with cancer [26]. Based on their guidance, factors to consider in selecting a frailty instrument are: (1) the feasibility of implementing the frailty instrument and its sustainability, and (2) specific clinical or research needs and considering limitations of the selected instrument. For example, if you are working in a busy clinic with a limited number of personnel, who are busy with many other tasks, selecting a self-reported frailty instrument might be more feasible for your practice than an instrument that requires interaction and time commitment between your staff and the patient.

Frailty and Health-Related Outcomes

While the association between frailty and clinical outcomes in different contexts has been established, in this section, we will focus on evidence suggestive of the relationship between frailty and cancer outcomes as many pelvic masses and surgeries may be conducted in the setting of oncologic diagnosis. Numerous studies have established a relationship between frailty and cancer outcomes [27–32]. A recent systematic review and meta-analysis of 71 studies demonstrated that frail patients are three times more likely, on average, to die within 30 days after surgery, and twice as likely to be discharged to locations other than their homes, experience postoperative complications, or have prolonged hospital stays [33]. They are also four times more likely to experience long-term mortality than fit patients.

In the surgery setting, a significant number of studies have used the modified frailty index [34], which is an 11-item instrument that includes 10 items related to a patient's comorbidities and one item related to functional independence. Because the modified frailty index is applied to a large dataset of the National Surgical Quality Improvement Program, studies that utilize the index have the advantage of a robust sample size, which allows for proper assessment of the relationship between frailty and surgical outcomes. For example, one study assessed the relationship between frailty and outcomes following gastrointestinal cancer surgery. They found that among 41,455 patients who had gastrointestinal cancer, frail patients were more likely to experience postoperative complications, prolonged hospital stays, and 30-day mortality compared to fit patients [35]. A similar finding was confirmed in another study of older women with ovarian cancer who underwent cytoreductive surgery [36]. A systematic review that evaluated seven studies showed that geriatric assessment is also associated with oncologic surgery outcomes. It demonstrated that impairments in basic and instrumental activities of daily living, as well as cognitive impairment, are associated with postoperative complications [37]. Another study of approximately 1000 patients over the age of 75 found that geriatric assessment is associated with six-month postoperative mortality [19].

Overall, these studies highlight the importance of considering frailty and conducting geriatric assessments in the context of oncologic or any high-risk surgery. They demonstrate that frailty is significantly associated with poor surgical outcomes, including postoperative complications, prolonged hospital stays, and mortality. By conducting proper assessments and taking appropriate precautions, healthcare professionals can better manage the care of frail cancer patients undergoing surgery.

Benefits of Frailty Assessment

Frailty assessment can be helpful in a variety of ways, including improving patient–physician communication. In fact, one study showed that performing geriatric assessment and sharing it with the oncology team leads to an improvement in communication, more discussion of aging-related issues in each encounter, and increased patient satisfaction with the care provided [38]. Another benefit of performing frailty assessment is a more accurate assessment of a patient's life expectancy, which can help in surgery decision-making. For example, many studies have shown that preoperative frailty of cancer patients is associated with both short- and long-term postoperative mortalities. Some patients after oncologic pelvic surgeries will be referred to the medical oncology team to make decisions on the risk/benefit of adjuvant treatment. To decide on administering adjuvant treatment, the medical oncology team should have a reasonable prediction of the benefits and risks of the proposed treatment. Therefore, a patient's lifespan plays an important role in this assessment. Assessing frailty allows the clinical teams to have a more accurate prediction of one's life expectancy. There are various life expectancy calculators available for use [39], which are suitable for patients with possible life expectancy of weeks (palliative prognostic index), 1 year (Gagne Index), four to 10 years (Lee Index), or 10 years (Suemoto Index) [40]. All these calculators have components of frailty and aging-related impairments. For example, the Lee Index [41] includes items related to comorbidities, basic and instrumental activities of daily living, and walking ability. Finally, the last yet not the least benefit of frailty assessment is the conversion of age as a nonmodifiable factor to frailty as a modifiable factor. Assessing a patient's frailty enables the cancer provider to provide more holistic care and not anchor on chronological age when making therapeutic decisions. Having frailty indexing tools readily available can help establish more person-centered care for older adults.

Interventions Following Frailty Assessment

Assessing frailty in older adults regardless of surgery procedure and/or type of comorbidities such as cancer is just the first step in providing person-centered care for these individuals. It is important to note that the frailty of a patient is dynamic and can potentially be improved with proper and timely interventions [42]. Referring frail patients to geriatricians and geriatric care providers is ideal when possible for further assessment and management of their aging-related impairments [43]. However, even in the absence of geriatricians, other interventions can be helpful in improving frailty and outcomes for these patients. Various guidelines for assessing and managing vulnerabilities of older adults are available [44]. According to the guideline, referring patients to physical or occupational therapy may be beneficial if they have fallen in the past or have impairment with basic and instrumental activities of daily living. Consultation with a pharmacist to assess for drug–drug interactions and possible de-prescribing may be helpful if the patient is taking too many medications. Active involvement by the patient's primary care provider and/or other subspecialists may be beneficial if the patient has multiple and severe comorbidities. Consultation with a social worker may be necessary to find proper community supportive services if the patient lives alone, has poor social support, or has difficulty with transportation. These interventions, either as a single intervention or as a bundle, can improve patient outcomes.

To improve perioperative outcomes of older adults with cancer, some have proposed a multiphase pathway that starts with frailty assessment and then proceeds to prehabilitation, collaboration with geriatricians, and interventions aimed at reducing the stress of surgery [45]. Over the past decade, prehabilitation has gained increasing attention as a potential strategy to address functional decline in older patients with or without cancer who undergo major surgeries. Such patients are often frail and may experience additional complications due to their comorbidities and surgery. Some studies have explored whether prehabilitation—which involves improving patients' physical condition before surgery—can be effective for older or frail adults. A systematic review of 33 studies, involving roughly 4000 patients who underwent elective abdominal cancer surgery, found that prehabilitation may lead to improvements in complication rates, hospital stays, and nutritional status [46]. However, additional studies are still needed, as some data remain mixed. For instance, a review of 10 studies on patients who underwent urological cancer procedures did not find any evidence that prehabilitation is associated with reduced surgical complications, hospital length of stay, or readmissions [47]. Other studies have examined the effects of preoperative geriatric assessments and identified high levels of distress or poor social support among patients, which could lead to increased utilization of mental health services in the postoperative period [48].

The Role of Geriatricians and Geriatric Care Providers

Geriatricians and geriatric care providers could play a crucial role in the care of older adults with or without cancer, given their expertise in assessing and managing aging-related impairments. In one care model, patients who screen positive for frailty by a short frailty instrument in the oncology clinic could be referred to a geriatric clinic for a more comprehensive assessment of aging-related impairments. Geriatricians can conduct a more thorough cognitive assessment, such as the Mini-Mental State Exam [9] or Montreal Cognitive Assessment [49], which is essential since several studies have indicated the possibility of cognitive decline during or after cancer treatment [50]. Having an accurate assessment of baseline cognitive function would enable the provision of support for those with cognitive impairment, as well as a more precise definition of the cognitive function trajectory during and after cancer treatment. Geriatricians and geriatric care providers could also be more cognizant of supportive services in the community and refer patients with various aging-related impairments to the appropriate resources.

In the hospital setting, geriatricians and geriatric care providers can assist in preventing, detecting early, and managing delirium. They can also engage in shared decision-making to assess the risk and benefits of treatment options based on the patient's frailty and overall goals of care. They can review the patient's medication list, particularly those dealing with polypharmacy, and assist cancer care providers in detecting drug–drug interactions, especially when one of the drugs is cancer-related treatment. Numerous studies have demonstrated that collaboration between geriatricians and other care providers improves outcomes for older adults, not only in cancer but also in other areas such as orthopedics. In the orthopedic setting, collaboration between geriatricians and orthopedic surgeons has resulted in significant improvements in postoperative outcomes for older adults.

A systematic review of 18 studies with approximately 9000 patients who underwent hip surgery demonstrated that geriatric comanagement was associated with a significant reduction in short- and long-term mortality and hospital length of stay [51]. A Cochrane review that primarily examined studies on geriatric comanagement for patients with hip fracture showed that geriatric comanagement reduced the likelihood of discharge to an elevated level of care [52]. One study assessed the impact of different models of geriatric comanagement on the outcomes of patients with hip fracture and discovered that all models of geriatric comanagement were similar in improving the outcomes of these patients [53].

In oncologic surgery, data are also emerging on the benefits of geriatric comanagement. A small study on older women with advanced ovarian cancer who underwent cytoreductive surgery showed that none of those patients died within 6 months of surgery [54]. Subsequently, a large retrospective study on approximately 1900 patients aged 75 and older who were either comanaged by the geriatric service or managed by a nongeriatrician team showed that geriatric comanagement was associated with a significant reduction in 90-day postoperative mortality [55]. A secondary data analysis of this study indicated that the benefit provided by geriatric comanagement could be irrespective of patients' frailty level in this relatively old age cohort of patients [56]. A pre–post geriatric comanagement implementation study demonstrated that geriatric comanagement was associated with a significant reduction in high-grade surgery complications and one-year readmission [57]. One study assessed the feasibility of geriatric comanagement in a prospective manner and found that geriatric comanagement was feasible in patients aged 75 and older who underwent radical cystectomy, and more importantly, the surgery team expressed their high level of satisfaction with such collaboration [58]. Due to this evidence, the American College of Surgery and the American Geriatrics Society have launched the Geriatric Surgery Verification Program to further advance the expansion of such programs [59].

Conclusion

We are facing an aging population. As we age, the likelihood of masses that are either symptomatic or found incidentally increases. The mainstay of treating majority of solid masses is surgery. Surgery in older patients is challenging. Those who are frail are at higher risk for adverse outcomes. Frailty assessment provides significant benefits for the patients, caregivers, and their cancer providers. Various interventions can be implemented with the aim of improving outcomes of these patients. High-quality data have emerged to support the benefit of frailty assessments and geriatric interventions, and it is very likely that soon, more data will emerge to further support this notion.

Financial Disclosure Nothing to disclose.

References

1. Baijal P, Periyakoil V. Understanding frailty in cancer patients. Cancer J. 2014;20(5):358–66.
2. Collard RM, et al. Prevalence of frailty in community-dwelling older persons: a systematic review. J Am Geriatr Soc. 2012;60(8):1487–92.
3. Chamberlain AM, et al. Frailty trajectories in an elderly population-based cohort. J Am Geriatr Soc. 2016;64(2):285–92.
4. Ofori-Asenso R, et al. Global incidence of frailty and Prefrailty among community-dwelling older adults: a systematic review and meta-analysis. JAMA Netw Open. 2019;2(8):e198398.
5. Khan SS, Singer BD, Vaughan DE. Molecular and physiological manifestations and measurement of aging in humans. Aging Cell. 2017;16(4):624–33.
6. López-Otín C, et al. The hallmarks of aging. Cell. 2013;153(6):1194–217.
7. Korc-Grodzicki B, Holmes HM, Shahrokni A. Geriatric assessment for oncologists. Cancer Biol Med. 2015;12(4):261–74.
8. Borson S, et al. The mini-cog as a screen for dementia: validation in a population-based sample. J Am Geriatr Soc. 2003;51(10):1451–4.
9. Creavin ST, et al. Mini-Mental State Examination (MMSE) for the detection of dementia in clinically unevaluated people aged 65 and over in community and primary care populations. Cochrane Database Syst Rev. 2016;2016(1):CD011145.
10. Hamaker ME, Wildes TM, Rostoft S. Time to stop saying geriatric assessment is too time consuming. J Clin Oncol. 2017;35(25):2871–4.
11. Shahrokni A, et al. Electronic rapid fitness assessment: a novel tool for preoperative evaluation of the geriatric oncology patient. J Natl Compr Cancer Netw. 2017;15(2):172–9.
12. Hurria A, et al. Reliability, validity, and feasibility of a computer-based geriatric assessment for older adults with cancer. J Oncol Pract. 2016;12(12):e1025–34.
13. McCleary NJ, et al. Feasibility of computer-based self-administered cancer-specific geriatric assessment in older patients with gastrointestinal malignancy. Oncologist. 2013;18(1):64–72.
14. Guerard E, et al. Electronic geriatric assessment: is it feasible in a multi-institutional study that included a notable proportion of older African American patients? (Alliance A171603). JCO Clin Cancer Inform. 2021;5:435–41.
15. Cuadra A, et al. Introducing the v-RFA, a voice assistant-based geriatric assessment. J Geriatr Oncol. 2022;13(8):1253–5.
16. Chen X, Mao G, Leng SX. Frailty syndrome: an overview. Clin Interv Aging. 2014;9:433–41.
17. Fried LP, et al. Frailty in older adults: evidence for a phenotype. J Gerontol A Biol Sci Med Sci. 2001;56(3):M146–56.
18. Rockwood K, Mitnitski A. Frailty defined by deficit accumulation and geriatric medicine defined by frailty. Clin Geriatr Med. 2011;27(1):17–26.
19. Shahrokni A, et al. Geriatric assessment, not ASA physical status, is associated with 6-month postoperative survival in patients with cancer aged ≥75 years. J Natl Compr Cancer Netw. 2019;17(6):687–94.
20. Cohen HJ, et al. Frailty as determined by a comprehensive geriatric assessment-derived deficit-accumulation index in older patients with cancer who receive chemotherapy. Cancer. 2016;122(24):3865–72.
21. de Vries J, et al. Association of Deficits Identified by geriatric assessment with deterioration of health-related quality of life in patients treated for head and neck cancer. JAMA Otolaryngol Head Neck Surg. 2021;147(12):1089–99.
22. Kenig J, et al. Cumulative deficit model of geriatric assessment to predict the postoperative outcomes of older patients with solid abdominal cancer. J Geriatr Oncol. 2015;6(5):370–9.
23. Clough-Gorr KM, et al. Older breast cancer survivors: geriatric assessment domains are associated with poor tolerance of treatment adverse effects and predict mortality over 7 years of follow-up. J Clin Oncol. 2010;28(3):380–6.

24. Hamaker ME, et al. Baseline comprehensive geriatric assessment is associated with toxicity and survival in elderly metastatic breast cancer patients receiving single-agent chemotherapy: results from the OMEGA study of the Dutch breast cancer trialists' group. Breast. 2014;23(1):81–7.
25. Apóstolo J, et al. Predicting risk and outcomes for frail older adults: an umbrella review of frailty screening tools. JBI Database System Rev Implement Rep. 2017;15(4):1154–208.
26. Huisingh-Scheetz M, Walston J. How should older adults with cancer be evaluated for frailty? J Geriatr Oncol. 2017;8(1):8–15.
27. Fagard K, et al. The impact of frailty on postoperative outcomes in individuals aged 65 and over undergoing elective surgery for colorectal cancer: a systematic review. J Geriatr Oncol. 2016;7(6):479–91.
28. Boakye D, et al. Impact of comorbidity and frailty on prognosis in colorectal cancer patients: a systematic review and meta-analysis. Cancer Treat Rev. 2018;64:30–9.
29. Ethun CG, et al. Frailty and cancer: implications for oncology surgery, medical oncology, and radiation oncology. CA Cancer J Clin. 2017;67(5):362–77.
30. Handforth C, et al. The prevalence and outcomes of frailty in older cancer patients: a systematic review. Ann Oncol. 2015;26(6):1091–101.
31. Abel GA, Klepin HD. Frailty and the management of hematologic malignancies. Blood. 2018;131(5):515–24.
32. Di Donato V, et al. Preoperative frailty assessment in patients undergoing gynecologic oncology surgery: a systematic review. Gynecol Oncol. 2021;161(1):11–9.
33. Shaw JF, et al. The Association of Frailty with outcomes after cancer surgery: a systematic review and Metaanalysis. Ann Surg Oncol. 2022;29(8):4690–704.
34. Tsiouris A, et al. A modified frailty index to assess morbidity and mortality after lobectomy. J Surg Res. 2013;183(1):40–6.
35. Vermillion SA, et al. Modified frailty index predicts postoperative outcomes in older gastrointestinal cancer patients. J Surg Oncol. 2017;115(8):997–1003.
36. Di Donato V, et al. Modified fragility index and surgical complexity score are able to predict postoperative morbidity and mortality after cytoreductive surgery for advanced ovarian cancer. Gynecol Oncol. 2021;161(1):4–10.
37. Feng MA, et al. Geriatric assessment in surgical oncology: a systematic review. J Surg Res. 2015;193(1):265–72.
38. Gilmore N, et al. Evaluating the association of frailty with communication about aging-related concerns between older patients with advanced cancer and their oncologists. Cancer. 2022;128(5):1101–9.
39. Rector T, et al. Life expectancy calculators. Washington, DC: Department of Veterans Affairs (US); 2016.
40. Verduzco-Aguirre HC, et al. Predicting life expectancy for older adults with cancer in clinical practice: implications for shared decision-making. Curr Oncol Rep. 2019;21(8):68.
41. Lee SJ, et al. Development and validation of a prognostic index for 4-year mortality in older adults. JAMA. 2006;295(7):801–8.
42. Marcucci M, et al. Interventions to prevent, delay or reverse frailty in older people: a journey towards clinical guidelines. BMC Med. 2019;17(1):193.
43. Cesari M, et al. The geriatric management of frailty as paradigm of "the end of the disease era". Eur J Intern Med. 2016;31:11–4.
44. Mohile SG, et al. Practical assessment and Management of Vulnerabilities in older patients receiving chemotherapy: ASCO guideline for geriatric oncology. J Clin Oncol. 2018;36(22):2326–47.
45. Montroni I, et al. Surgical considerations for older adults with cancer: a multidimensional, multiphase pathway to improve care. J Clin Oncol. 2021;39(19):2090–101.
46. Hijazi Y, Gondal U, Aziz O. A systematic review of prehabilitation programs in abdominal cancer surgery. Int J Surg. 2017;39:156–62.
47. Briggs LG, et al. Prehabilitation exercise before urologic cancer surgery: a systematic and interdisciplinary review. Eur Urol. 2022;81(2):157–67.
48. Trevino KM, et al. Is screening for psychosocial risk factors associated with mental health care in older adults with cancer undergoing surgery? Cancer. 2020;126(3):602–10.
49. Nasreddine ZS, et al. The Montreal cognitive assessment, MoCA: a brief screening tool for mild cognitive impairment. J Am Geriatr Soc. 2005;53(4):695–9.
50. Joly F, et al. Impact of cancer and its treatments on cognitive function: advances in research from the Paris international cognition and cancer task force symposium and update since 2012. J Pain Symptom Manag. 2015;50(6):830–41.
51. Grigoryan KV, Javedan H, Rudolph JL. Orthogeriatric care models and outcomes in hip fracture patients: a systematic review and meta-analysis. J Orthop Trauma. 2014;28(3):e49–55.
52. Eamer G, et al. Comprehensive geriatric assessment for older people admitted to a surgical service. Cochrane Database Syst Rev. 2018;1(1):CD012485.
53. Van Heghe A, et al. Effects of Orthogeriatric care models on outcomes of hip fracture patients: a systematic review and meta-analysis. Calcif Tissue Int. 2022;110(2):162–84.
54. Filippova OT, et al. Geriatric co-management leads to safely performed cytoreductive surgery in older women with advanced stage ovarian cancer treated at a tertiary care cancer center. Gynecol Oncol. 2019;154(1):77–82.
55. Shahrokni A, et al. Association of Geriatric Comanagement and 90-day postoperative mortality among patients aged 75 years and older with cancer. JAMA Netw Open. 2020;3(8):e209265.
56. McMillan S, et al. Association of frailty with 90-day postoperative mortality & geriatric comanagement

among older adults with cancer. Eur J Surg Oncol. 2022;48(4):903–8.
57. Giannotti C, et al. Effect of geriatric comanagement in older patients undergoing surgery for gastrointestinal cancer: a retrospective, before-and-after study. J Am Med Dir Assoc. 2022;23(11):1868.e9–1868.e16.
58. Letica-Kriegel AS, et al. Feasibility of a geriatric comanagement (GERICO) pilot program for patients 75 and older undergoing radical cystectomy. Eur J Surg Oncol. 2022;48(6):1427–32.
59. Cooper L, et al. Launching a geriatric surgery center: recommendations from the Society for Perioperative Assessment and Quality Improvement. J Am Geriatr Soc. 2020;68(9):1941–6.

Nutrition for the Surgical Patient

4

Richard A. Jacobson, Ankita Mishra, and Sean P. Dineen

Introduction

Patients undergoing pelvic operations are at high risk for nutritional morbidity owing to the nature of pelvic pathology, the operations, and adjuvant care required to treat them. This chapter will highlight the scope and scale of the issue of malnutrition before, during, and after pelvic surgery. We will review the consequences of malnutrition in surgical patients with benign and malignant diseases. Finally, we will detail recent trial data for interventions aimed at reducing the prevalence of perioperative malnutrition and mitigating its consequences.

Defining Malnutrition and Common Clinical Assessments

Patients requiring pelvic surgery have several risk factors for malnutrition related to disease status, including inflammatory and neoplastic pathology. The presence of obstructing masses, fistulae to the intestines, and cancer cachexia can exacerbate inadequate caloric intake over the course of weeks to months. Despite surgeons' knowledge of these risks, malnutrition was difficult to document and study for years, owing to the lack of (1) a concise and generalizable definition of the condition and (2) consensus biomarkers or laboratory values that identify malnutrition. Nutritional assessment is also quite dependent on the specific pathology further contributing to the need to individualize patient assessments [37].

Clinical assessments of malnutrition are the most rigorously validated measures in current clinical use. Traditional screening and assessment tools, such as the Subjective Global Assessment (SGA) [14, 15] and the Mini Nutritional Assessment [21, 22], rely on "snapshot" clinical metrics to assess the nutritional status of a patient [1]. These tools fail to recognize the importance of disease acuity and the contributions of inflammation and oxidative stress in deterioration of nutritional status and impaired utilization of feeding substrates [29]. Other validated tools, such as Nutrition Risk Score [14], the Nutritional Risk in the Critically Ill (NUTRIC) Score [24], and Global Leadership Initiative on Malnutrition (GLIM) [8], incorporate both nutritional status and disease severity. In these more modern metrics, nutritional status is determined by body mass index (BMI), percent weight loss, and reduced oral intake or the duration of hospitalization prior to being admitted to the ICU. Disease severity is determined by the Acute Physiologic and Chronic Health Evaluation (APACHE) II and Simplified Organ Failure Assessment scores [35].

R. A. Jacobson · A. Mishra · S. P. Dineen (✉)
GI Oncology, Moffitt Cancer Center,
Tampa, FL, USA
e-mail: sean.dineen@moffitt.org

M. Hoffman et al. (eds.), *Major Complications of Female Pelvic Surgery*,
https://doi.org/10.1007/978-3-031-66772-5_4

The tool most widely used clinically at our institution comes from the 2012 AND-ASPEN consensus statement for the identification and documentation of adult malnutrition. These guidelines define malnutrition as the presence of two of six clinical criteria listed in Table 4.1 in patients with chronic disease, with modifiers for acute illness. Severe malnutrition is defined as the presence of two or more factors listed in the second column [54]. Clinical malnutrition assessments such as these have outperformed circulating biomarkers in the identification of malnutrition amongst elective surgical patients [43]. The history and physical examination are a source for significant information regarding the risk of preoperative malnutrition. Recent weight loss, feeding difficulty or anorexia, and chronic infection are all important considerations for surgical planning. Additionally, BMI and percentage of weight loss are objective factors that are easily obtainable in all patients. Table 4.2 is a general comparison of commonly used nutritional screening and assessment tools.

Historically, serum albumin, prealbumin, and transferrin were used as biomarkers of nutritional risk status. The ease of using a laboratory panel was attractive for surgeons. However, these metrics have not been shown to correlate well with other nutritional parameters. The use of such markers may lead to underestimation of clinical malnutrition [43]. Albumin, prealbumin, and transferrin are negative acute-phase proteins, and

Table 4.1 Academy of Nutrition and Dietetics/American Society for Parenteral and Enteral Nutrition Consensus clinical characteristics supporting a diagnosis of malnutrition in patients with chronic disease

	Nonsevere		Severe	
Energy intake	<75% estimated requirement for 1 month		<50% estimated requirement for 1 month	
Weight loss	%	Months	%	Months
	5	1	>5	1
	7.5	3	>7.5	3
	10	6	>10	6
	20	12	>20	12
Loss of body fat	Mild		Severe	
Muscle mass	Mild		Severe	
Fluid accumulation	Mild		Severe	
Grip strength	NA		Measurably reduced	

Adapted from Ref. [54]

Table 4.2 Comparison of common clinical tools for the screening and assessment of malnutrition

Tool	Criteria	Use	Classifications
Subjective Global Assessment (SGA)	Nutritional intake, weight changes, gastrointestinal symptoms, functional capacity including fatigue, physical features including sarcopenia	Assessment	Well-nourished Mild/moderately malnourished Severely malnourished
Mini Nutritional Assessment (MNA)	Food intake, weight loss over 3 months, mobility, psychological stress, dementia, BMI	Screening and assessment	Protein-calorie malnutrition At risk Adequate nutrition
GLIM	Phenotypic: Weight loss, low BMI, decreased muscle mass Etiologic: Reduced intake, altered food absorption, inflammation (chronic or acute)	Screening and assessment	Moderate (Stage 1) Severe (Stage 2)
ASPEN/AND	Energy intake; weight loss; loss of body fat; muscle mass; fluid accumulation; grip strength	Assessment	Non severe Severe

their levels fall with any significant acute inflammation due to increased vascular permeability, change in hepatic protein synthesis (from homeostatic protein synthesis to production of acute-phase proteins such as fibrinogen and α-glycoprotein), and selective catabolism of albumin to make available cysteine for the glutathione antioxidant defense system [4, 35]. Similarly, once inflammation subsides, albumin and pre-albumin will rise regardless of nutritional therapy [17]. Trends in levels of prealbumin in combination with C-reactive protein can be helpful in assessment of nutritional therapy [12]. Additional markers, such as procalcitonin, interleukin-1, tumor necrosis factor, interleukin-6, and citrulline are surrogate markers of critical illness and possible bowel compromise, are still at an experimental stage [23, 52]. However, preoperative albumin levels have been shown to correlate with surgical outcomes. Hypoalbuminemia is associated with an increased risk for postoperative complications in many settings, including colorectal surgery [11]. Thus, preoperative albumin may still serve as a useful marker for predicting outcomes following pelvic surgery, even if not a significant predictor of malnutrition per se.

Emerging use of cross-sectional imaging may serve as important measures of lean body mass and appropriate tools to assess sarcopenia, a surrogate for malnutrition [16, 45]. Sarcopenia can be reliably measured on imaging, most commonly using the cross-sectional area of the psoas muscle at the level of the third lumbar vertebra. Sarcopenia defined as total psoas area normalized for height (<385 mm^2/m for females and <545 mm^2/m for males) was predictive of postoperative complications in colorectal surgery [26].

Prevalence of Preoperative Malnutrition in Pelvic Surgery

The underdiagnosis of malnutrition in cancer patients is a well-documented phenomenon [31, 42], and comparison of recently published administrative data to prospective investigation highlights this concept. A prospective study of 293 French patients admitted with genitourinary or colorectal cancer identified malnutrition in 32% and 31% of patients, respectively, using clinical criteria [44]. However, a retrospective study using National Inpatient Sample data to identify 17,010 patients undergoing surgery for rectal cancer between 2011 and 2017 found only 8% of patients carried a diagnosis of malnutrition at the time of surgery [32]. A NSQIP study of patients undergoing colorectal surgery between 2005 and 2017 identified 16% of the population as malnourished. All studies reached the conclusion that malnourished patients were more likely to suffer perioperative complications. However, these studies included patients treated prior to the wide dissemination of the AND-ASPEN criteria and highlight past struggles with under-identification of malnourished patients, particularly in administrative datasets.

General Consequences of Malnutrition in Pelvic Surgery

The consequences of malnutrition in patients undergoing pelvic surgery, like all surgery, are principally related to poor wound healing. Malnourished patients undergoing rectal resection are far more likely to suffer dehiscence of the colorectal anastomosis [3]. Ideally, this risk is appreciated preoperatively using clinical assessments and biomarkers such as albumin, and patients are diverted with a loop ileostomy to mitigate the consequences of anastomotic leak. However, as discussed below, the presence of an ileostomy comes with its own nutritional morbidity. Nondiverted patients who suffer leaks often require prolonged periods of nil per os and total parenteral nutrition, coupled with the metabolic stress of systemic sepsis. The unfortunate truth is that often in surgical patients, malnutrition begets malnutrition.

Malnutrition is associated with nongastrointestinal morbidity as well. A NSQIP study of 200,000 patients between 2005 and 2018 demonstrated a substantial increase in complications including bleeding, infection, VTE, and postoperative death in severely malnourished patients undergoing laparoscopic hysterectomy [51]. In a retrospective study, over 11,000 patients with malnutrition were propensity-score matched with nonmalnourished patients and found on multivariate analysis to have nearly twice the risk of postoperative mortality, along with increased hospital length of stay and associated costs [32]. Malnutrition is clearly associated with increased rates of postoperative fascial dehiscence and incisional hernia regardless of incision type or closure technique [34, 39]. Even patients undergoing minimally invasive operations have a higher hernia risk if malnourished [10].

In cancer patients, malnutrition is a marker of aggressive disease and immunocompromise. This concept is made clear in studies of oncologic outcomes after pelvic surgery in malnourished patients. Malnutrition was associated with recurrence of gynecologic malignancies in a retrospective review of 300 surgical patients [28]. Another retrospective study of 364 patients with locally advanced rectal cancer observed that preoperative malnutrition was associated with inferior 3-year overall survival (72% vs. 88% for nonmalnourished patients) after neoadjuvant chemoradiotherapy and resection [33]. Similar patterns were observed for patients with bladder cancer undergoing cystectomy [40]. Thus, malnutrition is a negative prognostic factor for postoperative outcomes but also for long-term outcomes—emphasizing the need for proper identification and treatment prior to surgery when possible.

Gastrointestinal Anatomic and Functional Alterations that Exacerbate Malnutrition

Ileostomies are frequently created in pelvic operations to divert the fecal stream, defunctionalizing the colon. The presence of an ileostomy puts patients at risk for dehydration, electrolyte disturbances, and malabsorption of protein, bile salts, and vitamin B12 [38]. Deficiencies are often exacerbated when patients alter their diet in specific ways to control the volume and character of stoma output, prioritizing convenience over nutrition [13]. These complications can be managed with rehydration, bulking agents, antimotility drugs and when appropriate, reversal of the ileostomy. Notably, diversion mitigates the consequences of colonic leak but does not prevent the leak from occurring outright, and healing of a "protected" distal anastomosis or injury must be documented before consideration of reversal. Patients with colostomies suffer far fewer nutritional morbidities than those with ileostomies; however, reversal is often technically more challenging and comes with higher risk of morbidity. In our experience with patients identified preoperatively as malnourished, end colostomy/ileostomy is likely a better strategy to mitigate complications rather than a colorectal anastomosis with proximal ileal diversion.

Any enteric resection, be it small bowel (including for cystectomy with ileal conduit) or colon, places patients at risk for future obstructions. Adhesive disease and anastomotic stricture can create obstructive episodes that put patients at risk for malnutrition and require surgical correction. Patients who undergo small bowel bypass for obstruction are left with defunctionalized bowel that is at risk for bacterial overgrowth [47]. Small intestinal bacterial overgrowth causes discomfort and diarrhea that may limit energy absorption along with vitamin B12 deficiency [20]. It is often treated with vitamin supplementation and nonabsorbed antibiotics.

(Neo)Adjuvant Therapy

Pelvic surgery is a frequency part of a multidisciplinary treatment sequence, and the impact of the nonsurgical components on nutritional status cannot be ignored. Chemotherapy toxicities such as nausea, vomiting, constipation, diarrhea, anorexia, malabsorption, taste and olfactory changes, and fatigue cause changes in ingestion and digestion, leading to malnutrition. Moreover, progressive malnutrition can be the cause of chemotherapy-related infection via increased gut permeability, impaired local mucosa-associated lymphoid tissue, and deficit of micronutrients to healthy nontumor tissue [41]. One study found the prevalence of moderate and severe malnutrition was 18.8% and 7.9%, respectively, in gynecological cancer patients during chemotherapy [49].

Radiation therapy is an important adjuvant in pelvic malignancy but one with significant nutritional morbidity. Up to 90% of patients develop a permanent change in their bowel habits after radiation [2]. Intestinal inflammation, oxidative stress, tissue damage, and edema lead to pain and functional changes that restrict dietary intake. Functional short bowel syndrome as a cause of protein-calorie malnutrition and micronutrient deficiencies is seen in chronic radiation enteritis [53]. Prior to starting pelvic radiation, up to 32% of patients have lost >5% of body weight suggesting high risk for malnutrition [36]. In the case of locally advanced rectal cancer requiring neoadjuvant therapy and proctectomy, neoadjuvant therapy contributes to preoperative malnutrition. A retrospective study of 49 patients with locally advanced rectal cancer in Japan identified malnutrition in 29% of patients at the time of surgery following chemoradiation [56].

Perioperative Nutrition and the Gut Microbiome

Particularly for cancer patients, the perioperative course of care has become increasingly protracted and complex with rounds of multimodality therapy. Patients undergoing colorectal resections endure periods of prolonged fasting and mechanical bowel preparation in the weeks before surgery, followed by IV and enteral antibiotics. While it decreases overall rates of surgical site infections, this course of events has been demonstrated to cause a profound and durable dysbiosis of the colonic microbiome [30]. Surgically induced dysbiosis is exacerbated by preexisting malnutrition [18]. Preoperative diet and the presence of dysbiosis are both mechanistically linked to complications such as anastomotic leak and surgical site infection [50]. Recent translational work suggests that the immune tolerance induced by diet-induced dysbiosis may permit the recurrence of gastrointestinal cancer [5, 55]. Cutaneous oncologists are leading the way in reducing antibiotic exposure in cancer patients out of concern for the negative impact of dysbiosis on cancer outcomes [7]. Multiple fecal microbial biomarkers are candidates for a targeted preoperative nutritional intervention designed to mitigate specific downstream effects of poor caloric intake [27]. Further translational work is necessary to determine whether the above findings apply to gastrointestinal and genitourinary pelvic surgery.

Potential Solutions: Evidence for Mitigation of Perioperative Malnutrition

Preoperative nutritional counseling in high-risk populations has been demonstrated to improve surgical outcomes in pelvic surgery patients. Generally, nutritional counseling has been employed in the trial setting as part of a preoperative bundle or pathway, so while its effect has not been isolated, strong evidence from randomized trials of bundles containing it supports its use [19]. Such sessions are generally performed by a multidisciplinary team of physicians and dieticians in the preoperative clinic.

Oral protein-calorie supplementation in the preoperative setting has demonstrated mixed results. Nonselective supplementation for the most part has not demonstrated a benefit on postoperative outcomes. However, in patients preoperatively identified as malnourished, supplementation with 250 mL daily protein-dense shakes reduced rates of surgical site infection compared to dietary counseling alone in a randomized controlled trial [6]. Protein-dense oral nutritional supplementation during postoperative chemotherapy decreased malnutrition observed in patients after cytoreductive surgery for ovarian cancer [46]. The effects of specialized immunonutrition supplements are mixed based on recent meta-analyses, and no conclusive recommendations can be made at this time. Preoperative probiotics, mostly cultures of *Lactobacillus* and *Bifidobacterium*, have shown promise in randomized trials in preventing surgical site infection and reducing length of stay [9].

An extensive and well-written review recently summarized available data on preoperative nutritional optimization for the cancer patient [5].

Postoperative patients, as a rule, benefit from feeding the gut as soon as safely feasible and parenteral nutrition used only when enteral nutrition is expected to be delayed for long periods. A recent trial randomized 87 patients with nasogastric tubes and continuous parenteral nutrition after pelvic exenteration to early trophic feeding versus standard of care suction. The results demonstrated that the incidence of postoperative ileus was significantly lower in participants who were enterally fed. Furthermore, regression analysis showed that the longer patients were restricted from an oral diet after surgery, the greater the time was to first bowel movement and the greater the postoperative complication rates [25]. In 2013, Roth et al. conducted a clinical trial with patients undergoing radical cystectomy/urinary detour procedures comparing two groups: first group had parenteral nutrition and oral supplements during the first five postoperative days and the other had only oral nutritional supplements. The first cohort was associated with more complications in general and infectious complications, adding to the wealth of data that supports parenteral nutrition only being used in cases of expected prolonged inadequate enteral nutrition [48]. There are occasions when the timing of surgery cannot be delayed, however. In instances of surgery on patients with or at high risk for malnutrition, consideration of early initiation of parenteral nutritional is justified. In a recent study of patients undergoing abdominal surgery, initiation of TPN at day 3 reduced infectious complications compared to initiation on day 8 [57].

Conclusions

Malnutrition is a significant modifiable risk factor in pelvic surgery across specialties. Patients and providers stand to gain from low-cost perioperative interventions that could improve surgical outcomes. Current data support the following practices: (1) Malnutrition needs to be recognized and measured in all patients prior to pelvic surgery using validated risk stratification tools. (2) If indicated, nutritional and physical prehabilitation should be implemented before surgery in a way that fits patients' means and abilities. (3) All patients should initiate enteral nutrition as early as possible in the postoperative period, with protein-calorie supplementation where needed. (4) Parenteral nutrition should be promptly initiated only in patients unable to receive adequate energy through the gut. Further study is required to use preoperative nutritional intervention, perhaps with prebiotics, to build resilience in the gut microbiome and prevent its attendant complications. Barriers to improving perioperative nutrition practices stem principally from poor transfer of information from the appropriate providers to patients during the perioperative period. Buy-in to dietary education from patients and multidisciplinary teams of providers is essential to improve surgical outcomes in the future.

References

1. Anthony PS. Nutrition screening tools for hospitalized patients. Nutr Clin Pract. 2008;23(4):373–82. https://doi.org/10.1177/0884533608321130.
2. Araujo IK, Munoz-Guglielmetti D, Molla M. Radiation-induced damage in the lower gastrointestinal tract: clinical presentation, diagnostic tests and treatment options. Best Pract Res Clin Gastroenterol. 2020;48-49:101707. https://doi.org/10.1016/j.bpg.2020.101707.
3. Asteria CR, Gagliardi G, Pucciarelli S, Romano G, Infantino A, La Torre F, Tonelli F, Martin F, Pulica C, Ripetti V, Diana G, Amicucci G, Carlini M, Sommariva A, Vinciguerra G, Poddie DB, Amato A, Bassi R, Galleano R, Veronese E, Mancini S, Pescio G, Occelli GL, Bracchitta S, Castagnola M, Pontillo T, Cimmino G, Prati U, Vincenti R. Anastomotic leaks after anterior resection for mid and low rectal cancer: survey of the Italian Society of Colorectal Surgery. Tech Coloproctol. 2008;12(2):103–10. https://doi.org/10.1007/s10151-008-0407-9.
4. Bernstein LH, Leukhardt-Fairfield CJ, Pleban W, Rudolph R. Usefulness of data on albumin and prealbumin concentrations in determining effectiveness of nutritional support. Clin Chem. 1989;35(2):271–4.
5. Brajcich BC, Stigall K, Walsh DS, Varghese TK, Barber AE, Kralovich KA, Wescott AB, Pockaj BA, Ko CY, Laronga C. Preoperative nutritional optimization of the oncology patient: a scoping review. J Am Coll Surg. 2022;234(3):384–94. https://doi.org/10.1097/XCS.0000000000000055.

6. Burden ST, Gibson DJ, Lal S, Hill J, Pilling M, Soop M, Ramesh A, Todd C. Pre-operative oral nutritional supplementation with dietary advice versus dietary advice alone in weight-losing patients with colorectal cancer: single-blind randomized controlled trial. J Cachexia Sarcopenia Muscle. 2017;8(3):437–46. https://doi.org/10.1002/jcsm.12170.
7. Cass RGW, Meng X, Sahasrabhojane P, Bassett RL, Shelburne S, Chang HY, Somaiya K, Mungovan K, Fisher SB, Lucci A, Lee JE, Ross MI, Gershenwald JE, Duncan S, Ajami NJ, Roland CL, Wargo JA, Keung EZ-Y. Evaluating the impact of perioperative antibiotic prophylaxis on the microbiome in patients with cutaneous malignancy. Abstract presented at JCO. J Clin Oncol. 2022;40(16 suppl):TPS9602.
8. Cederholm T, Jensen GL, Correia M, Gonzalez MC, Fukushima R, Higashiguchi T, Baptista G, Barazzoni R, Blaauw R, Coats AJS, Crivelli AN, Evans DC, Gramlich L, Fuchs-Tarlovsky V, Keller H, Llido L, Malone A, Mogensen KM, Morley JE, Muscaritoli M, Nyulasi I, Pirlich M, Pisprasert V, de van der Schueren MAE, Siltharm S, Singer P, Tappenden K, Velasco N, Waitzberg D, Yamwong P, Yu J, Van Gossum A, Compher C, Glim Core Leadership Committee GWG. GLIM criteria for the diagnosis of malnutrition—a consensus report from the global clinical nutrition community. J Cachexia Sarcopenia Muscle. 2019;10(1):207–17. https://doi.org/10.1002/jcsm.12383.
9. Chowdhury AH, Adiamah A, Kushairi A, Varadhan KK, Krznaric Z, Kulkarni AD, Neal KR, Lobo DN. Perioperative probiotics or Synbiotics in adults undergoing elective abdominal surgery: a systematic review and meta-analysis of randomized controlled trials. Ann Surg. 2020;271(6):1036–47. https://doi.org/10.1097/SLA.0000000000003581.
10. Coda A, Bossotti M, Ferri F, Mattio R, Ramellini G, Poma A, Quaglino F, Filippa C, Bona A. Incisional hernia and fascial defect following laparoscopic surgery. Surg Laparosc Endosc Percutan Tech. 2000;10(1):34–8.
11. Curran T. Perioperative nutritional considerations in colon and Rectal surgery. Clin Colon Rectal Surg. 2023;36(3):192–7. https://doi.org/10.1055/s-0043-1761152.
12. Davis CJ, Sowa D, Keim KS, Kinnare K, Peterson S. The use of prealbumin and C-reactive protein for monitoring nutrition support in adult patients receiving enteral nutrition in an urban medical center. JPEN J Parenter Enteral Nutr. 2012;36(2):197–204. https://doi.org/10.1177/0148607111413896.
13. de Oliveira AL, Boroni Moreira AP, Pereira Netto M, Goncalves Leite IC. A cross-sectional study of nutritional status, diet, and dietary restrictions among persons with an ileostomy or colostomy. Ostomy Wound Manage. 2018;64(5):18–29.
14. Detsky AS, McLaughlin JR, Baker JP, Johnston N, Whittaker S, Mendelson RA, Jeejeebhoy KN. What is subjective global assessment of nutritional status? JPEN J Parenter Enteral Nutr. 1987;11(1):8–13. https://doi.org/10.1177/014860718701100108.
15. Duerksen DR, Laporte M, Jeejeebhoy K. Evaluation of nutrition status using the subjective global assessment: malnutrition, cachexia, and sarcopenia. Nutr Clin Pract. 2021;36(5):942–56. https://doi.org/10.1002/ncp.10613.
16. Fazzini B, Markl T, Costas C, Blobner M, Schaller SJ, Prowle J, Puthucheary Z, Wackerhage H. The rate and assessment of muscle wasting during critical illness: a systematic review and meta-analysis. Crit Care. 2023;27(1):2. https://doi.org/10.1186/s13054-022-04253-0.
17. Fleck A. Clinical and nutritional aspects of changes in acute-phase proteins during inflammation. Proc Nutr Soc. 1989;48(3):347–54. https://doi.org/10.1079/pns19890050.
18. Gaines S, van Praagh JB, Williamson AJ, Jacobson RA, Hyoju S, Zaborin A, Mao J, Koo HY, Alpert L, Bissonnette M, Weichselbaum R, Gilbert J, Chang E, Hyman N, Zaborina O, Shogan BD, Alverdy JC. Western diet promotes intestinal colonization by Collagenolytic microbes and promotes tumor formation after colorectal surgery. Gastroenterology. 2020;158(4):958–970 e952. https://doi.org/10.1053/j.gastro.2019.10.020.
19. Gillis C, Buhler K, Bresee L, Carli F, Gramlich L, Culos-Reed N, Sajobi TT, Fenton TR. Effects of nutritional prehabilitation, with and without exercise, on outcomes of patients who undergo colorectal surgery: a systematic review and meta-analysis. Gastroenterology. 2018;155(2):391–410 e394. https://doi.org/10.1053/j.gastro.2018.05.012.
20. Grace E, Shaw C, Whelan K, Andreyev HJ. Review article: small intestinal bacterial overgrowth—prevalence, clinical features, current and developing diagnostic tests, and treatment. Aliment Pharmacol Ther. 2013;38(7):674–88. https://doi.org/10.1111/apt.12456.
21. Guigoz Y, Vellas B. The mini nutritional assessment (MNA) for grading the nutritional state of elderly patients: presentation of the MNA, history and validation. Nestle Nutr Workshop Ser Clin Perform Programme. 1999;1:3–11.; discussion 11–12. https://doi.org/10.1159/000062967.
22. Guigoz Y, Vellas B. Nutritional assessment in older adults : MNA(R) 25 years of a screening tool and a reference standard for care and research; what next? J Nutr Health Aging. 2021;25(4):528–83. https://doi.org/10.1007/s12603-021-1601-y.
23. Heper Y, Akalin EH, Mistik R, Akgoz S, Tore O, Goral G, Oral B, Budak F, Helvaci S. Evaluation of serum C-reactive protein, procalcitonin, tumor necrosis factor alpha, and interleukin-10 levels as diagnostic and prognostic parameters in patients with community-acquired sepsis, severe sepsis, and septic shock. Eur J Clin Microbiol Infect Dis. 2006;25(8):481–91. https://doi.org/10.1007/s10096-006-0168-1.

24. Heyland DK, Dhaliwal R, Jiang X, Day AG. Identifying critically ill patients who benefit the most from nutrition therapy: the development and initial validation of a novel risk assessment tool. Crit Care. 2011;15(6):R268. https://doi.org/10.1186/cc10546.
25. Hogan S, Reece L, Solomon M, Rangan A, Carey S. Early enteral feeding is beneficial for patients after pelvic exenteration surgery: a randomized controlled trial. JPEN J Parenter Enteral Nutr. 2022;46(2):411–21. https://doi.org/10.1002/jpen.2120.
26. Jones KI, Doleman B, Scott S, Lund JN, Williams JP. Simple psoas cross-sectional area measurement is a quick and easy method to assess sarcopenia and predicts major surgical complications. Color Dis. 2015;17(1):O20–6. https://doi.org/10.1111/codi.12805.
27. Jonkers DM. Microbial perturbations and modulation in conditions associated with malnutrition and malabsorption. Best Pract Res Clin Gastroenterol. 2016;30(2):161–72. https://doi.org/10.1016/j.bpg.2016.02.006.
28. Kathiresan AS, Brookfield KF, Schuman SI, Lucci JA 3rd. Malnutrition as a predictor of poor postoperative outcomes in gynecologic cancer patients. Arch Gynecol Obstet. 2011;284(2):445–51. https://doi.org/10.1007/s00404-010-1659-y.
29. Kondrup J. Nutritional-risk scoring systems in the intensive care unit. Curr Opin Clin Nutr Metab Care. 2014;17(2):177–82. https://doi.org/10.1097/MCO.0000000000000041.
30. Krezalek MA, Alverdy JC. The role of the microbiota in surgical recovery. Curr Opin Clin Nutr Metab Care. 2016;19(5):347–52. https://doi.org/10.1097/MCO.0000000000000299.
31. Lanctin DP, Merced-Nieves F, Mallett RM, Arensberg MB, Guenter P, Sulo S, Platts-Mills TF. Prevalence and economic Burden of malnutrition diagnosis among patients presenting to United States Emergency Departments. Acad Emerg Med. 2021;28(3):325–35. https://doi.org/10.1111/acem.13887.
32. Lee DU, Fan GH, Hastie DJ, Addonizio EA, Suh J, Prakasam VN, Karagozian R. The clinical impact of malnutrition on the postoperative outcomes of patients undergoing colorectal resection surgery for colon or rectal cancer: propensity score matched analysis of 2011–2017 US hospitals. Surg Oncol. 2021;38:101587. https://doi.org/10.1016/j.suronc.2021.101587.
33. Lin J, Peng J, Qdaisat A, Li L, Chen G, Lu Z, Wu X, Gao Y, Zeng Z, Ding P, Pan Z. Severe weight loss during preoperative chemoradiotherapy compromises survival outcome for patients with locally advanced rectal cancer. J Cancer Res Clin Oncol. 2016;142(12):2551–60. https://doi.org/10.1007/s00432-016-2225-1.
34. Makela JT, Kiviniemi H, Juvonen T, Laitinen S. Factors influencing wound dehiscence after midline laparotomy. Am J Surg. 1995;170(4):387–90. https://doi.org/10.1016/s0002-9610(99)80309-2.
35. McClave SA, DiBaise JK, Mullin GE, Martindale RG. ACG clinical guideline: nutrition therapy in the adult hospitalized patient. Am J Gastroenterol. 2016;111(3):315–34.; quiz 335. https://doi.org/10.1038/ajg.2016.28.
36. McGough C, Baldwin C, Frost G, Andreyev HJ. Role of nutritional intervention in patients treated with radiotherapy for pelvic malignancy. Br J Cancer. 2004;90(12):2278–87. https://doi.org/10.1038/sj.bjc.6601868.
37. McKenna NP, Bews KA, Al-Refaie WB, Colibaseanu DT, Pemberton JH, Cima RR, Habermann EB. Assessing malnutrition before major oncologic surgery: one size does not fit all. J Am Coll Surg. 2020;230(4):451–60. https://doi.org/10.1016/j.jamcollsurg.2019.12.034.
38. Moraes JT, Melo AFF, Araujo C, Faria R, Ferreira NR, Belo VS. Anthropometric and dietetic evaluation of people with ileostomies. Arq Gastroenterol. 2019;56(1):34–40. https://doi.org/10.1590/S0004-2803.201900000-07.
39. Nakayama M, Yoshimatsu K, Yokomizo H, Yano Y, Okayama S, Satake M, Matsumoto A, Fujimoto T, Usui T, Yamaguchi K, Shiozawa S, Shimakawa T, Katsube T, Naritaka Y. Incidence and risk factors for incisional hernia after open surgery for colorectal cancer. Hepato-Gastroenterology. 2014;61(133):1220–3.
40. Ornaghi PI, Afferi L, Antonelli A, Cerruto MA, Odorizzi K, Gozzo A, Mordasini L, Mattei A, Baumeister P, Cornelius J, Tafuri A, Moschini M. The impact of preoperative nutritional status on post-surgical complication and mortality rates in patients undergoing radical cystectomy for bladder cancer: a systematic review of the literature. World J Urol. 2021;39(4):1045–81. https://doi.org/10.1007/s00345-020-03291-z.
41. Ottery FD. Bidirectional interplay of nutrition and chemotherapy. Nestle Nutr Workshop Ser Clin Perform Programme. 2000;4:183–202.; discussion 203–186. https://doi.org/10.1159/000061815.
42. Paur I, Smedshaug GB, Haugum B, Bye A, Eliassen E, Flottorp TL, Juul HJ, Mowe M, Nakken T, Ore S, Sirevag GK, Sygnestveit K, Thoresen L, Aasen EB, Totland TH, Krogh HW. The Norwegian Directorate of Health recommends malnutrition screening tool (MST) for all adults. Clin Nutr ESPEN. 2022;52:28–31. https://doi.org/10.1016/j.clnesp.2022.09.029.
43. Portuondo JI, Probstfeld L, Massarweh NN, Le L, Wei Q, Chai CY, Taylor J, Awad SS, Tran Cao HS. Malnutrition in elective surgery: how traditional markers might be failing surgeons and patients. Surgery. 2020;168(6):1144–51. https://doi.org/10.1016/j.surg.2020.08.012.
44. Pressoir M, Desné S, Berchery D, Rossignol G, Poiree B, Meslier M, Traversier S, Vittot M, Simon M, Gekiere JP, Meuric J, Serot F, Falewee MN, Rodrigues I, Senesse P, Vasson MP, Chelle F, Maget B, Antoun

S, Bachmann P. Prevalence, risk factors and clinical implications of malnutrition in French comprehensive cancer Centres. Br J Cancer. 2010;102(6):966–71. https://doi.org/10.1038/sj.bjc.6605578.
45. Puthucheary ZA, McNelly AS, Rawal J, Connolly B, Sidhu PS, Rowlerson A, Moxham J, Harridge SD, Hart N, Montgomery HE. Rectus Femoris cross-sectional area and muscle layer thickness: comparative markers of muscle wasting and weakness. Am J Respir Crit Care Med. 2017;195(1):136–8. https://doi.org/10.1164/rccm.201604-0875LE.
46. Qin N, Jiang G, Zhang X, Sun D, Liu M. The effect of nutrition intervention with oral nutritional supplements on ovarian cancer patients undergoing chemotherapy. Front Nutr. 2021;8:685967. https://doi.org/10.3389/fnut.2021.685967.
47. Quigley EMM, Murray JA, Pimentel M. AGA clinical practice update on small intestinal bacterial overgrowth: expert review. Gastroenterology. 2020;159(4):1526–32. https://doi.org/10.1053/j.gastro.2020.06.090.
48. Roth B, Birkhauser FD, Zehnder P, Thalmann GN, Huwyler M, Burkhard FC, Studer UE. Parenteral nutrition does not improve postoperative recovery from radical cystectomy: results of a prospective randomised trial. Eur Urol. 2013;63(3):475–82. https://doi.org/10.1016/j.eururo.2012.05.052.
49. Sanguanwongthong K, Suprasert P. Prevalence of malnourishment and predictive factors associated with the nutritional status of gynecologic cancer patients undergoing chemotherapy: a cross-sectional analysis. Obstet Gynecol Sci. 2022;65(3):234–43. https://doi.org/10.5468/ogs.21298.
50. Shogan BD, Belogortseva N, Luong PM, Zaborin A, Lax S, Bethel C, Ward M, Muldoon JP, Singer M, An G, Umanskiy K, Konda V, Shakhsheer B, Luo J, Klabbers R, Hancock LE, Gilbert J, Zaborina O, Alverdy JC. Collagen degradation and MMP9 activation by enterococcus faecalis contribute to intestinal anastomotic leak. Sci Transl Med. 2015;7(286):286ra268. https://doi.org/10.1126/scitranslmed.3010658.
51. Soloff MA, Vargas MV, Wei C, Ohnona A, Tyan P, Gu A, Georgakopoulos B, Thomas CA, Quan T, Barishansky S, Moawad G. Malnutrition is associated with poor postoperative outcomes following laparoscopic hysterectomy. JSLS. 2021;25(1):e2020.00084. https://doi.org/10.4293/JSLS.2020.00084.
52. Thurnham DI. Interactions between nutrition and immune function: using inflammation biomarkers to interpret micronutrient status. Proc Nutr Soc. 2014;73(1):1–8. https://doi.org/10.1017/S0029665113003662.
53. Webb GJ, Brooke R, De Silva AN. Chronic radiation enteritis and malnutrition. J Dig Dis. 2013;14(7):350–7. https://doi.org/10.1111/1751-2980.12061.
54. White JV, Guenter P, Jensen G, Malone A, Schofield M. Consensus statement: academy of nutrition and dietetics and American Society for Parenteral and Enteral Nutrition. J Parenter Enter Nutr. 2012;36(3):275–83. https://doi.org/10.1177/0148607112440285.
55. Williamson AJ, Jacobson R, van Praagh JB, Gaines S, Koo HY, Lee B, Chan WC, Weichselbaum R, Alverdy JC, Zaborina O, Shogan BD. Enterococcus faecalis promotes a migratory and invasive phenotype in colon cancer cells. Neoplasia. 2022;27:100787. https://doi.org/10.1016/j.neo.2022.100787.
56. Yamano T, Yoshimura M, Kobayashi M, Beppu N, Hamanaka M, Babaya A, Tsukamoto K, Noda M, Matsubara N, Tomita N. Malnutrition in rectal cancer patients receiving preoperative chemoradiotherapy is common and associated with treatment tolerability and anastomotic leakage. Int J Color Dis. 2016;31(4):877–84. https://doi.org/10.1007/s00384-016-2507-8.
57. Zhu Z, Gao Z, Li K. Supplemental parenteral nutrition in patients undergoing abdominal surgery. JAMA Surg. 2022;157(10):966–7. https://doi.org/10.1001/jamasurg.2022.2654.

Part II

Lower Genital Tract

5 Uterine Surgery for Infertility

Jensen Reckhow and Zaraq Khan

Bleeding and Need for Hysterectomy

Background

Bleeding is one of the most significant risks of uterine surgery, as the uterus has a rich blood supply and uterine-sparing surgeries are often complex. Blood loss is of particular concern in more complex surgeries such as myomectomy, adenomyomectomy, and excision of deep infiltrating endometriosis, and excessive blood loss increases the risk of surgical site infection, transfusion, and reoperation [1]. Furthermore, significant blood loss at the time of myomectomy increases the risk for hysterectomy [2–5]. While there is currently no data on the risk of hysterectomy at the time of adenomyomectomy, this is likely to be a considerable risk as these procedures are technically challenging.

Bleeding is also the most common complication after transvaginal ultrasound-guided oocyte retrieval—the most frequently performed procedure by reproductive endocrinologists.

J. Reckhow
Department of Obstetrics and Gynecology, Mayo Clinic, Rochester, MN, USA
e-mail: reckhow.jensen@mayo.edu

Z. Khan (✉)
Division Chair for Reproductive Endocrinology and Infertility, Mayo Clinic, Rochester, MN, USA
e-mail: khan.zaraq@mayo.edu

Prevention

Medical optimization prior to surgery reduces complications. Preoperative anemia should be identified; pretreatment with oral or intravenous iron supplementation may reduce transfusion risk for patients undergoing procedures with a high anticipated blood loss [1]. Preoperative treatment with gonadotropin releasing hormone (GnRH) analogs should be considered in patients with leiomyomas or adenomyosis, as treatment can reduce uterine size and thereby help decrease intraoperative blood loss [6, 7]. Cumulative surgical complication risk is lower with laparoscopic myomectomy than open myomectomy and is notably associated with a fivefold reduction in blood transfusion risk [1, 8]. While the risk of any complication is currently lower with laparoscopic approach as compared to robotic approach, this difference is likely to be mitigated as robotic training becomes more widespread [9].

Minimizing intraoperative blood loss improves visualization and reduces risk of other surgical complications. When performing myomectomy through any approach, vasopressin injected into the cervix as well as the fibroids themselves helps reduce blood flow to the surgical field [10–12]. Transient occlusion of the uterine arteries (TOUA) and use of a uterine tourniquet have been shown to decrease blood loss during adenomyomectomy (Figs.5.1 and 5.2) [13]. Preoperative administration of miso-

M. Hoffman et al. (eds.), *Major Complications of Female Pelvic Surgery*,
https://doi.org/10.1007/978-3-031-66772-5_5

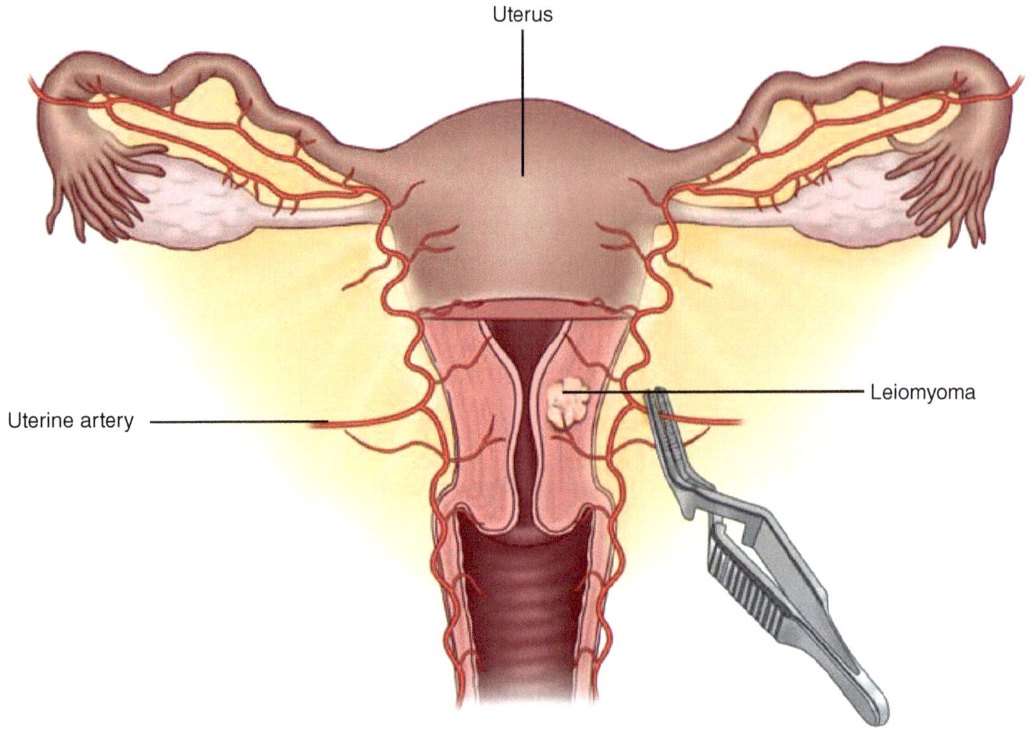

Fig. 5.1 A Bulldog clamp may be used to temporarily occlude the uterine vessels, decreasing the pulse pressure of blood flow to the uterus

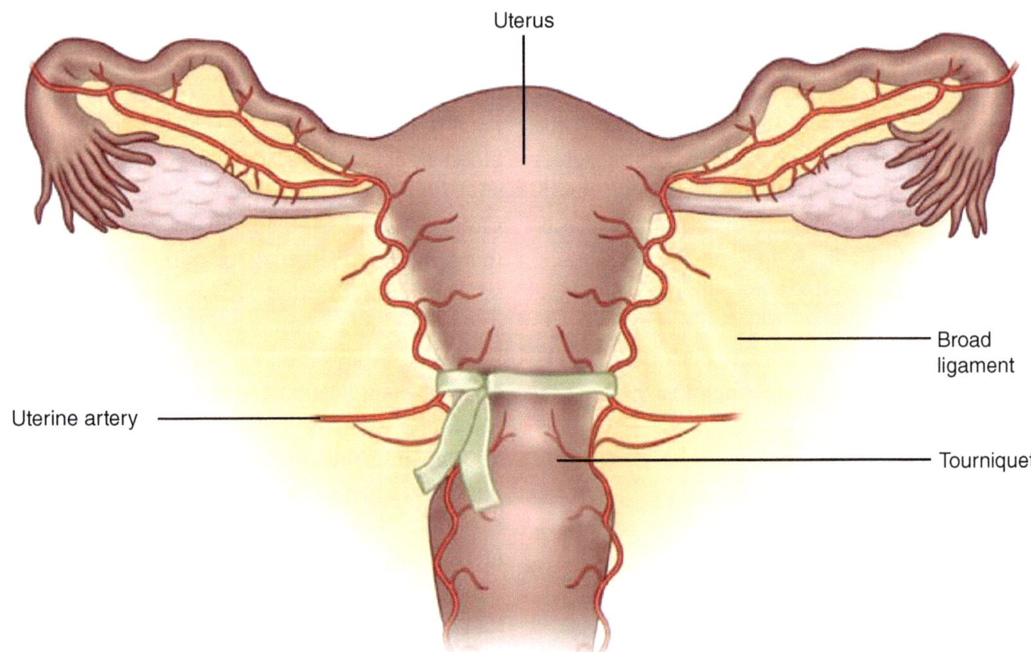

Fig. 5.2 A Penrose drain may be placed circumferentially around the cervix, passing it through the broad ligament on either side, to temporarily occlude the uterine vessels during uterine surgery

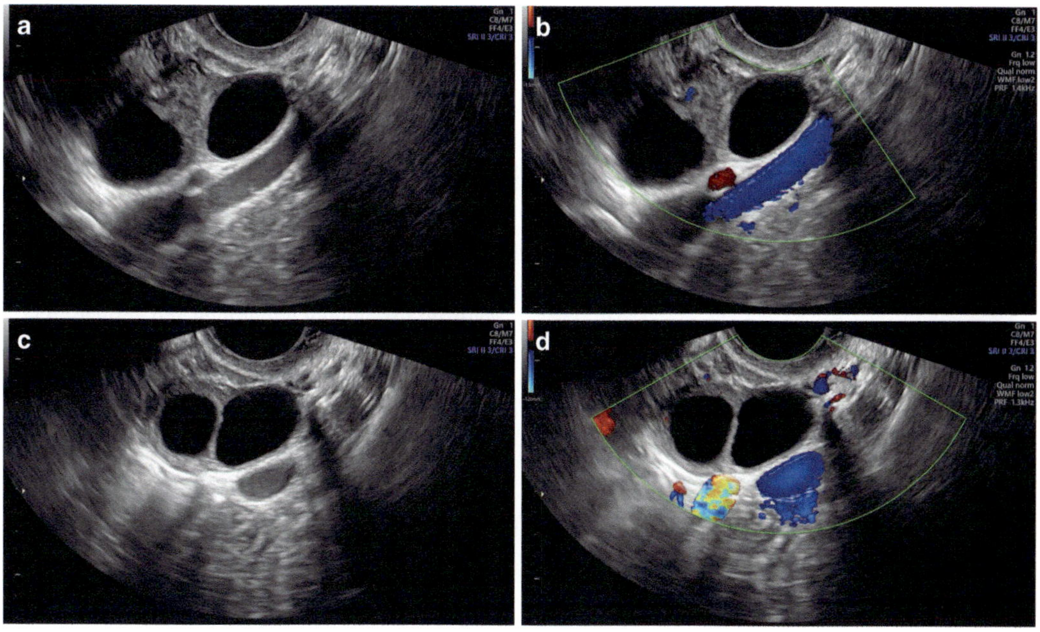

Fig. 5.3 (**a–d**) During transvaginal oocyte retrieval, significant hemorrhage can occur if the iliac vessels are mistakenly entered. (**a**) and (**b**) (without and with color doppler flow) show ovarian follicles in close proximity to the iliac vessels. In this plane, the vessels are readily distinguished from the follicles by shape. (**c**) and (**d**) (without and with color doppler flow) show the same follicles and the iliac vessels in cross section. In this view, the vessels may be mistaken for follicles. It is essential to note the difference in echogenicity between the follicles and the vessels, as this may be the main distinguishing feature between the two

prostol reduces blood flow to the uterus and may decrease blood loss for any uterine surgery [6]. Prophylactic administration of tranexamic acid is also associated with decreased intraoperative blood loss [13]. Intraoperative blood salvage is not recommended for routine use but may decrease the risk of blood transfusion in appropriately selected patients with a high burden of disease and when a prolonged, complex surgery is anticipated [14, 15].

Ultrasound guidance during oocyte retrieval allows the operator to stay clear of the iliac vessels upon which a stimulated ovary typically rests. In a certain plane, these large iliac vessels can be confused with a follicle. Closely watching for vessel movement with pulsation and turning the ultrasound probe to change the plane of view allows for differentiation of a large vessel from a stimulated follicle (Fig. 5.3a–d).

Recognition

A discussion of anticipated blood loss should take place prior to surgery with the full multidisciplinary surgical team so that a plan may be devised for intraoperative blood loss monitoring and resuscitation as needed. In hysteroscopic procedures, excess blood loss is easily recognized as the visual field is rapidly obscured by high-volume bleeds. In complex open or minimally invasive surgeries, intraoperative blood loss may be more insidious, and strict monitoring is needed. The surgeon should monitor for signs of uterine atony and evolving coagulopathy, which may develop in response to as well as precipitate further blood loss. Frequent closed-loop communication between the surgeon, nursing, and anesthesiology staff allows for timely response to blood loss with resuscitation with intravenous hydration, blood products, and vasopressor support to maintain hemodynamic stability. In these cases, it is essential to perform serial assessments of complete blood counts as well as coagulation profiles, as significant blood loss may precipitate coagulopathy or even disseminated intravascular coagulation (DIC), requiring judicious repletion of clotting factors [16, 17].

Management

In the event of hemorrhage, immediate direct pressure tamponade affords the surgeon time to plan management. If the source of the hemorrhage is visualized, the offending vessel may be tamponaded directly. If unable to identify the source of hemorrhage, temporary tamponade of the internal iliac vessels or even the common iliac vessels can afford the surgeon time to clear the surgical field to identify the source of bleeding. Vascular injuries should be repaired by an experienced surgeon. Minor low-volume oozing may be managed with direct pressure, cauterization of the vessel with monopolar or bipolar energy, suturing of the vessel, or application of hemostatic agents. Mechanical hemostatic agents come in a variety of forms (cloth, powder, foam, or sponge) and tend to be less costly than biologic agents. These agents work by establishing a scaffold for platelet adherence and activation [18, 19]. Biologic hemostatic agents act directly on the common pathway of the coagulation cascade to form a fibrin clot. These agents may require thawing or reconstitution by a trained operator prior to use [18, 20]. Table 5.1 outlines common hemostatic agents used in gynecologic surgery [18].

Most bleeding after oocyte retrieval is self-limited, and typically close observation with serial hemoglobin assessment is the primary management strategy in this scenario.

Table 5.1 Hemostatic Agents

Agent	Mechanism of action	Advantages	Limitations
Mechanical agents			
Oxidative regenerating cellulose	Scaffold for platelet aggregation Establishes acidic environment that induces local vasoconstriction Bactericidal	Pliable so can be passed through laparoscopic trocars Less expensive	Acidic environment inactivates biologic hemostatic agents, so this must be used alone or with other mechanical agents only Delayed absorption; can be mistaken for abscess or malignancy on imaging
Microfibrillar collagen	Scaffold for platelet adherence and activation	Less expensive Comes in multiple forms (powder, sheet)	Can be sticky and difficult to handle Increased risk of abscess formation Bovine-derived and may be immunogenic
Hydrocolloid gelatin matrix	Direct pressure from weight of the agent (absorb 35–45 times their weight in fluid)	May be used with biologic agents Less expensive	Porcine-derived and may be immunogenic Increased risk of abscess formation
Polysaccharide spheres	Absorbs water content from blood, increasing concentration of platelets and proteins to accelerate intrinsic clotting cascade	Powder form allows for diffuse application Not immunogenic Rapidly absorbed	Large doses (>50 g) may precipitate hyperglycemia

(continued)

Table 5.1 (continued)

Agent	Mechanism of action	Advantages	Limitations
Biologic agents			
Thrombin	Activates factors V, VIII, and XI Promotes platelet activation Converts fibrinogen to fibrin	Effect is immediate	Black box warning against repeated use of bovine-derived thrombin as it is highly immunogenic May transmit blood-borne disease
Thrombin + gelatin	Combined effects of thrombin and gelatin agents	Effect is immediate	Increased risk of small bowel obstruction (POD#5–9) Gentle irrigation is required to remove excess matrix after application to reduce adhesive disease formation Delayed absorption; can be mistaken for abscess or malignancy on imaging
Fibrin	Stabilizes clot by forming insoluble fibrin mesh scaffold for platelet organization	Effect is immediate	Expensive

Formation of Intrauterine Adhesive Disease

Background

The formation of intrauterine scar tissue is a dreaded complication after uterine instrumentation and curettage, particularly after management of first or second trimester pregnancy loss or retained placenta after delivery [21]. The true prevalence of intrauterine adhesive disease (IUA) and Asherman's syndrome (IUA formation after instrumentation of a gravid uterus) is unknown, as the condition may be asymptomatic [22]. The risk of scar tissue formation is highest after instrumentation of the postpartum uterus, with most risk occurring between the 2nd and 4th week postpartum (19–27%) [23–25] or after first trimester pregnancy loss (19%) [26]. Intrauterine adhesive disease may also develop after uterine septoplasty, extensive hysteroscopic myomectomy, and abdominal myomectomy with entry into the endometrial cavity [27]. Tissue ischemia secondary to uterine artery embolization or pelvic radiation may also induce intrauterine adhesion formation [28].

Prevention

When considering strategies to prevent intrauterine adhesion formation, it is important to consider both primary prevention as well as secondary prevention after surgical resection of existing adhesive disease. Unfortunately, the optimal approach to prevent IUA formation remains unknown [29, 30]. Hysteroscopic tissue resection for pregnancy loss or retained products of conception may decrease the risk of intrauterine adhesion formation (primary prevention) as compared to traditional blind curettage; however, data in this area remain mixed [31]. Secondary prevention after surgical resection of existing disease can be provided with placement of a solid barrier such as a Foley catheter balloon to prevent adhesion formation within the endometrium, although studies investigating the utility of this have not shown a clear reduction in intrauterine adhesion formation or subsequent pregnancy outcomes [32–34]. Limited evidence suggests that semisolid barriers such as hyaluronic acid gels or delayed absorbable adhesion barriers such as carboxymethylcellulose may decrease postoperative IUA formation [35, 36]. The role of hormonal treatments in reducing IUA formation remains to be determined [37, 38].

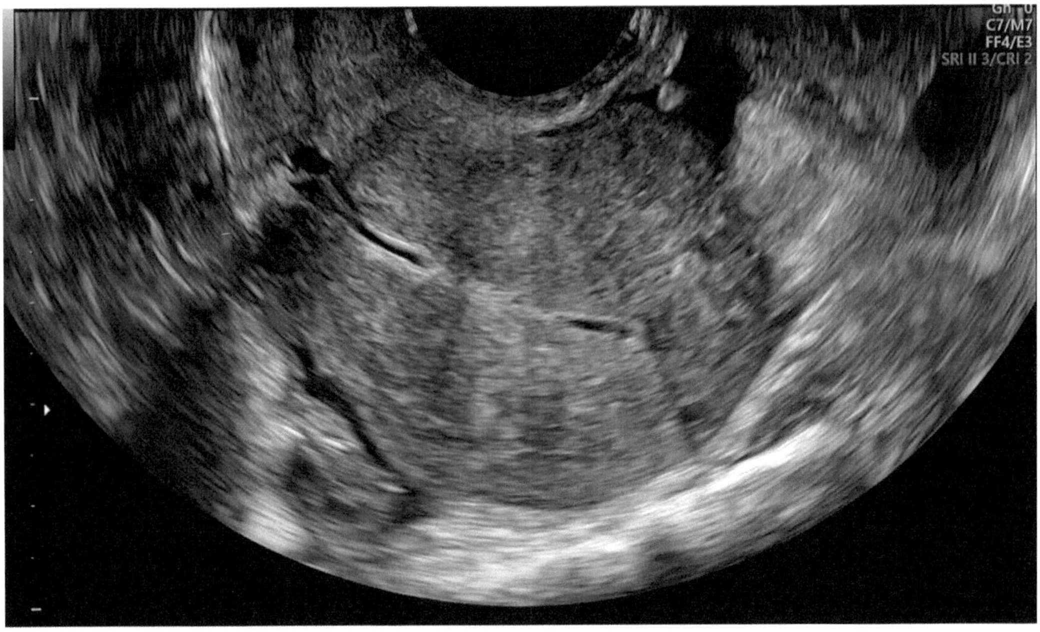

Fig. 5.4 Saline infusion sonohysterogram demonstrating intrauterine adhesive disease. Note that the uterine cavity does not distend uniformly with saline in these cases

Recognition

The presence of intrauterine adhesions may be suspected in patients who present with cyclic or chronic pelvic pain, amenorrhea, light menstrual bleeding or other menstrual irregularities, and infertility with or without recurrent pregnancy loss, particularly in those with a history of prior instrumentation of the endometrium [39]. A thin endometrial stripe may be noted on standard two-dimensional pelvic ultrasonography. Saline infusion sonohysterogram is the most sensitive imaging modality for identifying IUA (Fig. 5.4) [40, 41]. Definitive diagnosis requires direct visualization of intrauterine adhesions by hysteroscopy [42].

Management

Surgical management is indicated in symptomatic patients and may improve future fertility outcomes in those affected by infertility and/or recurrent pregnancy loss. Hysteroscopic lysis of adhesions, either in the office or outpatient surgical setting, is the gold standard treatment for intrauterine adhesive disease [43]. When lysing adhesions, the surgeon should use gentle blunt dissection when possible (for example, allowing distention of the uterus or the tip of the hysteroscope to break apart filmy adhesions) and favor the use of cold instruments such as hysteroscopic scissors to minimize the risk of injury to healthy endometrium [44]. Electrosurgical instruments should be used sparingly but may be essential for hemostasis in some cases. Hysteroscopic morcellator devices may be useful for the resection of excess tissue in patients with retained products of conception or endometrial polyps. In general, adhesiolysis should begin at the internal cervical os with careful progression towards the fundus, beginning with centrally located adhesions before progressing laterally and finally to the uterine cornua [21]. Filmy adhesions should be addressed first (Fig. 5.5a–b). Fluoroscopic or ultrasound guidance may be utilized in particularly challenging cases to minimize the risk of uterine perforation or entry into myometrial tissue [45].

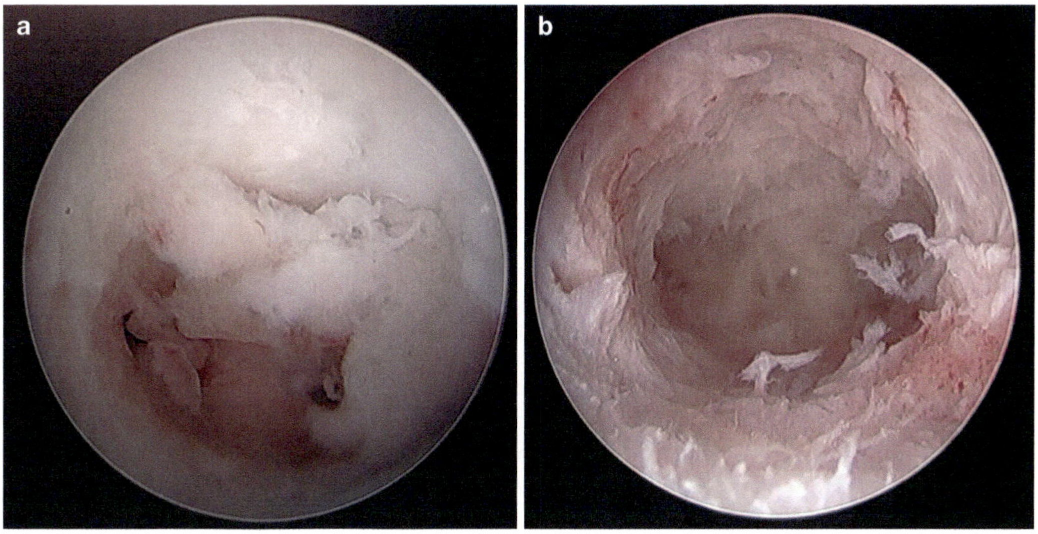

Fig. 5.5 (**a**–**b**) Hysteroscopic view of intrauterine adhesive disease before (**a**) and after (**b**) hysteroscopic adhesiolysis

Uterine Perforation

Background

Uterine perforation occurs in 0.1–4% of gynecologic procedures that involve instrumentation of the uterine cavity and may occur with the use of blunt, sharp, and heated instruments (Fig. 5.6a–b). The risk of perforation may be increased in cases of difficult entry, including in the setting of acute version and/or flexion of the uterus, cervical stenosis, nulliparity, and prior pelvic surgery or cervical procedures [46–48]. The recently gravid uterus may also be more susceptible to uterine perforation due to myometrial relaxation.

Prevention

Many cases of uterine perforation can be prevented by careful instrumentation. In cases where cervical stenosis is anticipated, preoperative misoprostol may decrease the risk of perforation during dilation of the cervix [49]. Deep intracervical injection of vasopressin in these cases decreases the force required for cervical dilation [47]. Finally, if the external cervical os is dilated, the hysteroscope can be utilized for hydrodilation under direct visualization to ensure that the appropriate path is taken. Transabdominal or transvaginal ultrasound guidance may also be utilized to prevent the formation of a false passage and uterine perforation. Electrosurgical instruments should only be activated when the operator has a clear view and control of the active instrument tip [48].

Recognition

Uterine perforation is often recognized by the tactile sensation of a loss of resistance or entry of an instrument beyond a reasonable depth. It may also be recognized visually with ultrasound or hysteroscopy. During hysteroscopy, rapid loss of visualization or collapse of the uterine cavity suggests perforation [50]. If the procedure is performed with the assistance of a fluid management system, a sudden increase in fluid deficit can also be seen in cases of uterine perforation.

Management

In the event of uterine perforation, a period of extended observation is appropriate to monitor for signs of possible bleeding, increased pain, and infection. When secondary to blunt instru-

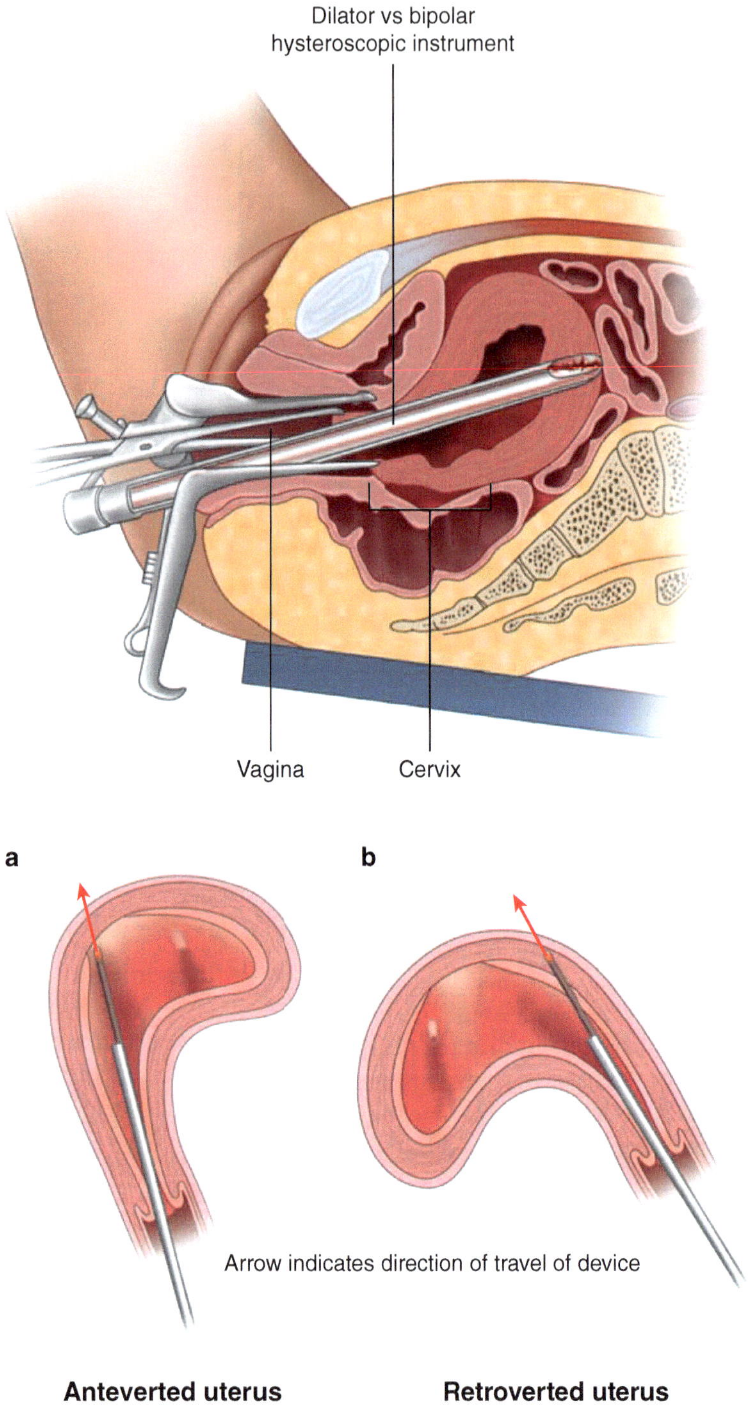

Fig. 5.6 (**a–b**) Uterine perforation occurs when an instrument passes through the wall of the uterus (**a**). Uterine perforation is most likely to occur through the posterior wall in the anteflexed uterus, and through the anterior well in the retroflexed uterus (**b**)

mentation there is a low risk of bleeding or visceral injury, and observation is typically sufficient. If there is concern for possible viscus or other intrabdominal injury, diagnostic laparoscopy should be performed to assess the abdominal cavity [51, 52]. If perforation occurred secondary to a sharp or heated instrument, diagnostic laparoscopy is recommended as the risk for intraabdominal bleeding, and visceral injury is higher with these instruments [46].

Uterine Rupture and Abnormal Placentation

Background

Uterine rupture and abnormal placentation are extremely rare but potentially catastrophic pregnancy complications that may occur as a result of myometrial thinning after surgical intervention as well as disruption of the junctional zone and scar tissue formation between the endometrium and myometrium following myomectomy or adenomyomectomy [53]. The risk of uterine rupture may be increased after myomectomy, adenomyomectomy, hysteroscopic curettage, and hysteroscopic septoplasty and is estimated to occur in 0.1–1% of these cases, consistent with the risk incurred after one or two low transverse Cesarean births [54]. The risk appears to be highest among patients who undergo laparoscopic as opposed to open myomectomy, and this is suspected to be due to less optimal closure of the myometrial defect with the minimally invasive approach [55, 56]. The risk for placenta accreta spectrum (PAS) is highest in patients with prior full-thickness uterine surgery, such as extensive myomectomy or adenomyomectomy but may be as high as 2% among patients who have undergone hysteroscopic intrauterine adhesiolysis [57]. Additionally, it is important to remember that the pathophysiology of adenomyosis, with the formation of fistula-like canals within the myometrium, may predispose to PAS as well [58].

Prevention

Proper surgical technique facilitates effective healing after invasive uterine surgery. Multilayer closure of the myometrium and judicious use of electrosurgery decrease the risk of uterine rupture after myomectomy and adenomyomectomy [59–61]. The Use of barbed suture helps with obtaining close reapproximation of the myoma bed, reducing hematoma formation and promoting efficient wound healing [3]. Planned late preterm Cesarean birth is recommended in pregnancies after extensive myomectomy, particularly if it is transmural or enters the endometrial cavity, and after adenomomectomy due to the increased risk of uterine rupture in these patients [62].

The prevention of catastrophic complications of uterine rupture and abnormal placentation relies on early recognition of these pathologies. Patients with a history of prior uterine surgery should undergo detailed obstetric ultrasonography to evaluate placentation in the second trimester. Further evaluation with MRI is recommended if PAS is suspected [63]. Screening should also be considered in patients with significant antepartum bleeding or uterine pain, as these symptoms may reflect abnormal placentation or thinning of the uterine wall [64]. Catastrophic complications of PAS, including life-threatening hemorrhage, uterine rupture, and need for emergent delivery with postpartum hysterectomy, can be prevented with judicious antepartum monitoring and planned medically indicated preterm birth at a facility with hysterectomy capabilities [65].

Recognition

The earliest sign of uterine rupture is usually fetal heart rate changes; however, suspicion should be raised in the event of loss of fetal station during labor, sudden onset severe abdominal pain with or without vaginal bleeding, and loss of intrauterine pressure [53]. As previously discussed, PAS is ideally identified in the antenatal period on imaging. If not previously recognized, it may be diagnosed at the time of delivery as the placenta will fail to separate and no plane will be appreciated between the placenta and the uterine wall. These cases may present with uterine atony and postpartum hemorrhage as well [53].

Management

Uterine rupture is an obstetric emergency and requires immediate birth via Cesarean delivery. Depending on patient stability and the extent of the rupture repair of the uterus may be possible, although hysterectomy is often required [66]. PAS is commonly managed by planned Cesarean hysterectomy (please see Chap. 30, Cesarean Hysterectomy, for additional details about this procedure). In appropriate cases, the placenta may be left in situ at the time of delivery with plan for close interim monitoring and interval removal after placental involution [67, 68].

Volume Overload with Hysteroscopic Procedures

Background

Modern-day hysteroscopy utilizes distension media for expansion of the uterine cavity to allow for visualization and targeted treatment of intrauterine pathology. Though generally considered a low-risk procedure, hysteroscopy can precipitate major hemodynamic complications, particularly in the setting of suboptimal fluid management.

Prevention

An automated fluid management system should be utilized to allow for objective tracking of absorption of distention media (Fig. 5.7). Procedures should be completed expeditiously by skilled surgeons and should be performed at the lowest possible fluid pressure that allows for adequate visualization (usually 60–80 mmHg) [48]. Intravascular hydration should be kept to a minimum during the procedure to minimize cumulative fluid intake. When a complex procedure is anticipated, intracervical injection of vasopressin may be considered as vasoconstriction may further decrease intravascular fluid absorption during the case [69].

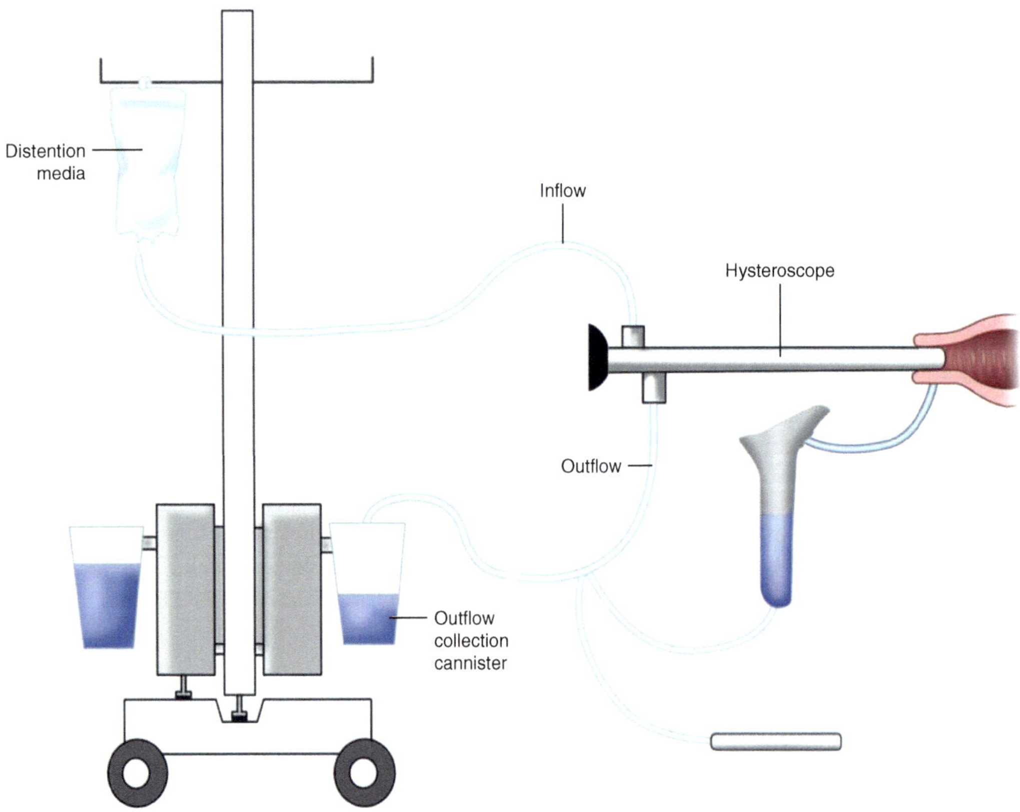

Fig. 5.7 Demonstration of a typical simple hysteroscopy fluid management system

Recognition

Pulmonary and cerebral edema may develop rapidly with overabsorption of distention media and are typically first detected by new onset ventilation difficulty, crackles or rales on pulmonary auscultation, brady- or tachyarrhythmias, altered mental status, and hypotension. These conditions frequently develop during or shortly after the procedure is completed or terminated [48, 70].

Management

Table 5.2 highlights management recommendations for complications that may arise with commonly used distention media.

Table 5.2 Media Selection and Considerations for Hysteroscopy

	Type of Media		
	Electrolyte-rich	Electrolyte-poor	Gaseous
Examples	Normal saline (isotonic) Lactated Ringer's (isotonic)	1.5% glycine (hypotonic) 2.5–5% sorbitol (hypotonic) 5% Mannitol (hypotonic) Dextran 70 (hypertonic)	CO_2
Uses	Diagnostic or operative hysteroscopy in which mechanical, laser, or bipolar energy sources are used	Operative hysteroscopy with monopolar electrosurgery only	Diagnostic hysteroscopy only, primarily in the office setting
Advantages	Low cost Readily available in most clinical settings Good electrical conductor so can be used with bipolar energy sources	Does not conduct electricity so can safely be used with monopolar energy sources Due to high viscosity, dextran does not readily spill into the peritoneal cavity or mix with blood Allows for better visualization in bleeding scenarios as blood does not mix with the distension medium	Low cost Conducts light well so provides optimal visualization Readily absorbed into bloodstream and removed via pulmonary ventilation so risk of accumulation is low
Disadvantages	Cannot be used with monopolar energy sources	Cannot be used with bipolar energy sources Allergy and contraindications are more common	Uneven distention of the uterine cavity, inability to clear secretions, and blood can result in poor visualization
Maximum fluid deficit	2500 cc. Consider terminating procedure at 2000 cc	1000 cc for hypotonic solutions. Consider terminating procedure at 750 cc. 500 cc for high-viscosity solutions. Consider terminating procedure at 300 cc.	N/A

(continued)

Table 5.2 (continued)

	Type of Media		
	Electrolyte-rich	Electrolyte-poor	Gaseous
Major risks	Excessive fluid absorption can cause isotonic volume overload, pulmonary edema, and congestive heart failure Air embolism is uncommon but may occur when ambient pressure is greater than diastolic venous pressure.	Excessive absorption can cause euvolemic hyponatremia and decreased serum osmolality, increasing the risk for seizures, cerebral edema, coma, and death. Glycine is metabolized into ammonia and glycol, which can cross the blood–brain barrier resulting in hyperammonemia. Sorbitol and mannitol have diuretic effects and may cause severe dehydration and subsequent hypotension and circulatory collapse	Gas embolism
Prevention	Volume overload: Prevent with continuous inflow–outflow monitoring Air embolism: Minimize duration and extent of Trendelenburg positioning; remove speculum once hysteroscope is inserted into the uterus and limit reinstrumentation to minimize exposure of the dilated cervix to the air; clear air from inflow tracts of hysteroscope	Prevent volume overload and rapid intravasation with continuous inflow–outflow monitoring. Consider intracervical injection of vasopressin to minimize intravascular fluid absorption.	Maintain low distention pressure (<100 mmHg) and minimize operative time. Never use a laparoscopic insufflator in place of a hysteroscopic insufflator as the flow rates differ between these devices.
Recognition	Volume overload: Decreasing oxygen saturation, crackles on pulmonary auscultation Air embolism: Chest pain and dyspnea, decreased end tidal CO_2, hypotension, tachycardia, mill-wheel murmur on cardiac auscultation	Hyponatremia: Muscle twitching, hypotension, tachycardia, seizures Hyperammonemia: Agitation, somnolence, dizziness, visual disturbances, vomiting, coma	Early signs: Cardiac arrhythmia, rising end-tidal CO_2, decreasing oxygen saturation Early symptoms: Chest pain, shortness of breath Late signs: Sudden drop in oxygen saturation, hypotension, pulmonary hypertension, hypercarbia, tachypnea

(continued)

Table 5.2 (continued)

	Type of Media		
	Electrolyte-rich	Electrolyte-poor	Gaseous
Management	Fluid restriction and diuretics	Hyponatremia: Fluid restriction and care by intensive care specialist for hyponatremia. Under the intensivists' care, slow correction with isotonic or hypertonic saline could be considered. Hyperammonemia: Consider administration of lactulose and/or rifaximin, consult internal medicine or critical care for assistance in management	Immediately terminate the procedure. With the assistance of anesthesia colleagues, place patient on mechanical ventilation with 100% FiO_2, place patient in left lateral decubitus position and in steep Trendelenburg to minimize gas embolism travel to the pulmonary circulation. Consider: IV fluid resuscitation with normal saline, placement of a central line to help remove air from the right atrium, pericardial thump to help break up larger gas bubbles

Diminished Ovarian Reserve and Loss of Ovary

Background

Surgery for infertility often includes intervention on the ovary so it is important to consider ovarian surgery when discussing complications of surgery for infertility. Common adnexal pathologies seen in reproductive-aged individuals include physiologic ovarian cysts, endometriomas, mature teratomas (dermoid tumors), and other benign ovarian neoplasms such as cystadenomas. Minimally invasive ovarian cystectomy is the gold standard for the management of these pathologies. In many cases, such as with endometriomas and dermoid tumors, disease may be bilateral or recurrent. This makes conservative surgery even more desirable, as future oophorectomy may be required [71]. While an initial decline in serum anti-mullerian hormone (AMH) is noted after surgery, levels return to normal within 3–6 months in most cases and within 12 months for endometriomas; ovarian cystectomy does not appear to have a meaningful long-term impact on ovarian reserve or live birth rates [72–77]. In patients with endometriosis who desire future fertility, removal of ovarian endometriomas >4 cm in size improves pregnancy rates [78]. This benefit may not be seen with excision of smaller endometriomas, and treatment of disease with coagulation or laser evaporation without pseudocapsule excision increases the risk of cyst recurrence and associated symptoms hence is not recommended [79].

Prevention

Benign lesions of the ovary should be removed via cystectomy performed by an appropriately skilled surgeon. Techniques to facilitate dissection of the cyst wall include the use of hydrodissection and injection of dilute vasopressin (0.1–1 unit/mL) once the plane of the cyst is identified [80]. If there is concern for oophorectomy, surgery should be performed by a skilled reproductive surgeon to maximize the likelihood of successful ovarian preservation [81].

Recognition

It is important to recognize that bleeding is expected during cystectomy and that ovarian cystectomy is a technically more complex procedure than oophorectomy in most cases [82].

Management

Preventing loss of ovarian function and loss of ovary at the time of ovarian surgery requires patience and judicious hemostasis. Hemostatic agents should be preferentially used for low-volume oozing of the cystectomy bed, and suture or electrosurgical techniques may be required to control higher volume bleeds [83]. The choice of hemostatic agent should be per provider preference as there is no difference in ovarian reserve outcomes with different agents [18, 84, 85]. Use of monopolar energy should be minimized as diffuse dispersion of energy throughout the ovary may result in injury to healthy tissue; bipolar or ultrasonic energy sources should be favored if electrosurgical hemostasis is required [73, 86]. Ovarian suturing for the purpose of hemostasis results in improved immediate post-operative ovarian function preservation, although long-term ovarian reserve outcomes are the same [87, 88]. If oophorectomy is required, the patient should be offered consultation with a reproductive endocrinologist to discuss options for fertility preservation, including ovarian tissue cryopreservation [89–94].

References

1. Kim T, Purdy MP, Kendall-Rauchfuss L, Habermann EB, Bews KA, Glasgow AE, et al. Myomectomy associated blood transfusion risk and morbidity after surgery. Fertil Steril. 2020;114(1):175–84.
2. Altgassen C, Kuss S, Berger U, Löning M, Diedrich K, Schneider A. Complications in laparoscopic myomectomy. Surg Endosc. 2006;20(4):614–8.
3. Tanos V, Berry KE, Frist M, Campo R, DeWilde RL. Prevention and Management of Complications in laparoscopic myomectomy. Biomed Res Int. 2018;2018:8250952.
4. Sizzi O, Rossetti A, Malzoni M, Minelli L, La Grotta F, Soranna L, et al. Italian multicenter study on complications of laparoscopic myomectomy. J Minim Invasive Gynecol. 2007;14(4):453–62.
5. Mirowska-Allen K, Kong K, Ang C. Unplanned hysterectomy following myomectomy at a tertiary institution: a case series and review of the literature. J Endometr Pelv Pain Disorder. 2018;10:228402651878366.
6. Lewis EI, Gargiulo AR. The role of Hysteroscopic and robot-assisted laparoscopic myomectomy in the setting of infertility. Clin Obstet Gynecol. 2016;59(1):53–65.
7. Lethaby A, Puscasiu L, Vollenhoven B. Preoperative medical therapy before surgery for uterine fibroids. Cochrane Database Syst Rev. 2017;11(11):Cd000547.
8. Simko S, Dallas K, Molina AL, Siedhoff MT, Wright KN, Anger JT, et al. Rates of complications and reoperation after myomectomy-the impact of surgical approach: a statewide population-based cohort study from 2005-2018. J Minim Invasive Gynecol. 2022;29(10):1157–64.
9. Zaritsky E, Le A, Tucker LY, Ojo A, Weintraub MR, Raine-Bennett T. Minimally invasive myomectomy: practice trends and differences between Black and non-Black women within a large integrated healthcare system. Am J Obstet Gynecol. 2022;226(6):826.e1–e11.
10. Alomar O, Abu-Zaid A, Jamjoom MZ, Almubarki AA, Alsehaimi SO, Alabdrabalamir S, et al. Prophylactic vasopressin to reduce intraoperative blood loss and associated morbidities during myomectomy: a systematic review and meta-analysis of 11 controlled trials. J Gynecol Obstet Hum Reprod. 2022;51(10):102485.
11. Barbosa PA, Villaescusa M, Andres MP, Fernandes LFC, Abrão MS. How to minimize bleeding in laparoscopic myomectomy. Curr Opin Obstet Gynecol. 2021;33(4):255–61.
12. Srivastava S, Mahey R, Kachhawa G, Bhatla N, Upadhyay AD, Kriplani A. Comparison of intramyometrial vasopressin plus rectal misoprostol with intramyometrial vasopressin alone to decrease blood loss during laparoscopic myomectomy: randomized clinical trial. Eur J Obstet Gynecol Reprod Biol. 2018;228:279–83.
13. Lu C, Corbett C, Elliott JE, Evans D. Fertility-sparing surgery for diffuse adenomyosis: a narrated, stepwise approach to the Osada procedure. Fertil Steril. 2022;118(3):588–90.
14. Wu H, Singh B, Yen TT, Maher J, Datta S, Chaves K, et al. Utilization and cost of cell salvage in minimally invasive myomectomy. Eur J Obstet Gynecol Reprod Biol. 2023;280:179–83.
15. Kumakiri J, Kikuchi I, Kitade M, Matsuoka S, Kono A, Takeda S. Retrospective analysis of the efficacy of perioperative use of the cell salvage and autologous blood recovery system during laparoscopic myomectomy. Arch Gynecol Obstet. 2012;285(4):1073–7.

16. Li XL, Wan XJ, Zhang Q, Zhu H, Zhou K, Yang XJ, et al. Laparoscopic myomectomy complicated by disseminated intravascular coagulation: a case report and review of the literature. Eur J Obstet Gynecol Reprod Biol. 2011;155(1):115–6.
17. Bar-Natan M, Hymes KB. Management of Intraoperative Coagulopathy. Neurosurg Clin N Am. 2018;29(4):557–65.
18. Cullifer RM, Makai G, Pacis M, Huynh T. Topical hemostatic and tissue-sealing agents in gynecologic surgery. Curr Opin Obstet Gynecol. 2020;32(4):285–91.
19. American College of Obstetricians and Gynecologists' Committee on Gynecologic Practice. Topical hemostatic agents at time of obstetric and gynecologic surgery: ACOG committee opinion, number 812. Obstet Gynecol. 2020;136(4):e81-e9.
20. Stachowicz AM, Whiteside JL. Topical hemostatic agents in gynecologic surgery for benign indications. Obstet Gynecol. 2020;135(2):463–8.
21. Khan Z, Goldberg JM. Hysteroscopic Management of Asherman's syndrome. J Minim Invasive Gynecol. 2018;25(2):218–28.
22. Yu D, Wong YM, Cheong Y, Xia E, Li TC. Asherman syndrome—one century later. Fertil Steril. 2008;89(4):759–79.
23. Poujade O, Grossetti A, Mougel L, Ceccaldi PF, Ducarme G, Luton D. Risk of synechiae following uterine compression sutures in the management of major postpartum haemorrhage. BJOG. 2011;118(4):433–9.
24. Rasheed SM, Amin MM, Abd Ellah AH, Abo Elhassan AM, El Zahry MA, Wahab HA. Reproductive performance after conservative surgical treatment of postpartum hemorrhage. Int J Gynaecol Obstet. 2014;124(3):248–52.
25. Schenker JG, Margalioth EJ. Intrauterine adhesions: an updated appraisal. Fertil Steril. 1982;37(5):593–610.
26. Hooker AB, Lemmers M, Thurkow AL, Heymans MW, Opmeer BC, Brolmann HA, et al. Systematic review and meta-analysis of intrauterine adhesions after miscarriage: prevalence, risk factors and long-term reproductive outcome. Hum Reprod Update. 2014;20(2):262–78.
27. Taskin O, Sadik S, Onoglu A, Gokdeniz R, Erturan E, Burak F, et al. Role of endometrial suppression on the frequency of intrauterine adhesions after resectoscopic surgery. J Am Assoc Gynecol Laparosc. 2000;7(3):351–4.
28. Mara M, Horak P, Kubinova K, Dundr P, Belsan T, Kuzel D. Hysteroscopy after uterine fibroid embolization: evaluation of intrauterine findings in 127 patients. J Obstet Gynaecol Res. 2012;38(5):823–31.
29. Healy MW, Schexnayder B, Connell MT, Terry N, AH DC, Csokmay JM, et al. Intrauterine adhesion prevention after hysteroscopy: a systematic review and meta-analysis. Am J Obstetr Gynecol. 2016;215(3):267–75.e7.
30. Bosteels J, Weyers S, D'Hooghe TM, Torrance H, Broekmans FJ, Chua SJ, et al. Anti-adhesion therapy following operative hysteroscopy for treatment of female subfertility. Cochrane Database Syst Rev. 2017;11(11):Cd011110.
31. Huchon C, Drioueche H, Koskas M, Agostini A, Bauville E, Bourdel N, et al. Operative hysteroscopy vs vacuum aspiration for incomplete spontaneous abortion: a randomized clinical trial. JAMA. 2023;329(14):1197–205.
32. Orhue AA, Aziken ME, Igbefoh JO. A comparison of two adjunctive treatments for intrauterine adhesions following lysis. Int J Gynaecol Obstet. 2003;82(1):49–56.
33. Lin XN, Zhou F, Wei ML, Yang Y, Li Y, Li TC, et al. Randomized, controlled trial comparing the efficacy of intrauterine balloon and intrauterine contraceptive device in the prevention of adhesion reformation after hysteroscopic adhesiolysis. Fertil Steril. 2015;104(1):235–40.
34. Lin X, Wei M, Li TC, Huang Q, Huang D, Zhou F, et al. A comparison of intrauterine balloon, intrauterine contraceptive device and hyaluronic acid gel in the prevention of adhesion reformation following hysteroscopic surgery for Asherman syndrome: a cohort study. Eur J Obstet Gynecol Reprod Biol. 2013;170(2):512–6.
35. Acunzo G, Guida M, Pellicano M, Tommaselli GA, Di Spiezio SA, Bifulco G, et al. Effectiveness of auto-cross-linked hyaluronic acid gel in the prevention of intrauterine adhesions after hysteroscopic adhesiolysis: a prospective, randomized, controlled study. Hum Reprod. 2003;18(9):1918–21.
36. Tsapanos VS, Stathopoulou LP, Papathanassopoulou VS, Tzingounis VA. The role of Seprafilm bioresorbable membrane in the prevention and therapy of endometrial synechiae. J Biomed Mater Res. 2002;63(1):10–4.
37. Farhi J, Bar-Hava I, Homburg R, Dicker D, Ben-Rafael Z. Induced regeneration of endometrium following curettage for abortion: a comparative study. Hum Reprod. 1993;8(7):1143–4.
38. Sanfilippo JS, Fitzgerald MR, Badawy SZ, Nussbaum ML, Yussman MA. Asherman's syndrome. A comparison of therapeutic methods. J Reprod Med. 1982;27(6):328–30.
39. Hanstede MM, van der Meij E, Goedemans L, Emanuel MH. Results of centralized Asherman surgery, 2003–2013. Fertil Steril. 2015;104(6):1561–8.e1.
40. Sylvestre C, Child TJ, Tulandi T, Tan SL. A prospective study to evaluate the efficacy of two- and three-dimensional sonohysterography in women with intrauterine lesions. Fertil Steril. 2003;79(5):1222–5.
41. Seshadri S, El-Toukhy T, Douiri A, Jayaprakasan K, Khalaf Y. Diagnostic accuracy of saline infusion sonography in the evaluation of uterine cavity abnor-

malities prior to assisted reproductive techniques: a systematic review and meta-analyses. Hum Reprod Update. 2015;21(2):262–74.
42. Dreisler E, Kjer JJ. Asherman's syndrome: current perspectives on diagnosis and management. Int J Women's Health. 2019;11:191–8.
43. Bougie O, Lortie K, Shenassa H, Chen I, Singh SS. Treatment of Asherman's syndrome in an outpatient hysteroscopy setting. J Minim Invasive Gynecol. 2015;22(3):446–50.
44. Sugimoto O. Diagnostic and therapeutic hysteroscopy for traumatic intrauterine adhesions. Am J Obstet Gynecol. 1978;131(5):539–47.
45. Thomson AJ, Abbott JA, Kingston A, Lenart M, Vancaillie TG. Fluoroscopically guided synechiolysis for patients with Asherman's syndrome: menstrual and fertility outcomes. Fertil Steril. 2007;87(2):405–10.
46. Richards EG, Rehmer JM, Falcone T. Perforation during gynecological procedures. JAMA. 2023;329(11):933–4.
47. Munro MG, Christianson LA. Complications of Hysteroscopic and uterine Resectoscopic surgery. Clin Obstet Gynecol. 2015;58(4):765–97.
48. Istre O. Managing bleeding, fluid absorption and uterine perforation at hysteroscopy. Best Pract Res Clin Obstet Gynaecol. 2009;23(5):619–29.
49. Al-Fozan H, Firwana B, Al Kadri H, Hassan S, Tulandi T. Preoperative ripening of the cervix before operative hysteroscopy. Cochrane Database Syst Rev. 2015;2015(4):Cd005998.
50. Agostini A, Cravello L, Bretelle F, Shojai R, Roger V, Blanc B. Risk of uterine perforation during hysteroscopic surgery. J Am Assoc Gynecol Laparosc. 2002;9(3):264–7.
51. Cholkeri-Singh A, Sasaki KJ. Hysteroscopy safety. Curr Opin Obstet Gynecol. 2016;28(4):250–4.
52. Driák D, Sehnal B, Jarošová L, Dvořáčková K. Uterine perforation during intrauterine procedures and its management. Ceska Gynekol. 2022;87(4):295–301.
53. Tanos V, Toney ZA. Uterine scar rupture - prediction, prevention, diagnosis, and management. Best Pract Res Clin Obstet Gynaecol. 2019;59:115–31.
54. Jansa V, Laganà AS, Ferrari F, Ghezzi F, Burnik Papler T, Vrtacnik Bokal E, et al. Uterine rupture in pregnancy after hysteroscopic septum resection: a 20-year retrospective analysis. Minim Invasive Ther Allied Technol. 2022;31(3):448–55.
55. Smith JG, Mertz HL, Merrill DC. Identifying risk factors for uterine rupture. Clin Perinatol. 2008;35(1):85–99. viii
56. Gil Y, Badeghiesh A, Suarthana E, Mansour F, Capmas P, Volodarsky-Perel A, et al. Risk of uterine rupture after myomectomy by laparoscopy or laparotomy. J Gynecol Obstet Hum Reprod. 2020;49(8):101843.
57. Silver RM, Branch DW. Placenta Accreta Spectrum. N Engl J Med. 2018;378(16):1529–36.
58. Jauniaux E, Jurkovic D, Hussein AM, Burton GJ. New insights into the etiopathology of placenta accreta spectrum. Am J Obstet Gynecol. 2022;227(3):384–91.
59. Parker WH, Einarsson J, Istre O, Dubuisson JB. Risk factors for uterine rupture after laparoscopic myomectomy. J Minim Invasive Gynecol. 2010;17(5):551–4.
60. Pistofidis G, Makrakis E, Balinakos P, Dimitriou E, Bardis N, Anaf V. Report of 7 uterine rupture cases after laparoscopic myomectomy: update of the literature. J Minim Invasive Gynecol. 2012;19(6):762–7.
61. Alvi FA, Glaser LM, Chaudhari A, Tsai S, Milad MP. New paradigms in the conservative surgical and interventional management of adenomyosis. Curr Opin Obstet Gynecol. 2017;29(4):240–8.
62. Landon MB, Lynch CD. Optimal timing and mode of delivery after cesarean with previous classical incision or myomectomy: a review of the data. Semin Perinatol. 2011;35(5):257–61.
63. Jauniaux E, Collins S, Burton GJ. Placenta accreta spectrum: pathophysiology and evidence-based anatomy for prenatal ultrasound imaging. Am J Obstet Gynecol. 2018;218(1):75–87.
64. Berkley EM, Abuhamad A. Imaging of placenta Accreta Spectrum. Clin Obstet Gynecol. 2018;61(4):755–65.
65. Horgan R, Abuhamad A. Placenta Accreta Spectrum: prenatal diagnosis and management. Obstet Gynecol Clin N Am. 2022;49(3):423–38.
66. Murphy DJ. Uterine rupture. Curr Opin Obstet Gynecol. 2006;18(2):135–40.
67. Cahill AG, Beigi R, Heine RP, Silver RM, Wax JR. Placenta Accreta Spectrum. Am J Obstet Gynecol. 2018;219(6):B2–b16.
68. Sentilhes L, Kayem G, Silver RM. Conservative Management of Placenta Accreta Spectrum. Clin Obstet Gynecol. 2018;61(4):783–94.
69. McGurgan PM, McIlwaine P. Complications of hysteroscopy and how to avoid them. Best Pract Res Clin Obstet Gynaecol. 2015;29(7):982–93.
70. Salazar CA, Isaacson KB. Office operative hysteroscopy: an update. J Minim Invasive Gynecol. 2018;25(2):199–208.
71. Pelusi G, Taroni B, Flamigni C. Benign ovarian tumors. Front Biosci. 1997;2:g5–7.
72. Sireesha MU, Chitra T, Subbaiah M, Nandeesha H. Effect of laparoscopic ovarian cystectomy on ovarian reserve in benign ovarian cysts. J Hum Reprod Sci. 2021;14(1):56–60.
73. Mansouri G, Safinataj M, Shahesmaeili A, Allahqoli L, Salehiniya H, Alkatout I. Effect of laparoscopic cystectomy on ovarian reserve in patients with ovarian cyst. Front Endocrinol (Lausanne). 2022;13:964229.
74. Moreno-Sepulveda J, Romeral C, Niño G, Pérez-Benavente A. The effect of laparoscopic endometrioma surgery on anti-müllerian hormone: a systematic review of the literature and meta-analysis. JBRA Assist Reprod. 2022;26(1):88–104.
75. Anh ND, Ha NTT, Tri NM, Huynh DK, Dat DT, Thuong PTH, et al. Long-term follow-up of anti-Mullerian hormone levels after laparoscopic Endometrioma cystectomy. Int J Med Sci. 2022;19(4):651–8.

76. Gomez R, Schorsch M, Gerhold-Ay A, Hasenburg A, Seufert R, Skala C. Fertility after ovarian cystectomy: how does surgery affect IVF/ICSI outcomes? Geburtshilfe Frauenheilkd. 2019;79(1):72–8.
77. Li H, Yan B, Wang Y, Shu Z, Li P, Liu Y, et al. The optimal time of ovarian reserve recovery after laparoscopic unilateral ovarian non-endometriotic cystectomy. Front Endocrinol (Lausanne). 2021;12:671225.
78. Beretta P, Franchi M, Ghezzi F, Busacca M, Zupi E, Bolis P. Randomized clinical trial of two laparoscopic treatments of endometriomas: cystectomy versus drainage and coagulation. Fertil Steril. 1998;70(6):1176–80.
79. Vercellini P, Chapron C, De Giorgi O, Consonni D, Frontino G, Crosignani PG. Coagulation or excision of ovarian endometriomas? Am J Obstet Gynecol. 2003;188(3):606–10.
80. Saridogan E, Becker CM, Feki A, Grimbizis GF, Hummelshoj L, Keckstein J, et al. Recommendations for the surgical treatment of endometriosis-part 1: ovarian endometrioma. Gynecol Surg. 2017;14(1):27.
81. Alammari R, Lightfoot M, Hur HC. Impact of cystectomy on ovarian reserve: review of the literature. J Minim Invasive Gynecol. 2017;24(2):247–57.
82. Tsiampa E, Spartalis E, Tsourouflis G, Dimitroulis D, Nikiteas N. Impact on ovarian reserve after minimally invasive single-port laparoscopic ovarian cystectomy in patients with benign ovarian cysts: a systematic review and meta-analysis. Int J Clin Pract. 2021;75(12):e14875.
83. Song T, Lee SH, Kim WY. Additional benefit of hemostatic sealant in preservation of ovarian reserve during laparoscopic ovarian cystectomy: a multi-center, randomized controlled trial. Hum Reprod. 2014;29(8):1659–65.
84. Choi C, Kim WY, Lee DH, Lee SH. Usefulness of hemostatic sealants for minimizing ovarian damage during laparoscopic cystectomy for endometriosis. J Obstet Gynaecol Res. 2018;44(3):532–9.
85. Kang JH, Kim YS, Lee SH, Kim WY. Comparison of hemostatic sealants on ovarian reserve during laparoscopic ovarian cystectomy. Eur J Obstet Gynecol Reprod Biol. 2015;194:64–7.
86. Xiao J, Zhou J, Liang H, Liu F, Xu C, Liang L. Impact of hemostatic methods on ovarian reserve and fertility in laparoscopic ovarian cystectomy. Exp Ther Med. 2019;17(4):2689–93.
87. Peters A, Rindos NB, Lee T. Hemostasis during ovarian cystectomy: systematic review of the impact of suturing versus surgical energy on ovarian function. J Minim Invasive Gynecol. 2017;24(2):235–46.
88. Shao M-J, Hu M, He Y-Q, Xu X-J. AMH trend after laparoscopic cystectomy and ovarian suturing in patients with endometriomas. Arch Gynecol Obstet. 2016;293(5):1049–52.
89. Cacciottola L, Donnez J, Dolmans MM. Ovarian tissue and oocyte cryopreservation prior to iatrogenic premature ovarian insufficiency. Best Pract Res Clin Obstet Gynaecol. 2022;81:119–33.
90. Practice Committee of American Society for Reproductive Medicine. Ovarian tissue cryopreservation: a committee opinion. Fertil Steril. 2014;101(5):1237–43.
91. Telfer EE, Andersen CY. In vitro growth and maturation of primordial follicles and immature oocytes. Fertil Steril. 2021;115(5):1116–25.
92. Bahroudi Z, Zarnaghi MR, Izadpanah M, Abedelahi A, Niknafs B, Nasrabadi HT, et al. Review of ovarian tissue cryopreservation techniques for fertility preservation. J Gynecol Obstet Hum Reprod. 2022;51(2):102290.
93. Dolmans MM, von Wolff M, Poirot C, Diaz-Garcia C, Cacciottola L, Boissel N, et al. Transplantation of cryopreserved ovarian tissue in a series of 285 women: a review of five leading European centers. Fertil Steril. 2021;115(5):1102–15.
94. Khattak H, Malhas R, Craciunas L, Afifi Y, Amorim CA, Fishel S, et al. Fresh and cryopreserved ovarian tissue transplantation for preserving reproductive and endocrine function: a systematic review and individual patient data meta-analysis. Hum Reprod Update. 2022;28(3):400–16.

6 Hysterectomy

Jessica Selle and John Gebhart

Introduction

Hysterectomy is one of the most common gynecologic procedures performed worldwide. Indications for benign hysterectomy include symptomatic uterine leiomyoma, abnormal uterine bleeding, postmenopausal bleeding, pelvic organ prolapse, endometriosis, pelvic pain, and pelvic mass [1, 2]. There are various approaches to hysterectomy including vaginal, laparoscopic, robotic, and open. While the vaginal route is preferred in the appropriate patient due to lower rates of complications and faster recovery times, appropriate selection is based on surgical indication, patient history, uterine access and size, concomitant procedures, surgical urgency, surgeon training and experience, available equipment, and patient wishes [3, 4].

Major complications of benign hysterectomy are rare but do occur and vary by approach. Understanding the pertinent anatomy, surgical steps, and ability to troubleshoot is crucial to prevention and managing intra- and postoperative complications. In this chapter, we review the major complications of hysterectomy in detail, along with prevention, recognition, and management strategies.

J. Selle (✉)
Department of OBGYN, Division of Urogynecology, Mayo Clinic, Rochester, MN, USA
e-mail: martin.jessica@mayo.edu

J. Gebhart
Department of OBGYN, Division Chair Urogynecology, Mayo Clinic, Rochester, MN, USA
e-mail: gebhart.john@mayo.edu

Hemorrhage

Background

Bleeding during benign hysterectomy is common and while some blood loss is expected, excessive blood loss constituting hemorrhage and requiring blood transfusion is rare. Given the potentially life-threatening nature of this complication, prevention and recognition are key. Rates of blood transfusion vary by approach and indication, with patient factors likely influencing the risk of excessive hemorrhage. A Cochrane review in 2015 reported lower risk of blood transfusion with a vaginal approach, but bleeding requiring a blood transfusion was overall low throughout all groups [5]. Other studies have found a rate of blood transfusion of 1.3% for minimally invasive hysterectomies, including vaginal, laparoscopic, and robotic approaches, while abdominal approaches reached 2.6% [6].

It is important to understand each patient's potential risk factors for excessive bleeding. Bleeding disorders, preoperative anemia, liver dysfunction, uterine abnormalities including patients with abnormal uterine bleeding, and surgical complexity all likely contribute to increased risk of blood transfusion [6].

M. Hoffman et al. (eds.), *Major Complications of Female Pelvic Surgery*,
https://doi.org/10.1007/978-3-031-66772-5_6

Prevention

Understanding the vascular anatomy and its relationship to the uterus and surrounding organs is crucial to preventing vascular injuries that can result in hemorrhage (Fig. 6.1). The major blood supply to the uterus includes the uterine and ovarian arteries and veins. The uterine artery originates from the anterior division of the internal iliac artery, while the ovarian artery arises from the aorta. The uterine artery and vein traverse the cardinal ligaments bilaterally, and the artery crosses obliquely over the ureter (water under the bridge) as it joins the uterus at the uterine–cervical junction [7]. The ovarian blood supply is equally important, traversing through the infundibulopelvic and utero-ovarian ligaments, supplying the ovaries and uterus. The ovarian vessels run anterior to the psoas in the retroperitoneum and cross the pelvic brim over the external iliac artery and vein as they supply the ovary. If an oophorectomy is being performed at the time of hysterectomy, identifying the ureter prior to securing the infundibulopelvic pedicle is vital due to their close relationship in this location, along with awareness of the external iliac vessels along the pelvic sidewall that are in close proximity.

Securing vascular pedicles can be performed with clamp/cut/tie techniques or with energy such as a bipolar device. The technique will depend on surgeon's preference and modality of surgery.

Other important prevention techniques include having appropriate exposure and retraction, lighting, instrumentation, and communication with the team [8].

Recognition

Early recognition is key in preventing significant morbidity or even death of a bleeding patient. Ideally, any significant bleeding is identified and managed intraoperatively.

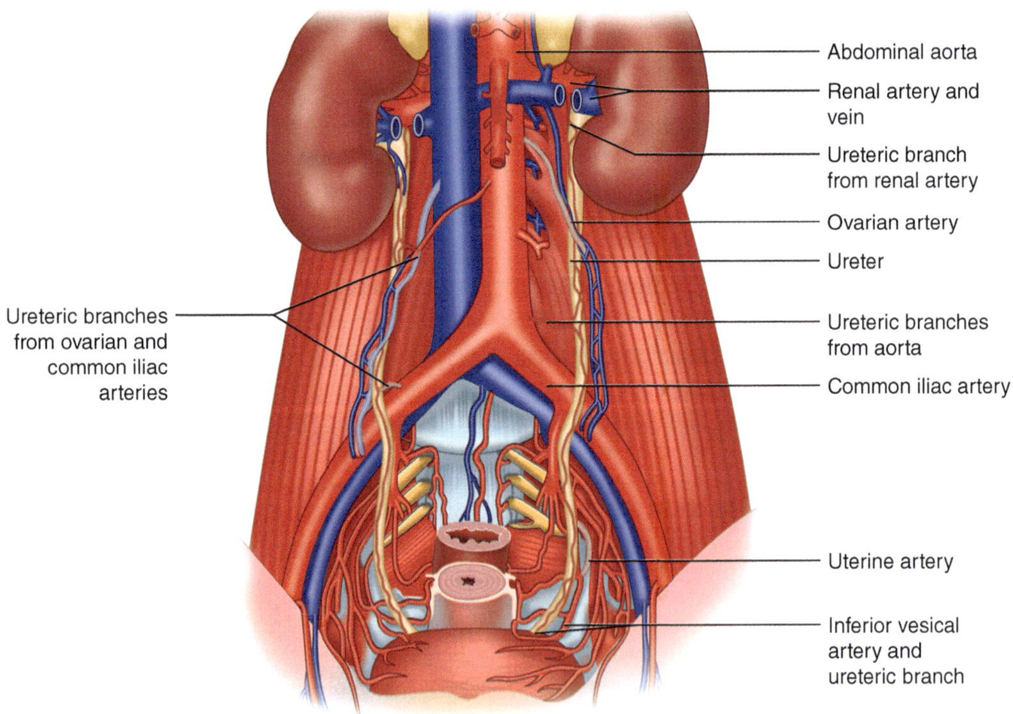

Fig. 6.1 Abdominopelvic vascular anatomy and ureteral anatomy. Highlighted areas denote highest risk of ureteral injury during hysterectomy

The most common sources of bleeding are from a vascular pedicle that has not been well secured or has retracted, which is why it is crucial to inspect each pedicle after removal of the uterus to ensure hemostasis. Additional sources of bleeding include any gaps between the utero-ovarian and cardinal pedicles. The posterior vaginal cuff and epithelium are often culprits and can easily be controlled with electrocautery or with suture ligature [4]. In the abdominal entry, bleeding should be cauterized as it is encountered. In laparoscopic or robotic surgery, injury to the inferior epigastric vessels or great vessels can also occur but this is beyond the scope of this chapter. Please see Chap. 23 for further details.

Postoperatively, hemorrhage may present as increased vaginal or abdominal bleeding, deterioration in vital signs (hypotension and/or tachycardia), abdominal or flank pain, abdominal distension, drop in hemoglobin/hematocrit, and light-headedness or syncopal episode. Any changes in patient status require immediate in-person assessment with a physical exam.

Management

If bleeding is identified intraoperatively, apply direct pressure and communicate with anesthesia to ensure the patient is vitally stable and not in need of immediate blood products. It is important to communicate with the operative team as well and use assistants and retractors for adequate exposure.

To manage bleeding, vessels must be isolated to avoid injury to surrounding structures. If a pedicle has loosened or retracted, it may be resecured with a suture ligature or vessel ligation device, keeping in mind the location of the ureter and other adjacent organs. Arterial bleeding may require surgical clips or fine suture ligature. Bleeding is common along cut edges, and cautery may be utilized.

Hemostatic agents can be particularly useful for small vessel venous bleeding and diffuse areas that ooze. There are several agents on the market that act on various aspects of the clotting cascade and differ in cost, consistency, and availability. Some examples include thrombin-soaked gel foam, oxidized regenerated cellulose, gelatin matrix–thrombin combination, microporous polysaccharide spheres, fibrin glue/sealant, tranexamic acid, and others [9]. Adverse effects and complications are typically uncommon.

If bleeding is identified postoperatively, imaging can be obtained in a stable patient with selective embolization by interventional radiology (Fig. 6.2). However, if a significant bleed is suspected, urgent return to the operating room is appropriate. Depending on the suspected site of bleeding and initial approach to surgery, a vaginal approach could be attempted, but laparotomy or laparoscopic evaluation may be warranted to better visualize and dissect out the vessel(s) from above [4, 10]. When large hemoperitoneum is expected, being prepared with two suction tips on the OR table, additional laparotomy sponges, and

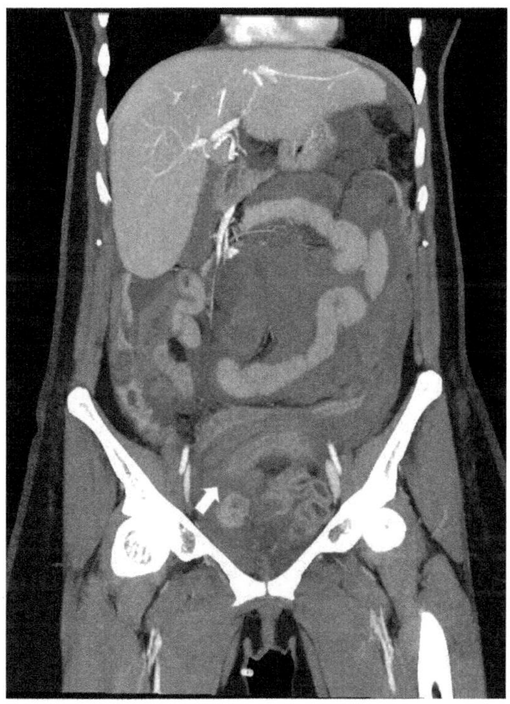

Fig. 6.2 Large hemoperitoneum requiring return to the operating room. Non-contrast CT can be obtained for rapid identification of hemoperitoneum, or CT with IV contrast can be performed to look for an active bleed. Blood products appear hyperdense to surrounding structures [30]. Used with permission of Mayo Foundation for Medical Education and Research, all rights reserved

saline solution for washout and identification of bleeding is helpful. Blood products should be replaced as needed, either traditionally or with blood salvage techniques.

The development of disseminated intravascular coagulation (DIC) is possible in the setting of excessive hemorrhage and is important to be aware of. These patients may warrant ICU admission and have clotting factors repleted. Protocols vary across hospitals but have historically been a 4:1 ratio of packed red cells to 1 of FFP or cryoprecipitate, while newer data reveal a 1:1:1 ratio (and include a platelet pack in cases of "massive" transfusion) can ultimately result in fewer products utilized [8].

Bladder Injury

Background

The risk of urinary tract injury is 1–2% for all gynecologic surgery [11]. The rates of cystotomy at the time of hysterectomy vary by approach. In a randomized trial of 1300 hysterectomies, bladder injury occurred 1% in the abdominal approach, 2.1% in the laparoscopic approach, and 1.2% in vaginal approach [11, 12]. This rate does vary amongst studies, and some report bladder injury more commonly occurring in vaginal hysterectomy with injury on anterior cul-de-sac entry.

Risk factors for bladder injury include previous cesarean section, endometriosis, pelvic inflammatory disease, cancer, and adhesions [11].

Prevention

Avoiding injury to the urinary tract requires anatomic knowledge of the relationships between the bladder and ureters to the uterus and its blood supply (Figs. 6.1 and 6.5). Identifying urinary tract structures at the time of surgery is essential. The bladder can be injured during lysis of adhesions, dissection of the vesicouterine space, and entry into the anterior cul-de-sac in vaginal hysterectomy [13]. In laparoscopic surgery, the bladder can also be injured during the introduction of a suprapubic trocar, so direct visualization is an important point of prevention.

To avoid bladder injury, some surgeons choose to continuously drain the bladder with a Foley catheter, intermittent drainage with an in and out catheter, or backfill the bladder with normal saline or sterile milk to delineate planes in patients with previous cesarean sections or difficult anatomy [13]. If identification is difficult, inserting a cystoscope can illuminate the bladder base. On abdominal entry, it is important to enter the peritoneum as cephalad as possible to avoid inadvertent bladder injury [14]. Proper use of assistants and retractors to help keep important structures out of the operative field is essential. In abdominal and laparoscopic/robotic surgeries, cephalad traction of the uterus helps to delineate the vesicouterine plane and mobilize the bladder away from the uterine arteries [15]. During abdominal hysterectomy, this can be accomplished with the use of Kocher clamps on the bilateral cornua and upward traction by the surgeon or assistant. In laparoscopic or robotic surgery, this can be achieved with the use of a uterine manipulator or the use of traction from a laparoscopic or robotic instrument from above. In vaginal hysterectomy, manual traction on the incised vaginal epithelium allows for easy dissection along the cervix and into the anterior cul-de-sac. Once the plane is achieved and caudad traction on the cervix is maintained, the use of an anterior Deaver retracts and protects the bladder.

Sharp dissection of the vesicovaginal space rather than blunt dissection is preferred as blunt dissection can distort planes and increase the risk of injury [4, 13]. The use of electrocautery should also be used cautiously near the bladder or ureters as delayed injury can result from a thermal spread injury [13].

Recognition

Although an area of controversy, the authors advocate for universal cystoscopy with hysterectomy as it increases the absolute recognition of bladder and ureteral injury. Due to the low incidence of ureteral injury, most studies do not show statistical significance in the use of routine cystoscopy [16]. However, cystoscopy has a sensitivity of 94.4% and 95.5% specificity in detecting ureteral injury [17]. Additionally, preoperative use of Pyridium or intraoperative use of indigo carmine, sodium fluorescein, or dextrose can assist in intraoperative detection of ureteral patency during cystourethroscopy with bilateral ureteral efflux [4, 14]. A recent cost analysis found preoperative Pyridium to be the most cost-effective agent, followed by intraoperative dextrose and use of IV agents if Pyridium and dextrose fail as primary agents [17].

Recognition of a cystostomy may be obvious (Figs. 6.3a and 6.4a), with extravasation of urine at the time of cystostomy. Or if the bladder is drained, may be less apparent and present as bladder thinning [4]. Bladder injuries are graded based on severity by the American Association for the Surgery of Trauma from 1 to 5 [13].

Postoperatively, suspicion of a bladder injury should be elevated with leakage of fluid from the vagina, oliguria or anuria, hematuria, abdominal pain/distension, fever, abdominal ascites with elevated fluid creatinine, and postoperative ileus. An easy diagnosis of cystotomy postoperatively is to backfill the bladder with 300ccs of normal saline and measure how much returns through the Foley catheter. No fluid return indicates extravasation of the fluid through a cystotomy [14]. Imaging can also be useful to identify a cystotomy and includes a CT cystogram.

Management

Depending on the size and location of the cystostomy, the bladder may or may not require surgical repair. An extraperitoneal laceration >2 cm or intraperitoneal laceration <2 cm generally requires surgical correction [13]. Cystotomies requiring repair should be identified and tagged, with subsequent repair after the hysterectomy is complete [14]. Exposure and visualization are particularly important before attempting repair, along with knowledge of the proximity of the injury to the ureter and trigone. A two-layer closure can be performed using either running non-locked technique or interrupted sutures. A second layer is typically performed in an imbricating fashion. A significant bladder injury >2 cm in size should be repaired in a tension-free two-layer closure for watertight repair (Figs. 6.3b and 6.4b). The authors use a combination of two 2-0 chromic gut sutures, but any delayed absorbable suture can be used. Barbed sutures are often used in laparoscopic and robotic cystotomy repairs as knot tying and keeping adequate tension can be difficult [18]. Avoidance of permanent suture is important as this will precipitate stone formation and could lead to fistula formation.

The cystostomy repair should be checked to ensure it is watertight. This can be done by backfilling the bladder with methylene blue-stained saline. The authors use 300ccs to adequately assess that the repair is watertight without putting undue stress on the repair.

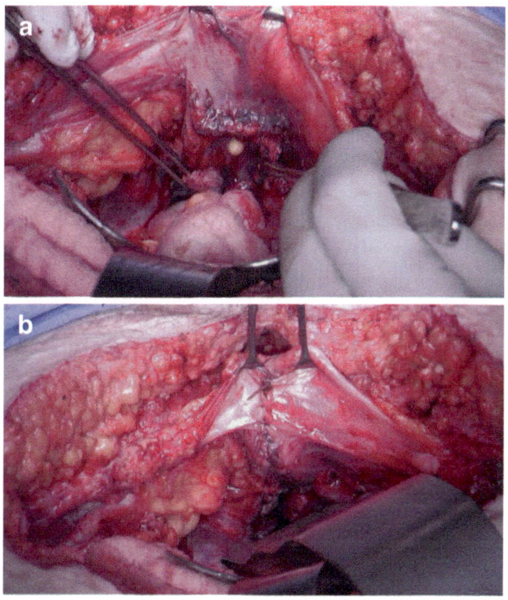

Fig. 6.3 (**a**) Large cystotomy with foley catheter visualized. Used with permission of Mayo Foundation for Medical Education and Research, all rights reserved. (**b**) After repair in 2 layer non-locked running closure with 2-0 chromic gut suture, the bladder is backfilled with 300 cc's of methylene blue stained fluid and showed no extravasation of contrast. Used with permission of Mayo Foundation for Medical Education and Research, all rights reserved

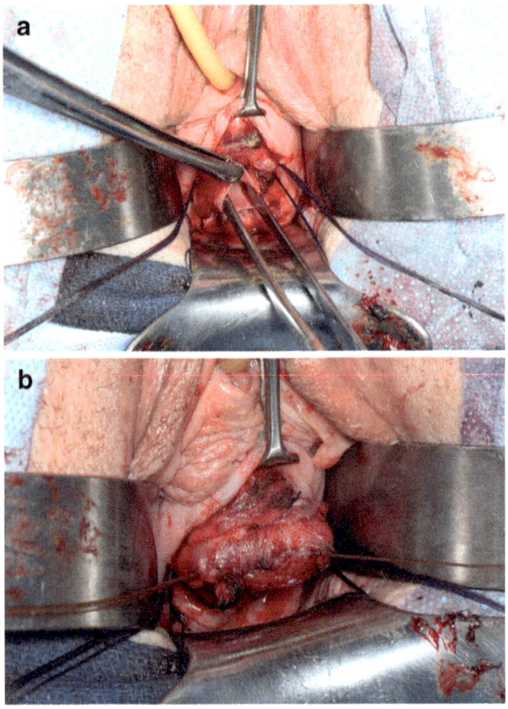

Fig. 6.4 (**a**) Vaginal cystotomy denoted by Russian forceps. Used with permission of Mayo Foundation for Medical Education and Research, all rights reserved. (**b**) Vaginal cystotomy repaired in 2 layer running non-locked closure and back filled with 300ccs of methylene blue stained fluid. Used with permission of Mayo Foundation for Medical Education and Research, all rights reserved

Postoperatively, the bladder should be decompressed with an indwelling Foley catheter. For a significant injury, we typically leave a catheter for 2–3 weeks, although there is no consensus on duration and this can range from 7 days to 3 weeks. Earlier removal decreases the risk of urinary tract infection and likely has similar cure rates. No prophylactic antibiotics are needed for short-term catheter use, although some studies suggest a dose of antibiotic at the time of catheter removal may decrease urinary tract infections [19]. There is controversy regarding the postoperative use of CT cystogram prior to Foley catheter removal [13]. In our experience, if it was an uncomplicated intraperitoneal repair, the Foley can be removed by the patient at home, but if there is any concern for healing it can be removed after ensuring no extravasation on CT cystogram.

Ureteral Injury

Background

Ureteral injury is reported more commonly in laparoscopic/robotic approaches to hysterectomy, and most frequently occurs at the site of uterine artery ligation (80%), followed by infundibulopelvic ligament, and vaginal cuff [4]. Ureteral injury has similar risk factors to bladder injury and includes prior pelvic surgery, hemorrhage, endometriosis, cancer, compromised exposure, pelvic organ prolapse, and obesity. Bladder and ureteral injuries can result in a genitourinary tract fistula, so identification and satisfactory repair are critical.

Recognition

The same principles apply in the identification of ureteral injury and include adequate exposure and identification prior to proceeding with the operation. In vaginal surgery, the ureters can be palpated prior to clamping the cardinal pedicles using an index finger through the anterior entry site against an antero-laterally placed Deaver [4]. If only posterior entry has been achieved, this palpation technique cannot be utilized, but taking small successive bites being sure to hug the uterus will keep the ureters out of the operative field. In robotic and laparoscopic surgeries, patients with risk factors for ureteral injury may warrant indocyanine green (ICG)injection into the bilateral ureters. ICG injection can be easily accomplished with cystoscopy and the advancement of a whistle-tip catheter into each ureter, advancing to 20 cm and injecting 5 mL of ICG. This allows the ureters to light up green with near infra-red robotic and laparoscopic optics. In open abdominal cases with anticipated difficult anatomy, the use of temporary ureteral stents can assist in identifying the ureters by palpation. It should be noted that routine use of stents for hysterectomy is not recommended as it has not been associated with a reduction in the incidence of ureteral injury and has its own associated risks [14].

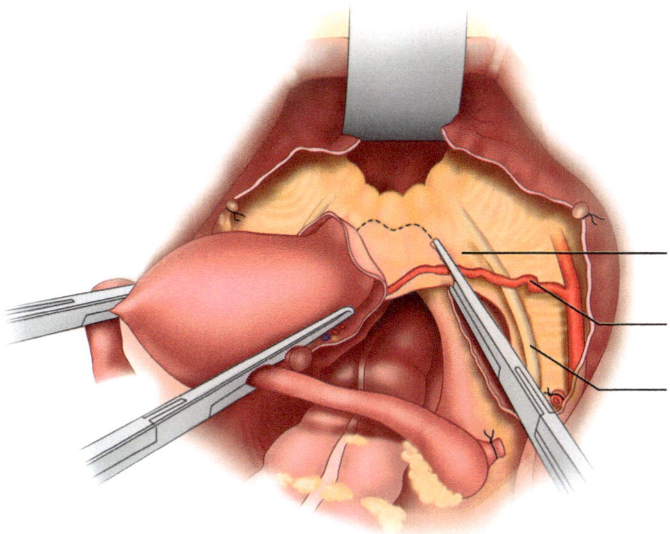

Fig. 6.5 Illustration of the ureter and its proximity to the uterine artery in an abdominal hysterectomy

Understanding ureteral anatomy is crucial to avoiding ureteral injury. The ureters pass over the bifurcation of the common iliac vessels, dive under the uterine arteries at the level of the cardinal ligament (water under the bridge), and pass lateral to the cervix (Figs. 6.1 and 6.5). In abdominal hysterectomy, the ureter is identified in the medial leaf of the broad ligament. In non-obese patients, the ureter can easily be identified transperitoneally as it crosses over the pelvic brim, distinguished by peristalsis. If the ureter is easily identified in laparoscopic or robotic approaches, some surgeons may opt to abandon opening the retroperitoneal space as is traditionally practiced. If bleeding is encountered, it is important to apply pressure and confirm the location of the ureter by dissecting it away from surrounding vessels rather than indiscriminately clamping or cauterizing.

Ureteral injuries are often more subtle than a bladder injury. They may be identified intraoperatively with extravasation of urine, indicating a transection injury and this can be more readily identified by giving the patient indigo carmine IV. On cystoscopy, an absence of efflux would indicate an obstruction and would be more readily apparent if pre-treated with Pyridium or intraoperatively with indigo carmine or sodium fluorescein.

If a ureteral injury is suspected postoperatively, the imaging of choice is a CT urogram with IV contrast.

Management

The management of ureteral injuries is beyond the scope of this chapter, but in general involves ureterolysis and ureteral stenting, with or without ureteral reimplantation or end-to-end anastomosis depending on the type and location of injury. On occasion, intentional cystotomy may be utilized to assist in stenting or to view the inside of the bladder if cystoscopy is not readily available [14]. Please see Chap. 17 for further details.

Bowel Injury

Background

Bowel injury as a result of benign hysterectomy is a rare but serious complication that can lead to serious morbidity and mortality if it goes unrecognized. In vaginal surgery, a rectal injury would be the most common GI injury and is rare, occurring 0.4% of the time and would most commonly occur on a difficult posterior entry [4]. A retrospective study showed an increased odds of bowel injury in laparoscopic hysterectomy (OR 2.06) and abdominal hysterectomy (OR 10.80) when compared to vaginal hysterectomy [20].

Major risk factors for bowel injury include older age, endometriosis, and abdominal surgical approach [20]. Others include the history of multiple abdominal surgeries and a lack of surgeon experience.

Prevention

In endoscopic surgery, the placement of an orogastric tube is important to decompress the stomach to help prevent gastric injury on entry and port placement. Bowel injury can occur during the insertion of a Veress needle, trocar placement, use of electrosurgery, suturing, or lysis of adhesions.

In laparoscopic and open approaches, most bowel injuries occur during abdominal entry [21]. Injury can occur in the form of laceration, perforation, thermal injury, crush injury, and vascular injury. Understanding the patient's surgical and medical history to be prepared for adherence of bowel to the anterior abdominal wall is critical. Thermal injuries tend to be very difficult to identify intraoperatively and are more commonly associated with a delay in diagnosis and treatment. Therefore, judicious use of electrocautery, with knowledge of how to effectively avoid inadvertent coupling and thermal spread, is crucial.

Recognition

Identification of injury at the time of surgery is critical but can be difficult especially as thermal injuries may be subtle or occur outside of the direct line of sight of the surgeon. Laceration resulting in spillage of stool is classic for bowel injury, although injuries are often not this obvious. If a bowel injury is encountered, always check for a "through and through" defect.

Delayed recognition can result in abscess, septic shock, fistula, and death. Signs of a bowel perforation include severe abdominal pain, nausea, and vomiting, fever or rise in body temperature, rise in white blood cell count, abdominal distension, and change in vitals, most notably tachycardia and hypotension. A high index of suspicion is crucial for prompt management. Workup includes serial abdominal examinations, lab work, upright abdominal X-ray, and CT scan with oral contrast. Delayed injury and perforation can occur between 24 h and up to 2–3 weeks postoperatively [22].

Management

Management of bowel injury is beyond the scope of this chapter but requires copious irrigation and involvement of a surgeon trained in bowel surgery, sometimes necessitating bowel resection or diversion. A small full-thickness or seromuscular enterotomy or colotomy is repaired in layers with gently approximating delayed absorbable suture.

Vaginal Cuff Dehiscence

Background

Vaginal cuff dehiscence is a rare but serious postoperative complication that can result in serious morbidity and mortality. It is defined as a partial or complete separation of the vaginal cuff margins after hysterectomy [23]. This complication ranges from several days to a few months postoperatively and can occur spontaneously but classically presents after direct trauma to the vaginal cuff with intercourse or straining with a bowel movement. Incidence ranges from 0.008 to 1.35% in several studies but has been reported as high as 5.8% [11, 24, 25]. Incidence varies by route of hysterectomy, with the highest rates occurring in laparoscopic (0.62–2.7%) and robotic hysterectomy (0.4–4.1%). Vaginal and abdominal hysterectomies come in with the lowest risk and have reported averages of 0.11% and 0.35%, respectively [26, 27]. Risk factors include constipation, smoking, immunosuppression, menopausal status, prior pelvic surgery, postoperative infection, and diabetes.

Prevention

There is no consensus on the best prevention strategy for vaginal cuff dehiscence. Several studies indicate that the incidence has increased after the introduction of laparoscopic and robotic surgery [23], although there is some thought that this may be due to inexperience and that this rate decreases significantly in experienced surgeons' hands [28]. Some advocate for a two-layer laparoscopic vaginal cuff closure, with one retrospective study showing 0.9% cuff complication rate versus 2.6% in a single-layer technique [25]. Barbed sutures have also been shown in retrospective studies to reduce the risk of dehiscence when compared to non-barbed sutures; however, out of 11 studies looking at this, only 2 found statistical significance [23]. Another strategy that has been implemented by many institutions has been delayed resumption of intercourse after laparoscopic or robotic cuff closure, our institution uses 9 weeks although data are lacking. The approach to colpotomy has been evaluated by looking at monopolar current versus cut cautery or cold knife, and no studies have been adequately powered to draw conclusions [23]. Another prevention technique has been to close the cuff vaginally after a laparoscopic or robotic procedure. Three studies evaluating this approach showed an increase in the risk of dehiscence with a transvaginal closure than laparoscopic closure (2.7% vs 1%; $p = 0.01$) [23, 29]. Some general strategies include adequate mobilization of the bladder to allow adequate cuff to suture, judicious use of cautery to minimize thermal damage, approximation of the cuff without strangulation, and, in selected cases, vertical closure.

Recognition

A delay in recognition and management can lead to life-threatening complications such as bowel perforation, peritonitis, sepsis, and even death [23]. The presentation includes postcoital bleeding, other vaginal bleeding or watery discharge, pelvic pressure or bulge, pelvic pain, and bowel evisceration (Fig. 6.6a–c). A high index of suspicion is critical with careful history taking and immediate physical examination to visually inspect and manually palpate the vaginal cuff.

Management

Although small or partial dehiscences may be safely managed with pelvic rest, a true vaginal cuff dehiscence is a surgical emergency and warrants a return to the operating room. If there is any delay in taking the patient to the operating room such as might occur if the patient needs to be transferred from an outside hospital, it should be requested that the patient remain supine or even in slight Trendelenburg with placement of a foley catheter and moist vaginal pack. If bowel is eviscerated, a moist sterile towel should be applied to cover the prolapsed bowel.

Cuff dehiscence can be closed vaginally when possible, but may require abdominal exploration (laparoscopy can be considered) in cases of bowel evisceration to thoroughly inspect the bowel and wash out the peritoneal cavity. If the bowel is able to be inspected vaginally, it can sometimes be reduced without trauma. However, if the bowel has become edematous and does not easily reduce, an exploratory laparotomy should be performed. Any necrotic bowel should be resected by a surgeon trained in bowel surgery.

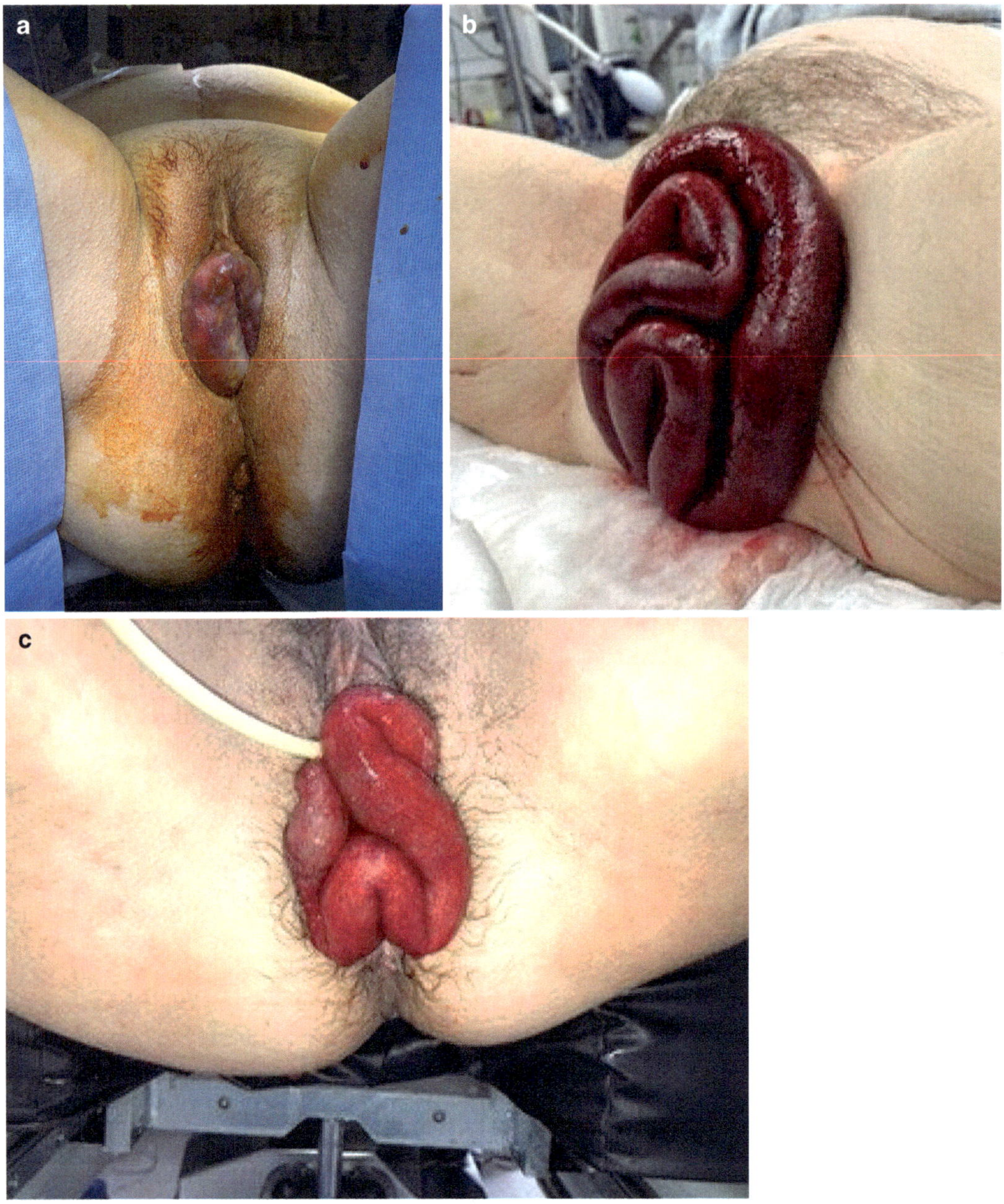

Fig. 6.6 (**a**) Vaginal bowel evisceration. She was taken to the OR and repair was able to be performed vaginally. Used with permission of Mayo Foundation for Medical Education and Research, all rights reserved. (**b**) Vaginal bowel evisceration with nonviable bowel, requiring resection. Copyright [2023] Journal of Gynecologic Surgery. (**c**) Vaginal bowel evisceration requiring laparoscopy with bowel reduction, abdominal washout, drain placement, and transvaginal closure. Copyright [2023] Journal of Gynecologic Surgery

References

1. Ramdhan RC, Loukas M, Tubbs RS. Anatomical complications of hysterectomy: a review. Clin Anat. 2017;30(7):946–52.
2. Hammer A, et al. Global epidemiology of hysterectomy: possible impact on gynecological cancer rates. Am J Obstet Gynecol. 2015;213(1):23–9.
3. Committee Opinion No. 701. Summary: choosing the route of hysterectomy for benign disease. Obstet Gynecol. 2017;129(6):1149–50.
4. Occhino JA, Gebhart JB. Vaginal hysterectomy. In: Le LV, Handa V, editors. Te Linde's operative gynecology. Wolters Kluwer Health; 2023.
5. Aarts JW, et al. Surgical approach to hysterectomy for benign gynaecological disease. Cochrane Database Syst Rev. 2015;2015(8):Cd003677.
6. Elfazari T, et al. Surgical indication and approach are associated with transfusion in hysterectomy for benign disease. JSLS. 2022;26(2)
7. Baggish MS, Karram MM. Atlas of pelvic anatomy and gynecologic surgery. 5th ed. Elsevier; 2021.
8. Hodges KR, Davis BR, Swaim LS. Prevention and management of hysterectomy complications. Clin Obstet Gynecol. 2014;57(1):43–57.
9. Tompeck AJ, et al. A comprehensive review of topical hemostatic agents: the good, the bad, and the novel. J Trauma Acute Care Surg. 2020;88(1):e1–e21.
10. Holub Z, Jabor A. Laparoscopic management of bleeding after laparoscopic or vaginal hysterectomy. JSLS. 2004;8(3):235–8.
11. Clarke-Pearson DL, Geller EJ. Complications of hysterectomy. Obstet Gynecol. 2013;121(3):654–73.
12. Johnson N, et al. Surgical approach to hysterectomy for benign gynaecological disease. Cochrane Database Syst Rev. 2006;2:Cd003677.
13. Zelivianskaia AS, Bradley SE, Morozov VV. Best practices for repair of iatrogenic bladder injury. AJOG Glob Rep. 2022;2(3):100062.
14. Matthews CA, Gebhart JB. Avoiding and managing lower urinary tract injuries during pelvic surgery. In: Walters & Karram Urogynecology and reconstructive pelvic surgery. Elsevier, Inc.; 2022. p. 386–98.
15. Glaser LM, Milad MP. Bowel and bladder injury repair and follow-up after gynecologic surgery. Obstet Gynecol. 2019;133(2):313–22.
16. AAGL Advancing Minimally Invasive Gynecology Worldwide. AAGL Practice Report: Practice guidelines for intraoperative cystoscopy in laparoscopic hysterectomy. J Minim Invasive Gynecol. 2012;19(4):407–11.
17. Askew AL, Myers ER, Dieter AA. Cost-effectiveness of agents used for evaluation of ureteral patency during intraoperative cystoscopy in gynecologic and urogynecologic surgery. Am J Obstet Gynecol. 2022;226(1):100.e1–6.
18. Shapiro R, et al. A comparative study of braided versus barbed suture for Cystotomy repair. Res Rep Urol. 2021;13:793–8.
19. Wolf JS Jr, et al. Best practice policy statement on urologic surgery antimicrobial prophylaxis. J Urol. 2008;179(4):1379–90.
20. Zhu CR, et al. Risk factors for bowel injury in hysterectomy for benign indications. Obstet Gynecol. 2020;136(4)
21. Elbiss HM, Abu-Zidan FM. Bowel injury following gynecological laparoscopic surgery. Afr Health Sci. 2017;17(4):1237–45.
22. Bhullar JS, et al. Delayed presentation of a bowel Bovie injury after laparoscopic ventral hernia repair. JSLS. 2013;17(3):495–8.
23. Uccella S, Zorzato PC, Kho RM. Incidence and prevention of vaginal cuff dehiscence after laparoscopic and robotic hysterectomy: a systematic review and meta-analysis. J Minim Invasive Gynecol. 2021;28(3):710–20.
24. Hur H-C, et al. Incidence and patient characteristics of vaginal cuff dehiscence after different modes of hysterectomies. J Minim Invasive Gynecol. 2007;14(3):311–7.
25. Peters A, et al. Two-layer compared with one-layer vaginal cuff closure at the time of Total laparoscopic hysterectomy to reduce complications. Obstet Gynecol. 2021;138(1):59–65.
26. Kho RM, et al. Incidence and characteristics of patients with vaginal cuff dehiscence after robotic procedures. Obstet Gynecol. 2009;114(2 Pt 1):231–5.
27. Hur HC, et al. Vaginal cuff dehiscence after different modes of hysterectomy. Obstet Gynecol. 2011;118(4):794–801.
28. Nezhat C, et al. Vaginal cuff dehiscence and evisceration: a review. Obstet Gynecol. 2018;132(4):972–85.
29. Uccella S, et al. Laparoscopic vs transvaginal cuff closure after total laparoscopic hysterectomy: a randomized trial by the Italian Society of Gynecologic Endoscopy. Am J Obstet Gynecol. 2018;218(5):500.e1–500.e13.
30. Gomez E, et al. CT of acute abdominopelvic hemorrhage: protocols, pearls, and pitfalls. Abdom Radiol NY. 2022;47(1):475–84.

7 Genital Tract Prolapse

Brittany L. Roberts and Rebecca G. Rogers

Intraoperative Injuries

General complications of surgery apply to pelvic reconstructive surgeries as well. Overall, intraoperative complications are rare; however, it is important to understand how to identify and manage complications. We will discuss hemorrhage and injury to the urinary tract, gastrointestinal tract, and nervous system specific to the most common pelvic reconstructive surgeries.

Vascular Injury

Background

Hemorrhage related to pelvic organ prolapse surgery is uncommon and estimated to be 1.5% [1]. Although rare, excessive blood loss requiring transfusion or formation of a hematoma may occur in any pelvic reconstructive surgery. Hemorrhage risk varies between procedures with the highest risk of severe hemorrhage occurring with sacrospinous ligament fixation and sacral colpopexy. The incidence of life-threatening hemorrhage related to sacrospinous ligament fixation ranges from 0.2% to 2% [2, 3]. During a sacrospinous ligament fixation, severe hemorrhage most commonly occurs with dissection superior to the coccygeus muscle or lateral to the ischial spine in the ischiorectal fossa. The inferior gluteal artery and its coccygeal branch are most susceptible to injury [4, 5]. During sacrocolpopexy, the mesh is attached to the sacral promontory. This is defined as the most superior point on the anterior surface of S1 into the anterior longitudinal ligament. Figure 7.1 demonstrates the presacral space and the proximity of vital structures. The reported hemorrhage or transfusion rate for abdominal sacral colpopexies is 4.4% [6]. There are several potential hemorrhage sources when dissecting the presacral space including presacral vessels/venous complexes, the middle sacral vessels, and the left common iliac vein.

Prevention

As the sacrospinous ligament dissection is typically performed without visualization, hemorrhage during the procedure may be difficult to control. Since life-threatening hemorrhage is rare, there are few guidelines on how to manage hemorrhage. Utilization of the Capio device or passage of the needle tip downward into the ischiorectal space rather than passing the needle tip superior toward vasculature is preferred [7].

B. L. Roberts · R. G. Rogers (✉)
Department of Obstetrics and Gynecology, Division of Urogynecology and Reconstructive Pelvic Surgery Albany Medical Center, Albany, NY, USA
e-mail: robertb5@amc.edu; rogersr2@amc.edu

M. Hoffman et al. (eds.), *Major Complications of Female Pelvic Surgery*,
https://doi.org/10.1007/978-3-031-66772-5_7

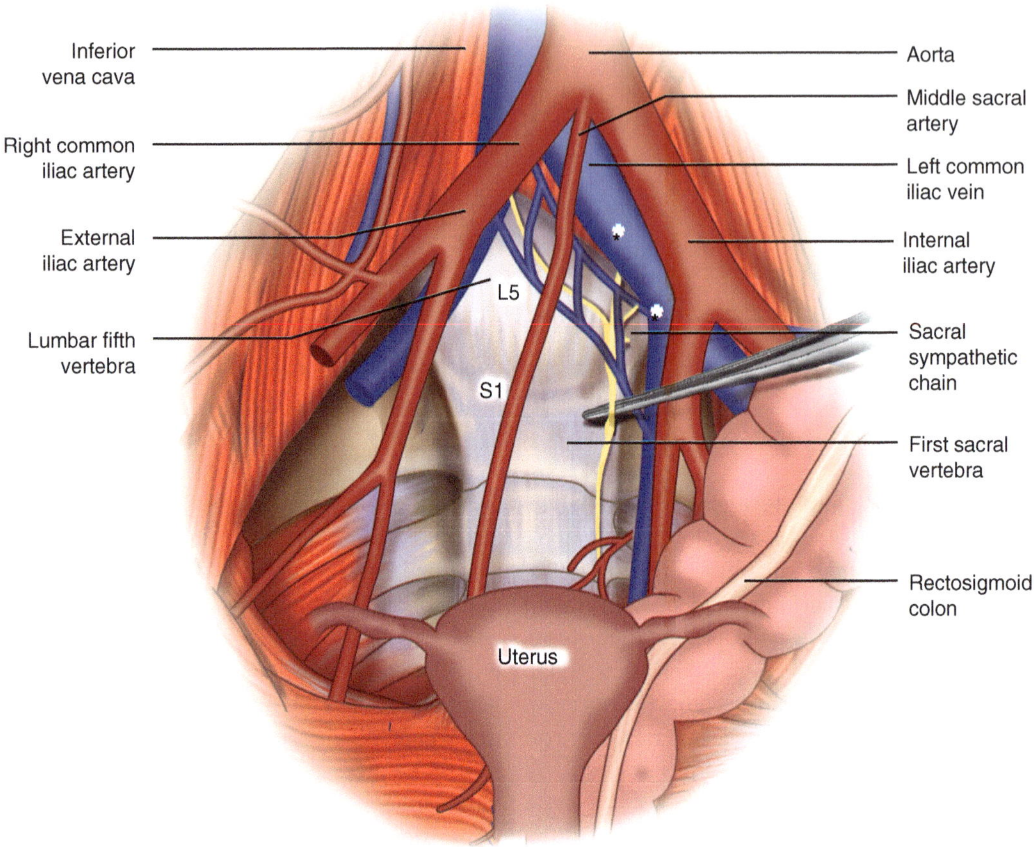

Fig. 7.1 Presacral dissection: Dissection of the presacral space with surrounding organs, vasculature and nerves

A recent study was performed evaluating the relationship of critical structures to the sacral suture during a robotic sacrocolpopexy [8]. A vascular clip was placed at the level of the sacral suture and 6 weeks later, patients underwent imaging to evaluate the anatomy relative to the sacral suture. The left common iliac vein was an average of 26 mm away from the sacral suture, while the right common iliac artery was 18 mm away. It is important to be mindful of the proximity of these structures when performing the sacral dissection and placement of sacral sutures.

Recognition

During sacrospinous ligament fixation, sudden significant bleeding may be encountered during the dissection or following placement of the sacrospinous sutures. Hemorrhage is most likely to occur at the time of dissection of the presacral space during sacrocolpopexy. When bleeding occurs at the presacral vessels, hemostasis can be difficult to achieve because of the venous network both beneath and on the surface of the periosteum. Vessels retract beneath the surface of the anterior sacrum and recede into the bone, including sacral foramina.

Management

Initial management of hemorrhage includes compression of the sacrospinous ligament. This is performed by applying pressure with a sponge on the sacrospinous ligament at the insertion of the ischial spine. Although there is limited evidence on the length of time to hold pressure, a minimum compression time of 10 min has been suggested [9]. If bleeding continues, application of hemostatic agents can be applied. This is most helpful for venous bleeding or capillary oozing. If despite these measures bleeding continues, a narrow malleable or Breisky retractor may be used to attempt visualization of the injured vessel. If visualized, suture ligation or placement of vascular clips may be performed. Conversion to laparotomy is not recommended as does not allow for visualization of the hemorrhage source.

Packing of the presacral space may temporarily control bleeding, but it may recur once packing is removed. Packing must be done cautiously and without undue pressure to avoid tearing the delicate venous network. Agents for hemostasis may include sutures, metallic clips, cautery, and bone wax. If not successful, stainless steel thumbtacks can be placed on a retracted bleeding presacral vein or into the associated foramen to treat a life-threatening hemorrhage [10]. If performing a laparoscopic or robotic sacrocolpopexy, conversion to laparotomy may be performed depending on the vasculature injured, poor control of the hemorrhage, or inadequate visualization.

Urinary Tract Injury

Background

Urinary tract injury at the time of prolapse surgery varies depending on the procedure being performed. Cystotomy and ureteral injuries are often diagnosed at the time of surgical procedures secondary to the utilization of intraoperative cystoscopy [11]. Specific to pelvic reconstructive surgery, the rate of cystotomy is around 3.2% [12] and ureteral obstruction and/or injury ranges from 0.3 to 11% of cases [13, 14]. Uterosacral ligament suspension (USLS) is the most common procedure associated with ureteral injury [15]. One of the most common complications associated with uterosacral ligament suspension is ureteral injury or kinking (risk up to 11% [13]). This risk is high because of ureteral proximity to the uterosacral ligament. The ureter may also be injured directly with the placement of the stitch. This injury is typically identified following the needle placement with leakage of urine into the posterior cul-de-sac. It is often helpful to administer phenazopyridine in the preoperative period versus methylene blue for easy identification.

Prevention

The ureter is located lateral and ventral to the uterosacral ligament along its course. The distance from the ureter to the uterosacral ligament is estimated to be 0.9 cm in the cervical portion, 2.3 cm in the intermediate portion, and 4.1 cm in the sacral portion. [16] The optimal fixation site is the intermediate portion of the uterosacral ligament, 1 cm posterior to its most anterior palpable margin, at the level of the ischial spine or above [16]. Identification of the uterosacral ligament is paramount in performing this procedure safely. If a USLS is being performed at the time of the vaginal hysterectomy, keeping the ligament tagged at the time of suture ligation is useful to aid in later identification. Adequate visualization of the pelvis is then achieved with the packing of the bowel and use of retractors. An Allis or Babcock clamp may then be placed at the vaginal portion of the uterosacral ligament, and gentle traction is utilized to aide in identification. If this is performed in a patient who is post-hysterectomy, the clamps may be placed at 4 and 8 o clock [17]. The sutures should be placed from ventral to dorsal, avoiding peritoneum lateral to the ligament, to minimize the risk of ureteral entrapment or kinking.

Recognition

It is imperative to perform an intraoperative cystoscopy to ensure ureteral patency with these procedures. If ureteral efflux is weak or not observed, the suspension on that side should be removed suture by suture with repetitive re-evaluation.

Management

As the ureter is in closest proximity to the uterosacral ligament distally, the distal suture on the ipsilateral side of the suspension should be removed first (lateral to medial). The suture can be replaced more medially.

Bowel Injury

Background

Bowel injury during general gynecologic surgery is rare and ranges from 0.13 to 0.54% [18]. The majority of these injuries occur during vaginal or abdominal entry and adhesiolysis [18, 19]. Bowel injuries in pelvic reconstructive surgery are similar, and the same general principles of early diagnosis and repair apply. Sacrospinous ligament fixation and sacrocolpopexy have features that may elicit bowel injury specific to these reconstructive procedures. The global rate of rectal injury during sacrospinous ligament fixation is 0.4% [20]. Injury to the rectum is higher if a previous colporrhaphy was performed [21].

The incidence of bowel injury during sacrocolpopexy ranges from 0 to 1.6% [22–24]. As with general gynecologic surgery, injuries typically occur with entry. Rectal injury may occur during the development of the rectovaginal space, especially in patients with cul-de-sac adhesions.

Prevention

Although rare, rectal injury is most likely to occur during entry of the ischiorectal fossa while gaining access to the sacrospinous ligament. If retractors are necessary to aid in visualization of the ligament or to increase the space of dissection, careful placement is necessary to avoid rectal injury. This may be accomplished by displacing the rectum with a finger and placing the retractor over your finger.

During sacrocolpopexy, utilization of an endoanal sizer may aid in delineation of the rectum and development of the rectovaginal space.

Recognition

A rectal examination should be performed after placement of the sutures because of the close proximity of the rectum to the sacrospinous ligament [7].

Management

If a rectal injury is identified during sacrospinous ligament fixation, it can be repaired transvaginally.

Limited evidence exists on whether or not a mesh sacrocolpopexy should be completed following a bowel injury. A recent review of the literature utilizing the Delphi process recommended that if there is an uncomplicated small bowel injury, the sacrocolpopexy should be completed. If a large bowel injury occurs, the sacrocolpopexy should be deferred [25]. Alternatively, consideration can be given to completing the procedure with native tissue such as rectus fascia.

Nerve Injury

Background

The incidence of postoperative neuropathy in pelvic surgery is estimated to range from 1.1 to 1.9% [26–28]. The procedure with the highest risk of nerve related injury in prolapse surgery is sacrospinous ligament fixation. An estimated 55–84% of patients experience some gluteal or thigh pain immediately postop [29,

30]. This decreases to around 3–16% by 6 weeks [2, 29, 30].

Although rare, nerve injuries can occur with USLS [31]. There have been conflicting literature describing the anatomy of the uterosacral ligaments. Several studies have demonstrated that the uterosacral ligaments insert directly into the sacrum [16, 32], while others have demonstrated that most of the ligaments insert into the sacrospinous and coccygeus muscle complex [33]. Cadaveric studies have demonstrated that entrapment of S1–S4 nerves is most likely implicated in neuropathic pain after USLS [34–36].

Prevention

Postoperative pain is secondary to the proximity of the sciatic nerve to the sacrospinous ligament. Cadaver studies have demonstrated that branches from S3 and/or S4 course between the sacrospinous and sacrotuberous ligaments and are most likely to be affected in this procedure [37]. Figure 7.2 demonstrates the sacrospinous ligament and the proximity to vital structures. To minimize entrapment, it is recommended that the sutures be placed 2–3 cm from the ischial spine at the mid-section of the ligament [38].

The anatomic studies also indicate that there may be significant variability in the anatomy of the uterosacral ligament. One theory is that nerve entrapment most likely occurs when the uterosacral suture is placed too lateral and deep [31].

Recognition

Nerve injury at the time of pelvic reconstructive surgery is rare and is typically not diagnosed in the operating room. Injuries are identified postoperatively based on patient symptoms. If there is severe or persistent pain following a sacrospinous ligament fixation, this may indicate a pudendal nerve entrapment. USLS nerve entrapment from the S1 to S4 distribution may include sharp pain radiating from the buttocks into the posterior leg, resulting in difficulty sitting and walking [39].

Nerve injuries related to position should be considered in any surgery. For pelvic organ prolapse surgery, the patients are positioned in the dorsal lithotomy or high lithotomy position. The

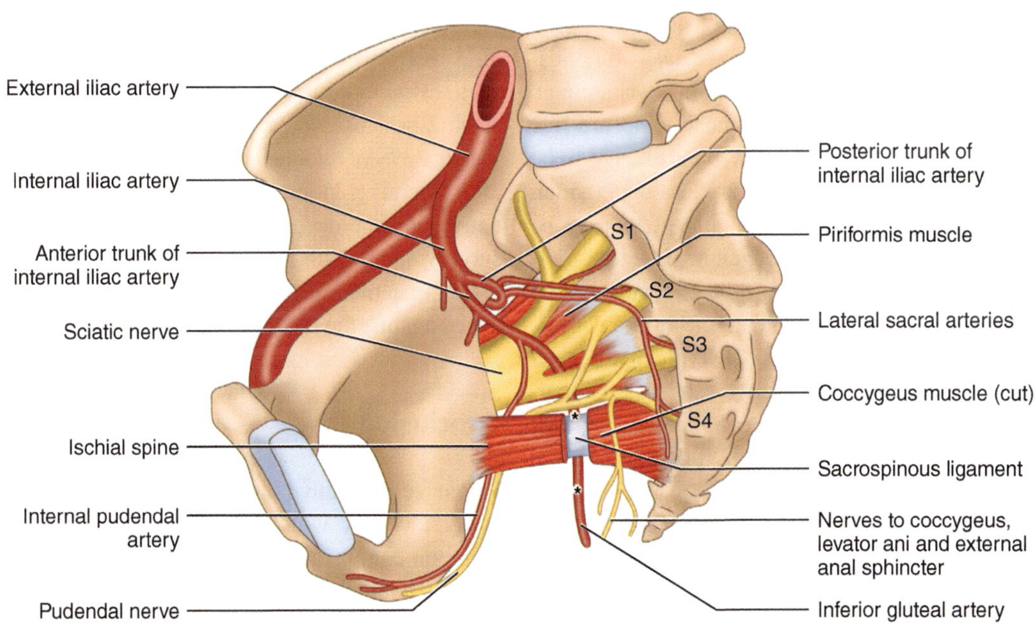

Fig. 7.2 Sacrospinous anatomy: Depiction of the sacrospinous ligament and important surrounding structures

most common injuries include the common peroneal and femoral nerves. Positional injuries may be avoided by ensuring padding over bony prominences and avoiding excessive flexion and external rotation of the hip.

Management

In such instances, prompt suture removal should be considered [40]. Uterosacral nerve entrapment may be managed similarly to that of sacrospinous neuropathy. Conservative management may include physical therapy, stretching exercises, and medical management with neuroleptics, such as Gabapentin. If not alleviated by conservative management, surgical intervention with suture removal should be considered.

Postoperative Considerations

Postoperative complications of pelvic reconstructive surgery are rare and may consist of infection, urinary retention, bleeding, and pain. For the purposes of this chapter, we will discuss specific complications in the most common prolapse surgeries.

The treatment of mesh complications is unique in pelvic reconstructive surgery. Mesh complications may include exposure, pain, dyspareunia, infection, and erosion. The mesh exposure rate for abdominal sacrocolpopexy is estimated to be 3% [41]. If mesh exposures are less than 0.5 cm and the patient is asymptomatic, they may be managed with topical estrogen or observation. If the patient is symptomatic, the exposure is persistent, or a multifilament mesh was used, removal is recommended [42]. Typically, vaginal excision of the visualized mesh may be performed. If infected, the recommendation is for the removal of the entire mesh. If there is concern for an infection, a pelvic MRI to evaluate the entire length of the mesh and the sacral promontory is recommended. If a patient complains of persistent back pain, an MRI to evaluate the promontory should be performed to evaluate for osteomyelitis. While the incidence is less than 1/1000 sacrocolpopexy cases [43], the sequelae from this can be devastating. Mesh erosion into the bowel or bladder is extremely rare and is typically managed with an interdisciplinary team depending on the organ affected.

Reperitonealization following sacrocolpopexy is often recommended to hypothetically prevent small bowel obstruction. Recent studies have found that bowel complications are similar in women who undergo reperitonealization of mesh versus those who do not [44, 45].

Prolapse Recurrence

Approximately 11% of women will undergo surgery for prolapse or stress urinary incontinence in their lifetime [46]. Unfortunately, one of the most common complications related to prolapse repair is recurrent prolapse. Reoperation for prolapse recurrence ranges from 2.2 to 4.4% for sacrocolpopexy [47, 48] and 3–6.5% for native tissue repair [49, 50] at 2 years postoperatively. Epidemiologic studies report that a 20-year risk of repeat operation is 11% overall with younger (<50 years of age) women having higher risk of repeat surgery compared to women >/= 50 (26.9% vs.10.1%) [51]. Recurrent prolapse as measured by POPQ criteria is more common after native tissue than mesh augmented repairs, such as sacrocolpopexy. Defined as recurrent stage 2 prolapse on pelvic examination, an estimated 23% of women have recurrent prolapse after sacral colpopexy and around 41% after native tissue procedures at 1–2 years following surgery [41]. Although the recurrence rate is higher in native tissue procedures, this risk is balanced against the risk of mesh complications.

Conclusion

Pelvic reconstructive surgery procedures are generally low risk with low morbidity. The most common complication is recurrence of prolapse. Other complications of these surgeries are rare, although if not managed appropriately can be catastrophic.

References

1. Alshankiti H, Houlihan S, Robert M, Calgary Women's Pelvic Health Research G. Incidence and contributing factors of perioperative complications in surgical procedures for pelvic organ prolapse. Int Urogynecol J. 2019;30(11):1945–53.
2. Sze E, Karram M. Transvaginal repair of vault prolapse: a review. Obstet Gynecol. 1997;89(3):466–75.
3. Monk B, Ramp J, Montz F, Lebherz T. Sacrospinous ligament fixation for vaginal vault prolapse: complications and results. J Gynecol Surg. 1991;7(2):87–92.
4. Thompson J, Gibb J, Genadry R, Burrows L, Lambrou N, Buller L. Anatomy of pelvic arteries adjacent to the sacrospinous ligament: importance of the coccygeal branch of the inferior gluteal artery. Obstet Gynecol. 1991;94(6):973–7.
5. Barksdale P, Elkins T, Sanders C, Jaramillo F, Gasser R. An anatomic approach to pelvic hemorrhage during sacrospinous ligament fixation of the vaginal vault. Obstet Gynecol. 1998;91(5 Pt 1):715–8.
6. Sutton G, Addison W, Cr L, a. Life-threatening hemorrhage complicating sacral colpopexy. Am J Obstet Gynecol. 1981;140:836–7.
7. Walters M, Karram M. Urogynecology and reconstructive pelvic surgery. 3rd ed. Philadelphia: Mosby Inc; 2007.
8. Crisp C, Herfel C, Pauls R, Westermann L, Kleeman S. Critical anatomy relative to the sacral suture. Female Pelvic Med Reconstr Surg. 2016;22(1):33–6.
9. Pahwa A, Arya L, Andy U. Management of arterial and venous hemorrhage during sacrospinous ligament fixation: cases and review of the literature. Int Urogynecol J. 2016;27:387–91.
10. Chen C, Paraiso M. Open abdominal sacral colpopexy. In: Female urology. Philadelphia: Saunders; 2008. p. 724–8.
11. Gustilo-Ashby AM, Jelovsek JE, Barber MD, Yoo E-H, Paraiso MFR, Walters MD. The incidence of ureteral obstruction and the value of intraoperative cystoscopy during vaginal surgery for pelvic organ prolaps. Am J Obstet Gynecol. 2006;194(5):1478–85.
12. Saguan D, Northington G, Chinthakanan O, a. Iatrogenic lower urinary tract injury at the time of pelvic reconstructive surgery: does previous pelvic surgery increase the risk? Int Urogynecol J. 2014;25(8):1041–6.
13. Barber M, Visco A, Weidner A, Amundsen C, Bump R. Bilateral uterosacral ligament vaginal vault suspension with site-specific endopelvic fascia defect repair for treatment of pelvic organ prolapse. Am J Obstet Gynecol. 2000;183:1402–11.
14. Stanhope C, Wilson T, Utz W, Smith L, O'Brien P. Suture entrapment and secondary ureteral obstruction. Am J Obstet Gynecol. 1991;164:1513–9.
15. Sheyn D, Gupta A, Boyd S, Wu X, Shoag J, Bretschneider CE. Incidence and risk factors for genitourinary tract injury within 1 year after surgery for pelvic organ prolapse. Urogynecology. 2022;28(8):506–17.
16. Buller JL, Thompson JR, Cundiff GW, Sullivan LK, Schön Ybarra MA, Bent AE. Uterosacral ligament: description of anatomic relationships to optimize surgical safety. Obstet Gynecol. 2001;97(6):873–9.
17. Manodoro S, Frigerio M, Milani R, a. Tips and tricks for uterosacral ligament suspension: how to avoid ureteral injury. Int Urogynecol J. 2018;29:161–3.
18. Bhattee G, Rahman J, Rahman M. Bowel injury in gynecologic operations: analysis of 110 cases. Int Surg. 2006;91:336–40.
19. Llarena N, Shah A, Milad M. Bowel injury in gynecologic laparoscopy: a systematic review. Obstet Gynecol. 2015;125:1407–17.
20. David-Montefiore E, Garbin O, Hummel M, Nisand I. Sacro-spinous ligament fixation peri-operative complications in 195 cases: visual approach versus digital approach of the sacro-spinous ligament. Eur J Obstet Gynecol Reprod Biol. 2004;116(1):71–8.
21. Sauer H, Klutke C. Transvaginal Sacrospinous ligament fixation for treatment of vaginal prolapse. J Urol. 1995;154(3):1008–12.
22. Whitehead W, Bradley C, Brown M, et al. Gastrointestinal complications following abdominal sacrocolpopexy for advanced pelvic organ prolapse. Am J Obstet Gynecol. 2007;197(1):78.
23. Warner W, Vora S, Alonge A, Welgoss J, Hurtado E, von Pechmann W. Intraoperative and postoperative gastrointestinal complications associated with laparoscopic Sacrocolpopexy. Female Pelvic Med Reconstr Surg. 2012;18(6):321–4.
24. Nygaard I, McCreery R, Brubaker L, et al. Abdominal sacrocolpopexy: a comprehensive review. Obstet Gynecol. 2004;104:805–23.
25. Costantini E, Brubaker L, Cervigni M, et al. Sacrocolpopexy for pelvic organ prolapse: evidence-based review and recommendations. Eur J Obstet Gynecol Reprod Biol. 2016;205:60–5.
26. Hoffman MS, Roberts WS, Cavanagh D. Neuropathies associated with radical pelvic surgery for gynecologic cancer. Gynecol Oncol. 1988;31:462–6.
27. Cardosi RJ, Cox CS, Hoffman MS. Postoperative neuropathies after major pelvic surgery. Obstet Gynecol. 2002;100:240–4.
28. Bohrer JC, Walters MD, Park A, Polston D, Barber MD. Pelvic nerve injury following gynecologic surgery: a prospective cohort study. Am J Obstet Gynecol. 2009;201(5):531.e531–7.
29. Unger C, Walters M. Gluteal and posterior thigh pain in the postoperative period and the need for intervention after sacrospinous ligament colpopexy. Female Pelvic Med Reconstr Surg. 2014;20:208–11.
30. Mowat A, Wong V, Goh J, Krause H, Pelecanos A, Higgs P. A descriptive study on the efficacy and complications of the Capio (Boston Scientific) suturing device for sacrospinous ligament fixation. Aust N Z J Obstet Gynaecol. 2018;58(1):119–24.

31. Flynn MK, Weidner AC, Amundsen CL. Sensory nerve injury after uterosacral ligament suspension. Am J Obstet Gynecol. 2006;195(6):1869–72.
32. Campbell R. The anatomy and histology of the sacrouterine ligaments. Am J Obstet Gynecol. 1950;59:1–12.
33. Umek WH, Morgan DM, Ashton-Miller JA, DeLancey JO. Quantitative analysis of uterosacral ligament origin and insertion points by magnetic resonance imaging. Obstet Gynecol. 2004;103:447–51.
34. Siddique SA, Gutman RE, Schön Ybarra MA, Rojas F, Handa VL. Relationship of the uterosacral ligament to the sacral plexus and to the pudendal nerve. Int Urogynecol J Pelvic Floor Dysfunct. 2006;17:642–5.
35. Wieslander CK, Roshanravan SM, Wai CY, Schaffer JI, MM C. Uterosacral ligament suspension sutures: anatomic relationships in unembalmed female cadavers. Am J Obstet Gynecol. 2007;197(672):e671–6.
36. Schön Ybarra MA, Gutman RE, Rini D, VL H. Etiology of post-uterosacral suspension neuropathies. Int Urogynecol J Pelvic Floor Dysfunct. 2009;20:1067–71.
37. Florian-Rodriguez M, Hare A, Chin K, Phelan J, Ripperda C, Corton M. Inferior gluteal and other nerves associated with sacrospinous ligament: a cadaver study. Am J Obstet Gynecol. 2016;215(5):646.e641–6.
38. Hefni M, El-Toukhy T. Sacrospinous colpopexy at vaginal hysterectomy: method, results and follow up in 75 patients. J Obstet Gynaecol. 2000;20(1):59–62.
39. Chung Christopher P, Kuehl TJ, Larsen WI, Yandell PM, Shull BL. Recognition and Management of Nerve Entrapment Pain after Uterosacral Ligament Suspension. Obstet Gynecol. 2012;120:292–5.
40. Vodegel EV, vDK, Nuboer CHC, Kowalik CR, Roovers JWR. Surgical management of pudendal nerve entrapment after sacrospinous ligament fixation. BJOG. 2022;129(11):1908–15.
41. Maher C, Feiner B, Baessler K, Christmann-Schmid C, Haya N, Brown J. Surgery for women with apical vaginal prolapse. Cochrane Database Syst Rev. 2016;10(10):CD012376.
42. No Authors Listed. Management of mesh and graft complications in gynecologic surgery. Female Pelvic Med Reconstr Surg. 2017;23(3):171–6.
43. Stork AM, Giugale LE, Bradley MS, Zyczynski HM. Incidence of sacral osteomyelitis and discitis after minimally invasive Sacrocolpopexy. Female Pelvic Med Reconstr Surg. 2021;27(11):672–5.
44. Mueller MG, Jacobs KM, Mueller ER, Abernethy MG, Kenton KS. Outcomes in 450 women after minimally invasive abdominal Sacrocolpopexy for pelvic organ prolapse. Female Pelvic Med Reconstr Surg. 2016;22(4):267–71.
45. Glass Clark SM, Shannon MB, Gill E, Clark MD, Lamb E, Carroll A. Complications after Reperitonealization of mesh at time of Sacrocolpopexy: a retrospective cohort study. Female Pelvic Med Reconstr Surg. 2020;26(2):116–9.
46. Olsen AL. Epidemiology of surgically managed pelvic organ prolapse and urinary incontinence. Obstet Gynecol. 1997;89(4):501–6.
47. Diwadkar GB, Barber MD, Feiner B, Maher C, Jelovsek JE. Complication and reoperation rates after apical vaginal prolapse surgical repair: a systematic review. Obstet Gynecol. 2009;113(2 Part 1):367–73.
48. Nygaard I, Brubaker L, Zyczynski HM, et al. Long-term outcomes following abdominal sacrocolpopexy for pelvic organ prolapse. JAMA. 2013;309(19):2016–24.
49. Silva W, Pauls R, Segal J, Rooney C, Kleeman S, Karram M. Uterosacral ligament vault suspension: five-year outcomes. Obstet Gynecol. 2006;108:255–63.
50. Karram M, Goldwasser S, Kleeman S, Steele A, Vassallo B, Walsh P. High uterosacral vaginal vault suspension with fascial reconstruction for vaginal repair of enterocele and vaginal vault prolapse. Am J Obstet Gynecol. 2001;185:1339–42.
51. Løwenstein E, Møller LA, Laigaard J, et al. Reoperation for pelvic organ prolapse: a Danish cohort study with 15–20 years' follow-up. Int Urogynecol J. 2018;29:119–24.

Part III

Lower Urinary Tract

Operations for Stress Urinary Incontinence

8

Lauren M. Conroy and O. Lenaine Westney

Introduction

Stress urinary incontinence (SUI) is a common condition affecting up to 50% of women at some point in their lives [1]. It is characterized by the involuntary loss of urine with increased abdominal pressure or physical exertion and is caused by urethral hypermobility and/or intrinsic sphincter deficiency (ISD) [2].

While the initial treatments for SUI are conservative, such as pelvic floor exercises, many women seek surgical intervention for persistently bothersome symptoms. Surgeries aim to support the urethra and bladder neck, improving urethral coaptation. They include urethral injections, slings (synthetic or autologous), and retropubic suspensions. The optimal procedure selection depends on several patient factors, such as the characterization and severity of their incontinence and their ability to tolerate invasive procedures.

In addition, each procedure is associated with complications, with the most prevalent being transient urinary retention and new-onset irritative voiding symptoms, such as urgency and frequency. Complications vary between techniques, and clinicians must weigh these risks when counseling patients on optimal surgical management.

L. M. Conroy
Department of Urology, University of Texas Health Science Center at Houston, Houston, TX, USA
e-mail: lauren.m.conroy@uth.tmc.edu

O. L. Westney (✉)
Department of Urology, University of Texas—MD Anderson Cancer Center, Houston, TX, USA
e-mail: owestney@mdanderson.org

Injectable Therapy

An Overview

Urethral injection therapy represents a minimally invasive option to treat SUI, ideal for patients who may not tolerate or desire surgical interventions or who have SUI primarily driven by suboptimal sphincter activity [3]. A urethral bulking agent (UBA) is injected into the submucosa of the proximal urethra using endoscopy (Fig. 8.1). The agent is injected with a needle, either transurethrally through a scope or periurethrally. These techniques are reported to be similarly effective. However, the periurethral route is associated with higher rates of early complications [4].

There are two prevailing types of UBAs. The first are gels with suspended macroparticles (e.g., Macroplastique), and the second group is homogeneous gels that provide a bulking effect through volume alone (e.g., Bulkamid) [5]. There are limited data to support any one agent over another [6]. The agents are believed to increase the central filling volume of the urethra, thus increasing the power of the urethral sphincter with contraction and decreasing urinary leakage [7].

M. Hoffman et al. (eds.), *Major Complications of Female Pelvic Surgery*,
https://doi.org/10.1007/978-3-031-66772-5_8

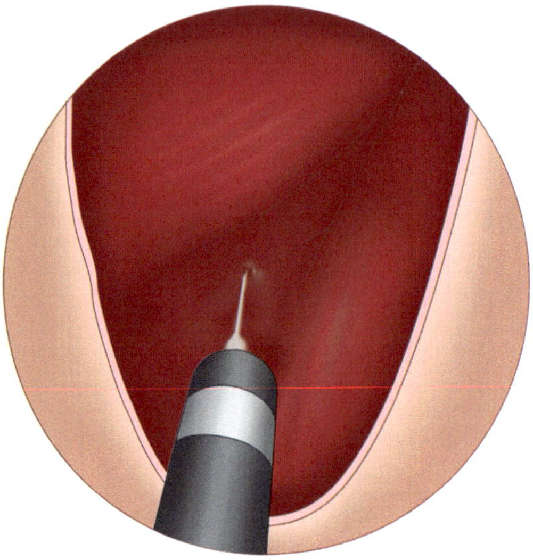

Fig. 8.1 Picture of transurethral injection

Complications

Retention

One of the most common postoperative complications associated with UBAs is urinary retention. A review of 117 articles, including case reports, found that amongst 6462 patients, 542 incidents of retention were reported [8]. The retention duration needed to be clarified in this review. However, several prospective studies with extended follow-up periods have shown this retention to be primarily transient [9, 10]. Hoe et al. reported that of five incidents of acute urinary retention requiring catheterization, four spontaneously resolved the following day [10]. Postoperative transient urinary retention rates are higher when injecting via the periurethral route [4].

De Novo Irritative Voiding Symptoms

UBAs are also associated with new-onset urgency, frequency, and urge incontinence. de Vries et al. found that amongst 6462 patients, 452 reported urinary issues such as these [8]. While symptom duration was not reported in this review, another study noted that 3 years postinjection of Macroplastique, the rate of de novo irritative voiding symptoms was 1.2% [9]. Notably, urinary tract infections (UTIs) are common with UBAs, occurring in 10% of patients postoperatively and presenting with similar urinary symptoms [11].

Mid-Urethral Slings (MUS)

An Overview

Mid-urethral slings (MUS) are the current gold standard surgical treatment for SUI in women [6]. In an MUS procedure, a sling is placed under the urethra at the level of the mid-urethra. The sling works by compressing and securing the posterior wall of the urethra with increased intra-abdominal pressure, thus preventing urinary leakage [1, 12]. The slings are made of a polypropylene monofilament, macroporous mesh [12].

Tension-Free Vaginal Tape (TVT)

One of the initial MUS procedures developed was a tension-free vaginal tape (TVT), also known as a retropubic mid-urethral sling. In this procedure, a tape is inserted through the retropubic space. Two techniques are utilized: a bottom-up approach and a top-down approach. In the bottom-up technique, a trocar with an attached sling is inserted through the vagina on one side of the urethra, elevated through the retropubic space, and out the suprapubic skin. This is performed contralaterally, leaving the tape suspended beneath the urethra. In the top-down technique, trocars are inserted into the suprapubic skin and exit in the vagina [12, 13]. The bottom-up approach is more effective and associated with fewer adverse effects [1].

Transobturator Tape (TOT)

The transobturator tape (TOT) procedure was developed to minimize the morbidity associated with TVT and the risk of injury to local structures. In this procedure, a tape is inserted horizontally between the bilateral obturator foramens, avoiding the retropubic space [12] (Fig. 8.2). Two techniques are utilized: outside-to-inside and inside-to-outside. Using the outside-to-inside method, a trocar is placed through the adductor longus tendon and rotated inward through the

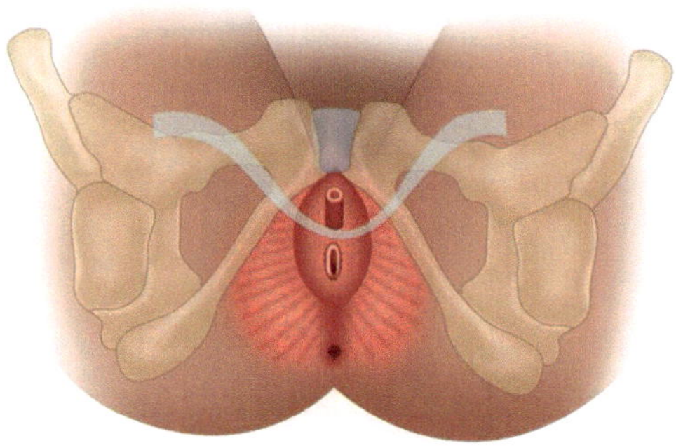

Fig. 8.2 Pelvic diagram with TOT in place

vagina bilaterally. A tape is then attached to the trocars and withdrawn with them through the thigh incisions, remaining suspended beneath the urethra. In the inside-to-outside technique, trocars are inserted into the vagina and exit through the adductor longus tendon [12–14]. These techniques have similar effectiveness; however, the outside-to-inside approach is associated with a higher risk of vaginal perforation and erosion [15].

Single-Incision Slings (SIS)

The most recently developed mid-urethral slings are single-incision slings (SIS) or mini-slings. These were designed to reduce further morbidity associated with slings and provide a less invasive, potentially outpatient option to treat SUI [16]. In this procedure, the sling consists of a piece of mesh positioned between two anchoring ends. A single incision is made in the vaginal epithelium, and the device is pushed under the mid-urethra [12]. Different SIS are associated with other anchoring mechanisms [17].

Complications

Mesh Erosion

In 2011, the Food and Drug Administration (FDA) released a safety communication reporting severe complications associated with transvaginal placement of mesh for pelvic organ prolapse (POP) repair. While MUS were not included in this communication, media attention and increased litigation raised concerns surrounding the use of synthetic mesh in the treatment of incontinence [18]. Since then, several studies have investigated the risk of mesh eroding into the urethra and vagina in patients who have undergone an MUS procedure. Overall, mesh erosion is uncommon and not more common in one type of MUS over another, as seen in two recent meta-analyses. A Cochrane review found that mesh erosion occurred in 2.0% of TVT procedures vs. 2.2% of TOT procedures (Table 8.1) [1]. These results were supported by Brazzelli et al., who found similar erosion rates [19]. Notably, most of the studies reviewed in these meta-analyses had short follow-up periods. One study, which followed patients for more than 10 years, found that the rates of sling erosion with TOT increased after 10 years; however, the rate of erosion at this time was 2.4% [20]. The limited studies comparing MUS and SIS indicate that the erosion rates are similar [19].

Risk factors associated with mesh erosion include age, current smoking status, diabetes mellitus, vaginal incision >2 cm, and a history of prior surgery for incontinence or POP. Studies have shown that older age is associated with erosion, likely secondary to increased urogenital atrophy and resulting thinner tissue. However, other studies have shown that younger age and increased sexual activity may also be associated with an increased erosion risk. Increased incision size and a history of a prior surgery with scar tissue are related to vascular damage and diminished tissue perfusion [9].

Bladder Injury

Blind passage of trocars through the retropubic space with TVT puts patients at risk of bladder perforation and vascular, nerve, and bowel injuries [21]. As a result, bladder perforation is significantly more common with TVT than with TOT. A Cochrane review found that the risk of bladder or urethral injury was 4.9% with TVT vs. 0.6% with TOT [1].

Pain

Groin pain is a common complication associated with TOT, as the exit point of the trocars is the

Table 8.1 TOT compared to TVT for SUI in women

Outcomes	Illustrative comparative risks* (95% CI)		Relative effect (95% CI)	No of participants (studies)	Quality of the evidence (GRADE)	Comments
	Assumed risk	Corresponding risk				
	Retropubic (RPR) route	Transobturator (TOR)				
Subjective cure (Short term <1 year)	Study population		RR 0.98 (0.96–1.00)	5514 (36 RCTs)	⊕⊕⊕⊖ MODERATE [1]	
	844 per 1000	827 per 1000 (810–844)				
	Mean control group risk across studies					
	833 per 1000	816 per 1000 (800–833)				
Subjective cure (medium term, 1–5 years)	Study population		RR 0.97 (0.92–1.03)	683 (5 RCTs)	⊕⊕⊖⊖ LOW [2,3]	
	881 per 1000	854 per 1000 (810–907)				
	Mean control group risk across studies					
	869 per 1000	843 per 1000 (799–895)				
Subjective cure (long term, >5 years)	Study population		RR 0.95 (0.87–1.04)	714 (4 RCTS)	⊕⊕⊕⊖MODERATE [4]	
	707 per 1000	671 per 1000 (615–735)				
	Mean control group risk across studies					
	843 per 1000	801 per 1000 (733–877)				
Bladder or urethral perforation	Study population		RR 0.13 (0.08–0.20)	6372 (40 RCTs)	⊕⊕⊕⊖ MODERATE[5]	
	49 per 1000	6 per 1000 (4–10)				
	Mean control group risk across studies					
	25 per 1000	3 per 1000 (2–5)				
Voiding dysfunction (short and medium term, up to 5 years)	Study population		RR 0.53 (0.43–0.65)	6217 (37 RCTs)	⊕⊕⊕⊖ MODERATE[6]	
	72 per 1000	38 per 1000 (31–47)				
	Mean control group risk across studies					
	55 per 1000	29 per 1000 (24–36)				
De novo urgency or urgency incontinence (short term, up to 12 months)	Study population		RR 0.98 (0.82–1.17)	4923 (31 RCTs)	⊕⊕⊕⊖ MODERATE[7]	
	82 per 1000	80 per 1000 (67–96)				
	Mean control group risk across studies					
	83 per 1000	81 per 1000 (68–97)				

Groin pain	Study population		RR 4.62 (3.09–6.92)	3226 (18 RCTs)	⊕⊕⊕⊖ MODERATE[8]	
	14 per 1000	66 per 1000 (44–99)				
	Mean control group risk across studies					
	45 per 1000	208 per 1000 (139–311)				
Suprapubic pain	Study population		RR 0.29 (0.11–0.78)	1105 (4 RCTs)	⊕⊕⊕⊖ MODERATE[9]	
	29 per 1000	8 per 1000 (3–23)				
	Mean control group risk across studies					
	18 per 1000	6 per 1000 (2–14)				
Vaginal tape erosion (short and medium term, up to 5 years)	Study population		RR 1.13 (0.78–1.65)	4743 (31 RCTs)	⊕⊕⊕⊖ MODERATE [10]	
	20 per 1000	22 per 1000 (15–32)				
	Mean control group risk across studies					
	21 per 1000	24 per 1000 (16–34)				
Repeat incontinence surgery (short term, within 12 months)	Study population		RR 1.64 (0.85–3.16)	1402 (9 RCTs)	⊕⊕⊕⊖ MODERATE [11]	
	19 per 1000	31 per 1000 (16–60)				
	mean control group across studies					
	24 per 1000	39 per 1000 (20–76)				
Repeat incontinence surgery (long term, > 5 years)	Study population		RR 8.79 (3.36–23.00)	695 (4 RCTs)	⊕⊕⊖⊖LOW [12,13]	
	11 per 1000	100 per 1000 (38–262)				
	Mean control group across studies					
	67 per 1000	589 per 1000 (225–1000)				

Modified from a Cochrane review

medial thigh. The pain is often transient and resolves in the post-op period [22]; however, in rare cases, it can persist and become chronic [22]. This chronic pain is associated with damage to the obturator nerve as the trocar traverses the obturator foramen [12]. Not surprisingly, groin pain is significantly more common with TOT than with TVT. A recent meta-analysis has reported the rate of groin pain to be 6.3% with TOT versus 1.3% with TVT [19]. These findings are primarily based on studies conducted within 1-year post-op. One study, which evaluated outcomes after 13 years, found 1 of 168 patients to have persistent groin pain, not requiring analgesics [20].

SIS was developed in part to reduce the risk of developing postoperative pain. A meta-analysis of 14 studies found the immediate post-operative pain rate to be 6.8% with SIS versus 19.2% with TVT [19]. There is limited data to show the long-term comparison of pain with SIS and standard MUS.

Voiding Dysfunction

While an MUS functions to compress the urethra, patients risk obstruction and resulting voiding dysfunction if the tape is placed with too much tension around the urethra or too close to the bladder neck [12]. This is more commonly found with TVT, where the tape is placed at a more vertical angle, resulting in increased obstruction [23]. Within the first 5 years postoperatively, the risk of voiding dysfunction is 7.2% with TVT vs. 3.8% with TOT [1]. This is often transient, however, as long-term dysfunction necessitating surgery or permanent catheterization is rare. One randomized controlled trial (RCT) found that the risk of requiring these measures was 2.7% with TVT vs. 0% with TOT [23].

De Novo Irritative Voiding Symptoms

One of the most common complications after an MUS surgery is new-onset irritative bladder symptoms, such as increased urinary urgency or detrusor overactivity (DO). Meta-analyses revealed no significant difference in these symptoms between TVT and TOT (8.2% vs. 8%) [1] or TVT and SIS (9.2% vs. 9.5%) (Brazzelli 2019) in the first 12 months post-operation [1].

Recurrent Incontinence

It is not uncommon for patients to require multiple procedures to manage their SUI adequately. At 12 months post-operation, 3.6% of patients with TOT vs. 2.2% with TVT will require repeat continence surgery. After 1–5 years, 18.3% of patients with TOT will require repeat surgery (vs. 0.5% with TVT) [1]. Limited data demonstrate the long-term need for repeat surgery following an SIS surgery. However, current data indicate that in the short term, the need is greater than for standard MUS [1, 17].

Recurrent or persistent SUI following an MUS surgery may also be due to various factors, including the wrong choice of the initial procedure, patient characteristics, and the natural history of incontinence. When deciding between TVT and TOT, many factors must be considered. Some evidence indicates that TOT is less effective in patients with SUI, primarily caused by intrinsic sphincter deficiency or more severe initial SUI [23, 24]. Other factors, such as patient weight and age, may also impact surgery success [12]. Finally, with time, the pelvic floor weakens, and the intrinsic sphincter function declines, worsening SUI naturally [3].

Pubovaginal Slings (PVS)

An Overview

Before the widespread use of synthetic slings, the traditional slings used to treat SUI were pubovaginal slings (PVS) composed of autologous fascia. Today, this type of sling is still widely used for patients when synthetic materials are not desired or contraindicated, such as with patients at risk of poor wound healing, immunocompromise, or regularly require clean intermittent catheterization (CIC) [6, 25, 26]. Furthermore, there is a belief that these slings are more compressive and, thus, are more appropriate for patients with worse incontinence [26].

PVS are placed at the bladder neck, compressing the proximal urethra and bladder neck with increased abdominal stress, providing bladder outlet resistance and thus preventing urinary leakage [26] (Fig. 8.3). Fascial slings are most

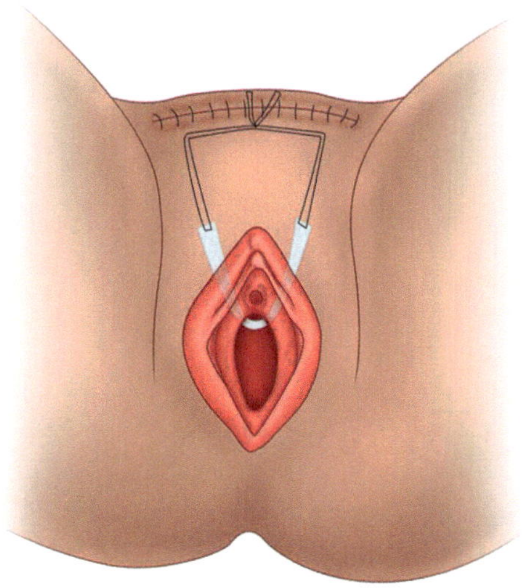

Fig. 8.3 Diagram with an implanted pubovaginal sling

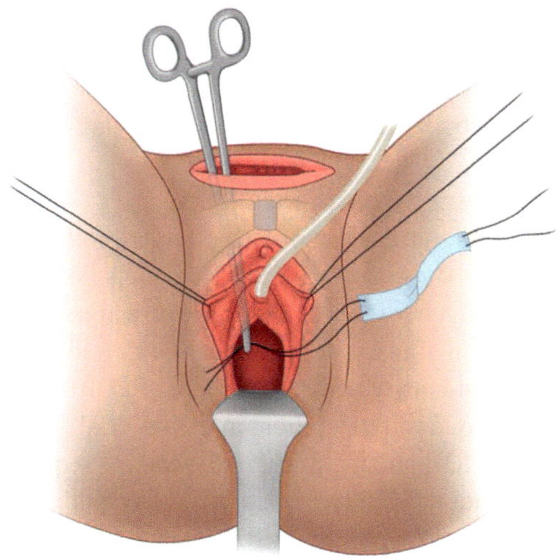

Fig. 8.4 Diagram demonstrating passage of sling sutures using a Sarot clamp

commonly composed of rectus abdominis fascia from the abdominal wall or fascia lata from the lateral thigh [27]. In a PVS procedure, following the harvesting of fascia, the vaginal epithelium is dissected under the mid-urethra and bladder neck. The endopelvic fascia is perforated using this dissection, and the retropubic space is developed on either side of the urethra. Clamps or needles are then passed from the abdomen, through the previously developed plane, into the vaginal incision, where they grasp a suture tied to the harvested fascial sling (Fig. 8.4). The ends of the graft suture are then brought out of the abdominal incision bilaterally, leaving the fascia suspended beneath the bladder neck. Finally, the suture is tied down over the rectus fascia to secure the sling and provide adequate tensioning [12, 26].

Complications

Bladder Perforation

The PVS procedure requires blind passage of instruments through the retropubic space, putting patients at risk of bladder perforation. The American Urological Association (AUA) guideline meta-analysis reported a perforation rate of 4% [28]. Patients with previous pelvic surgeries are at an increased risk of perforation [26].

Urinary Retention

The placement of a PVS at the bladder neck, as well as the tensioning of the sling, puts patients at risk of bladder outlet obstruction, resulting in urinary retention [27]. Studies have shown a voiding dysfunction rate of up to 14% [26]. Several studies investigated the duration of urinary retention. Mock et al. found that 4.4% of patients who received a PVS developed voiding dysfunction, 1.1% required long-term CIC, and 3.3% resolved spontaneously within 1 month of surgery [25]. Athanasopoulos et al. found that 10.6% of patients developed voiding dysfunction, with most of these cases resolving within 2 months and 1.9% eventually requiring surgical resolution [29].

De Novo Irritative Voiding Symptoms

One of the most common complications of PVS is postoperative irritative voiding symptoms, possibly related to a degree of bladder outlet obstruction created by the sling [29]. Studies have shown a rate of de novo urgency of up to 18.5% [25, 26, 29]. Kim et al. found an increase in irritative voiding symptoms with increased time from sling placement, likely secondary to worsening detrusor function with age rather than a long-term consequence of the sling [30].

Recurrent Incontinence

The need for repeat continence surgery following primary or secondary PVS placement is minimal. However, only some studies have investigated the long-term efficacy of PVS. Khan et al. found that of 61 patients who received PVS, after 10 years, none required reoperation, and Kim et al. found that of 83 patients, after 14.5 years, 2 required reoperation [30, 31]. Other studies have indicated up to an 84% absence of SUI symptoms 10 years following a PVS surgery [32]; however, after this extended period, it is unclear whether repeat symptoms are due to operation failure or age-related changes [30, 32].

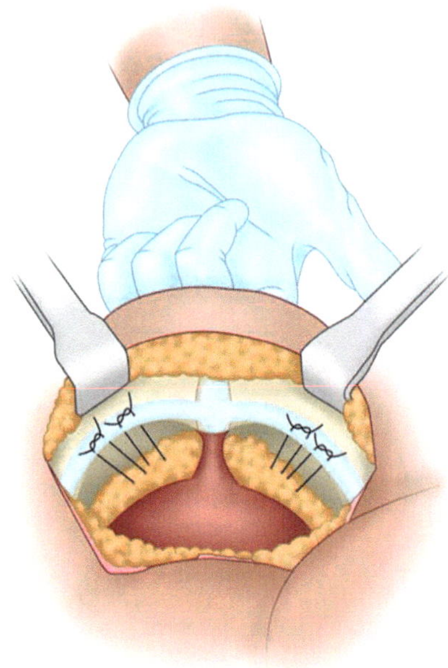

Fig. 8.5 Diagram demonstrating the location of Burch suspension sutures

Retropubic Suspensions

An Overview

Retropubic suspensions involve lifting the tissue surrounding the bladder neck and proximal urethra into the pelvis behind the anterior pubic bones [33]. These procedures have largely been replaced by less invasive procedures, such as slings. They are now mostly reserved for patients for whom synthetic materials are contraindicated or who are undergoing concomitant pelvic surgery [6]. They are used to treat patients with SUI primarily caused by urethral hypermobility [33].

There are several variations of retropubic suspensions, with Burch colposuspension being the most common. In a Burch procedure, the anterior vaginal wall at the bladder neck level is elevated and sutured to the iliopectineal ligament [34] (Fig. 8.5). This is believed to aid in continence by stabilizing the bladder, neck, and urethra and restoring them to their original retropubic position [33]. This procedure can be performed either open or laparoscopically, with similar efficacy [35].

Another common variation is the Marshall–Marchetti–Krantz (MMK) procedure, where the bladder neck is suspended onto the periosteum of the pubic symphysis. Minimal data favor Burch to MMK in effectively treating SUI [36].

Complications

Voiding Dysfunction

Voiding dysfunction or urinary retention is rare following retropubic suspension, especially compared to slings, the gold standard SUI treatment. Data show almost no risk of developing voiding dysfunction following retropubic suspension [36–38].

Recurrent Incontinence

Compared to slings, the trade-off associated with reduced morbidity of retropubic suspensions is at a lesser degree of treatment "success." Brubaker et al. found that 5 years following Burch, 12% of patients required surgical retreatment, and Albo et al. found that 2 years following Burch, 11% needed surgical retreatment [37, 38].

Conclusions

Several procedures are available to treat SUI, each with varying risk profiles. Clinicians should consider these risks and counsel patients based on their unique needs when making recommendations regarding the optimal procedure.

References

1. Ford AA, Rogerson L, Cody JD, Aluko P, Ogah JA. Mid-urethral sling operations for stress urinary incontinence in women. Cochrane Database Syst Rev. 2017;7(7):CD006375. https://doi.org/10.1002/14651858.CD006375.pub4.
2. Ford AA, Ogah JA. Retropubic or transobturator mid-urethral slings for intrinsic sphincter deficiency-related stress urinary incontinence in women: a systematic review and meta-analysis. Int Urogynecol J. 2016;27(1):19–28. https://doi.org/10.1007/s00192-015-2797-3.
3. Elmelund M, Sokol ER, Karram MM, Dmochowski R, Klarskov N. Patient characteristics that may influence the effect of urethral injection therapy for female stress urinary incontinence. J Urol. 2019;202(1):125–31. https://doi.org/10.1097/JU.0000000000000176.
4. Kirchin V, Page T, Keegan PE, Atiemo KO, Cody JD, McClinton S, et al. Urethral injection therapy for urinary incontinence in women. Cochrane Database Syst Rev. 2017;7(7):CD003881. https://doi.org/10.1002/14651858.CD003881.pub4.
5. Itkonen Freitas AM, Mentula M, Rahkola-Soisalo P, Tulokas S, Mikkola TS. Tension-free vaginal tape surgery versus polyacrylamide hydrogel injection for primary stress urinary incontinence: a randomized clinical trial. J Urol. 2020;203(2):372–8. https://doi.org/10.1097/JU.0000000000000517.
6. Kobashi KC, Albo ME, Dmochowski RR, Ginsberg DA, Goldman HB, Gomelsky A, et al. Surgical treatment of female stress urinary incontinence: AUA/SUFU guideline. J Urol. 2017;198(4):875–83. https://doi.org/10.1016/j.juro.2017.06.061.
7. Klarskov N, Lose G. Urethral injection therapy: what is the mechanism of action? Neurourol Urodyn. 2008;27(8):789–92. https://doi.org/10.1002/nau.20602.
8. de Vries AM, Wadhwa H, Huang J, Farag F, Heesakkers JPFA, Kocjancic E. Complications of urethral bulking agents for stress urinary incontinence: an extensive review including case reports. Female Pelvic Med Reconstr Surg. 2018;24(6):392–8. https://doi.org/10.1097/SPV.0000000000000495.
9. Serati M, Soligo M, Braga A, Cantaluppi S, Coluccia AC, Di Dedda MC, et al. Efficacy and safety of polydimethylsiloxane injection (Macroplastique®) for the treatment of female stress urinary incontinence: results of a series of 85 patients with ≥3 years of follow-up. BJU Int. 2019;123(2):353–9. https://doi.org/10.1111/bju.14550.
10. Hoe V, Yao HH, Gough K, O'Connell HE. Long-term outcomes of polyacrylamide hydrogel treatment in women with stress urinary incontinence. BJU Int. 2022;130(Suppl 1):22–4. https://doi.org/10.1111/bju.15717.
11. Siddiqui ZA, Abboudi H, Crawford R, Shah S. Intraurethral bulking agents for the management of female stress urinary incontinence: a systematic review. Int Urogynecol J. 2017;28(9):1275–84. https://doi.org/10.1007/s00192-017-3278-7.
12. Gomelsky A, Dmochowski A. Slings: autologous, biologic, synthetic, and mid-urethral. Campbell-Walsh-Wein urology. 12th ed. Elsevier Inc.; 2021. p. 2830–76.
13. Wolter CE. Tension-free vaginal tape/Suprapubic Midurethral Sling. Hinman's atlas of urologic surgery. 4th ed. Elsevier Inc.; 2019. p. 754–8.
14. Kit LC. Transobturator midurethral sling. In: Hinman's atlas of urologic surgery. 4th ed. Elsevier Inc.; 2019. p. 759–63.
15. Fusco F, Abdel-Fattah M, Chapple CR, Creta M, La Falce S, Waltregny D, et al. Updated systematic review and meta-analysis of the comparative data on colposuspensions, pubovaginal slings, and midurethral tapes in the surgical treatment of female stress urinary incontinence. Eur Urol. 2017;72(4):567–91. https://doi.org/10.1016/j.eururo.2017.04.026.
16. White AB, Kahn BS, Gonzalez RR, Rosamilia A, Anger JT, Eilber KS, et al. Prospective study of a single-incision sling versus a transobturator sling in women with stress urinary incontinence: 3-year results. Am J Obstet Gynecol. 2020;223(4):545.e1–e11. https://doi.org/10.1016/j.ajog.2020.03.008.
17. Nambiar A, Cody JD, Jeffery ST, Aluko P. Single-incision sling operations for urinary incontinence in women. Cochrane Database Syst Rev. 2017;7(7):CD008709. https://doi.org/10.1002/14651858.CD008709.pub3.
18. Bretschneider CE, Geynisman-Tan J, Mueller MG, Collins SA, Lewicky-Gaupp C, Kenton K. Rates of Sling procedures and revisions-a National Surgical Quality Improvement Program Database Study. Female Pelvic Med Reconstr Surg. 2021;27(6):e559–e62. https://doi.org/10.1097/SPV.0000000000000995.
19. Brazzelli M, Javanbakht M, Imamura M, Hudson J, Moloney E, Becker F, et al. Surgical treatments for women with stress urinary incontinence: the ESTER systematic review and economic evaluation. Health Technol Assess. 2019;23(14):1–306. https://doi.org/10.3310/hta23140.
20. Serati M, Braga A, Caccia G, Torella M, Ghezzi F, Salvatore S, et al. TVT-O for treatment of pure

urodynamic stress urinary incontinence: efficacy and adverse effects at 13-years follow-up. Neurourol Urodyn. 2020;39(5):1423–9. https://doi.org/10.1002/nau.24358.
21. Kokanali MK, Doğanay M, Aksakal O, Cavkaytar S, Topçu HO, Özer İ. Risk factors for mesh erosion after vaginal sling procedures for urinary incontinence. Eur J Obstet Gynecol Reprod Biol. 2014;177:146–50. https://doi.org/10.1016/j.ejogrb.2014.03.039.
22. de Leval J. Novel surgical technique for the treatment of female stress urinary incontinence: transobturator vaginal tape inside-out. Eur Urol. 2003;44(6):724–30. https://doi.org/10.1016/j.eururo.2003.09.003.
23. Richter HE, Albo ME, Zyczynski HM, Kenton K, Norton PA, Sirls LT, et al. Retropubic versus transobturator midurethral slings for stress incontinence. N Engl J Med. 2010;362(22):2066–76. https://doi.org/10.1056/NEJMoa0912658.
24. Schierlitz L, Dwyer PL, Rosamilia A, Murray C, Thomas E, De Souza A, et al. Three-year follow-up of tension-free vaginal tape compared with transobturator tape in women with stress urinary incontinence and intrinsic sphincter deficiency. Obstet Gynecol. 2012;119(2 Pt 1):321–7. https://doi.org/10.1097/AOG.0b013e31823dfc73.
25. Mock S, Angelle J, Reynolds WS, Osborn DJ, Dmochowski RR, Gomelsky A. Contemporary comparison between retropubic midurethral sling and autologous pubovaginal sling for stress urinary incontinence after the FDA advisory notification. Urology. 2015;85(2):321–5. https://doi.org/10.1016/j.urology.2014.10.017.
26. Plagakis S, Tse V. The autologous pubovaginal fascial sling: an update in 2019. Low Urin Tract Symptoms. 2020;12(1):2–7. https://doi.org/10.1111/luts.12281.
27. Niknejad K, Plzak LS, Staskin DR, Loughlin KR. Autologous and synthetic urethral slings for female incontinence. Urol Clin North Am. 2002;29(3):597–611. https://doi.org/10.1016/s0094-0143(02)00074-5.
28. Dmochowski RR, Blaivas JM, Gormley EA, Juma S, Karram MM, Lightner DJ, et al. Update of AUA guideline on the surgical management of female stress urinary incontinence. J Urol. 2010;183(5):1906–14. https://doi.org/10.1016/j.juro.2010.02.2369.
29. Athanasopoulos A, Gyftopoulos K, McGuire EJ. Efficacy and preoperative prognostic factors of autologous fascia rectus sling for treatment of female stress urinary incontinence. Urology. 2011;78(5):1034–8. https://doi.org/10.1016/j.urology.2011.05.069.
30. Kim S, Wong DG, Lee D, Christie AL, Zimmern PE. Very long-term follow-up of autologous pubovaginal fascia slings in women with stress urinary incontinence. Int Urogynecol J. 2022;33(4):821–8. https://doi.org/10.1007/s00192-021-04737-7.
31. Khan ZA, Nambiar A, Morley R, Chapple CR, Emery SJ, Lucas MG. Long-term follow-up of a multicentre randomised controlled trial comparing tension-free vaginal tape, xenograft and autologous fascial slings for the treatment of stress urinary incontinence in women. BJU Int. 2015;115(6):968–77. https://doi.org/10.1111/bju.12851.
32. Sharifiaghdas F, Mirzaei M, Daneshpajooh A, Narouie B. Long-term results of tension-free vaginal tape and pubovaginal sling in the treatment of stress urinary incontinence in female patients. Clin Exp Obstet Gynecol. 2017;44(1):44–7.
33. Hartigan SM, Chapple CR, Dmochowski RR. Retropubic suspension surgery for incontinence in women Campbell-Walsh-Wein urology. 12th ed. Elsevier Inc.; 2021. p. 2756–75.
34. Burch JC. Urethrovaginal fixation to Cooper's ligament for correction of stress incontinence, cystocele, and prolapse. Am J Obstet Gynecol. 1961;81:281–90. https://doi.org/10.1016/s0002-9378(16)36367-0.
35. Freites J, Stewart F, Omar MI, Mashayekhi A, Agur WI. Laparoscopic colposuspension for urinary incontinence in women. Cochrane Database Syst Rev. 2019;12(12):CD002239. https://doi.org/10.1002/14651858.CD002239.pub4.
36. Lapitan MCM, Cody JD, Mashayekhi A. Open retropubic colposuspension for urinary incontinence in women. Cochrane Database Syst Rev. 2017;7(7):CD002912. https://doi.org/10.1002/14651858.CD002912.pub7.
37. Brubaker L, Richter HE, Norton PA, Albo M, Zyczynski HM, Chai TC, et al. 5-year continence rates, satisfaction and adverse events of burch urethropexy and fascial sling surgery for urinary incontinence. J Urol. 2012;187(4):1324–30. https://doi.org/10.1016/j.juro.2011.11.087.
38. Albo ME, Richter HE, Brubaker L, Norton P, Kraus SR, Zimmern PE, et al. Burch colposuspension versus fascial sling to reduce urinary stress incontinence. N Engl J Med. 2007;356(21):2143–55. https://doi.org/10.1056/NEJMoa070416.

Urethral Diverticulectomy

9

Richard Lee and Leo Dreyfuss

Pathophysiology of a Urethral Diverticulum (UD)

The exact etiology of a urethral diverticulum is unclear. While there are reports of congenital urethral diverticula in females and males, it is accepted that most urethral diverticula are acquired in adulthood [1, 2]. Urethral diverticula are thought to arise from the periurethral glands, located in the posterolateral mid- to distal urethra. The pathophysiologic process behind the formation of urethral diverticula is likely related to infection, which can lead to abscess formation within the periurethral glands. Recurrent infection causes submucosal tracking of the abscess within the periurethral fascia, which eventually ruptures into the urethral lumen, creating the characteristic ostium.

The most common location of urethral diverticula is the distal two-thirds of the ventral urethra. This corresponds to the location of most periurethral glands, supporting the aforementioned pathophysiologic hypothesis (Fig. 9.1). One-third of diverticula, however, are found in the proximal portion of the urethra, and expansion of the diverticula can occur anteriorly or extend circumferentially [3].

Surgical pathology following excision most often reveals a benign histology, although inflammatory changes are common. Premalignant changes can be seen in 10–20% of specimens. Malignancy within a urethral diverticulum is rare. Adenocarcinoma is the most common malignant pathology seen, in contrast to urethral carcinoma, where squamous cell carcinoma is more common [4, 5]. Urethral diverticula may contain stones caused by urinary stasis. Their size and location are variable; urethral diverticula can extend anywhere within the periurethral fascia, and may extend circumferentially or in a horseshoe orientation. Multiple diverticula may be present [5, 6].

R. Lee (✉) · L. Dreyfuss
Department of Urology, Weill Cornell Medical College, New York Presbyterian Hospital, New York, NY, USA
e-mail: ril9010@med.cornell.edu; ldd9009@nyp.org

M. Hoffman et al. (eds.), *Major Complications of Female Pelvic Surgery*,
https://doi.org/10.1007/978-3-031-66772-5_9

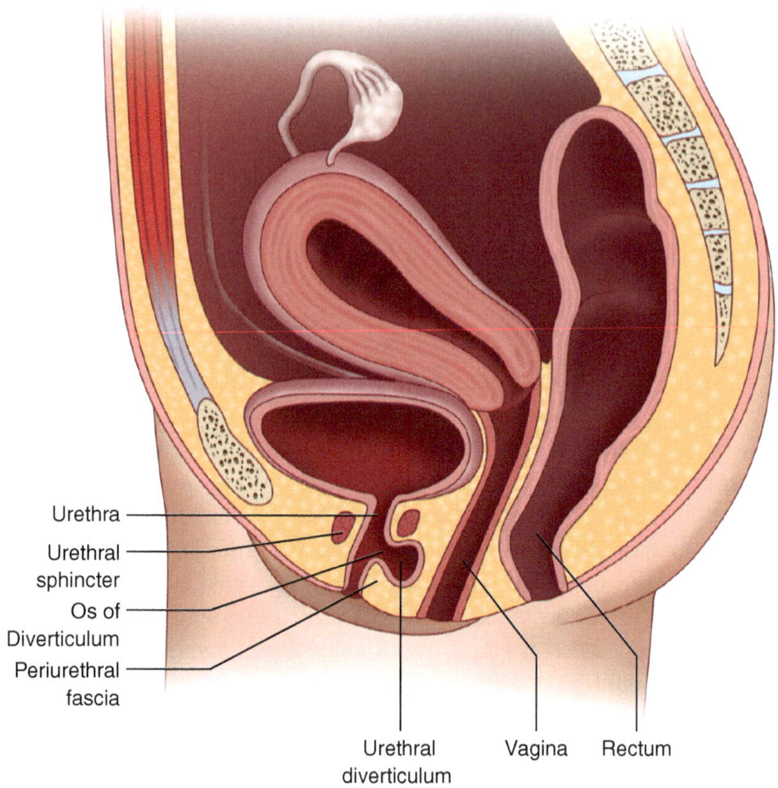

Fig. 9.1 Sagittal view of the female pelvis with the urethral diverticulum distal to the urethral sphincter. Adapted from EAU 2016 [51]

Prevalence and Presentation

Presentation is variable. Patients tend to be in the third to sixth decade of life. Incidence is estimated to be between 1 and 6% [7, 8]. The most common presenting symptoms are a vaginal lump, pain in the area of the diverticulum, dysuria, and dyspareunia. Post-void dribbling, recurrent urinary tract infections (UTIs), and urethral discharge can also be present [9, 10]. The classic "three D's" (discharge, dyspareunia, and dribbling) are found in only 5% of patients [11].

Diagnosis

According to Davis and Telinde, "The most important single diagnostic instrument for the discovery of suburethral diverticula is a high index of suspicion" [12]. Patients presenting with the above symptoms should undergo a thorough history and physical exam. Physical exam may reveal a fluctuant bulge over the anterior vaginal wall. Occasionally, firm palpation of this mass may result in expression of purulent debris from the urethra. Urine studies should be obtained and sent for culture to guide perioperative antimicrobial coverage. Cystourethroscopy can be performed to visualize the ostium of the diverticulum. Multiple ostia may be present and are commonly located posterolaterally at the 4 and 8 o'clock position but can be visualized in a minority of patients.

Numerous imaging studies have been employed in the diagnosis of urethral diverticula. Double balloon positive pressure urethrography (PPU) is considered the historic gold standard for diagnosis and characterization of UDs but is rarely used. If the patient is able to void, a voiding cystourethrogram (VCUG) can be used to diagnose the presence of a UD, which will opacify with contrast during voiding. Transvaginal ultrasound can provide useful information regarding the size and location of a UD but is operator-dependent and does not produce detailed images. Magnetic resonance imaging (MRI) is commonly employed as the standard imaging modality for diagnosis of UDs with good performance compared to the gold standard PPU [13].

Differential Diagnosis

Periurethral masses that may be mistaken for urethral diverticula include vaginal leiomyoma, Skene's gland abnormalities, Gartner duct abnormalities, vaginal wall cysts, urethral prolapse, urethral caruncle, or periurethral bulking agents. Careful history and physical exam can help differentiate urethral diverticula from these distinct entities [3].

Indications for Repair

Excision of urethral diverticula may be offered to symptomatic patients who desire surgical intervention. It is important to counsel patients whose primary complaint is pain that concurrent conditions, particularly pelvic floor dysfunction or lower urinary tract symptoms (LUTSs), may exist and may not resolve following diverticulectomy. While progression to carcinoma has been reported, it is considered a rare entity; prophylactic urethral diverticulectomy in an asymptomatic patient for the sole intent of avoiding a malignancy is not necessary. However, patients who desire nonoperative management must be counseled on the low risk of malignancy, which may not be seen on diagnostic imaging [4, 5, 14]. Conservative management is an option for patients with UDs; recurrent UTIs and stress urinary incontinence (SUI) can be managed with prophylactic antibiotics and pelvic floor physical therapy (PFPT), respectively, but no guidance exists for periodic screening of patients with urethral diverticula for malignancy.

Surgical Management

Multiple surgical techniques for the management of urethral diverticula have been reported [15–18]. Currently, the two most widely used techniques are transvaginal marsupialization and excision and reconstruction, with the latter being far more common. Despite the overwhelming popularity of this technique, there is insufficient evidence to compare differences in outcomes and complications between various procedures [19].

Transvaginal marsupialization is an option for distal urethral diverticula. Originally described by Spence and Duckett, marsupialization may be faster and lead to less blood loss than excision and reconstruction. Briefly, the procedure involves placement of one blade of a Metzenbaum scissors into the urethra and incision into the diverticulum and anterior vaginal wall to create a "generous meatotomy" [16]. However, extension of the incision too far proximally may lead to damage of the external sphincter and cause incontinence or to development of a "pseudoseptum" between the urethra and anterior bladder wall. This may cause dyspareunia and limit the classic marsupialization technique to the distal diverticula in patients who are not sexually active. Recently, a variation of the Spence and Duckett procedure has been described for distal diverticula involving an incision directly on the diverticular ostium followed by marsupialization, allowing the area to drain into the vagina. This technique may offer the benefits of the traditional Spence and Duckett technique while minimizing the risks of long-term dyspareunia or incontinence [20].

For patients with complicated urethral diverticula, such as those undergoing repeat surgeries, or for those with complex or circumferential diverticula, variations in surgical technique have been described with favorable results. These include use of xenogenic grafts, lateral vaginal flaps, urethroplasty with remnants of the diverticular sac, end-to-end urethroplasty following diverticulectomy, and the transabdominal robot-assisted laparoscopic approach [21–24].

Excision and Reconstruction

Excision and reconstruction is the most commonly used technique for excision of urethral diverticula, although there is insufficient evidence to compare the rates of complications and outcomes between different techniques [19]. Basic surgical principles can be employed to optimize outcomes and minimize complications; vaginal wall flaps dissected out with preserved blood supply, periurethral fascia preserved as separate layer, and the ostium neck and diverticulum wall completely excised. Closure should be performed in a watertight manner with minimal overlapping of sutures. Topical estrogen can be administered for 4–6 weeks preoperatively if the patient is postmenopausal to improve vascular supply to the tissue. Preoperative, culture-specific antibiotics should be given if the patient has a history of recurrent urinary tract infections.

The procedure is carried out in the dorsal lithotomy position with a Foley catheter placed. An inverted-U incision is made with special consideration to make the proximal portion of the "U" (toward the bladder neck) wide to preserve proximal blood supply. During dissection, the periurethral facia should be preserved as it is an essential layer to close with following removal of diverticular sac. Once the periurethral tissue plane around the diverticulum is developed, a horizontal incision can be made on the diverticulum taking care to not violate the sac. The diverticulum is then dissected free of the periurethral tissue to the ostium origin on the urethra and then excised. The entire mucosal surface of the diverticulum should be removed in order to prevent recurrence. Following excision, the Foley catheter can be seen through the defect and a tension-free closure is performed using multiple layers of absorbable sutures (Fig. 9.2). Following

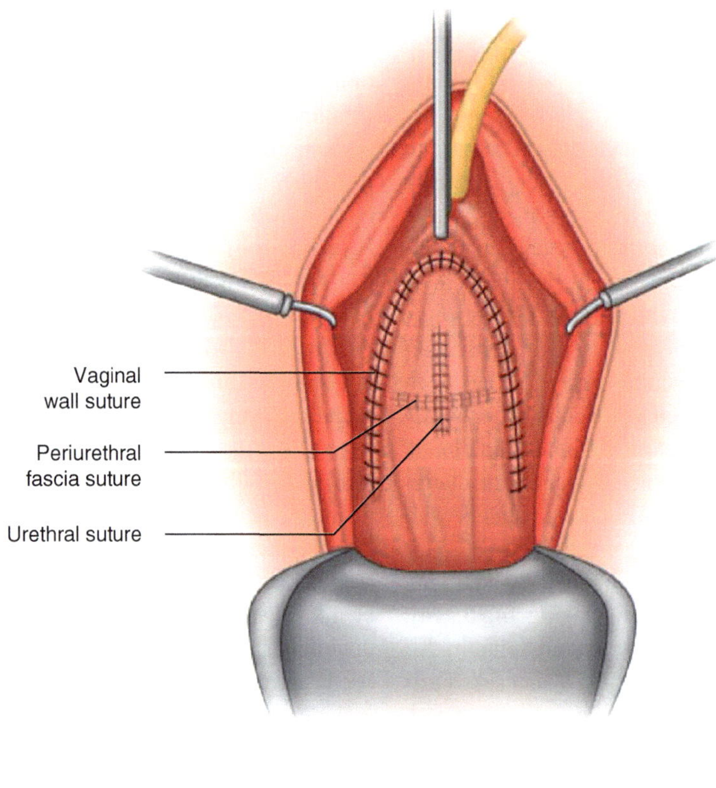

Fig. 9.2 Diagram of a multilayered closure of (from deep to superficial) a urethral defect, the periurethral fascia, and the vaginal epithelium. The minimal overlapping of suture lines should be noted. Adapted from Ref. [52]

closure, the Foley catheter is removed and diluted methylene blue is gently injected into the urethra with a catheter tip syringe to ensure watertight closure.

It is essential to avoid dead space by securing the periurethral fascial flaps. Deep to the vaginal wall, fibrofatty labial flaps can be used to prevent risk of wound breakdown or fistula with a low rate of complication. Use of a Martius flap is safe but can result in pain, dyspareunia, hematoma, or abscess requiring drainage [25–27].

Complications Following Urethral Diverticulectomy

Short-term complications (<30 days) following urethral diverticulectomy include urinary tract infections (1–10%), soft tissue infections (<1%), and bleeding requiring transfusion (<1%) [28–30].

Long-term complications include lower urinary tract symptoms (frequency, dysuria, 10%) and pain (11%). There have been reports of an overactive bladder following urethral diverticulectomy, which can be managed with medical therapy [29, 31]. De novo SUI can occur in up to 17% of patients following urethral diverticulectomy [10, 32]. Vesicovaginal fistulas and urethral strictures are rare outcomes following surgery [23, 30, 33]. Residual or recurrent urethral diverticula are found at rates as high as 10–16% postoperatively, and this is related to the complexity of the diverticulum [3, 6, 34–36].

Stress Urinary Incontinence

Stress urinary incontinence deserves special attention in the context of UD as one of the hallmark symptoms of UD, post-void dribbling can easily be mistaken for SUI. SUI can also be diagnosed as a separate entity during preoperative evaluation. It can also arise de novo as a complication of diverticulectomy. It is important to discuss SUI separately in the context of each of these distinct presentations.

Concurrent SUI with a Urethral Diverticulum

For patients who present with SUI in the setting of a urethral diverticulum, an accurate diagnosis is important, as leakage of accumulated urine from the diverticulum can be mistaken for SUI. Diagnosticians can manually empty out the diverticulum and ask the patient to cough as a means of elucidating the presence of SUI [37].

Urodynamic evaluation can be conducted preoperatively to delineate symptomatology in patients with a urethral diverticulum. Video urodynamics (VUD) is preferred as a voiding cystourethrogram (VCUG) can allow for visualization of the diverticulum. SUI can be found during urodynamic evaluation in up to 50% of patients presenting with a urethral diverticulum [29, 38].

Patients who present preoperatively with SUI may be offered anti-incontinence surgery at the time of diverticulectomy. It is also reasonable to defer treatment of SUI and reevaluate symptoms following diverticulectomy. A retrospective analysis by Greiman et al. showed that 8 of 15 patients who underwent urethral diverticulectomy without simultaneous placement of an autologous pubovaginal sling saw resolution of SUI following surgery, compared to 20 of 24 patients who had simultaneous sling placement [39]. The staged approach can be particularly helpful for patients for whom differentiation between SUI and urethral post-void dribbling cannot be achieved. Caution should be taken for placement of slings for proximal diverticula as increased intraurethral pressure with Valsalva can cause rupture of the suture line leading to fistula formation.

De Novo SUI

De novo SUI following urethral diverticulectomy can occur in up to 17% of patients. A recent prospective series of 100 patients who underwent video urodynamics prior to diverticulectomy with modified Martius interposition has found the rate of de novo SUI to be 16% [10, 32]. Risk factors for de novo SUI include diverticulum size (>30 mm), proximal location, and complex configuration of the diverticulum on preoperative imaging [9, 40, 41]. Limited contemporary data suggest that simultaneous autologous sling placement at the time of diverticulectomy is safe and may reduce the risk of post-procedural SUI [39]. The decision to offer concurrent SUI treatment should be balanced with the risk of complications such as urinary retention, urinary urgency, and recurrent UTIs [31, 39, 42, 43]. Importantly, concomitant use of synthetic mid-urethral slings should be avoided due to the risk of erosion of the graft into the urethra [44]. Additionally, it has been advised that concomitant sling surgery should be avoided in patients with contraindications to pubovaginal slings, including pure urgency incontinence, primary bladder neck obstruction, urethral stricture, and a poorly contractile or acontractile bladder with urinary retention [45].

Management of de novo SUI can be either conservative or interventional. Conservative management of postoperative SUI includes pelvic floor muscle training (PFMT), and it can be expected that the majority of patients who develop de novo SUI following diverticulectomy will improve without the need for surgical intervention [32]. In the series published by Barratt et al., 12 of 16 patients with de novo SUI saw resolution of symptoms with 3 months of pelvic floor physical therapy [10]. The remaining four patients underwent video urodynamics (VUDS), demonstrating distal stricture in one patient, detrusor overactivity in one patient, and SUI in two patients.

Surgical management of de novo SUI may be necessary for a minority (4–10%) of patients who undergo diverticulectomy [9, 32, 46]. Treatment options include bulking agents or autologous fascia mid-urethral slings. It must be stressed again that synthetic materials should never be used in management of patients with SUI following urethral diverticulectomy due to the risk of urethral erosion [44]. It is unknown whether the risk of erosion decreases with time or whether synthetic materials may be used in patients with a remote history of urethral diverticulectomy.

Urethrovaginal Fistula

Fistula formation following diverticulectomy is reported in 0–6% of patients. Risk factors for fistula formation include surgery on a recurrent diverticulum, complexity of the diverticulum, overlapping suture lines, tension on the incision, poor mobilization of flaps, or poor tissue quality [6, 47]. Urethrovaginal fistula formation distal to the external urinary sphincter can be mildly symptomatic, presenting with double voiding or vaginal voiding. Urethrovaginal fistulae proximal to the external urinary sphincter may result in continuous leakage of urine (Fig. 9.3) [33]. Repair of fistula should be delayed until at least 3–6 months following index surgery to allow time for tissue regrowth [48]. Use of fibrofatty labial (Martius) flaps is recommended at the time of repair. As discussed earlier, a Martius flap may be used at the time of urethral diverticulectomy and may reduce the risk of fistula

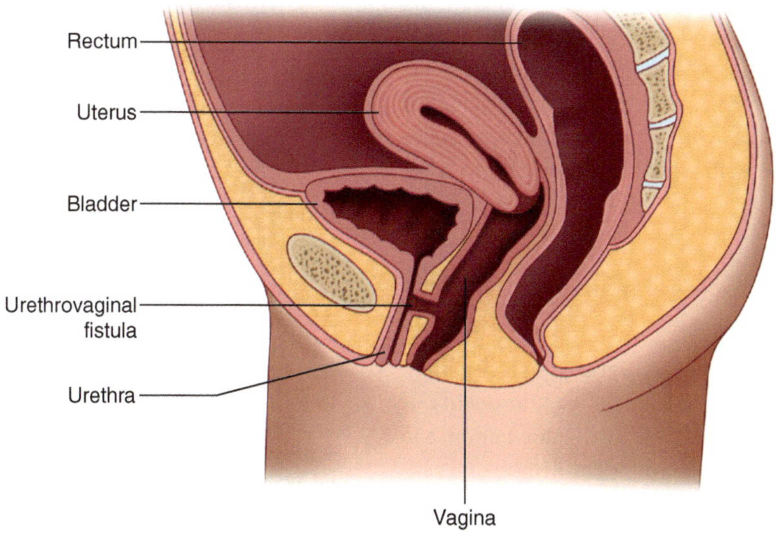

Fig. 9.3 Sagittal view of the female pelvis with a ureterovesical fistula. Adapted from Ref. [53]

formation with minimal added postoperative risk [25–27].

Urethral Stricture

Urethral stricture is a rare complication following diverticulectomy and is found in 0–2% of patients postoperatively. It may be associated with excision of complex diverticula, particularly if end-to-end urethroplasty is performed [23]. Presenting symptoms include slow stream, high post-void residual, or recurrent UTIs. Urethral strictures can be managed with balloon dilation, meatotomy, or urethroplasty or conservatively with clean intermittent catheterization [6, 33, 49].

Recurrent Urethral Diverticulum

Many patients will experience temporary symptoms following urethral diverticulectomy, including pain, dysuria, urgency, and urinary leakage. The majority of these patients will improve spontaneously without intervention [9]. Persistent symptoms following diverticulectomy should raise concern for a residual or recurrent diverticulum and prompt repeat imaging.

Diverticular recurrence is common and can be found in 2–16% of patients postoperatively [6, 9, 30, 49]. Recurrences are believed to arise from residual dead space or incomplete excision of the diverticular sac [50], and recurrence rates are higher for patients with a history of prior urethral diverticulectomy. Ingber reported 122 patients with urethral diverticulectomy that underwent excision and found that, of the 110 patients without prior urethral diverticulectomy, the rate of recurrence was 9.1%, compared to 25% (3 of 12) of patients who were undergoing surgery for a recurrence. Patients with a history of any pelvic surgery were also more likely to experience residual or recurrent diverticula ($p < 0.001$) [35].

It is believed that the complexity of the diverticulum affects outcomes. Han et al. report a series of 30 women with simple or complex (C- or U-shaped) diverticula. Notably, 0/17 patients with simple diverticula experienced recurrence and 7/13 patients with complex diverticula recurred [34]. Conversely, a series of 43 patients that underwent diverticulectomy for simple ($n = 32$) or complex ($n = 11$) diverticula found no difference in the rates of recurrent diverticula between the two groups [49]. Recurrent diverticula can be managed similarly to de novo diverticula; asymptomatic recurrences can be managed with observation while symptomatic recurrences can be treated with repeat diverticulectomy with good results [9].

Conclusions

Urethral diverticula represent a benign condition with potential morbid implications for quality of life. When indicated, surgical intervention can lead to resolution of symptoms. However, complications can arise. With a careful surgical technique and proper selection, complications can be minimized and outcomes improved.

References

1. Marshall S. Urethral diverticula in young girls. Urology. 1981;17(3):243–5.
2. Ortlip SA, Gonzalez R, Williams RD. Diverticula of the male urethra. J Urol. 1980;124(3):350–5.
3. Rovner ES. Bladder and female urethral diverticula. In: Partin AW, editor. Campbell walsh wein urology. Elsevier; 2021.
4. Rajan N, Tucci P, Mallouh C, Choudhury M. Carcinoma in female urethral diverticulum: case reports and review of management. J Urol. 1993;150(6):1911–4.
5. Thomas AA, Rackley RR, Lee U, Goldman HB, Vasavada SP, Hansel DE. Urethral diverticula in 90 female patients: a study with emphasis on neoplastic alterations. J Urol. 2008;180(6):2463–7.
6. Ljungqvist L, Peeker R, Fall M. Female urethral diverticulum: 26-year followup of a large series. J Urol. 2007;177(1):219–24. discussion 24
7. Aldridge CW, Beaton JH, Nanzig RP. A review of office urethroscopy and cystometry. Am J Obstet Gynecol. 1978;131(4):432–7.
8. El-Nashar SA, Bacon MM, Kim-Fine S, Weaver AL, Gebhart JB, Klingele CJ. Incidence of female urethral diverticulum: a population-based analysis and literature review. Int Urogynecol J. 2014;25(1):73–9.
9. Stav K, Dwyer PL, Rosamilia A, Chao F. Urinary symptoms before and after female urethral diverticulectomy--can we predict de novo stress urinary incontinence? J Urol 2008; 180(5): 2088–2090.
10. Barratt R, Malde S, Pakzad M, Hamid R, Ockrim J, Greenwell T. The incidence and outcomes of urodynamic stress urinary incontinence in female patients with urethral diverticulum. Neurourol Urodyn. 2019;38(7):1889–900.
11. Baradaran N, Chiles LR, Freilich DA, Rames RA, Cox L, Rovner ES. Female urethral diverticula in the contemporary era: is the classic triad of the "3Ds" still relevant? Urology. 2016;94:53–6.
12. Davis HJ, Telinde RW. Urethral diverticula: an assay of 121 cases. J Urol. 1958;80(1):34–9.
13. Portnoy O, Kitrey N, Eshed I, Apter S, Amitai MM, Golomb J. Correlation between MRI and double-balloon urethrography findings in the diagnosis of female periurethral lesions. Eur J Radiol. 2013;82(12):2183–8.
14. Chung DE, Purohit RS, Girshman J, Blaivas JG. Urethral diverticula in women: discrepancies between magnetic resonance imaging and surgical findings. J Urol. 2010;183(6):2265–9.
15. Spencer WF, Streem SB. Diverticulum of the female urethral roof managed endoscopically. J Urol. 1987;138(1):147–8.
16. Spence HM, Duckett JW. Diverticulum of the female urethra: clinical aspects and presentation of a simple operative technique for cure. J Urol. 1970;104(3):432–7.
17. Saito S. Usefulness of diagnosis by the urethroscopy under anesthesia and effect of transurethral electrocoagulation in symptomatic female urethral diverticula. J Endourol. 2000;14(5):455–7.
18. Mizrahi S, Bitterman W. Transvaginal, periurethral injection of polytetrafluoroethylene (polytef) in the treatment of urethral diverticula. Br J Urol. 1988;62(3):280.
19. Bodner-Adler B, Halpern K, Hanzal E. Surgical management of urethral diverticula in women: a systematic review. Int Urogynecol J. 2016;27(7):993–1001.
20. Welch EK, Dengler KL, Welgoss JA. Urethral diverticulum marsupialization with modified Spence-Duckett procedure. Urology. 2023;
21. Clyne OJ, Flood HD. Giant urethral diverticulum: a novel approach to repair. J Urol. 2002;167(4):1796.
22. Woodhouse CR, Flynn JT, Molland EA, Blandy JP. Urethral diverticulum in females. Br J Urol. 1980;52(4):305–10.
23. Rovner ES, Wein AJ. Diagnosis and reconstruction of the dorsal or circumferential urethral diverticulum. J Urol. 2003;170(1):82–6. discussion 6
24. Sivarajan G, Glickman L, Faber K, Kim M, Fromer D, Munver R. Transabdominal robot-assisted laparoscopic urethral diverticulectomy of a complex anterior horseshoe diverticulum of the proximal urethra. J Endourol Case Rep. 2015;1(1):33–5.
25. Malde S, Sihra N, Naaseri S, Spilotros M, Solomon E, Pakzad M, et al. Urethral diverticulectomy with Martius labial fat pad interposition improves symptom resolution and reduces recurrence. BJU Int. 2017;119(1):158–63.
26. Dmochowski R. Urethral diverticula: evolving diagnostics and improved surgical management. Curr Urol Rep. 2001;2(5):373–8.

27. Romanzi LJ, Groutz A, Blaivas JG. Urethral diverticulum in women: diverse presentations resulting in diagnostic delay and mismanagement. J Urol. 2000;164(2):428–33.
28. Raup VT, Hess DS, Hanske J, Schmid M, Varda B, Das A, et al. Patient characteristics and perioperative outcomes of female urethral diverticulectomy (UD): analysis of a multi-institutional prospective database. Urology. 2015;86(4):712–5.
29. Ganabathi K, Leach GE, Zimmern PE, Dmochowski R. Experience with the management of urethral diverticulum in 63 women. J Urol. 1994;152(5 Pt 1):1445–52.
30. Reeves FA, Inman RD, Chapple CR. Management of symptomatic urethral diverticula in women: a single-Centre experience. Eur Urol. 2014;66(1):164–72.
31. Swierzewski SJ, McGuire EJ. Pubovaginal sling for treatment of female stress urinary incontinence complicated by urethral diverticulum. J Urol. 1993;149(5):1012–4.
32. Lee UJ, Goldman H, Moore C, Daneshgari F, Rackley RR, Vasavada SP. Rate of de novo stress urinary incontinence after urethal diverticulum repair. Urology. 2008;71(5):849–53.
33. Kim HW, Lee JZ, Shin DG. Pathophysiology and Management of Long-term Complications after Transvaginal Urethral Diverticulectomy. Int Neurourol J. 2021;25(3):202–9.
34. Han DH, Jeong YS, Choo MS, Lee KS. Outcomes of surgery of female urethral diverticula classified using magnetic resonance imaging. Eur Urol. 2007;51(6):1664–70.
35. Ingber MS, Firoozi F, Vasavada SP, Ching CB, Goldman HB, Moore CK, et al. Surgically corrected urethral diverticula: long-term voiding dysfunction and reoperation rates. Urology. 2011;77(1):65–9.
36. Lee RA. Diverticulum of the urethra: clinical presentation, diagnosis, and management. Clin Obstet Gynecol. 1984;27(2):490–8.
37. Sun Y, Peng B, Wu J, Li Q. Stress urinary incontinence after urethral diverticulum repair without concomitant anti-incontinence procedure. Urology. 2022;160:229.
38. Bass JS, Leach GE. Surgical treatment of concomitant urethral diverticulum and stress incontinence. Urol Clin North Am. 1991;18(2):365–73.
39. Greiman A, Rittenberg L, Freilich D, Rames R, El-Zawahry A, Koski M, et al. Outcomes of treatment of stress urinary incontinence associated with female urethral diverticula: a selective approach. Neurourol Urodyn. 2018;37(1):478–84.
40. Kim JH, Lee KW, Kim JM, Kim ME, Kim YH. Risk factors for de novo mixed urinary incontinence and stress urinary incontinence following surgical removal of a urethral diverticulum. Low Urin Tract Symptoms. 2013;5(3):154–8.
41. Malde S, Naaseri S, Kavia R, Pakzad M, Hamid R, Ockrim J, et al. Preliminary report on the effect of urethral diverticulum magnetic resonance imaging configuration on the incidence of new onset urodynamic stress urinary incontinence following excision. Urol Ann. 2017;9(4):321–3.
42. Enemchukwu E, Lai C, Reynolds WS, Kaufman M, Dmochowski R. Autologous pubovaginal sling for the treatment of concomitant female urethral diverticula and stress urinary incontinence. Urology. 2015;85(6):1300–3.
43. Bradley SE, Leach DA, Panza J, Sassani J, Escobar C, Ogorek J, et al. A multicenter retrospective cohort study comparing urethral diverticulectomy with and without pubovaginal sling. Am J Obstet Gynecol. 2020;223(2):273.e1–e9.
44. Kobashi KC, Albo ME, Dmochowski RR, Ginsberg DA, Goldman HB, Gomelsky A, et al. Surgical treatment of female stress urinary incontinence: AUA/SUFU guideline. J Urol. 2017;198(4): 875–83.
45. Wein AJ. Re: autologous Pubovaginal sling for the treatment of concomitant female urethral diverticula and stress urinary incontinence. J Urol. 2016;195(4 Pt 1):1040–1.
46. Chavez JA, Fuentes JL, Christie AL, Alhalabi F, Carmel ME, Lemack GE, et al. Stress urinary incontinence after urethral diverticulum repair without concomitant anti-incontinence procedure. Urology. 2021;154:103–8.
47. Crescenze IM, Goldman HB. Female urethral diverticulum: current diagnosis and management. Curr Urol Rep. 2015;16(10):71.
48. Greiman AK, Rolef J, Rovner ES. Urethral diverticulum: a systematic review. Arab J Urol. 2019;17(1):49–57.
49. Nickles SW, Ikwuezunma G, MacLachlan L, El-Zawahry A, Rames R, Rovner E. Simple vs complex urethral diverticulum: presentation and outcomes. Urology. 2014;84(6):1516–9.
50. Aspera AM, Rackley RR, Vasavada SP. Contemporary evaluation and management of the female urethral diverticulum. Urol Clin North Am. 2002;29(3):617–24.
51. Working-Group E. Primary urethral cancer 2016. Available from: https://patients.uroweb.org/cancers/primary-urethral-cancer/.
52. Raz S. Excision of urethral diverticula. In: Atlas of vaginal reconstructive surgery. New York, NY: Springer; 2015.
53. Lue K, Heinsimer K, Madiraju SK, Rideout D, Wiegand L. Urologic trauma from vaginal dilation for congenital vaginal stenosis: a newly-described and challenging complication. Urol Case Rep. 2020;28:101075.

Segmental or Total Female Urethrectomy

10

Kirolos N. Meilika and Jaspreet S. Sandhu

Urethrectomy for Urethral Malignancies

Female urethrectomy could be performed for various benign and malignant diseases; the decision to perform segmental or total urethrectomy is based on the pathology and extent of the urethral lesion. Female primary urethral cancers (PUCs) are rare, and most of the published studies mainly focus on oncological and survival outcomes [13, 19, 27, 39]. The female urethra is about 4 cm long and is divided based on the cellular lining or its relation to the surrounding anatomical structures, mainly the urethral sphincters. Histologically, the proximal third is lined by urothelial cells, and the distal two-thirds are lined by the squamous epithelium. The Skene (paraurethral) glands surround the urethra, and their ducts open near the external meatus. Anatomically, the female urethra is divided into the distal one-third (anterior segment) and the proximal two-thirds (posterior segment). The former can be resected without affecting the urinary sphincter. In all, 28%–45% of female primary urethral cancers (PUCs) are urothelial carcinomas and arise from the proximal urethra. Squamous cell carcinoma arises from the distal urethra and accounts for 19%–29% of female PUCs. Adenocarcinoma arises from the Skene glands, which are located alongside the entire urethra, and represents 28%–38% of female PUCs [9, 39] (Fig. 10.1).

Distal urethral cancers occur in about one-third of patients; the remainder have proximal or panurethral tumors—30%–50% of females with PUC present with locally advanced disease [20]. A multimodal approach is usually utilized for female PUC treatment and includes surgery, radiation therapy, and chemotherapy alone or in combination [39].

Urethra-sparing surgery or segmental urethrectomy is a valid therapeutic approach in women with localized anterior carcinomas [16]. Segmental urethrectomy aims to achieve cancer control without compromising the voiding function. Compared to minimally invasive approaches such as transurethral resection (TUR) or laser ablation, distal urethrectomy achieved higher local cancer control and better cancer-specific survival rates [10]. Distal urethrectomy is usually performed via a transvaginal approach, which is feasible for tumors in the urethral meatus or the distal third of the urethra. Transvaginal distal urethrectomy (Fig. 10.2) should also include removing part of the anterior vaginal wall and achieving a negative proximal urethral margin on intraoperative frozen section pathology [27]. Dimarco

K. N. Meilika
Department of Urology, University of Rochester Medical Center, Rochester, NY, USA
e-mail: kirolos_meilika@urmc.rochester.edu

J. S. Sandhu (✉)
Department of Surgery, Memorial Sloan Kettering Cancer Center, New York, NY, USA
e-mail: sandhuj@mskcc.org

M. Hoffman et al. (eds.), *Major Complications of Female Pelvic Surgery*,
https://doi.org/10.1007/978-3-031-66772-5_10

Fig. 10.1 Female urethra

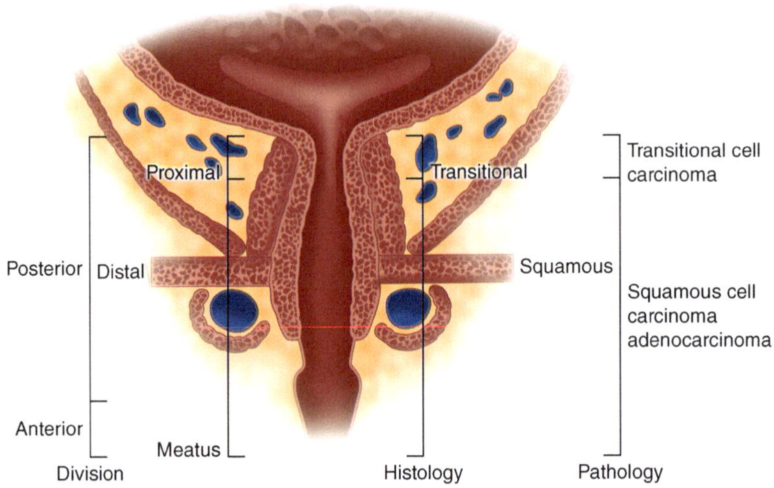

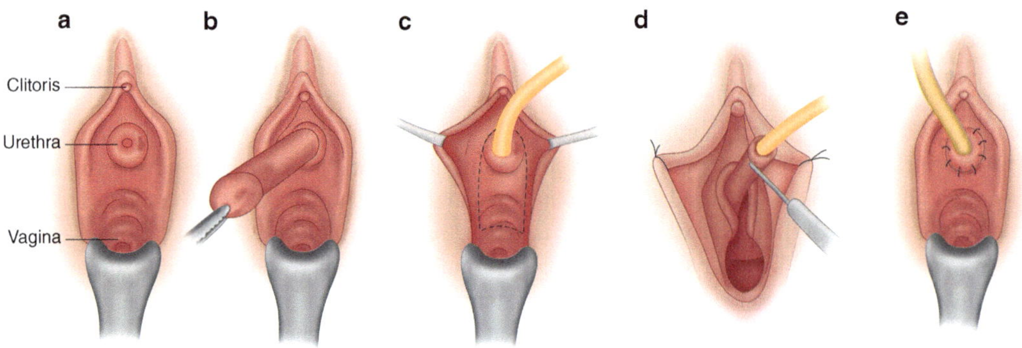

Fig. 10.2 Surgical steps for transvaginal distal urethrectomy: (**a**) The external genital anatomy of the female is observed to be within normal limits. (**b**) A circumferential incision is made around the external urethral meatus, followed by careful dissection and mobilization of the distal urethra. (**c**) Alternatively, an inverted U-shaped incision can be made on the anterior vaginal wall to facilitate the dissection and mobilization of the distal urethra. (**d**) Consider removing a section of the anterior vaginal wall to achieve a negative proximal urethral margin on intraoperative frozen section pathology. (**e**) The healthy urethra is then sutured to the anterior vaginal wall using simple interrupted absorbable sutures to establish a new urethral meatus

et al. studied the outcome of partial urethrectomy in 26 patients and found that the main complication was stress urinary incontinence (SUI) in 11 of them (42%). Additionally, two (8%) patients developed urinary retention. One patient (4%) developed urge incontinence [10].

In cases of higher-stage urethral cancers where it is impossible to achieve negative margins with partial urethrectomy, primary radical urethrectomy (Fig. 10.3) is the recommended approach to achieve a local cure. This surgical procedure entails removing the periurethral tissue completely, including both bulbospongiosus muscles. Moreover, the excision should extend superiorly up to the pubic symphysis and posteriorly to the anterior vaginal wall, ensuring thorough tumor removal while preserving the bladder neck. Following the procedure, bladder neck closure is performed and urinary diversion is accomplished by creating a

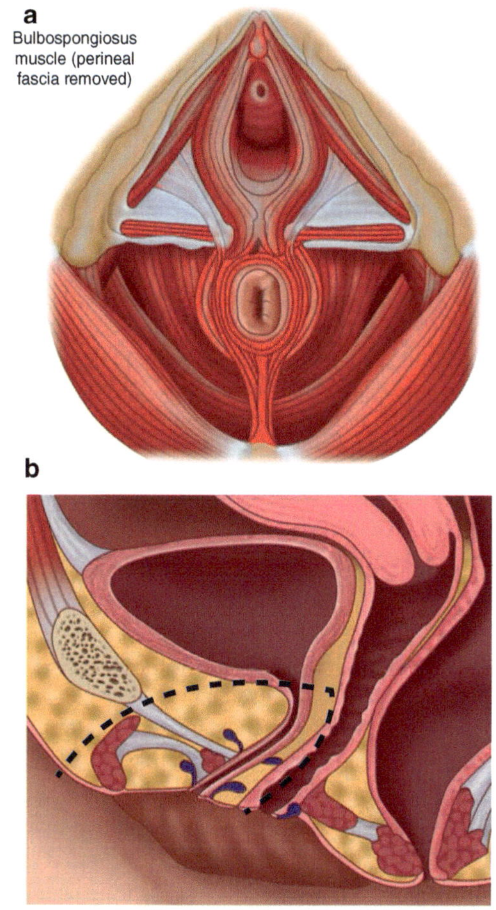

Fig. 10.3 Radical (total) urethrectomy excision margins. (**a**) The bulbocavernosus (bulbospongiosus) muscles on both sides delineate the lateral margins for a radical urethrectomy. (**b**) The dotted line represents the anteroposterior and cephalocaudal margins for a radical urethrectomy

catheterizable continent stoma [10]. The complications following radical urethrectomy and stoma creation include superficial wound infections, urine leakage (fistula formation between the bladder neck and the perineum), pelvic abscesses, and sepsis.

Locally advanced female urethral carcinomas, particularly those situated proximally, tend to be of a high stage and may exhibit infiltration into the bladder and vagina. A comprehensive treatment approach combining chemotherapy, radiation therapy, and surgery is recommended to manage such cases effectively [7]. Surgical intervention for locally advanced female urethral cancer often involves anterior pelvic exenteration, accompanied by lymphadenectomy in both the inguinal and pelvic regions. When the tumor extends into the external genitalia, additional excision of the vaginal and labial tissues may be necessary to ensure negative surgical margins. The potential complications associated with pelvic exenteration and urinary diversion will be addressed in a separate chapter of this book.

Segmental and total female urethrectomy can also be performed during the excision of vulvar and vaginal cancers. The complications of surgical excision of vulvar and vaginal cancers will be discussed in the corresponding chapters.

Urethrectomy for Noncancerous Diseases

Female urethrectomy can also be performed for the treatment of benign conditions, commonly urethral diverticula, urethral caruncle [6, 38], or a Skene gland cyst [15, 36]. Other less common benign diseases are Bartholin duct cysts and abscesses [41], Gartner's duct cysts [29], and leiomyomas [40]. The complications of urethral diverticulectomy are addressed in a separate chapter of this book. This chapter will present the complications commonly seen after partial or total urethrectomy, including distal (meatal) urethral stricture and stress or total urinary incontinence.

Meatal Stenosis and Distal Urethral Stricture After Partial Urethrectomy

Meatal stenosis (Fig. 10.4) and distal urethral stricture in females are generally rare, and only 1% of women who present with voiding complaints are found to have urethral stenosis [1]. Symptoms of meatal stenosis include varying degrees of obstructive and irritative lower urinary tract symptoms (LUTSs), such as urinary frequency, urgency, weak urinary stream, urinary incontinence, and recurrent urinary tract infections. Occasionally, meatal stenosis may present with urinary retention [25], renal failure, hydronephrosis, or pyelonephritis [34]. Diagnostic workup for meatal stenosis entails urinary flow studies, post-void residual urine, flexible urethroscopy, and video urodynamics [1].

Meatal stenosis can be avoided by performing wide ventral spatulation before suturing the urethral edge to the vagina. The role of meatal dilation using urethral sounds (Fig. 10.5) is feasible in mild meatal stenosis [1]. The success rate of urethral dilation is 47% at a mean follow-up of 43 months [30]. Other authors do not recommend meatal dilation, especially for recurrent cases [11] [18].

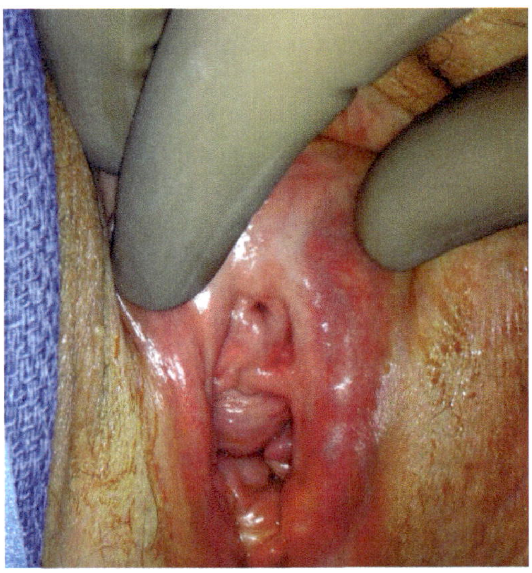

Fig. 10.4 Meatal stenosis

Meatotomy

Urethral meatotomy in females is performed for short segment distal and superficial strictures by making an endoscopic dorsal incision [35]. Alternatively, a 1-cm open incision on the ventral aspect of the distal urethra can be made followed by suturing the urethral mucosa to the vagina using a 4–0 Vicryl in a "V"-shaped manner [11]. The long-term functional outcomes of meatotomy are generally unsatisfactory, and additional procedures such as circumferential, distal urethrectomy and advancement meatoplasty are required in the future.

Distal Urethrectomy and Advancement Meatoplasty

Surgical reconstruction has the highest success rate if compared to less invasive procedures such as dilations and meatotomy. The minimally invasive procedure should be reserved for short urethral stenosis in women with high comorbidity [12]. The **initial step of** distal urethrectomy with advancement meatoplasty is identifying a healthy proximal tissue, followed by placement of circumferential stay sutures to prevent retraction, sparing as much of the healthy mucosa as possible. The fibrotic tissue is then completely excised, and the healthy urethral mucosa is sewn to the healthy vaginal mucosa with interrupted absorbable sutures [35] (Fig. 10.6). Vulvar cancers are typically not estrogen-dependent [37], so local estrogen can be safely applied postoperatively to promote healing and prevent stricture recurrence [14].

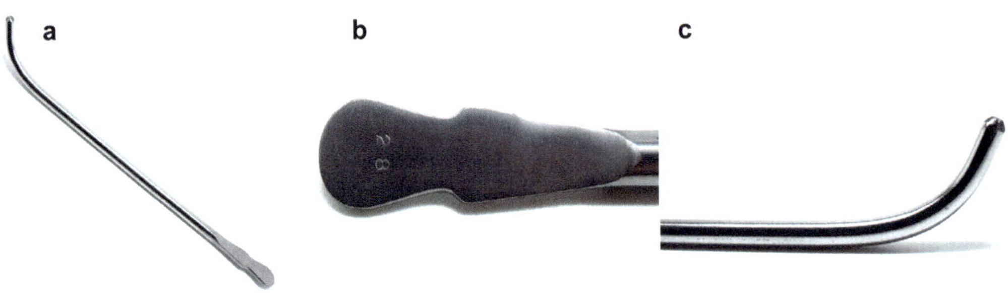

Fig. 10.5 Urethral sounds. (**a**) Van Buren urethral sounds are characterized by their distinctive J-shaped or curved design. (**b**) The sound diameter (in French size) usually found on the handle. (**c**) The urethral sound tip

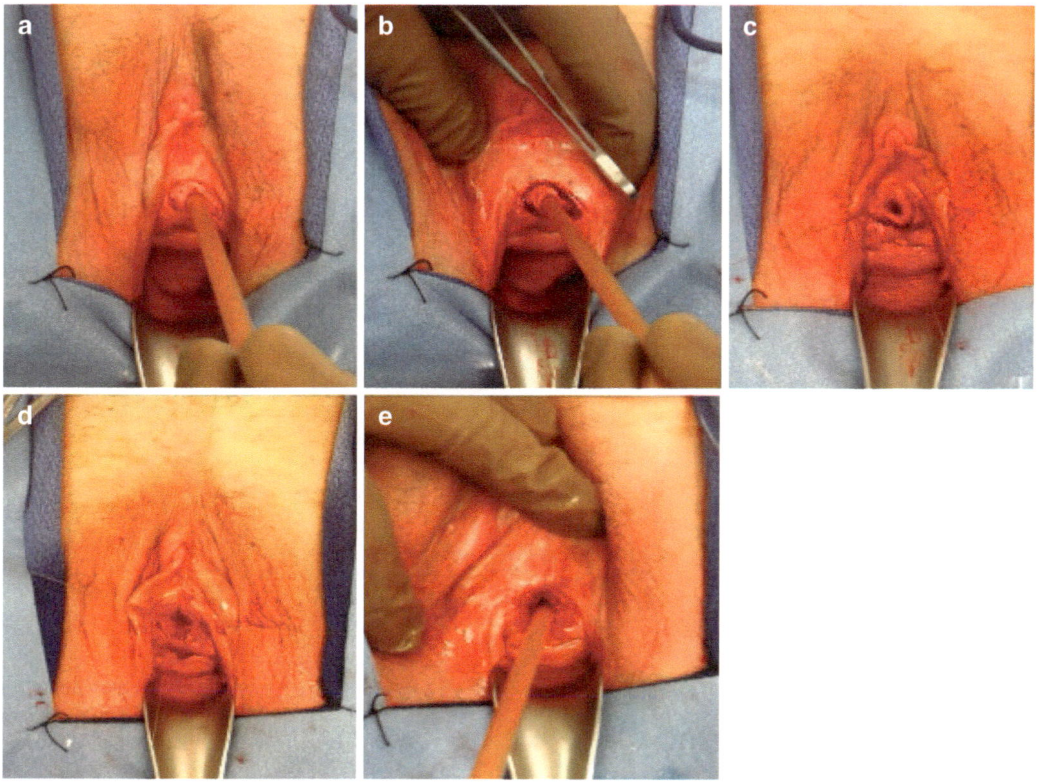

Fig. 10.6 Surgical steps for distal urethrectomy and advancement meatoplasty. (**a**) A circumferential incision is performed around the external urethral meatus. (**b**) Healthy urethral tissue proximal to the fibrotic segment is identified. (**c**) Circumferential stay sutures are placed to prevent tissue retraction, preserving as much healthy mucosa as possible. (**d**) The fibrotic urethra is completely excised. (**e**) Interrupted absorbable sutures are used to attach the healthy urethral mucosa to the healthy vaginal mucosa, establishing a new urethral meatus

Stress Urinary Incontinence (SUI) After Partial Urethrectomy

The female urethral sphincteric mechanism is complex with multiple contributing factors; the external sphincter is composed of circular and longitudinal striated muscles (Figs. 10.7 and 10.8).

Additionally, a healthy urethral mucosa tends to stay coapted, and the spongy, vascular nature of the submucosal layer adds more support to the urethral wall (Fig. 10.9).

The middle third of the urethra is supported posteriorly by the anterior vaginal wall and the endopelvic fascia, which is firmly connected to the arcus tendon fascia pelvis and the levator ani muscle (Fig. 10.10). These pubourethral ligaments prevent the transmission of intra-abdominal pressure to the distal urethra during straining (Fig. 10.11).

The incidence of stress urinary incontinence (SUI) after partial urethrectomy is variable. de Mooij et al. compared the SUI outcome between 2 groups of patients with vulvar cancer: 18 patients with vulvar cancer affecting the urethra, treated with radical vulvectomy and partial urethrectomy, and 17 patients treated with vulvectomy alone without partial urethrectomy. After 6 months of follow-up, they found that partial resection of 1–1.5 cm of the distal urethra during radical local excision for vulvar cancer does not lead to a significant increase in the frequency of urinary incontinence when compared to vulvar cancer patients who did not undergo partial urethrectomy [8]. The incidence of new or worsening SUI after partial urethrectomy is about 24–40% [10, 33]. The incidence of urge incontinence after partial urethrectomy is about 4%, and it usually responds to medical treatment [10, 33].

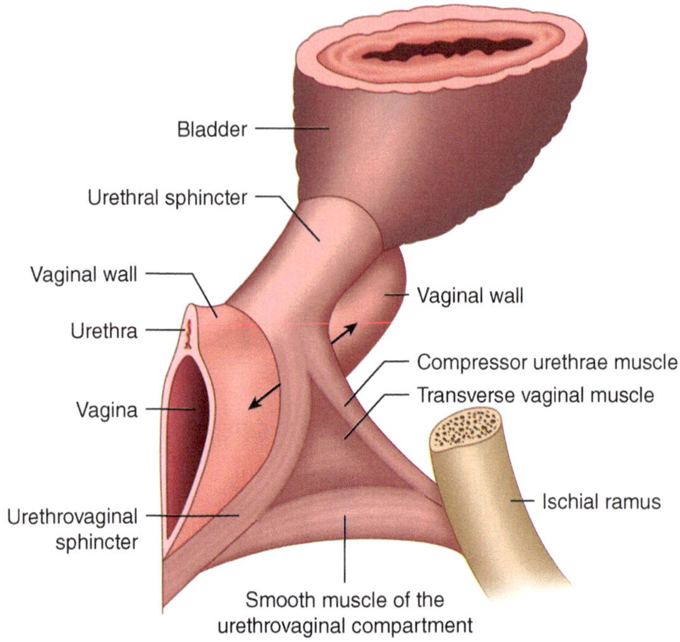

Fig. 10.7 Anatomy of the urethral sphincter muscle. Bladder, urethral sphincter, vaginal wall, urethra, vagina, compressor urethrae muscle, transverse vaginal muscle, ischial ramus, urethrovaginal sphincter, smooth muscle of the urethrovaginal compartment

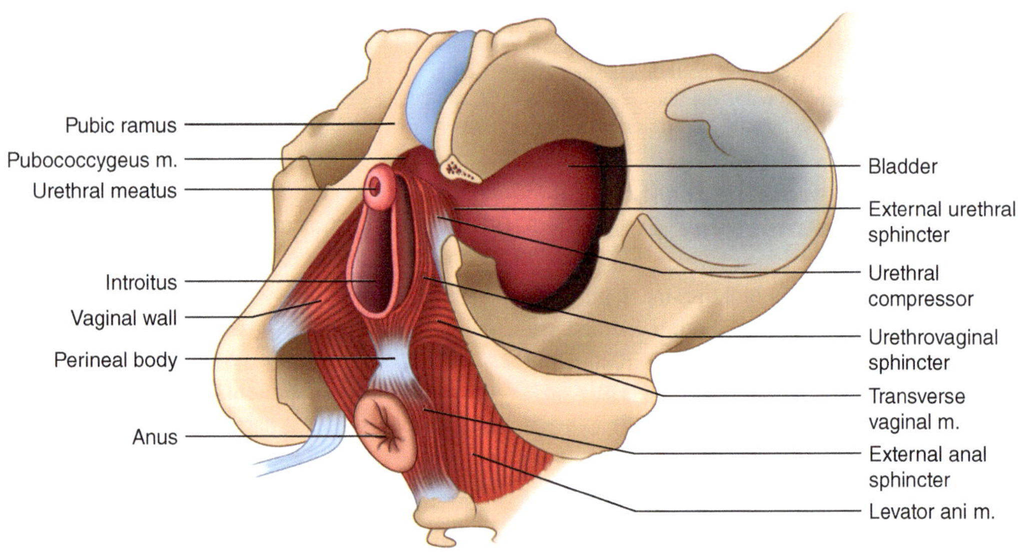

Fig. 10.8 Anatomy of the urethral sphincter muscle

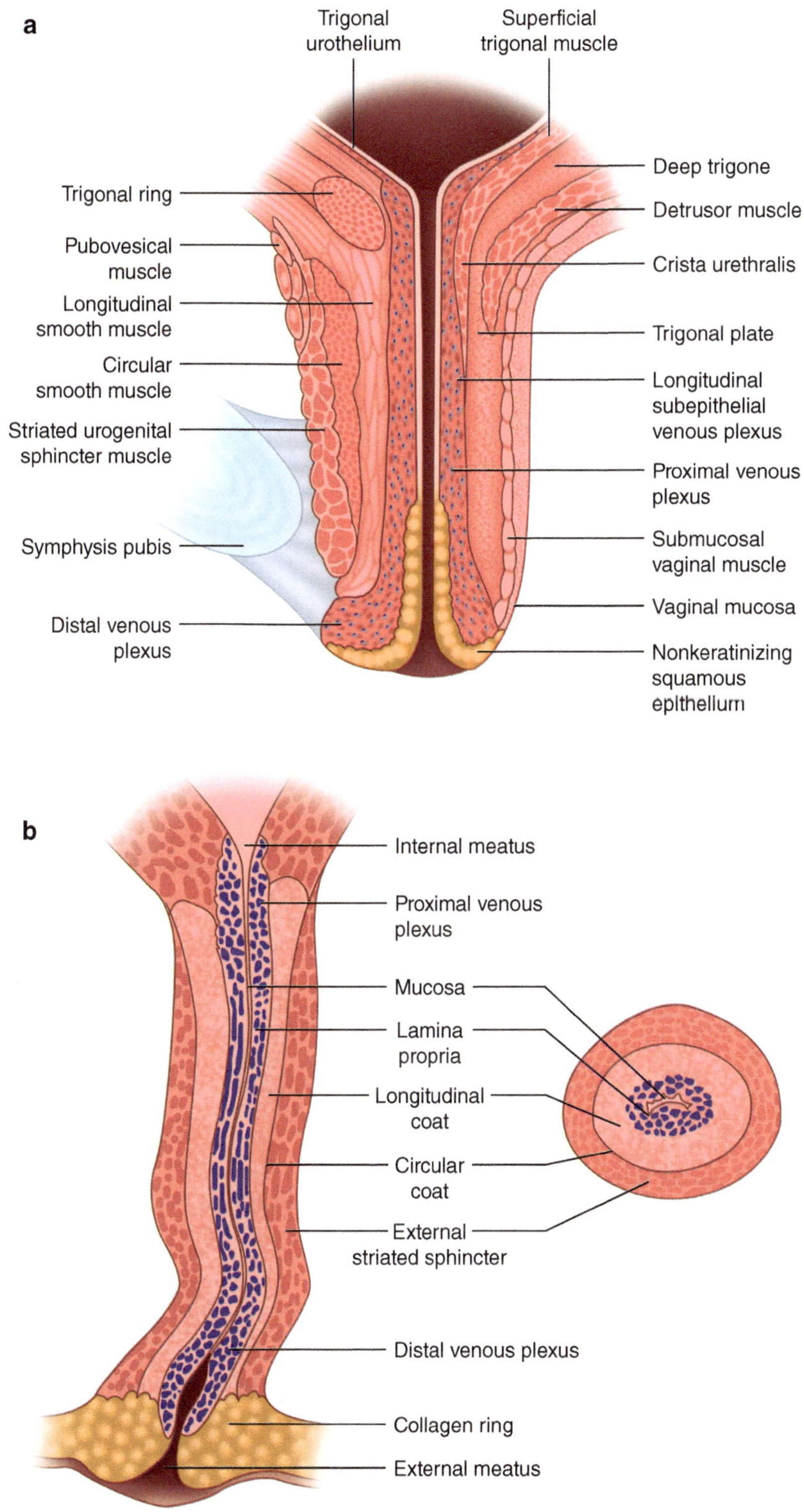

Fig. 10.9 The urethral mucosa and submucosal layers

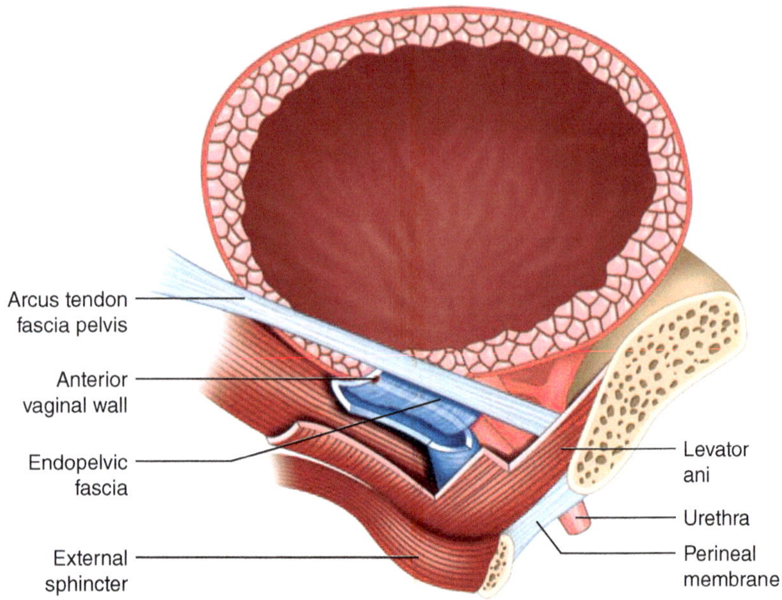

Fig. 10.10 Posterior urethral support

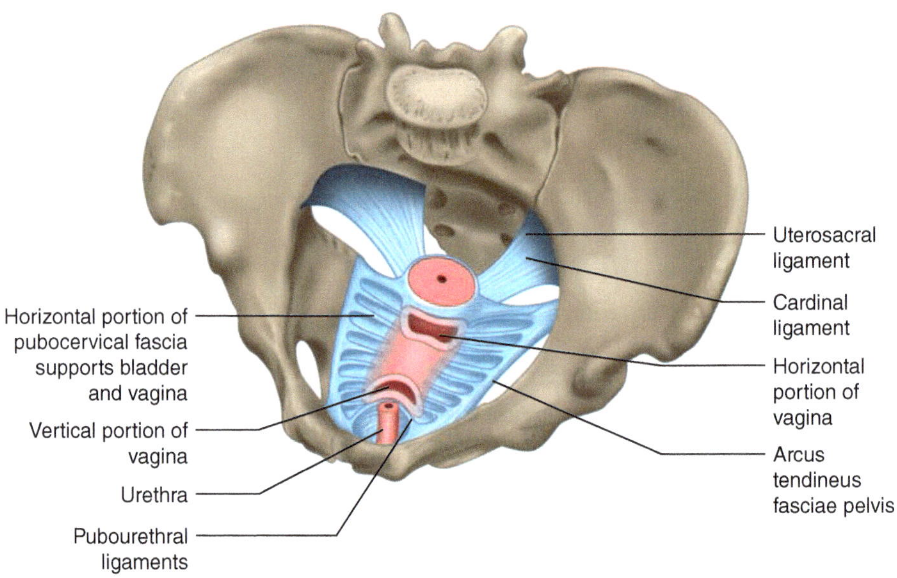

Fig. 10.11 Ligaments and fascial support to the urethra

Treatment of Post-Urethrectomy Stress Urinary Incontinence in Women

Mid-urethral slings are ineffective in treating SUI after partial urethrectomy due to the short urethra, vaginal wall retraction, and fibrosis [22]. Both a transurethral Macroplastique injection (Fig. 10.12) and a pubovaginal sling (PVS) (Fig. 10.13) are effective in treating SUI after partial urethrectomy [24].

A transurethral Macroplastique injection is a minimally invasive approach. It has a success rate of about 40%, but the drawback of this modality

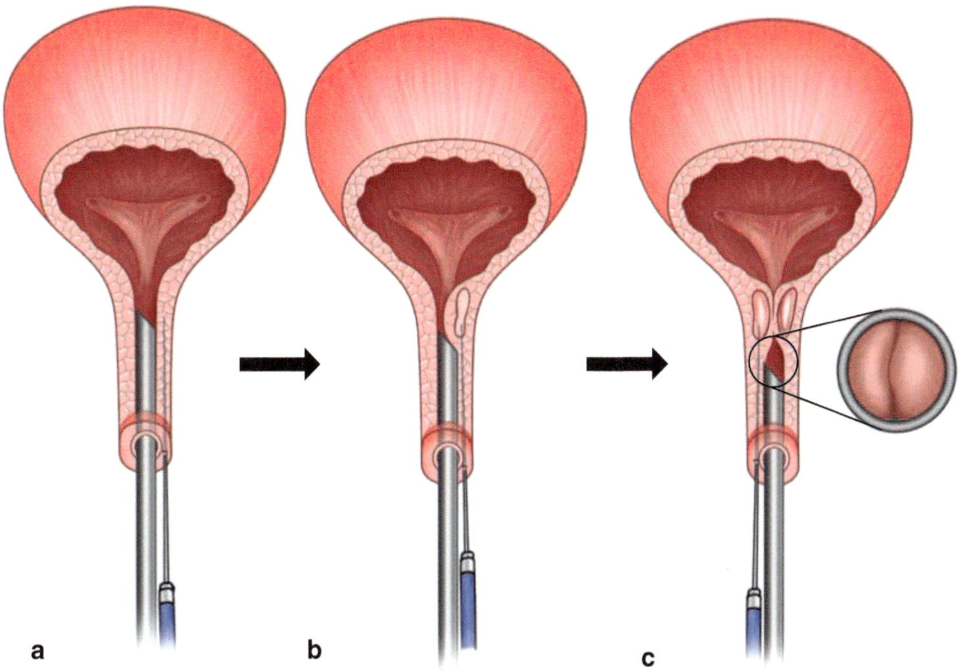

Fig. 10.12 A transurethral Macroplastique injection

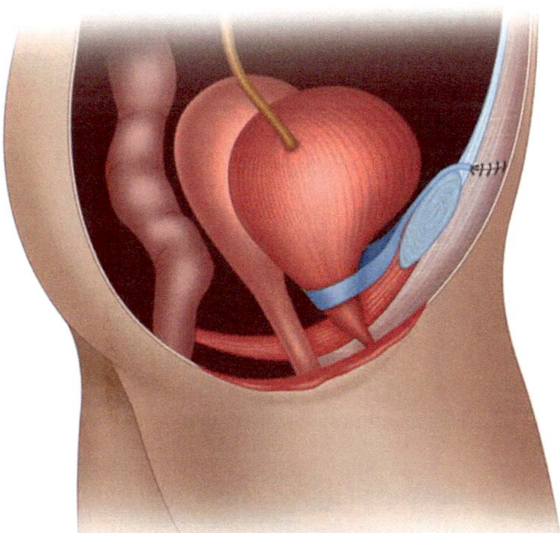

Fig. 10.13 Diagram showing the location of the pubovaginal sling

is the need for subsequent injections and its higher costs [24, 32]. Massive urethral prolapse is reported after transurethral Coaptite injection [21, 23, 31] (Fig. 10.14).

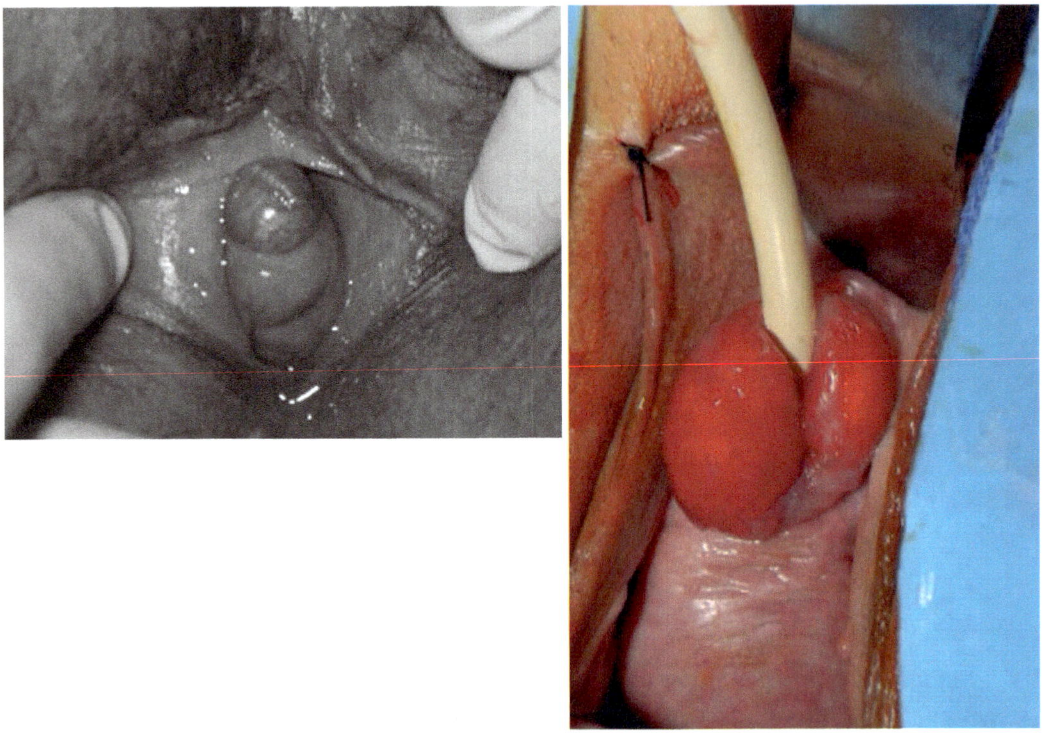

Fig. 10.14 Urethral prolapse after transurethral bulking agent injection

Pubovaginal Slings (PVSs)

Compared to mid-urethral slings, pubovaginal slings yield superior continence results owing to their strategic placement at the bladder neck, taking advantage of unique anatomical factors. Among various sling materials, autologous fascia pubovaginal slings are considered the benchmark, excelling in terms of performance. While the autologous sling exhibits reduced urethral perforation rates, it requires longer operative time, and patients may experience heightened postoperative pain and extended hospital stays compared to procedures involving biological or synthetic grafts [28].

The most commonly used tissues for autologous PVSs are the fascia lata (Fig. 10.15) and the rectus sheath (Fig. 10.16).

The success rates of pubovaginal slings range from 31% to 97%. Morgan et al. reported a cure rate of 85% in 247 patients after a mean of 51 months of follow-up. In all, 92% of the

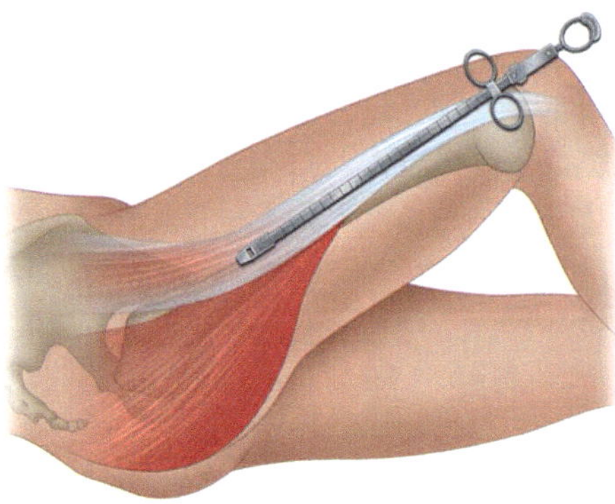

Fig. 10.15 The autologous fascia lata

patients in this study reported high satisfaction and overall improvement in their quality of life [26].

Iatrogenic bladder injury is a common complication after a PVS surgery, leading to urinary urgency, bladder outlet obstruction, and urinary retention. Urinary urge incontinence is reported in 20% of patients who received a PVS. Complete urinary obstruction and retention are reported in

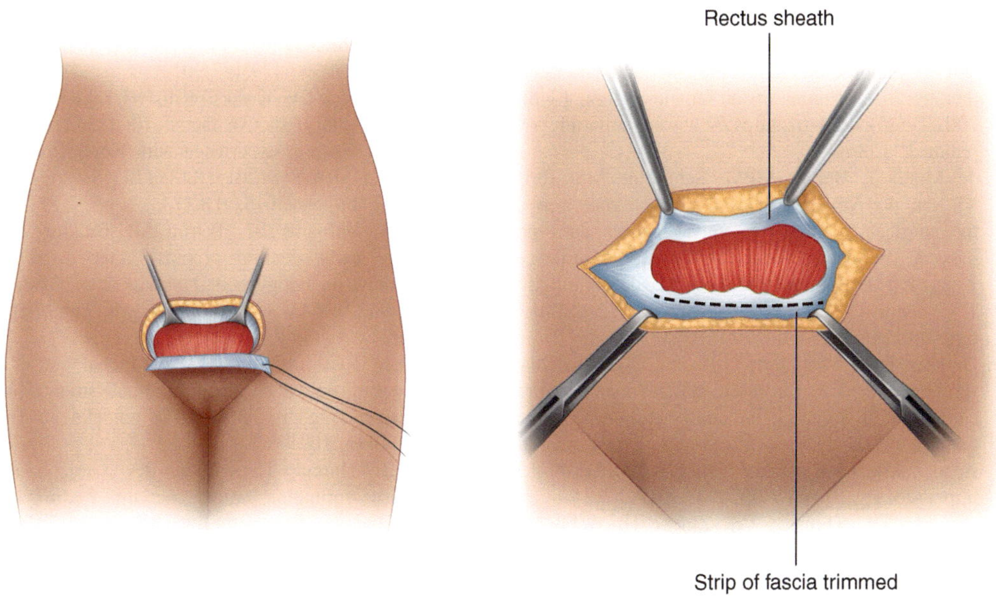

Fig. 10.16 The autologous rectus sheath

about 5% of patients. Brubaker et al. reported a new onset of urinary urgency and urge incontinence in 1.2% and persisted urinary retention in 2.4% of 243 patients who received a PVS after a mean of 60 months of follow-up. In all, 83% of the patients in this study reported high satisfaction and overall improvement in their quality of life [4].

Pubovaginal Sling Erosion

The incidence of PBS sling erosion and exposure mainly depends on the sling material. Sling perforation occurs 15 times more in synthetic slings than in autologous slings [3]. Only a few cases of autologous sling perforation have been reported in the literature [17]. The management of sling perforation includes the removal of the sling and simple urethral repair. In all, 44%–100% of patients developed recurrent SUI after removing the perforated sling [2, 5]. Urethral bulking agents and PVSs can be used to treat SUI after removing the perforated sling. Higher incontinence rates are observed after secondary treatments if the perforation affects the bladder neck [3].

References

1. Ackerman AL, Blaivas J, Anger JT. Female urethral reconstruction. Curr Bladder Dysfunct Rep. 2010;5(4):225–32. https://doi.org/10.1007/s11884-010-0071-6.
2. Amundsen CL, Flynn BJ, Webster GD. Urethral erosion after synthetic and nonsynthetic pubovaginal slings: differences in management and continence outcome. J Urol. 2003;170(1):134–7.; discussion 137. https://doi.org/10.1097/01.ju.0000064442.45724.af.
3. Blaivas JG, Sandhu J. Urethral reconstruction after erosion of slings in women. Curr Opin Urol. 2004;14(6):335–8. https://doi.org/10.1097/00042307-200411000-00007.
4. Brubaker L, Richter HE, Norton PA, Albo M, Zyczynski HM, Chai TC, Zimmern P, Kraus S, Sirls L, Kusek JW, Stoddard A, Tennstedt S, Gormley EA, Urinary Incontinence Treatment Network. 5-year continence rates, satisfaction and adverse events of burch urethropexy and fascial sling surgery for urinary incontinence. J Urol. 2012;187(4):1324–30. https://doi.org/10.1016/j.juro.2011.11.087.
5. Clemens JQ, DeLancey JO, Faerber GJ, Westney OL, Mcguire EJ. Urinary tract erosions after synthetic pubovaginal slings: diagnosis and management strategy. Urology. 2000;56(4):589–94. https://doi.org/10.1016/s0090-4295(00)00740-8.
6. Conces MR, Williamson SR, Montironi R, Lopez-Beltran A, Scarpelli M, Cheng L. Urethral caruncle: clinicopathologic features of 41 cases. Hum Pathol. 2012;43(9):1400–4. https://doi.org/10.1016/j.humpath.2011.10.015.

7. Dalbagni G, Donat SM, Eschwège P, Herr HW, Zelefsky MJ. Results of high dose rate brachytherapy, anterior pelvic exenteration and external beam radiotherapy for carcinoma of the female urethra. J Urol. 2001;166(5):1759–61. https://www.ncbi.nlm.nih.gov/pubmed/11586218.
8. de Mooij Y, Burger MPM, Schilthuis MS, Buist M, van der Velden J. Partial urethral resection in the surgical treatment of vulvar cancer does not have a significant impact on urinary continence. A confirmation of an authority-based opinion. Int J Gynecol Cancer. 2007;17(1):294–7. https://doi.org/10.1111/j.1525-1438.2007.00788.x.
9. Derksen JW, Visser O, de la Rivière GB, Meuleman EJ, Heldeweg EA, Lagerveld BW. Primary urethral carcinoma in females: an epidemiologic study on demographical factors, histological types, tumour stage and survival. World J Urol. 2013;31(1):147–53. https://doi.org/10.1007/s00345-012-0882-5.
10. Dimarco DS, Dimarco CS, Zincke H, Webb MJ, Bass SE, Slezak JM, Lightner DJ. Surgical treatment for local control of female urethral carcinoma. Urol Oncol. 2004;22(5):404–9. https://doi.org/10.1016/S1078-1439(03)00174-1.
11. Elliott CS. Female urethral stricture management: the initial experience of an female pelvic medicine and reconstructive surgery-trained urologist. Female Pelvic Med Reconstr Surg. 2021;27(4):e516–20. https://doi.org/10.1097/SPV.0000000000000969.
12. Escribano Patiño G, Husillos Alonso A, Rodriguez Fernandez E, Cancho Gil MJ, Hernandez Fernandez C. Urethral stricture in women. Arch Esp Urol. 2014;67(1):129–37. https://www.ncbi.nlm.nih.gov/pubmed/24531681.
13. Fagan GE, Hertig AT. Carcinoma of the female urethra; review of the literature; report of eight cases. Obstet Gynecol. 1955;6(1):1–11. https://www.ncbi.nlm.nih.gov/pubmed/14394542.
14. Faiena I, Koprowski C, Tunuguntla H. Female urethral reconstruction. J Urol. 2016;195(3):557–67. https://doi.org/10.1016/j.juro.2015.07.124.
15. Foster J, Lemack G, Zimmern P. Skene's gland cyst excision. Int Urogynecol J. 2016;27(5):817–20. https://doi.org/10.1007/s00192-015-2872-9.
16. Gakis G, Witjes JA, Compérat E, Cowan NC, De Santis M, Lebret T, Ribal MJ, Sherif AM, European Association, of Urology. EAU guidelines on primary urethral carcinoma. Eur Urol. 2013;64(5):823–30. https://doi.org/10.1016/j.eururo.2013.03.044.
17. Golomb J, Groutz A, Mor Y, Leibovitch I, Ramon J. Management of urethral erosion caused by a pubovaginal fascial sling. Urology. 2001;57(1):159–60. https://doi.org/10.1016/s0090-4295(00)00887-6.
18. Greenwell TJ, Castle C, Andrich DE, MacDonald JT, Nicol DL, Mundy AR. Repeat urethrotomy and dilation for the treatment of urethral stricture are neither clinically effective nor cost-effective. J Urol. 2004;172(1):275–7. https://doi.org/10.1097/01.ju.0000132156.76403.8f.
19. Johnson DE, O'Connell JR. Primary carcinima of female urethra. Urology. 1983;21(1):42–5. https://doi.org/10.1016/0090-4295(83)90120-6.
20. Kang M, Jeong CW, Kwak C, Kim HH, Ku JH. Survival outcomes and predictive factors for female urethral cancer: long-term experience with Korean patients. J Korean Med Sci. 2015;30(8):1143–9. https://doi.org/10.3346/jkms.2015.30.8.1143.
21. Ko EY, Williams BF, Petrou SP. Bulking agent induced early urethral prolapse after distal urethrectomy. Int Urogynecol J Pelvic Floor Dysfunct. 2007;18(12):1511–3. https://doi.org/10.1007/s00192-007-0439-0.
22. Kobashi KC, Vasavada S, Bloschichak A, et al. Updates to surgical treatment of female stress urinary incontinence (SUI): AUA/SUFU guideline. J Urol. 2023;209(6):1091–8.
23. Lai HH, Hurtado EA, Appell RA. Large urethral prolapse formation after calcium hydroxylapatite (Coaptite) injection. Int Urogynecol J Pelvic Floor Dysfunct. 2008;19(9):1315–7. https://doi.org/10.1007/s00192-008-0604-0.
24. Maher CF, O'Reilly BA, Dwyer PL, Carey MP, Cornish A, Schluter P. Pubovaginal sling versus transurethral Macroplastique for stress urinary incontinence and intrinsic sphincter deficiency: a prospective randomised controlled trial. BJOG. 2005;112(6):797–801. https://doi.org/10.1111/j.1471-0528.2005.00547.x.
25. Merimsky E. Case profile: retention secondary to urethral stricture in the female. Urology. 1985; https://pascal-francis.inist.fr/vibad/index.php?action=getRecordDetail&idt=8673464.
26. Morgan TO Jr, Westney OL, McGuire EJ. Pubovaginal sling: 4-YEAR outcome analysis and quality of life assessment. J Urol. 2000;163(6):1845–8. https://doi.org/10.1016/s0022-5347(05)67557-x.
27. Narayan P, Konety B. Surgical treatment of female urethral carcinoma. Urol Clin North Am. 1992;19(2):373–82. https://www.ncbi.nlm.nih.gov/pubmed/1574827.
28. Niknejad K, Plzak LS 3rd, Staskin DR, Loughlin KR. Autologous and synthetic urethral slings for female incontinence. Urol Clin North Am. 2002;29(3):597–611. https://doi.org/10.1016/s0094-0143(02)00074-5.
29. Niu S, Didde RD, Schuchmann JK, Zoorob D. Gartner's duct cysts: a review of surgical management and a new technique using fluorescein dye. Int Urogynecol J. 2020;31(1):55–61. https://doi.org/10.1007/s00192-019-04091-9.
30. Osman NI, Mangera A, Chapple CR. A systematic review of surgical techniques used in the treatment of female urethral stricture. Eur Urol. 2013;64(6):965–73. https://doi.org/10.1016/j.eururo.2013.07.038.
31. Palma PCR, Riccetto CLZ, Martins MHT, Herrmann V, de Fraga R, Billis A, Netto NR Jr. Massive prolapse of the urethral mucosa following periurethral

injection of calcium hydroxylapatite for stress urinary incontinence. Int Urogynecol J Pelvic Floor Dysfunct. 2006;17(6):670–1. https://doi.org/10.1007/s00192-005-0038-x.
32. Plotti F, Zullo MA, Palaia I, Angioli R, Panici PB. Urinary incontinence after radical vulvectomy treated with Macroplastique implantation. J Minim Invasive Gynecol. 2008;15(1):113–5. https://doi.org/10.1016/j.jmig.2007.08.607.
33. Reid GC, DeLancey JO, Hopkins MP, Roberts JA, Morley GW. Urinary incontinence following radical vulvectomy. Obstet Gynecol. 1990;75(5):852–8. https://www.ncbi.nlm.nih.gov/pubmed/2325969.
34. Romero Pérez P, Mira Llinares A. Renal and ureteral complications of urethral stenosis. Actas Urol Esp. 1995;19(6):432–40. https://europepmc.org/article/med/8571802.
35. Rosenblum N, Nitti VW. Female urethral reconstruction. Urol Clin North Am. 2011;38(1):55–64., vi. https://doi.org/10.1016/j.ucl.2010.12.008.
36. Shah SR, Biggs GY, Rosenblum N, Nitti VW. Surgical management of Skene's gland abscess/infection: a contemporary series. Int Urogynecol J. 2012;23(2):159–64. https://doi.org/10.1007/s00192-011-1488-y.
37. Sherman KJ, Daling JR, McKnight B, Chu J. Hormonal factors in vulvar cancer. A case-control study. J Reprod Med. 1994;39(11):857–61. https://www.ncbi.nlm.nih.gov/pubmed/7853273.
38. Shim JS, Oh MM, Lee JG, Bae JH. Anterior urethrectomy for primary carcinoma of the female urethra mimicking a urethral caruncle. Int Neurourol J. 2013;17(4):197–9. https://doi.org/10.5213/inj.2013.17.4.197.
39. Sui W, RoyChoudhury A, Wenske S, Decastro GJ, McKiernan JM, Anderson CB. Outcomes and prognostic factors of primary urethral cancer. Urology. 2017;100:180–6. https://doi.org/10.1016/j.urology.2016.09.042.
40. Surabhi VR, Menias CO, George V, Siegel CL, Prasad SR. Magnetic resonance imaging of female urethral and periurethral disorders. Radiol Clin North Am. 2013;51(6):941–53. https://doi.org/10.1016/j.rcl.2013.07.001.
41. Wechter ME, Wu JM, Marzano D, Haefner H. Management of Bartholin duct cysts and abscesses: a systematic review. Obstet Gynecol Surv. 2009;64(6):395–404. https://doi.org/10.1097/OGX.0b013e31819f9c76.

11 Transurethral Bladder Surgery

Joshua J. Meeks

Introduction

Bladder cancer (BCa) is the ninth-most common cancer in the USA, with 82,290 new diagnoses annually, including 19,870 women [4]. The significant risk factors for BCa in women are early menopause and cigarette smoking [5, 6]. Despite a lower incidence, women are diagnosed with BCa at a more advanced stage and have a higher risk of death from BCa [7]. The causes of increased aggressiveness of BCa in women are not understood, but potential mechanisms include decreased detection of early-stage BCa or biologically more lethal tumor subtypes [7].

The first symptom for most BCas is gross or microscopic hematuria evaluated by imaging and cystoscopy [2]. After identifying a bladder mass, the next step is surgical removal of the tumor. Transurethral resection of a bladder tumor (TURBT) is the most frequently performed surgery for BCa, with nearly all patients having at least one TURBT [8]. Among urologic procedures, TURBT is the third most frequent procedure after catheterization and cystoscopy [8]. While TURBT is a routine urologic surgery, the complication rate is 4–6%, with a 30- and 90-day mortality rate of 1.3% and 3.3%, respectively [9].

J. J. Meeks (✉)
Departments of Urology and Biochemistry, Feinberg School of Medicine, Northwestern University, Chicago, IL, USA
e-mail: joshua.meeks@northwestern.edu

During transurethral resection of a bladder tumor (TURBT), the surgeon uses an endoscopic resectoscope with a cautery loop directing monopolar or bipolar energy to resect the tumor [10]. Surgery is usually performed in an outpatient setting under anesthesia [11]. The guideline-directed goal of nearly every TURBT is to resect the tumor completely and obtain a pathologic stage that includes sampling the detrusor [12, 13]. While most BCas are stage I or less, called non-muscle-invasive BCa (NMIBC), a precise pathologic evaluation of the detrusor muscle is essential for staging. In this chapter, we discuss the most common complications of TURBT, highlight their incidence in women, and describe their recognition and management.

Bladder Perforation

Background The bladder is comprised of four layers: the urothelium (in direct contact with urine), the lamina propria, the detrusor, and the fat outside the bladder. Anatomically, the bladder is located in the space of Retzius in the retroperitoneum, but the peritoneum covers the dome and posterior bladder. Thus, perforation of the bladder can result in an opening to the peritoneal or retroperitoneal space, depending on the location of the perforation. The overall risk of perforation is between 0.5% and 1% [3] and is directly related to tumor size [14]. Yet, in a prospective

M. Hoffman et al. (eds.), *Major Complications of Female Pelvic Surgery*,
https://doi.org/10.1007/978-3-031-66772-5_11

cohort of 36 patients in whom a cystogram was routinely performed, 21 (58%) were found to have perforations [14]. Perforation has been reported at a threefold higher rate in females in some series (female and male, 7.2% and 2.6%, respectively, $p < 0.001$) [15]. More than 80% of perforations are extraperitoneal [16]. The bladder wall has a thickness that can vary from millimeters to centimeters, depending on the age and gender of the patient, with most women having a thinner bladder wall.

Prevention In patients with an extremely thin bladder wall, it can be challenging to prevent bladder perforation, and complications after TURBT are inversely associated with body mass index (BMI) [17]. Yet, there are technical and anesthetic maneuvers to decrease the risk of perforation. For each tumor resection or "swipe" of the electrocautery loop, the surgeon should attempt to identify the location of the normal bladder wall. Commonly, perforations occur when the loop is inadvertently extended past a tumor and touches the posterior wall. Perforations encountered during resection of lateral BCa are often caused by obturator nerve reflex and can be mitigated by paralysis or careful resection with a "staccato" or tap-tap technique [18]. The staccato tapping of the cutting cautery can halt a resection that is deeper than anticipated, preventing a larger perforation. We recommend this stop-and-start or staccato technique to adjust the resection depth during each transurethral resection (TUR) swipe. Anterior perforations, secondary to bladder movement during breathing, can be prevented by stabilizing the bladder with the nondominant hand or controlling breathing with intubation. The thickness of the bladder, and therefore the depth of resection, can be managed by performing the resection under limited bladder filling to decrease the wall tension. During a re-resection, in which a prior tumor area is mostly composed of scar tissue, perforation can be avoided by starting the swipe in a normal bladder area outside of the scar. Resection experience has been associated with a higher risk of complications, with TURBT performed by residents often associated with greater frequency. Finally, the use of bipolar energy has been associated with a lower risk of perforation (0.6% and 0.3%, odds ratio (OR) 0.57) [19] but not necessarily obturator reflex [20].

Recognition Visual identification of the fat layer beyond the detrusor is the first recognition of perforation. The fat layer can be either white or yellow but has a glistening appearance. In some cases, the muscle layer can have a fat layer, which may mistook for perforation. Once a bladder perforation is recognized, the next step is performing an intraoperative cystogram to confirm the perforation and identify the location as either intraperitoneal or extraperitoneal. Finally, manual palpation of the abdomen and pelvis can be performed to determine if irrigation has escaped the bladder and is palpable as ascites. Once a perforation is identified, the procedure should be stopped once hemostasis is achieved to avoid further extravasation of irrigation into the abdomen. A significant advantage of bipolar over monopolar resection is using normal saline for irrigation in bipolar cautery, which will have less risk of hyponatremia if perforation occurs. Unrecognized injuries can cause abdominal pain, urinary ascites, and increased serum creatinine values [21].

Management The management of bladder perforation is determined by the size of the perforation and its location [21]. Extraperitoneal perforations can be managed conservatively with a Foley catheter to drain the bladder for 7–10 days before repeated testing with a cystogram to confirm healing [22]. Intraperitoneal bladder perforations are usually treated with repair by laparotomy or laparoscopy. Due to the larger volume of irrigation fluids used during a transurethral resection, removal of this fluid is often necessary. If a laparotomy is not necessary, a drain may be placed by the surgeon or interventional radiology to remove the irrigation fluid.

Bleeding and Reoperation/Transfusion

Background It is nearly impossible to accurately measure blood loss during TURBT because of the large amount of irrigation fluid used for visualization. The complication rate of bleeding is 1.1% [3]. Bleeding during TURBT occurs during resection of the vascular tumor and/or resection into the bladder wall for staging. Most of the larger blood vessels in the bladder are found in the detrusor layer and may be encountered during muscle resection. During TURBT, the blood vessels are sealed with fulguration and cautery [10]. Hypothesized mechanisms of postoperative bleeding include stretching of the bladder fibers from urinary retention, increased abdominal pressure from straining, or decreased clotting from anti-coagulation medications. Since TURBT is an outpatient procedure, blood counts are not measured, and, for most patients, the change in hemoglobin is not significant. The rate of transfusion after TURBT varies between 0.6% and 2.9% depending on the size of the tumor [23]. Yet, postoperative bleeding is a significant complication requiring hospitalization and return to the operating room to control it. Bleeding is the common cause of reoperation after TURBT, occurring in 1.5% of resections [9] with readmission to the hospital in 3.7% [9].

Prevention Risk factors for postoperative bleeding include use of blood thinners and antiplatelet medications and broad and deep tumor resections [24]. Because of comorbid conditions, use of blood-thinning medications cannot be prevented. After resection of the tumor, hemostasis is achieved by coagulating the resection area and surrounding epithelium. Bleeding can be decreased by technical attention to each resection site and evaluation under lower hydrostatic pressure by underfilling the bladder. Stretching of the bladder fibers can be limited by the use of a postoperative catheter. Bladder irrigation, run through a three-way catheter, can decrease the formation of clots in patients after surgery and prevent catheter obstruction. Preventing post-TUR straining to avoid elevations in pelvic venous pressure is also important for preventing bleeding. Avoidance of heavy lifting or strenuous activity should be emphasized. Commonly, post-resection bleeding will occur after the patient strains to have a bowel movement. Liberal use of periprocedural laxatives and stool softeners can help avoid this complication.

Recognition Bleeding during TURBT can occur at any time but can often be managed technically. Starting a resection at one edge of the tumor and then progressing to the other side is a surgical strategy to decrease bleeding from the tumor bed. Achieving hemostasis is more challenging if the specimen is resected in multiple areas. A rollerball electrode, applied with pressure in a rolling motion over the base of the tumor, can be applied after a resection to ensure hemostasis is obtained. After the TURBT, either a voiding trial or a postoperative period of catheter observation allows for identifying any hematuria. While light pink- to blush-colored urine is normal after TURBT, identifying dark, "merlot"-colored urine and/or passing clots implies higher amounts of bleeding.

Management During surgery, every effort should be made to decrease surgical bleeding at the resection site of the tumor. This involves multiple evaluations of the tumor bed. Postoperatively, a three-way irrigating catheter can be used for continuous bladder irrigation (CBI) if bleeding is identified. This often decreases the risk of clot formation but requires 23-h hospitalization. If bleeding does not improve with CBI or continues after CBI, the patient will likely need to return to the operating room for clot evacuation and fulguration of bleeding. In a patient with a perforation, if bleeding occurs, CBI is not possible and return to the operation room is necessary. Unfortunately, tranexamic acid has not decreased the risk of bleeding or complications after TUR procedures [25]. During clot evacuation, we favor gentle pressure to remove clots rather than forceful piston irrigation. This decreases the risk of perforation. The bleeding site is often a blood vessel in the muscle layer that requires further coagulation. Most patients are then observed overnight to ensure that no further bleeding occurs.

Cystitis: Infection/Urinary Tract Infection (UTI)

Background The most common cause of 30-day complications are associated with infections representing almost 70% of all complications after TURBT [9] occurring in 2% [3]. Infection can occur before, during, and after the procedure. Before surgery, patients may be colonized and/or at risk of recurrent UTIs. Men are more likely to be catheter-dependent, but the rate of asymptomatic bacteriuria is greater in women. During surgery, contaminated instruments or infections from proximity to the perianal flora can be the source of bacterial infection. After surgery, using catheters, compromised bladder emptying, and necrotic tissue can be a nidus for persistent infection. UTIs can result in delayed recovery from surgery, causing the postponement of intravesical therapy. Disseminated infection from sepsis is rare after TURBT.

Prevention UTIs may be prevented by routine preoperative urinalysis. Every hospital system has a different policy on routine preoperative urine cultures for patients with uncompromised immune systems and no prior UTIs [26]. Patients with indwelling catheters should be changed before surgery, and a urine culture should be sent within 72 h before surgery. If significant bacteria are identified, the patient can be treated before surgery with an oral antibiotic, admitted for intravenous (IV) antibiotics, or treated preoperatively with culture-directed antibiotics. Prevention of sepsis can be managed by early intervention with antibiotics.

Recognition The identification of post-operative UTIs can be made by discussing symptoms with the patient or routine urine culture. For patients with a catheter for >72 h, sending a urine culture from the catheter before removal is reasonable. Unfortunately, the symptoms of a UTI overlap heavily with the expected bladder urgency and dysuria after TURBT. In patients with symptoms possibly consistent with UTI, we send the urine for culture to determine whether an infection is present.

Management Culture-directed antibiotics usually decrease lower urinary tract symptoms if a UTI is detected. In patients with persistent and/or recurrent UTIs after TUR, evaluation of the bladder by cystoscopy and measurement of post-void residual are the next steps. Cystoscopy can identify necrotic scar after TURBT that can be a nidus for infection and be brushed from the bladder epithelium. The post-void residual can be measured to ensure that the bladder is completely emptied to prevent recurrent infections.

Noninfective Cystitis and Voiding Discomfort

Background Irritative bladder symptoms can affect patients' quality of life after TURBT with a frequency of 17% [27]. These symptoms often include burning (dysuria), urgency, frequency, bladder, and penile pain. Dysuria is secondary to irritation of the bladder mucosa from extensive resection or surgical manipulation of the bladder and urethra. The bladder can be further irritated by postoperative intravesical therapy with chemotherapy, a guideline-recommended treatment for patients with newly diagnosed bladder cancers [27]. These symptoms, often heard but challenging to treat by the surgeon, significantly impact the quality of life of patients with BCa and can delay intravesical therapy.

Prevention The cause of noninfective cystitis and discomfort after TURBT is unknown and therefore challenging to prevent. One method to decrease symptoms can be a preoperative discussion with the patient about expectations and potential voiding symptoms after surgery to establish expectations.

Recognition Most patients will have at least mild urinary symptoms after TURBT, and discussions with physicians and members of the urology team can improve communication to help decrease symptoms.

Management Most irritative voiding symptoms will improve with time and resolve by 3–4 weeks after surgery. The most common symptom of urgency can be treated with anticholinergic or overactive bladder medications [28]. Dysuria may be improved by phenazopyridine. Anti-inflammatory medications can also reduce the inflammatory symptoms after surgery.

Summary

Transurethral resection of a bladder tumor is a frequently performed surgery to diagnose and manage BCa [8]. The overall complication rate ranges from 4 to 6%. Complications range from mild, irritative symptoms to bladder perforation, resulting in laparotomy. Early identification and management of these complications can improve recovery and clinical outcomes for patients with BCa.

References

1. Hollenbeck BK, Miller DC, Taub D, Dunn RL, Khuri SF, Henderson WG, et al. Risk factors for adverse outcomes after transurethral resection of bladder tumors. Cancer. 2006;106:1527–35. https://doi.org/10.1002/cncr.21765.
2. Sharma S, Ksheersagar P, Sharma P. Diagnosis and treatment of bladder cancer. Am Fam Physician. 2009;80:717–23.
3. Gregg JR, McCormick B, Wang L, Cohen P, Sun D, Penson DF, et al. Short term complications from transurethral resection of bladder tumor. Can J Urol. 2016;23(2):8198–203.
4. Siegel RL, et al. Cancer statistics, 2023. CA Cancer J Clinic. 2023;73(1):17–48. Wiley Online Library. [cited 1 Jul 2023]. Available: https://acsjournals.onlinelibrary.wiley.com/doi/10.3322/caac.21763.
5. Freedman ND, Silverman DT, Hollenbeck AR, Schatzkin A, Abnet CC. Association between smoking and risk of bladder cancer among men and women. JAMA. 2011;306:737–45. https://doi.org/10.1001/jama.2011.1142.
6. McGrath M, Michaud DS, De Vivo I. Hormonal and reproductive factors and the risk of bladder cancer in women. Am J Epidemiol. 2006;163:236–44. https://doi.org/10.1093/aje/kwj028.
7. Matulewicz RS, Demzik AL, DeLancey JO, Popescu O, Makarov DV, Meeks JJ. Disparities in the diagnostic evaluation of microhematuriaand implications for the detection of urologic malignancy. Urol Oncol. 2019;37(300):e1–300.e7. https://doi.org/10.1016/j.urolonc.2019.01.007.
8. Lee F, Patel HRH, Emberton M. The "top 10" urological procedures: a study of hospital episodes statistics 1998–99. BJU Int. 2002;90:1–6. https://doi.org/10.1046/j.1464-410x.2002.02833.x.
9. Pereira JF, Pareek G, Mueller-Leonhard C, Zhang Z, Amin A, Mega A, et al. The perioperative morbidity of transurethral resection of bladder tumor: implications for quality improvement. Urology. 2019;125:131–7. https://doi.org/10.1016/j.urology.2018.10.027.
10. Herr HW. Surgical factors in the treatment of superficial and invasive bladder cancer. Urol Clin North Am. 2005;32:157–64. https://doi.org/10.1016/j.ucl.2005.02.003.
11. Kim LHC, Patel MI. Transurethral resection of bladder tumour (TURBT). Transl Androl Urol. 2020;9:3056–72. https://doi.org/10.21037/tau.2019.09.38.
12. Flaig TW, Spiess PE, Abern M, Agarwal N, Bangs R, Boorjian SA, et al. NCCN Guidelines® insights: bladder cancer, version 2.2022. J Natl Compr Cancer Netw. 2022;20:866–78. https://doi.org/10.6004/jnccn.2022.0041.
13. Chang SS, Boorjian SA, Chou R, Clark PE, Daneshmand S, Konety BR, et al. Diagnosis and treatment of non-muscle invasive bladder cancer: AUA/SUO guideline. J Urol. 2016;196:1021–9. https://doi.org/10.1016/j.juro.2016.06.049.
14. Balbay MD, Cimentepe E, Unsal A, Bayrak O, Koç A, Akbulut Z. The actual incidence of bladder perforation following transurethral bladder surgery. J Urol. 2005;174:2260–2., discussion 2262–2263. https://doi.org/10.1097/01.ju.0000181811.61199.35.
15. Herkommer K, Hofer C, Gschwend JE, Kron M, Treiber U. Gender and body mass index as risk factors for bladder perforation during primary transurethral resection of bladder tumors. J Urol. 2012;187:1566–70. https://doi.org/10.1016/j.juro.2011.12.114.
16. Collado A, Chéchile GE, Salvador J, Vicente J. Early complications of endoscopic treatment for superficial bladder tumors. J Urol. 2000;164:1529–32.
17. Poletajew S, Krajewski W, Gajewska D, Sondka-Migdalska J, Borowik M, Buraczyński P, et al. Prediction of the risk of surgical complications in patients undergoing monopolar transurethral resection of bladder tumour—a prospective multicentre observational study. Arch Med Sci. 2019;16:863–70. https://doi.org/10.5114/aoms.2019.88430.

18. Panagoda PI, Vasdev N, Gowrie-Mohan S. Avoiding the Obturator jerk during TURBT. Curr Urol. 2018;12:1–5. https://doi.org/10.1159/000447223.
19. Sugihara T, Yasunaga H, Horiguchi H, Matsui H, Nishimatsu H, Nakagawa T, et al. Comparison of perioperative outcomes including severe bladder injury between Monopolar and bipolar transurethral resection of bladder tumors: a population based comparison. J Urol. 2014;192:1355–9. https://doi.org/10.1016/j.juro.2014.05.100.
20. Ozer K, Horsanali MO, Gorgel SN, Ozbek E. Bladder injury secondary to obturator reflex is more common with plasmakinetic transurethral resection than monopolar transurethral resection of bladder cancer. Cent European J Urol. 2015;68:284–8. https://doi.org/10.5173/ceju.2015.565.
21. Corriere JN, Sandler CM. Management of the ruptured bladder: seven years of experience with 111 cases. J Trauma. 1986;26:830–3. https://doi.org/10.1097/00005373-198609000-00009.
22. Anderson RE, Keihani S, Moses RA, Nocera AP, Selph JP, Castillejo Becerra CM, et al. Current Management of Extraperitoneal Bladder Injuries: results from the multi-institutional Genito-urinary trauma study (MiGUTS). J Urol. 2020;204:538–44. https://doi.org/10.1097/JU.0000000000001075.
23. Matulewicz RS, Sharma V, McGuire BB, Oberlin DT, Perry KT, Nadler RB. The effect of surgical duration of transurethral resection of bladder tumors on post-operative complications: an analysis of ACS NSQIP data. Urol Oncol. 2015;33(338):e19–338.e24. https://doi.org/10.1016/j.urolonc.2015.05.011.
24. Konishi T, Washino S, Nakamura Y, Ohshima M, Saito K, Arai Y, et al. Risks and complications of transurethral resection of bladder tumors in patients receiving antiplatelet and/or anticoagulant therapy: a retrospective cohort study. BMC Urol. 2017;17:118. https://doi.org/10.1186/s12894-017-0309-0.
25. Pranata FH, Kloping YP, Hidayatullah F, Rahman ZA, Yogiswara N, Rahman IA, et al. The role of tranexamic acid in reducing bleeding during transurethral resection of the prostate: an updated systematic review and meta-analysis of randomized controlled trials. Indian J Urol. 2022;38:258–67. https://doi.org/10.4103/iju.iju_98_22.
26. Lightner DJ, Wymer K, Sanchez J, Kavoussi L. Best practice statement on urologic procedures and antimicrobial prophylaxis. J Urol. 2020;203:351–6. https://doi.org/10.1097/JU.0000000000000509.
27. Filson CP, Montgomery JS, Dailey SM, Crossley HS, Lentz H, Tallman CT, et al. Complications associated with single-dose, perioperative mitomycin-C for patients undergoing bladder tumor resection. Urol Oncol. 2014;32(40):e1–8. https://doi.org/10.1016/j.urolonc.2013.04.006.
28. Sun K, Wang D, Wu G, Ma J, Wang T, Wu J, et al. Mirabegron improves the irritative symptoms caused by BCG immunotherapy after transurethral resection of bladder tumors. Cancer Med. 2021;10:7534–41. https://doi.org/10.1002/cam4.4278.

Partial Cystectomy

12

Óscar Rodríguez Faba, Alberto Breda,
and Joan Palou

Introduction

Partial cystectomy (PC) is a urological surgical technique in which only a portion of the bladder is resected for benign and/or oncological conditions [1].

The advantages include preservation of a functional and continent urinary reservoir, and potency in men [2].

Classic indications for PC include treatment of bladder cancer (BC), specifically, primary, solitary, and muscle-invasive or high-grade tumors in a region of the bladder that allows complete excision with adequate margins, in a patient with biopsy-proved absence of carcinoma in situ (CIS) in the remaining bladder [3].

Other indications for PC include [3]:

1. The inability to resect tumors by an endoscopic approach because of their size or location.
2. A need for adequate biopsy of the full thickness of the bladder wall.
3. Radiation-induced ulcerations.
4. A tumor overlying a ureteral orifice with the need for ureteral reimplantation.
5. Palliation of severe local symptoms.
6. Excision of a bladder tumor in a patient who refuses urinary diversion.
7. A very-high-risk patient in whom urinary diversion is deemed inappropriate.
8. Excision of a bladder diverticulum.
9. A patient with colon cancer invading the bladder.

The reality is that the real incidence is very low, and it is used mainly only in patients with tumor in a bladder diverticulum or a partial cystectomy in fragile patients to avoid cystectomy.

Relative and absolute contraindications for PC include the presence of multiple tumors, carcinoma in situ (CIS), prostatic and/or trigone involvement, inability to resect with secure margins, prior radiation therapy, inability to maintain an adequate bladder volume after resection, evidence of extravesical tumor extension, and generally unfit patients for surgery.

The indication of PC ranges from 7 to 10% of all the cystectomies performed according to studies of the National Cancer Database [4]. Nevertheless, some specific studies have assessed that PC for BC may be overperformed, at a rate of 14% versus the commonly accepted 5–6% [5].

Ó. R. Faba · A. Breda · J. Palou (✉)
Urology Department, Universitat Autònoma de Barcelona, Fundació Puigvert, Barcelona, Spain
e-mail: jpalou@fundacio-puigvert.es

M. Hoffman et al. (eds.), *Major Complications of Female Pelvic Surgery*,
https://doi.org/10.1007/978-3-031-66772-5_12

Preoperative Workup

All candidates should be discussed in multidisciplinary committee with the same work-up for muscle-invasive bladder cancer. This comprises a complete blood test, a CT scan of the abdomen and pelvis with intravenous contrast, and thoracic CT. If there is any suspicious for bone metastasis, then a bone scan should also be indicated. Random bladder biopsies should also be performed priory to surgery to exclude multifocal disease and/or CIS. Moreover, a cystoscopy might be part of the preoperative workup to assess the location of the tumor and the bladder capacity.

Special consideration should be taken in the diagnosis and management of urachal tumors as it can be difficult to distinguish between urachal and nonurachal bladder adenocarcinomas. While various criteria have been established to rule-out in this differentiation, a practical approach was reported by Johnson et al. The clinic and pathologic characteristics required for a diagnosis include an enteric-type adenocarcinoma in the midline of the bladder, location within the bladder wall, sharp demarcation between tumor and normal urothelium, and exclusion of a primary adenocarcinoma located elsewhere that has spread secondarily to the bladder [6]. Urachal cancers may express detectable serum levels of tumor markers as carcinoembryonic antigen (CEA), cancer antigen (CA) 125, and cancer antigen (CA) 19-9, especially in the setting of locally advanced or peritoneal carcinomatosis [7, 8].

Surgical Technique

The surgical technique for an open PC has been well-described in the literature over the years by different authors [3]. A lower midline incision is made from the pubic symphysis to the level of the umbilicus. PC may be performed either transperitoneally or extraperitoneally. Dissection progresses down through the fascia, after which the peritoneum and the Retzius space are opened. To open the surgical field, the vascular pedicles might be divided on one side. The colon is partially mobilized on each side to partially expose the retroperitoneum. The ureters are carefully identified and swept medially. A surgical retractor of the surgeon's choice is recommended to be placed at this point. The pelvic lymph nodes should be removed from the obturator fossa to the common iliac vessels. After the lymphadenectomy, the bladder tumor is resected. The bladder is opened away from the site of the tumor, preferably on the anterior bladder wall. The tumor is identified intravesically and then excised with a 1–2-cm margin. Alternatively, a flexible cystoscope can be inserted to identify the location of the tumor or perform first step endoscopic approach to delineate endoscopically the location of the tumor. Next, the bladder is closed in two layers and filled to confirm that the closure is watertight. A closed suction drain is placed, and the abdominal incision is closed [9].

Robotic surgery has some advantages over open and laparoscopic surgery. It provides the surgeon with superior optics with three-dimensional visualization of the surgical field as well as improved dexterity that allows for precise intracorporeal suturing. Furthermore, patients who undergo robot-assisted PC (RAPC) could potentially benefit from earlier postoperative recovery, improved postoperative cosmesis, and reduced postoperative pain [10]. But it has been reported the increased risk of cell seeding and implantation in urothelial cell carcinoma [11].

Partial Cystectomy for Urachal Tumors

The open surgical approach for urachal adenocarcinoma proceeds in much the same way as it does for urothelial carcinoma. However, because the urachus may be involved with the tumor anywhere along its course, an "en bloc" resection of the entire urachus as well as umbilicus is required.

There is not much evidence on how to manage urachal tumors in an adult population. When a urachal mass is detected incidence of malignancy ranges from 51 to 64% [12]. The surgical technique for treating a symptomatic urachal remnant includes excision of the urachus and its tract, including the portion that is attached to the bladder dome. Open partial cystectomy is the most widely used technique for urachal disease. Robotic partial cystectomy has been described for the management of both pediatric and adult urachal disease with good results [13].

The advantage of complete excision of the urachal tract, including umbilectomy to achieve a negative surgical margin, has been described to be an important oncological aspect. The failure to perform umbilectomy is an independent predictor of increased cancer-specific mortality [14]. In other reports, the authors did not find umbilectomy to be a statistically significant factor associated with survival [15] (Figs. 12.1 and 12.2).

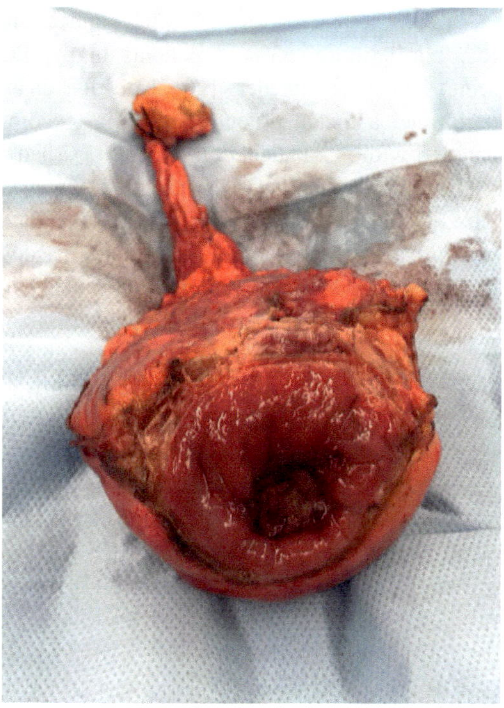

Fig. 12.1 Partial cystectomy for urachal tumor

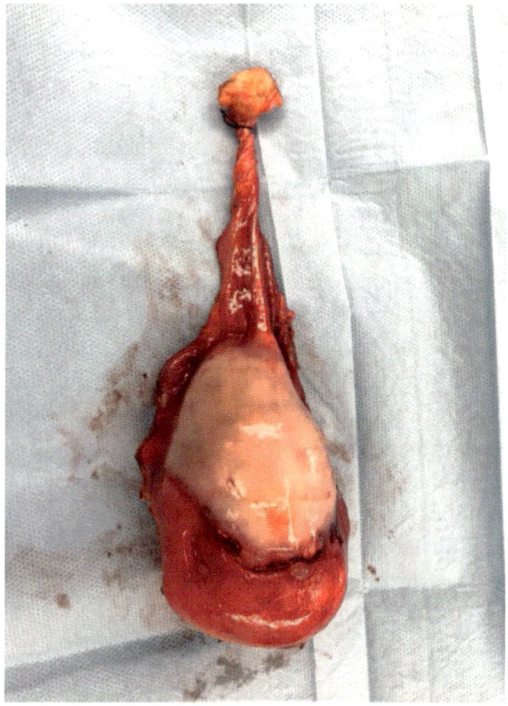

Fig. 12.2 Partial cystectomy for urachal tumor

Complications

Apart from oncological issues (recurrence, progression), the complication rate of PC ranges from 11–29% [1]. It is important to consider that lower complication and mortality rates have been reported at high-volume centers. Specifically, no cases of intrahospital mortality were identified among hospitals performing at least five PC procedures in a year [5]. Kates et al. [5] analyzed more than 10, 000 patients who underwent PC for BC (2002–2008). PC represented 13.9% of all cystectomies performed. The complications rate was 15.8%, with a mortality rate of 1.8%. Results revealed that patients who died had higher comorbidity status and were significantly older when compared to patients undergoing radical cystectomy (74.1 vs. 70.4 years; $P < 0.001$), and therefore likely represent a population. It is important to consider that a complication rate of

15.8% is markedly decreased when compared to that of radical cystectomy; 67% of radical cystectomy patients experienced an in-hospital complication and 13% had Clavien grade 3–5 complications [16].

Common complications of partial cystectomy include bleeding, infection, reduction of bladder capacity, and urinary fistula. Less commonly, some patients develop fistulas (vesicocutaneous, vesicovaginal, colovesical). Other complications include those that are possible in any major surgery: myocardial infarction, pulmonary embolus, congestive heart failure, upper gastrointestinal hemorrhage, and death [3].

The implementation of laparoscopic and robotic surgical approaches to PC represents a significant advancement and promises to further reduce the length of hospital stay, surgical morbidity, and complication rates [17]. Robotic PC results have been reported in small, single-center studies, including a heterogenous patient population. Global results report a median hospital length of stay of 1 day and an overall 90-day complication rate of 24.1% (all Clavien grades I–II) [1, 18]. Complications of robotic PC for muscle-invasive BC have been explained in detail in a retrospective series of 35 patients. Any grade complications (ileus, pneumonia, and urethral stricture) were reported in 4 patients. After 1 year, seven patients presented with recurrence; five of those patients died of their disease, and the other two died of unrelated causes [10].

Oncological Outcomes

There are not randomized trials comparing radical and partial cystectomy in the contemporary literature. Nevertheless, the retrospective data report that in selected patients who fit the profile, PC may be a good alternative.

Capitanio et al. analyzed PC and RC after matching at a ratio of 1:4 for tumor grade, pT stage, pN stage, age, race, and year of surgery. A second matched analysis was performed after adding the number of removed lymph nodes to the matching criteria. In the first analysis, the overall survival (OS) and cause-specific survival (CSS) estimates at 5 years were 57.2% and 76.4%, respectively, for PC patients and 50.2% and 65.8%, respectively, for RC patients ($P < 0.001$). In the second analysis, the OS and CSS estimates were 56.0% and 73.5%, respectively, for PC patients and 50.9% and 67.5%, respectively, for RC patients ($P = 0.03$ and $P < 0.001$ for both). When the number of removed lymph nodes was included in the third analysis, the 5-year OS and CSS estimates were 57.2% and 70.3%, respectively, for PC patients and 54.6% and 69.2%, respectively, for RC patients [19].

To assess the role of neoadjuvant chemotherapy in this field, 60 patients who achieved cT0 after receiving MVAC (methotrexate, vinblastine, doxorubicin, and cisplatin) chemotherapy followed by transurethral resection of a bladder tumor (TURBT) were studied. Fifteen of these patients subsequently underwent PC and 17 underwent RC. The 10-year metastasis-free survival (MFS) was 73% for those who underwent PC and 65% for those who underwent RC. Furthermore, 53% of patients in the PC group had intact bladders [20]. Knoedler et al. performed a matched-control analysis to compare RC with PC. Patients submitted to PC had a single tumor without CIS. They were matched based on age, gender, pathological stage, and neoadjuvant chemotherapy. The results revealed that patients undergoing PC were less likely to have multifocal bladder tumors on the final pathology as compared to those undergoing RC (15.1% vs. 32.9%). In all, 38% of patients who underwent PC developed intravesical recurrence. Five percent of PC patients experienced pelvic recurrence. At a mean follow-up of 6.2 years, 81% of patients maintained an intact bladder. Most significantly, no differences existed between PC and RC with regard to 10-year MFS (61% vs. 66%), CSS (58% vs. 63%), and OS (36% vs. 36%) [21].

Koga et al. developed a much stricter protocol. Patients received as first step a debulking TURBT with random biopsy and were subsequently considered for PC if they had intravesical circumscribed tumors ≤25% of the bladder area and no involvement of the bladder neck or trigone. They

Table 12.1 Oncological outcomes PC

Author	N (PC)	F-U (months)	Outcomes (y; %)	Characteristics
Capitanio [19]	1573	64	DSS(5y): 76.4 OS(5y):57.2	SEER database T1-4, N0-2, M0; RC vs.PC
Herr [20]	15	120	MFS (10y): 73	Neoadj MVAC RC vs. PC (T0)
Knoedler [21]	86	74	MFS (10y):61 DSS (10y):58 OS (10y);36	RC vs.PC
Koga [22]	46	45	MFS (10y): 100 DSS(5y):100	Pior TURBT
Golombos [18]	29	37	RFS (5y): 68 OS (5y): 79	Robotic

DSS Disease free survival, *OS* Overall Survival, *RFS* Recurrence free survival, *MFS* Metastasis free survival

were then submitted to radiotherapy and two cycles of cisplatin, before being restaged 4–6 weeks later. To be included as a PC candidate, the restaged TURBT must show no evidence of disease or small residual non-muscle-invasive disease. Of their initial cohort of 183 patients, 65 met the criteria, of which 46 underwent PC. Seven patients developed intravesical recurrence, all of which was superficial. Five-year CSS for this cohort was 100% [22].

One of the largest robotic PC series included 29 patients who underwent robotic PC. With a median follow-up of 37 months, the 5-year OS and recurrence-free survival (RFS) rates were 79% and 68%, respectively. Seven patients (24%) had a recurrence, three of which were local and four of which were regional or distant. Two local recurrences were managed with TURBT because there was no muscle invasion. The third local recurrence was muscle-invasive and was thus managed with a cystectomy [18] (Table 12.1).

Conclusions

- Approximately 5.8–18.9% of patients with muscle-invasive bladder cancer are suitable candidates for partial cystectomy.
- PC is indicated in patients with a normally functioning bladder with good capacity and a solitary tumor located where a 1–2-cm resection margin is possible.
- For high-risk tumors, a multimodal approach with neoadjuvant or adjuvant chemotherapy and possible radiotherapy may be needed.
- Absolute contraindications include carcinoma in situ (CIS) elsewhere in the bladder and multifocal tumors.
- After surgery, ongoing surveillance, including imaging, cystoscopy, and cytology, is important because the local recurrence rate is high (37–78%).
- Patients who have undergone partial cystectomy for bladder cancer should have cystoscopy and urinary cytological examination every 3 months for at least 2 years. Regular CT scans of the pelvis and abdomen are recommended in the first several years of follow-up.
- With proper patient selection, long-term, bladder-sparing survival rates with partial cystectomy range from 35 to 70%.

References

1. Knoedler J, Frank I. Organ-sparing surgery in urology: partial cystectomy. Curr Opin Urol. 2015;25:111–5.
2. Holzbeierlein JM, Lopez-Corona E, Bochner BH, Herr HW, Donat SM, Russo P, et al. Partial cystectomy: a contemporary review of the Memorial Sloan-Kettering Cancer Center experience and recommendations for patient selection. J Urol. 2004;172:878–81.
3. Sweeney P, Kursh ED, Resnick MI. Partial cystectomy. Urol Clin North Am. 1992;19:701–11.

4. Gray PJ, Fedewa SA, Shipley WU, Efstathiou JA, Lin CC, Zietman AL, et al. Use of potentially curative therapies for muscle-invasive bladder cancer in the United States: results from the National Cancer Data Base. Eur Urol. 2013;63:823–9.
5. Kates M, Gorin MA, Deibert CM, Pierorazio PM, Schoenberg MP, McKiernan JM, et al. In-hospital death and hospital-acquired complications among patients undergoing partial cystectomy for bladder cancer in the United States. Urol Oncol. 2014;32(53):e9–14.
6. Johnson DE, Hodge GB, Abdul-Karim FW, Ayala AG. Urachal carcinoma. Urology. 1985;26:218–21.
7. Kikuno N, Urakami S, Shigeno K, Shiina H, Igawa M. Urachal carcinoma associated with increased carbohydrate antigen 19-9 and carcinoembryonic antigen. J Urol. 2001;166:604.
8. Guarnaccia S, Pais V, Grous J, Spirito N. Adenocarcinoma of the urachus associated with elevated levels of CA 125. J Urol. 1991;145:140–1.
9. Peak TC, Hemal A. Partial cystectomy for muscle-invasive bladder cancer: a review of the literature. Transl Androl Urol. 2020;9:2938–45.
10. Alanee S, El-Zawahry A. Robotic-assisted partial cystectomy for muscle invasive bladder cancer: contemporary experience. Int J Med Robot. 2022;18:e2390.
11. Carrion A, Huguet J, Garcia-Cruz E, Izquierdo L, Mateu L, Musquera M, et al. Intraoperative prognostic factors and atypical patterns of recurrence in patients with upper urinary tract urothelial carcinoma treated with laparoscopic radical nephroureterectomy. Scand J Urol. 2016;50:305–12.
12. Ashley RA, Inman BA, Routh JC, Rohlinger AL, Husmann DA, Kramer SA. Urachal anomalies: a longitudinal study of urachal remnants in children and adults. J Urol. 2007;178:1615–8.
13. Kim DK, Lee JW, Park SY, Kim YT, Park HY, Lee TY. Initial experience with robotic-assisted laparoscopic partial cystectomy in urachal diseases. Korean J Urol. 2010;51:318–22.
14. Ashley RA, Inman BA, Sebo TJ, Leibovich BC, Blute ML, Kwon ED, et al. Urachal carcinoma: clinicopathologic features and long-term outcomes of an aggressive malignancy. Cancer. 2006;107:712–20.
15. Siefker-Radtke AO, Gee J, Shen Y, Wen S, Daliani D, Millikan RE, et al. Multimodality management of urachal carcinoma: the M. D. Anderson cancer center experience. J Urol. 2003;169:1295–8.
16. Shabsigh A, Korets R, Vora KC, Brooks CM, Cronin AM, Savage C, et al. Defining early morbidity of radical cystectomy for patients with bladder cancer using a standardized reporting methodology. Eur Urol. 2009;55:164–74.
17. Bailey GC, Frank I, Tollefson MK, Gettman MT, Knoedler JJ. Perioperative outcomes of robot-assisted laparoscopic partial cystectomy. J Robot Surg. 2018;12:223–8.
18. Golombos DM, O'Malley P, Lewicki P, Stone BV, Scherr DS. Robot-assisted partial cystectomy: perioperative outcomes and early oncological efficacy. BJU Int. 2017;119:128–34.
19. Capitanio U, Isbarn H, Shariat SF, Jeldres C, Zini L, Saad F, et al. Partial cystectomy does not undermine cancer control in appropriately selected patients with urothelial carcinoma of the bladder: a population-based matched analysist. Urology. 2009;74:858–64.
20. Herr HW, Bajorin DF, Scher HI. Neoadjuvant chemotherapy and bladder-sparing surgery for invasive bladder cancer: ten-year outcome. J Clin Oncol. 1998;16:1298–301.
21. Knoedler JJ, Boorjian SA, Kim SP, Weight CJ, Thapa P, Tarrell RF, et al. Does partial cystectomy compromise oncologic outcomes for patients with bladder cancer compared to radical cystectomy? A matched case-control analysis. J Urol. 2012;188:1115–9.
22. Koga F, Kihara K, Yoshida S, Yokoyama M, Saito K, Masuda H, et al. Selective bladder-sparing protocol consisting of induction low-dose chemoradiotherapy plus partial cystectomy with pelvic lymph node dissection against muscle-invasive bladder cancer: oncological outcomes of the initial 46 patients. BJU Int. 2012;109:860–6.

Complications of Radical Cystectomy

13

Kelly R. Pekala and Bernard H. Bochner

Introduction

Radical cystectomy in women (with hysterectomy, bilateral salpingectomy, +/− oophorectomy, +/− anterior vaginectomy and urethral excision) and pelvic lymphadenectomy with subsequent urinary diversion are the gold-standard operation for women with invasive bladder cancer [1]. When performed for bladder cancer the average age of women undergoing cystectomy is 68 years, with two thirds having a prior history of extensive smoking. Owing to advanced age, multiple comorbidities, and the extent of the procedure, complications are common. In a series of 1142 radical cystectomy patients at a large cancer center, in which complications were recorded prospectively, 64% of patients were observed to have a complication of any grade (1–5) at 90-days. Approximately two thirds experienced a complication during the initial hospital admission and 58% following postoperative discharge. Importantly, of these complications, only 13% were of high grade (grades 3–5) with a 30-day mortality rate of 1.5% [2]. These are consistent with more contemporary series, in which the rate of grade 3–5 complications was 14.4% at 30 days and 21.7% at 90 days [3].

K. R. Pekala · B. H. Bochner (✉)
Urology Service, Department of Surgery, Memorial Sloan Kettering Cancer Center, New York, NY, USA
e-mail: bochnerb@mskcc.org

There is retrospective evidence that women undergoing radical cystectomy may experience more complications than men in patients undergoing radical cystectomy for reasons other than bladder cancer. In one analysis of the National Surgical Quality Improvement Program Database, after propensity matching, there was an increased risk of readmission, superficial surgical wound infection, and transfusion in women compared with men. The addition of organ sparing to radical cystectomy in women did not increase the complication rates [4].

Herein, we review the common complications following radical cystectomy.

Surgical Approach

Historically, the majority of radical cystectomy series encompassed patients undergoing open surgery. The use of robotic cystectomy, with intra- or extracorporeal diversion, is increasing, with a recent analysis of the national cancer database revealing that 40.6% of cystectomies were performed robotically in 2015 [5]. There have been several randomized controlled trials (RCTs) comparing robotic with open cystectomy. The MSKCC trial was the initial RCT, with a primary endpoint of 90-day complication rates of open versus robotic techniques. The robotic group underwent robotic extirpative surgery and the diversion was performed as open surgery. Overall

M. Hoffman et al. (eds.), *Major Complications of Female Pelvic Surgery*,
https://doi.org/10.1007/978-3-031-66772-5_13

complications of 62% and 66% were observed in the robot-assisted radical cystectomy (RARC) and open radical cystectomy (ORC) patients respectively ($p = 0.7$). Operative time was longer with RARC but resulted in a lower intraoperative blood loss. The RAZOR trial had a primary endpoint of 3-year cancer recurrence. Similar to the MSKCC study, it compared open and robotic approaches with extracorporeal diversion and found no difference in rates of overall complications or rates of major grade 3–5 complications. There were higher rates of urinary tract infection (35% vs 26%) and similar rates of postoperative ileus (22% vs 20%) in the robotic group versus the open group [6]. The recently published iROC study, a randomized controlled trial that compared robotic cystectomy plus intracorporeal diversion with open radical cystectomy found no differences in overall complications, or high-grade complications. Closer evaluation of specific categories of complications found that wound complications (17.3% vs 5.6%) and thromboembolic events (8.3% vs 1.9%) showed a higher trend in the open surgical groups. Readmission rates of 32% in the open and 22% in the robotic cohort were observed; however, most readmissions were short with a median readmission time of 0 days [7].

Table 13.1 Early and overall complications within 90 days following radical cystectomy and urinary diversion

30-day complications (*N* = 149)		Overall complications within 90 days (*N* = 199)	
GU	24%	GU	28%
Infectious	20%	Infectious	23%
Pulmonary	11%	GI	9%
Cardiac	10%	Cardiac	9%
DVT/PE	9%	Pulmonary	9%

Reproduced with permission from Ref. [2]
GU genitourinary, *GI* gastrointestinal, *DVT* deep vein thrombosis, *PE* pulmonary embolism

Complications by Category

The most common complications by category following radical cystectomy include genitourinary, infectious, gastrointestinal, cardiac, and pulmonary complications (Table 13.1).

Genitourinary

There is an 11% rate of genitourinary (GU) complications found in ORC and RARC patients undergoing cystectomy [2, 7]. The most common GU complications are typically urinary diversion related and include ureteral obstruction, renal failure, and urine leaks. The iROC study found that there were higher rates of ureteroenteric anastomotic strictures (2.5% vs 0.6%) and urine leakage (4.3% vs 2.6%) amongst the robotic group [7]. Renal failure occurred in 5–7% of patients in the iROC study [7] and 11–13% in the RAZOR trial [6]. However, these data contradict rates of new renal failure or worsening of CKD, which was noted to be ~3% in an MSKCC prospectively recorded database that included over 1100 patients [2]. Renal failure can be managed expectantly postoperatively by assessment for the presence or absence of hydronephrosis and subsequent placement of appropriate nephrostomy tubes, with concomitant management of electrolyte disturbances.

Infection

Infectious complications are another major category of complications and are seen in one quarter to one third of all patients undergoing ORC [2]. Randomized trial data demonstrated rates of infection of 24–38% and 29–33% in the RARC vs ORC cohorts in the iROC and MSKCC studies [7, 8]. Rates of infection types were similar, with the exception of wound infections, seen more frequently in the open cohorts of both trials [7, 8]. Common sources of infection are urinary (pyelonephritis, urosepsis, urinary tract infections), abdominal fluid collections, wound infections, or rarer infections such as pulmonary, bowel leaks, or osteomyelitis of the pubic bone.

Careful assessment and treatment of preoperative positive urine cultures and administration of antibiotics that cover likely organisms to include skin flora, *S. aureus*, Gram-negative rods, possibly *Enterococcus*, and anaerobic coverage is recommended by American Urological Association guidelines, depending on the type of planned urinary diversion and use of the small or large bowel [9].

Gastrointestinal

As radical cystectomy is accompanied by a urinary diversion using a segment of the gastrointestinal tract, gastrointestinal complications are a common postoperative complication. The most common gastrointestinal complications include ileus or small bowel obstruction. Less common gastrointestinal-associated complications include anastomotic bowel leak and gastrointestinal bleeding. In the randomized controlled trials of open versus robotic cystectomy, the MSKCC trial found 23% vs 29% gastrointestinal complications in ORC versus RARC, whereas the iROC study found similar rates of gastrointestinal complications within 90 days of 28%, similar rates of ileus of around 10%, and small bowel obstruction of 3% [7]. These findings are echoed by smaller real world series that report that ileus is the most common reason for readmission within 30 days (11%), whereas small bowel obstruction was a common reason for readmissions within 90 days (5%). [10]

There have been several efforts to improve on gastrointestinal complications over the years. The enhanced recovery after surgery (ERAS) approach, originally designed for colorectal surgery, has been adopted for radical cystectomy and is detailed in another chapter in this textbook. ERAS typically consists of alterations to historical management in the preoperative phase (bowel preparation, preoperative fasting), intraoperative phase (intravenous fluid management, alterations to analgesia with minimization of opioids), and postoperative phase (alteration of diet advancement and use of nasogastric tubes). There have been three randomized controlled trials of ERAS for cystectomy. Two trials found no difference in 30-day postoperative complications [11, 12], with improved time to bowel function and length of stay group in the ERAS group. One trial found that patients who received alvimopan (Entereg) had a statistically significantly faster recovery of bowel function than those who received placebo (5.5 days vs 6.8 days), shorter length of stay (7.4 vs 10.1 days), and fewer postoperative ileus-related morbidity (8.4% vs 29.1%) [13]. A systematic review and meta-analysis performed a multivariable analysis of individual ERAS factors associated with length of stay and found that omitting the nasogastric tube (−8.7 days) and the use of local anesthetic blocks (−3.29 days) reduced the duration of hospital stay [14].

Cardiopulmonary

Cardiopulmonary complications such as cardiac arrhythmia, congestive heart failure, hypertension, hypotension, myocardial infarction, atelectasis, pleural effusion, pneumothorax, and pneumonia are relatively rare but certainly possible in patients with pre-existing comorbidities. In these cases, postoperative cardiac monitoring should be performed, at least in the initial perioperative setting, with early evaluation by Cardiology as indicated. Pre- and postoperative use of incentive spirometry and early ambulation can reduce the risk of pulmonary complications.

Bleeding/Thromboembolic

Although bleeding is a common surgical risk for radical cystectomy, prospective series demonstrate average intraoperative blood loss of 500 vs 680 cc (MSKCC), 300 vs 700 cc (RAZOR), 200 vs 550 cc (iROC) for robotic versus open respectively [6–8]. Transfusion rates in large open series of approximately 8% have been reported [2]. Open versus robotic comparisons have consistently noted a lower estimated blood loss (EBL) in RARC-treated patients; however, this is not necessarily associated with a lower transfusion rate of 12% vs 7% in the iROC study. Still, major bleeding complications (0.6%), wound hematomas (0%), and postoperative bleeding (0%) remain rare amongst both the open and robotic cohorts. Other clinical characteristics associated with increased EBL come from real-world data using the NSQIP database. Propensity matching and multivariable analysis note that women were twice as likely to require postoperative blood transfusion for anemia (53% vs 38%) [4].

In one, the largest radical cystectomy analysis of complications, there was a 8% risk of thromboembolic events, with deep vein thrombosis (5%) and pulmonary embolism (3%) the most common events. This was confirmed by the RAZOR trial, which found a 8% versus 5% thromboembolic event rate (deep vein thrombosis, DVT) in open versus robotic and similar rates of pulmonary embolism (PE; 3%). These data contrast with the iROC study, in which thromboembolic events such as DVT (0.6% vs 0%), PE (7.1% vs 1.9%) were higher in the open cohort [7].

Postoperative thromboembolic prevention is a mainstay for patients undergoing major abdominal and pelvic surgery, with a large Cochrane review that demonstrated a reduction of thromboembolic events from 13.2% to 5.3%, without an associated increase in bleeding complications or mortality [15]. In the cystectomy setting, it typically consists of sequential compression devices, early ambulation, pre- and post-operative administration of subcutaneous heparin during the perioperative inpatient hospital stay and discharge with 30 days of anticoagulation (commonly subcutaneous enoxaparin), with emerging evidence for the use of oral anticoagulation with apixaban [16].

Neurological

Cerebrovascular Accident/Stroke

Cerebrovascular accident/stroke are uncommon complications following radical cystectomy (<1%) [2], but are more common in older patients. Octogenarians have a significantly higher rate of neurological complications than patients aged <80 years (10.3% vs 3.9%) [17].

Delirium/Agitation

As radical cystectomy patients have an average age of 68 years old and spend several days in the hospital recovering, they are at particular risk of hospital-induced delirium, with disturbed sleep/wake cycles. There was a 2% rate of delirium in the MSKCC series and similar rates of delirium of approximately 3% in both the open and robotic cohorts in the iROC study [7]. Efforts to reduce delirium, such as reduced night-time sleep disruptions for unnecessary vital signs, ensuring adequate sunlight during the day, and efforts to reorient patients, are recommended to reduce the risk of hospital-induced delirium. There are also low-risk pharmacological interventions, such as melatonin or ramelteon, that can be used at night, and in a recent systematic review of randomized controlled trials significantly reduced hospital delirium by 49% in surgical patients [18].

Miscellaneous

Lymphocele

Pelvic lymph node dissection performed for radical cystectomy is associated with a risk of lymphocele of approximately 3% that has been reported in randomized controlled trials [6]. These can present with lower-extremity swelling, DVT, or abdominal fluid collections. Management may consist of needle aspiration or drain placement in selected cases, depending on whether or not there are signs of infection or other related symptoms. Extending the pelvic lymphadenectomy to the level of the aortic bifurcation can increase the risk of lymphocele formation [19].

Unique Complications for Women

The concept of radical cystectomy for women has evolved over time with uterus-, fallopian tube-, ovary-, and vagina-sparing cystectomy entering the treatment paradigm to maintain the oncological outcomes while attempting to preserve gynecological organs of importance to women for endocrine and sexual function [20]. Patients must be appropriately selected for pelvic organ sparing, taking into consideration bimanual examination, tumor location, gynecological history, and relevant cervical cancer screening, menopausal status, sexual function, and family history (*BRCA 1 or 2* mutation or Lynch syndrome) [21].

Organ-Sparing Cystectomy (Uterus-, Fallopian Tube-, Ovary-Sparing)

The rationale for organ-sparing approaches includes the low incidence of involvement of gynecological organs by direct extension, with a rate of 2.5–7.5%, improved sexual function, reduction in neobladder–vaginal fistula, and improved voiding for the neobladder. [22] Series have demonstrated that in the well-selected patient, there are equivalent oncological outcomes and excellent urinary and sexual functional outcomes [21].

Ovary Removal Risks (Bone Loss, Fracture Risk, Cardiac Events, Cognitive Decline, Mortality)

Bilateral oophorectomy has been based on the risk of bladder cancer presence or recurrence within the ovaries and risk of ovarian primary malignancy. However, ovarian involvement of cancer is rare, with one retrospective study that found 4% ovarian involvement and 2.5% involvement of the fallopian tubes with urothelial carcinoma and no primary gynecological malignancies [23]. After excluding patients with advanced disease, women with ≤pT2 had a 0% rate of ovarian involvement.

There have been several large prospective studies that have found that women who undergo bilateral salpingo-oophorectomy as part of a hysterectomy had a 13% increase in overall mortality [24], particularly in women up to the age of 50–65, where the risk of mortality related to oophorectomy was similar to other competing risks [25, 26]. Even in the postmenopausal setting, ovaries continue to secrete hormones, which has a variety of benefits, including cardiac, cognitive, bone, sexual, and health [27–31]. Gynecologists recognizing the benefits of leaving the ovary in situ in younger women, have adopted a practice of prophylactic bilateral salpingectomies as there is evidence that most ovarian cancers originate in the fallopian tubes [32, 33].

Vaginal Complications

There are many possible vaginal complications following removal of the anterior vaginal wall and subsequent closure, including vaginal prolapse, fistula, dyspareunia, cuff dehiscence, and subsequent bowel evisceration. In a study that evaluated SEER-Medicare, which includes patients 65 and older including 481 women, there was a 20% rate of vaginal complications within 2 years of radical cystectomy. They found that cuff dehiscence was the most common vaginal complication (10.2%), followed by fistula (6.9%), prolapse (4.5%), and dyspareunia (2.3%). However, only 26% of these women went on to have an intervention [34]. In a systematic review that reviewed the same topic with an inclusive cohort that included younger patients, a neobladder vaginal fistula rate of 3–6% at high-volume centers with risk factors for fistula such as poor vascularity, overlapping suture lines, prior radiation, and tumor recurrence [35]. There are several techniques to counter the potential for neobladder vaginal fistula including organ preservation of the uterus and omental interposition.

References

1. Brown KG, Solomon MJ, Latif ER, et al. Urological complications after cystectomy as part of pelvic exenteration are higher than that after cystectomy for primary bladder malignancy. J Surg Oncol. 2017;115(3):307–11. https://doi.org/10.1002/jso.24511.
2. Shabsigh A, Korets R, Vora KC, et al. Defining early morbidity of radical cystectomy for patients with bladder cancer using a standardized reporting methodology. Eur Urol. 2009;55(1):164–74. https://doi.org/10.1016/j.eururo.2008.07.031.
3. Knorr JM, Ericson KJ, Zhang JH, et al. Comparison of major complications at 30 and 90 days following radical cystectomy. Urology. 2021;148:192–7. https://doi.org/10.1016/j.urology.2020.08.038.
4. Bukavina L, Mishra K, Mahran A, et al. Gender disparity in cystectomy postoperative outcomes: propensity score analysis of the National Surgical Quality Improvement Program Database. Eur Urol Oncol. 2021;4(1):84–92. https://doi.org/10.1016/j.euo.2019.04.004.
5. Elshabrawy A, Wang H, Dursun F, et al. Diffusion of robot-assisted radical cystectomy: Nationwide trends, predictors, and association with continent urinary

diversion. Arab J Urol. 2022;20(3):159–67. https://doi.org/10.1080/2090598x.2022.2032562.
6. Parekh DJ, Reis IM, Castle EP, et al. Robot-assisted radical cystectomy versus open radical cystectomy in patients with bladder cancer (RAZOR): an open-label, randomised, phase 3, non-inferiority trial. Lancet, 2018. 391(10139):2525–36. https://doi.org/10.1016/s0140-6736(18)30996-6.
7. Catto JWF, Khetrapal P, Ricciardi F, et al. Effect of robot-assisted radical cystectomy with intracorporeal urinary diversion vs open radical cystectomy on 90-day morbidity and mortality among patients with bladder cancer: a randomized clinical trial. JAMA. 2022;327(21):2092–103. https://doi.org/10.1001/jama.2022.7393.
8. Bochner BH, Dalbagni G, Sjoberg DD, et al. Comparing open radical cystectomy and robot-assisted laparoscopic radical cystectomy: a randomized clinical trial. Eur Urol. 2015;67(6):1042–50. https://doi.org/10.1016/j.eururo.2014.11.043.
9. Lightner DJ, Wymer K, Sanchez J, Kavoussi L. Best practice statement on urologic procedures and antimicrobial prophylaxis. J Urol. 2020;203(2):351–6. https://doi.org/10.1097/ju.0000000000000509.
10. Stimson CJ, Chang SS, Barocas DA, et al. Early and late perioperative outcomes following radical cystectomy: 90-day readmissions, morbidity and mortality in a contemporary series. J Urol. 2010;184(4):1296–300. https://doi.org/10.1016/j.juro.2010.06.007.
11. Frees SK, Aning J, Black P, et al. A prospective randomized pilot study evaluating an ERAS protocol versus a standard protocol for patients treated with radical cystectomy and urinary diversion for bladder cancer. World J Urol. 2018;36(2):215–20. https://doi.org/10.1007/s00345-017-2109-2.
12. Lin T, Li K, Liu H, et al. Enhanced recovery after surgery for radical cystectomy with ileal urinary diversion: a multi-institutional, randomized, controlled trial from the Chinese bladder cancer consortium. World J Urol. 2018;36(1):41–50. https://doi.org/10.1007/s00345-017-2108-3.
13. Lee CT, Chang SS, Kamat AM, et al. Alvimopan accelerates gastrointestinal recovery after radical cystectomy: a multicenter randomized placebo-controlled trial. Eur Urol. 2014;66(2):265–72. https://doi.org/10.1016/j.eururo.2014.02.036.
14. Williams SB, Cumberbatch MGK, Kamat AM, et al. Reporting radical cystectomy outcomes following implementation of enhanced recovery after surgery protocols: a systematic review and individual patient data meta-analysis. Eur Urol. 2020;78(5):719–30. https://doi.org/10.1016/j.eururo.2020.06.039.
15. Felder S, Rasmussen MS, King R, et al. Prolonged thromboprophylaxis with low molecular weight heparin for abdominal or pelvic surgery. Cochrane Database Syst Rev. 2019;8(8):Cd004318. https://doi.org/10.1002/14651858.CD004318.pub5.
16. Westerman ME, Bree KK, Msaouel P, et al. Apixaban vs enoxaparin for post-surgical extended-duration venous thromboembolic event prophylaxis: a prospective quality improvement study. J Urol. 2022;208(4):886–95. https://doi.org/10.1097/ju.0000000000002788.
17. Donat SM, Siegrist T, Cronin A, Savage C, Milowsky MI, Herr HW. Radical cystectomy in octogenarians--does morbidity outweigh the potential survival benefits? J Urol. 2010;183(6):2171–7. https://doi.org/10.1016/j.juro.2010.02.015.
18. Khaing K, Nair BR. Melatonin for delirium prevention in hospitalized patients: a systematic review and meta-analysis. J Psychiatr Res. 2021;133:181–90. https://doi.org/10.1016/j.jpsychires.2020.12.020.
19. Gschwend JE, Heck MM, Lehmann J, et al. Extended versus limited lymph node dissection in bladder cancer patients undergoing radical cystectomy: survival results from a prospective, Randomized Trial. Eur Urol. 2019;75(4):604–11. https://doi.org/10.1016/j.eururo.2018.09.047.
20. Koie T, Hatakeyama S, Yoneyama T, Hashimoto Y, Kamimura N, Ohyama C. Uterus-, fallopian tube-, ovary-, and vagina-sparing cystectomy followed by U-shaped ileal neobladder construction for female bladder cancer patients: oncological and functional outcomes. Urology. 2010;75(6):1499–503. https://doi.org/10.1016/j.urology.2009.08.083.
21. Truong H, Maxon V, Goh AC. Robotic female radical cystectomy. J Endourol. 2021;35(S2):S106–s115. https://doi.org/10.1089/end.2020.1190.
22. Niver BE, Daneshmand S, Satkunasivam R. Female reproductive organ-sparing radical cystectomy: contemporary indications, techniques and outcomes. Curr Opin Urol. 2015;25(2):105–10. https://doi.org/10.1097/mou.0000000000000146.
23. Taylor BL, Matrai CE, Smith AL, et al. Gynecologic organ involvement during radical cystectomy for bladder cancer: is it time to routinely spare the ovaries? Clin Genitourin Cancer. 2019;17(1):e209–15. https://doi.org/10.1016/j.clgc.2018.10.009.
24. Parker WH, Feskanich D, Broder MS, et al. Long-term mortality associated with oophorectomy compared with ovarian conservation in the nurses' health study. Obstet Gynecol. 2013;121(4):709–16. https://doi.org/10.1097/AOG.0b013e3182864350.
25. Parker WH, Broder MS, Liu Z, Shoupe D, Farquhar C, Berek JS. Ovarian conservation at the time of hysterectomy for benign disease. Obstet Gynecol. 2005;106(2):219–26. https://doi.org/10.1097/01.Aog.0000167394.38215.56.
26. Rush KS, Ma X, Newton MA, Rose SL. A revised markov model evaluating oophorectomy at the time of hysterectomy for benign indication age 65 years revisited. Obstet Gynecol. 2022;139(5).
27. Rivera CM, Grossardt BR, Rhodes DJ, et al. Increased cardiovascular mortality after early bilateral oophorectomy. Menopause. 2009;16(1):15–23. https://doi.org/10.1097/gme.0b013e31818888f7.
28. Fogle RH, Stanczyk FZ, Zhang X, Paulson RJ. Ovarian androgen production in postmenopausal women. J Clin Endocrinol Metab. 2007;92(8):3040–3. https://doi.org/10.1210/jc.2007-0581.

29. Melton LJ 3rd, Khosla S, Malkasian GD, Achenbach SJ, Oberg AL, Riggs BL. Fracture risk after bilateral oophorectomy in elderly women. J Bone Miner Res. 2003;18(5):900–5. https://doi.org/10.1359/jbmr.2003.18.5.900.
30. Shoupe D, Parker WH, Broder MS, Liu Z, Farquhar C, Berek JS. Elective oophorectomy for benign gynecological disorders. Menopause. 2007;14(3 Pt 2):580–5. https://doi.org/10.1097/gme.0b013e31803c56a4.
31. Rocca WA, Grossardt BR, Maraganore DM. The long-term effects of oophorectomy on cognitive and motor aging are age dependent. Neurodegener Dis. 2008;5(3–4):257–60. https://doi.org/10.1159/000113718.
32. Society gynecology oncology clinical practice statement: salpingectomy for ovarian cancer prevention (SGO, November 2013). 2013.
33. Kurman RJ, Shih IM. The origin and pathogenesis of epithelial ovarian cancer: a proposed unifying theory. Am J Surg Pathol. 2010;34(3):433–43. https://doi.org/10.1097/PAS.0b013e3181cf3d79.
34. Richter LA, Osazuwa-Peters OL, Routh JC, Handa VL. Vaginal complications after cystectomy: results from a Medicare sample. J Urol. 2022;207(4):789–96. https://doi.org/10.1097/ju.0000000000002336.
35. Richter LA, Egan J, Alagha EC, Handa VL. Vaginal complications after radical cystectomy for bladder cancer: a systematic review. Urology. 2021;156:e20–9. https://doi.org/10.1016/j.urology.2021.07.001.

Complications in Orthotopic Neobladders

14

Kathrin Meisterhofer, Bastian Amend, and Arnulf Stenzl

Introduction

In women, radical cystectomy includes removal of the urinary bladder, distal ureters, uterus, proximal two-thirds of the vaginal anterior wall, both ovaries, and pelvic lymph nodes. Depending on tumor location, patients' age, and indication, the vaginal anterior wall and ovaries may be preserved.

The most common indication for cystectomy in women is cancer of the urinary bladder. Other indications for bladder removal are gynecological tumors or colon carcinoma, although orthotopic bladder replacement is usually not an option in these cases due to the locally advanced growth. Nononcological indications for cystectomy are a small-capacity bladder, post-radiogenic cystitis, and interstitial cystitis.

Urinary diversions are divided into continent and incontinent (ileal conduit, ureterocutaneostomy) solutions. Continent urinary diversions can be subdivided into orthotopic and heterotopic (catheterizable pouches) approaches. This chapter focuses on complications of orthotopic ileal neobladders.

K. Meisterhofer · B. Amend · A. Stenzl (✉)
Department of Urology, University Hospital of Tuebingen, Eberhard Karls University, Tuebingen, Germany
e-mail: kathrin.meisterhofer@med.uni-tuebingen.de; bastian.amend@med.uni-tuebingen.de; uro@stenzl.net

Over time, many different forms of neobladders have been described and modified by surgeons. The variants of neobladders differ in terms of folding techniques of the bowel and refluxing or nonrefluxing implantation of the ureters. Cystectomy with urinary diversion can be performed either by open surgery or robot-assisted laparoscopy. The complication rate, oncological outcome, and quality of life are all similar for both robotic and open approaches. The surgeon's experience and institutional volume are more important for the outcome than the technique [1]. Therefore, the procedure should only be performed at specialized centers.

The perioperative mortality rate after radical cystectomy is 2.1–3.2% at 30 days and 3.4–8% at 90 days [2, 3]. Complications can be categorized as early postoperative complications and long-term complications. Therefore, a lifelong follow-up is needed after a neobladder reconstruction.

This chapter summarizes the complications of orthotopic ileal neobladders and their management.

Early Postoperative Complications

Perioperative Bleeding Intraoperative bleeding may occur during cystectomy in women, especially at the vaginal venous plexus. It corresponds to the prostatic venous plexus in men.

M. Hoffman et al. (eds.), *Major Complications of Female Pelvic Surgery*,
https://doi.org/10.1007/978-3-031-66772-5_14

Various hemostyptics can be used. In case of increased blood loss and coagulation disorders, transfusion of red blood cells, platelets, fresh frozen plasma, and specific coagulation factors—depending on specific diagnostics—should be considered. In case of unmanageable intraoperative bleeding, “packing” of the surgical area and a second-look surgery within 72 h can be performed.

If postoperative bleeding is suspected, due to hemodynamic instability, increased bloody drainage volumes, drop in hemoglobin, or free fluid in sonographic examination, CT scanning should be performed to localize the hemorrhage. Before immediate surgical revision, the possibility of angiographic embolization of the bleeding should be evaluated.

Ileus or Bowel Obstruction An ileus is described in up to 26.9% of cases after radical cystectomy [4]. It may be caused by peritoneal irritation due to peritonitis or urine leakage, adhesion formation, or herniation of intestinal loops. Enteral and parenteral bowel stimulation by indirect parasympathomimetic drugs is essential in the early postoperative period. If an inserted nasogastric tube is used, it should be removed as early as possible because its irritation might have a negative influence on bowel recovery. The diagnosis of ileus is made clinically or by imaging. Paralytic ileus can be treated conservatively with forced bowel stimulation and reinsertion of a gastric tube. If a mechanical obstruction is highly probable, a surgical revision is indicated.

Insufficiency of Intestinal Anastomosis There are different techniques for performing intestinal anastomosis. While stapled side-to-side or end-to-side anastomosis is technically faster and easier to perform, handsewn end-to-end anastomosis preserves the straight flow of the intestinal contents and should therefore be preferred.

Insufficiency of intestinal anastomosis is clinically manifested by acute abdominal pain. In addition, air or even stool appears in the drainage. An immediate surgical revision is indispensable in this potentially lethal complication (Fig. 14.1).

Insufficiency of Urological Anastomosis and Suture Lines The various urological anastomoses include the sutures between the ureter and neobladder and the urethra and neobladder or those of the neobladder itself. Clinically, suture insufficiency is manifested by an increased flow rate of the drainage. Therefore, the creatinine level in the drainage should be compared to the serum level. If the levels are identical, a major insufficiency is unlikely. In addition, a radiographic exclusion of leakage (conventional cys-

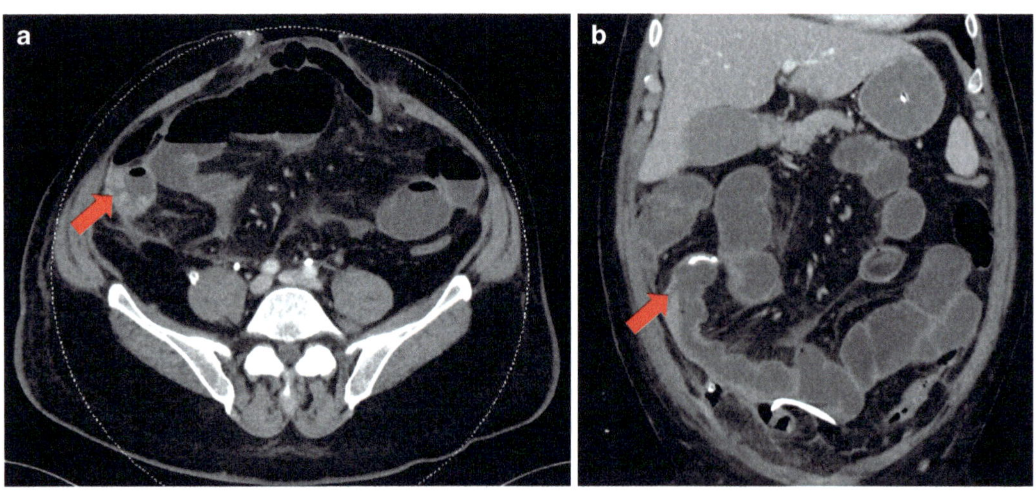

Fig. 14.1 Insufficiency of intestinal anastomosis

togram) should be performed before removing the inserted catheter.

In case of insufficiency, a conservative approach with low-pressure drainage should be pursued. If necessary, stents that have already been removed (e.g., catheter, ureteric stents, or additionally nephrostomies) must be reinserted. Surgical revision is rarely required. However, suture insufficiency leads to an increased risk of tubular stricture (Fig. 14.2).

Vesicovaginal Fistula To avoid a fistula between the vagina and neobladder or anastomosis, the suture lines should be kept distant. In addition, an omental flap is usually created and placed around the lowest part of the neobladder. This prevents fistula formation and suspends the neobladder floor, reducing the risk of urinary retention by preventing ileal fold formation, as mentioned below (Fig. 14.3).

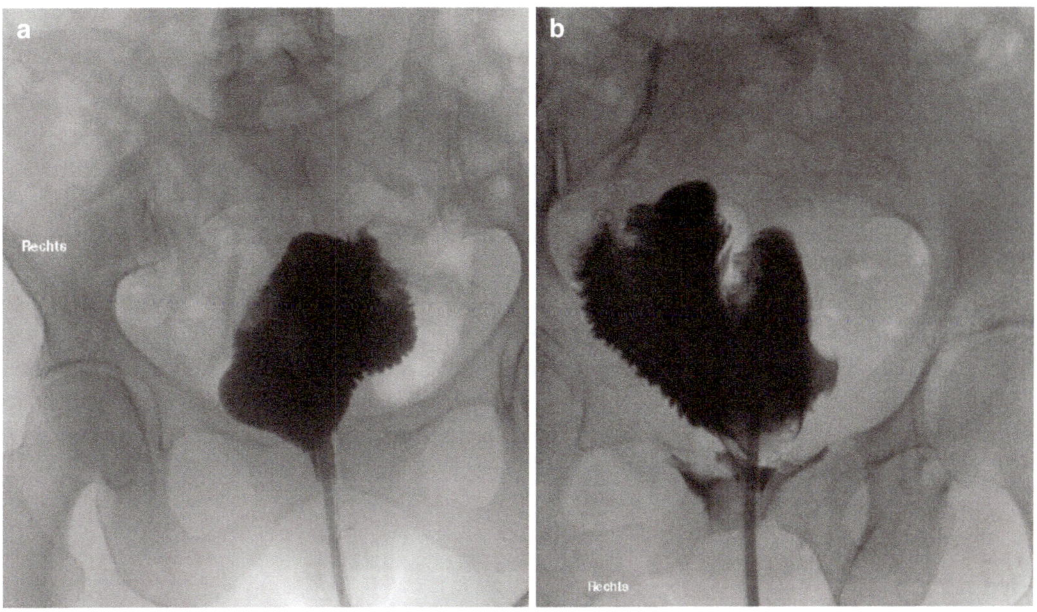

Fig. 14.2 An inconspicuous cystogram (**a**). Insufficiency of the ureteroileal anastomosis (**b**)

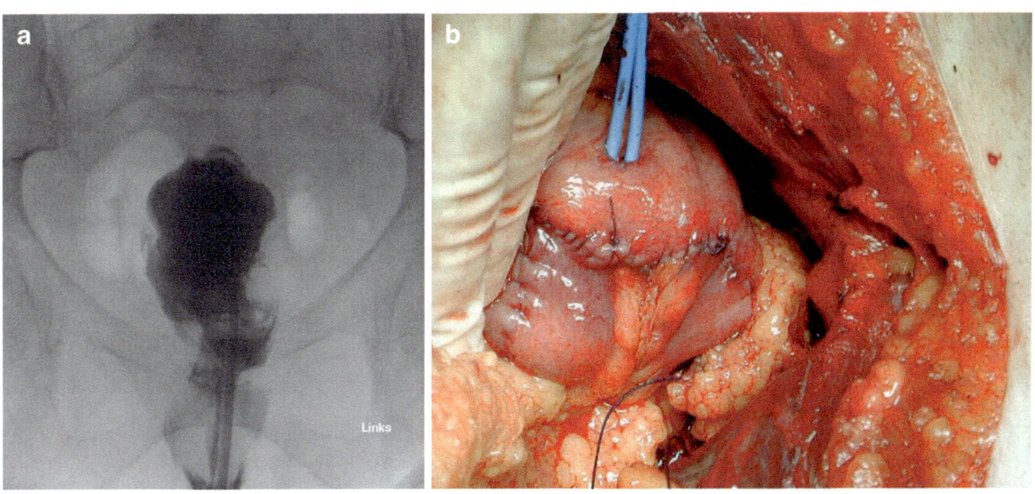

Fig. 14.3 To avoid a vesicovaginal fistula (**a**), an omental flap should be placed around the neobladder (**b**)

Urinary Tract Infections (UTIs) Urinary tract infections (UTIs) are one of the most common problems in urinary diversions. They should be first ruled out before reconstructive urological surgery. In addition, it is recommended to check for significant bacteriuria before removing catheters or stents to reduce the risk of febrile UTI, which can be life-threatening.

Long-Term Complications

Urinary Incontinence Daytime and nighttime continence rates in women with an orthotopic neobladder range from 82 to 95% and from 72 to 86% and are comparable to male patients [5].

For a good functional result, intraoperative preservation of the autonomic nerve fibers is mandatory. While the external urinary sphincter is innervated by the pudendal nerve, the proximal urethra is also innervated by sympathetic nerves. The sympathetic nerves originate from the sympathetic trunk and reach the pelvis through the superior and inferior hypogastric plexus, with additional fibers arising directly from the sacral nerves. The fibers run in front of the common iliac artery and medial to the ureter. If acceptable from an oncological point of view, it is important to preserve these fibers, especially when performing a pelvic lymphadenectomy.

Furthermore, dissection of the bladder neck is essential for preservation of continence. If the urethra is cut too short, there is a deficit of sphincter tissue, resulting in stress urinary incontinence. However, leaving a too long urethral segment might result in urinary retention. Therefore, the urethra should be dissected 5 mm below the bladder neck (Fig. 14.4).

To assess incontinence, a medical history (preexisting incontinence increases the risk), physical examination, and sonography (differential diagnosis is overflow incontinence due to urinary retention) should be performed first. In patients with an orthotopic neobladder, in whom the surgical principles of detubularization and reconfiguration to achieve a low-pressure reservoir were not adhered to, urodynamic diagnostics can determine the increased pressures and thus the indication for revision surgery.

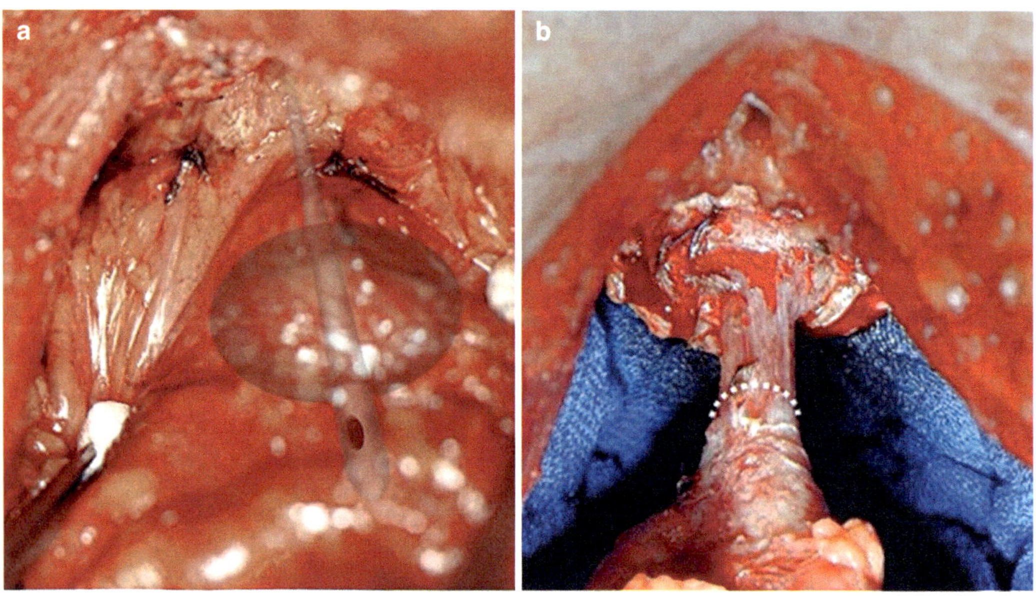

Fig. 14.4 Bladder neck dissection: A Foley catheter (virtually superimposed) helps identify the bladder neck (**a**). Dissection 5 mm below the bladder neck (**b**) (with permission from John Wiley and Sons [6])

Conservative treatment options for incontinence are pelvic floor exercises with or without biofeedback and electric stimulation. However, the improvement depends on the patient's compliance. Duloxetine, a serotonin and noradrenaline reuptake inhibitor, is currently the only pharmaceutical treatment option for incontinence. There are only limited surgical options available for treating stress urinary incontinence in women who have undergone orthotopic neobladder replacement. While bulking agents may provide temporary relief, the use of tension-free vaginal tapes is associated with a high risk of perforation. In cases of refractory stress urinary incontinence, diversion into an ileal conduit or a catheterizable continent reservoir may be the last option.

Urinary Retention Various causes of post-void residual urine have been identified in patients with neobladders (Fig. 14.5). Ileal folds, anastomotic strictures, tumor recurrence, and prolapse can lead to outlet obstruction. The nerve-sparing approach and dissection of the urethra have already been described above. Preservation of urethral vascularization in bladder neck dissection is also mandatory. To avoid kinking of the reservoir outlet, a separate buttonhole should be created at the most caudal point of the pouch for the ureteroileal anastomosis while creating the neobladder. Cystoscopy is a main component in the diagnosis of bladder emptying disorders. Strictures and intestinal folds can be transurethrally resected. Urinary retention may cause recurrent UTIs and cystolithiasis and can damage the upper urinary tract with impairment of the renal function. Urinary retention often results in long-term intermittent aseptic catheterization. The rate of residual urine with an indication for intermittent aseptic catheterization is more common in female patients (0–53%) than in men (4–33%) [7] (Fig. 14.6).

Ureteric Strictures Ureteral strictures usually occur distal to the implantation in the neobladder and were reported in 2.7–3.8% of cases [5]. To avoid ureteric strictures, it is essential to maintain the vascular and nerve supply of the ureters (Fig. 14.7). As already described above, suture insufficiency at the ureteral implantation site increases the risk of strictures. In case of hydronephrosis, renal scintigraphy should be performed to differentiate between chronic ectasia without urodynamic problems and significant hydronephrosis. If an obstructive outflow is detected, a double J (DJ) stent or a nephrostomy tube (in patients with challenging retrograde instrumentation) should be inserted, to protect the upper urinary tract from further damage. The only way to cure the stricture would be a surgical revision.

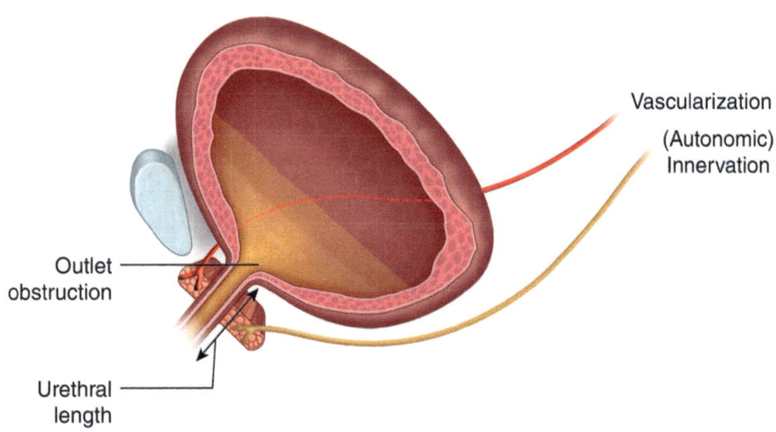

Fig. 14.5 Causes of urinary retention

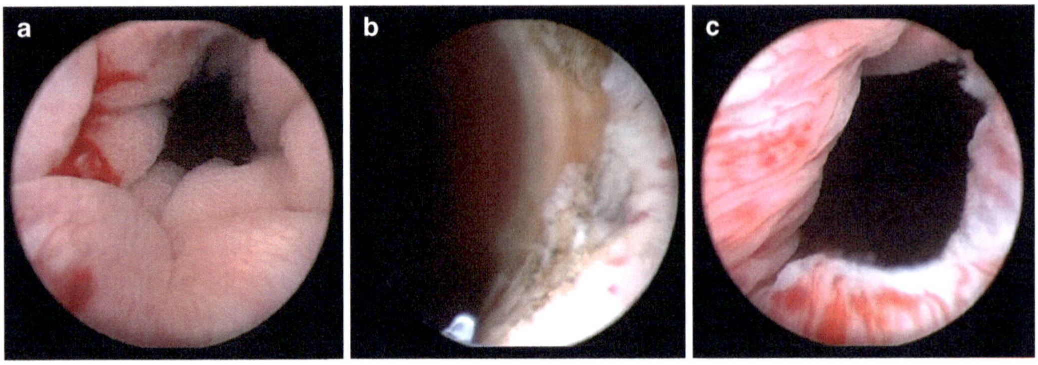

Fig. 14.6 An obstructive ileal fold (**a**). Transurethral resection of the fold (**b**). Postoperative result with a wide outlet of the neobladder (**c**)

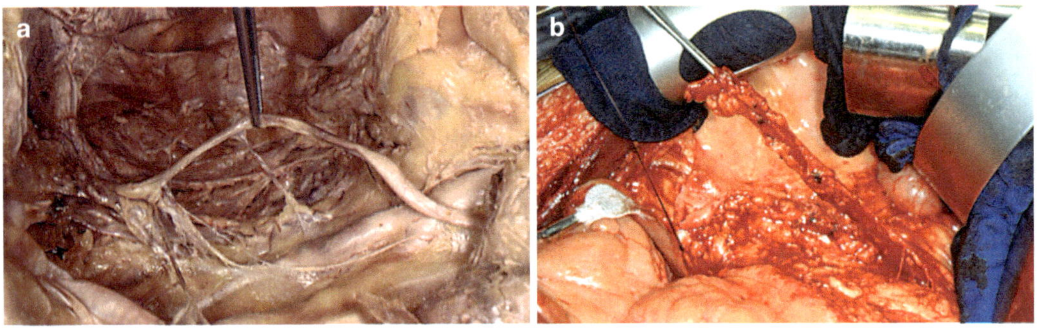

Fig. 14.7 To avoid ureteric strictures (**a**), it is essential to maintain the vascular and nerve supply of the ureters (**b**) (specimen from K. Colleselli)

Sexual Dysfunctions Sexual dysfunctions include decreased desire, decreased lubrication of the vagina, decreased ability to achieve an orgasm, and dyspareunia. The disorders were reported at rates of 49%, 9.5%, 39%, and 25%, respectively, after cystectomy [8].

Devascularization of the surrounding neurovascular bundles of the vagina and clitoris and shortening of the vaginal length cause sexual dysfunction after cystectomy. Therefore, preservation of autonomic nerve fibers is not only important for continence but also for sexual function. The nerve-sparing approach has already been described above. Radical cystectomy includes resection of the uterus and part of the anterior wall of the vagina. A longitudinal re-tubularization of the vagina increases the depth of the vagina compared to a transversal closing but may result in a narrow lumen, causing dyspareunia. In benign indications for cystectomy, a genital-preserving technique can be offered. The incidence of sexual dysfunction was reported in 10% of patients receiving sexual organ- or nerve-sparing cystectomy and in 59% receiving radical cystectomy [8]. In addition, bilateral removal of the ovaries leads to impairment of sexual functions, especially in young patients. Accordingly, preservation of an ovary should be discussed preoperatively; the removal of the fallopian tube, including the fimbrial funnel, is recommended with regard to the prevention of ovarian carcinoma (opportunistic salpingectomy).

Pelvic Organ Prolapse The incidence of vaginal prolapse after cystectomy is 6–12% [9]. Patients may experience vaginal bulging, pelvic pressure, difficulty emptying the bowel or bladder, or sexual dysfunction. Management includes conservative therapy such as vaginal pessaries or surgery with transabdominal or transvaginal suspension with or without mesh. However, there is

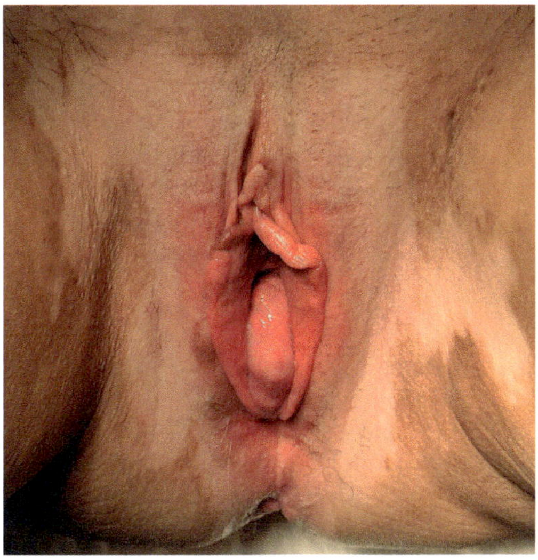

Fig. 14.8 Vaginal prolapse after cystectomy with neobladder replacement

no standardized recommendation for pelvic organ prolapse with an orthotopic neobladder. The combination of colpectomy and colpocleisis represents a last resort in older patients who do not wish to have sexual intercourse (Fig. 14.8).

Urinary Tract Infections Patients with a neobladder do not have typical dysuric symptoms of an UTI. A common symptom is increased mucus production. Residual urine often leads to UTIs and stone formation, which, in turn, leads to recurrent UTIs. In case of urinary diversions, the infections are defined as complicated UTIs. Therefore, microbiological examinations should be performed, and patients should be treated with antibiotic therapy in sufficient dosage and duration (usually 7 days).

Metabolic Imbalance Reabsorption of urine through the intestinal mucosa of the neobladder may lead to metabolic imbalance. It depends on the length of the used intestinal segment, the length of time the urine remains in the neobladder, and the pH and osmolarity of the urine. Metabolic imbalance occurs mostly in the early time period after catheter removal. Due to atrophy of the mucosa, reabsorption decreases over time. Nevertheless, some patients have metabolic problems even after years. Metabolic imbalance causes symptoms like lethargy, confusion, muscular weakness, fatigue, nausea, vomiting, or abdominal pain. Therefore, blood gas analysis should be performed regularly.

Patients who have an ileal reservoir tend to develop hypochloremic acidosis, while those with colonic segments tend to develop hyperchloremic acidosis. Acidosis can be treated with sodium bicarbonate. In cases of hyperchloremic acidosis, patients may require potassium supplementation. Chronic metabolic acidosis may cause bone demineralization and therefore osteoporosis.

Malabsorption Reduced intestinal absorption of vitamin D and calcium following ileal resection may also affect bone metabolism in urinary diversions.

Vitamin B12 is absorbed in the terminal ileum. Extensive use of this small intestinal part can lead to decreased absorption. Deficiency may lead to anemia or severe and irreversible neurological diseases (e.g., peripheral polyneuropathy, dementia, spinal cord degeneration, optic atrophy). In people consuming a balanced diet, vitamin B12 is stored in sufficient amounts in the liver. Hence, deficiency may not become apparent for several years. Screening for vitamin B12 deficiency is therefore recommended throughout life, and, if a deficiency is confirmed, parenteral supplementation is extremely important.

Bile acids are reabsorbed in the terminal ileum. A shortened ileum can lead to chologenic diarrhea. In this case cholestyramine bind bile acids thereby relieving these symptoms.

Short Bowel Syndrome In addition to malabsorption, the use of a long bowel segment for urological reconstruction can result in faster bowel transit time. This can lead to increased stool frequency and diarrhea. Loperamide or opium tincture can improve the amount and frequency of diarrhea (Fig. 14.9).

Psychological Effects Surgery can also have psychological effects on patients, especially when they experience complications or have difficulties in adjusting to their neobladder. Symptoms may include anxiety, depression, or

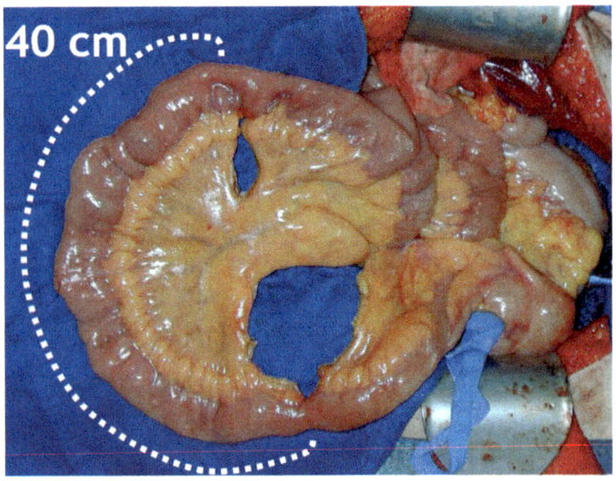

Fig. 14.9 The use of a long bowel segment for neobladder reconstruction increases the risk of short bowel syndrome. The I-Pouch neobladder requires only 40 cm of the terminal ileum, whereas other techniques require up to 70 cm of the intestine [10, 11]

feelings of isolation or frustration. Treatment options may include therapy or medication to manage symptoms as well as support from relatives or support groups.

Conclusions

In summary, to avoid all these early and long-term risks and complications, after cystectomy and orthotopic bladder replacement, patients benefit from standardized perioperative management and need a close and lifelong follow-up.

The use of a fast-track program reduces morbidity and improves early recovery [12]. This concept includes, e.g., sufficient pain management, including epidural anesthesia, early mobilization, and early removal of the gastric tube for bowel recovery. The drainages and catheter should be removed after exclusion of leakage, as described above. In addition, a prophylaxis of thrombosis and pulmonary embolism is essential in the early postoperative time.

During follow-up, the anamnesis should cover drinking and voiding behavior as well as catheterization frequency if performed. In addition, sexual anamnesis and questions about quality of life should be included, to recognize psychological problems at an early stage.

Blood tests should focus on hemoglobin, creatinine, electrolytes, vitamin B12, and venous blood gas analysis to detect anemia, increased renal function, vitamin deficiency, and metabolic imbalance. If an UTI is suspected, a urine culture should be obtained. Ultrasound should be performed to exclude residual urine and hydronephrosis. CT scans or MRI should be performed according to the oncological follow-up plan in case of an underlying malignancy.

References

1. EAU Guidelines. Edn. presented at the EAU Annual Congress Milan 2023. ISBN 978-94-92671-19-6.
2. Bochner BH, et al. Comparing open radical cystectomy and robot-assisted laparoscopic radical cystectomy: a randomized clinical trial. Eur Urol. 2015;67:1042.
3. Mossanen M, et al. Examining the relationship between complications and perioperative mortality following radical cystectomy: a population-based analysis. BJU Int. 2019;124:40.
4. Nutt M, Scaief S, Dynda D, Alanee S. Ileus and small bowel obstruction after radical cystectomy for bladder cancer: analysis from the Nationwide inpatient sample. Surg Oncol. 2018;27(3):341–5.
5. Stenzl A, Sherif H, Kuczyk M. Radical cystectomy with orthotopic neobladder for invasive bladder cancer: a critical analysis of long term oncological, functional and quality of life results. Int Braz J Urol. 2010;36(5):537–47.
6. Schilling D, Horstmann M, Nagele U, Sievert KD, Stenzl A. Cystectomy in women. BJU Int. 2008;102(9 Pt B):1289–95.
7. World Health Organization (WHO) Consensus Conference on Bladder Cancer, Hautmann RE, Abol-Enein H, Hafez K, Haro I, Mansson W, Mills RD, Montie JD, Sagalowsky AI, Stein JP, Stenzl A, Studer UE, Volkmer BG. Urinary diversion. Urology. 2007;69(1 Suppl):17–49.
8. Zahran MH, Fahmy O, El-Hefnawy AS, Ali-El-Dein B. Female sexual dysfunction post radical cystectomy and urinary diversion. Climacteric. 2016;19(6):546–50.
9. Voigt M, Hemal K, Matthews C. Influence of simple and radical cystectomy on sexual function and pelvic organ prolapse in female patients: a scoping review of the literature. Sex Med Rev. 2019;7(3):408–15.
10. Gakis G, Abdelhafez MF, Stenzl A. The "I-Pouch": results of a new ileal neobladder technique. Scand J Urol. 2015;49(5):400–6.
11. Hautmann RE, Egghart G, Frohneberg D, Miller K. The ileal neobladder. J Urol. 1988;139(1): 39–42.
12. Pruthi RS, Nielsen M, Smith A, Nix J, Schultz H, Wallen EM. Fast track program in patients undergoing radical cystectomy: results in 362 consecutive patients. J Am Coll Surg. 2010;210(1):93–9.

15 Continent Cutaneous Urinary Diversion in Women

Jakob Klemm, Malte W. Vetterlein, and Margit Fisch

Introduction

To reestablish urinary passage after removal of the bladder, there are various options for urinary diversion (UD), including conduits, cutaneous ureterostomy, orthotopic neobladder, and continent cutaneous urinary diversion (CCUD). Aside from bladder cancer, which represents a common malignancy with an incidence rate of 2.4/100,000 in women worldwide in 2020 [1], UD is also used in the management of advanced or recurrent pelvic malignancies, as well as for benign indications as a salvage treatment strategy [2–4]. However, radical cystectomy, which is the standard of care for nonmetastatic muscle-invasive bladder cancer, is associated with significant perioperative morbidity and is the most common indication for UD [5, 6]. In general, incontinent UDs are used more frequently with an increasing trend in recent years [7]. An ileal conduit is the most common form of incontinent UD across both genders, whereas an orthotopic neobladder is the most frequent variant of continent UD [8, 9]. Although it has been shown that an orthotopic neobladder is feasible in women under certain conditions, it is performed significantly more often in men [10]. For this reason, CCUD represents an important alternative, particularly in women, offering the benefit of patients being dry immediately after surgery [11, 12]. In this chapter, we aim to provide a comprehensive overview of the history, different techniques, outcomes, and complications of CCUDs in women.

J. Klemm · M. W. Vetterlein · M. Fisch (✉)
Department of Urology, University Medical Center Hamburg-Eppendorf, Hamburg, Germany
e-mail: j.klemm@uke.de; m.vetterlein@uke.de; m.fisch@uke.de

History, Techniques, and Outcomes for CCUD Reservoirs

Many of the earliest descriptions of various CCUD techniques date back to the years 1890–1920. However, due to high complication rates and poor functional outcomes, these approaches were abandoned [11]. Decades later, the techniques were revived and refined as a result of progressive medical advancements, particularly the advent of antimicrobial treatment and antacids [11].

In general, all techniques involve a reservoir into which the ureters are implanted, as well as an efferent segment with a continence mechanism that connects the reservoir to the skin. The reservoir is emptied intermittently by self-catheterization through the efferent segment. In the following, we provide a brief overview of the history, techniques, and outcomes of the most common surgical approaches for CCUDs.

M. Hoffman et al. (eds.), *Major Complications of Female Pelvic Surgery*,
https://doi.org/10.1007/978-3-031-66772-5_15

Ileocecal Reservoirs

The first descriptions of an ileocecal reservoir were published between 1900 and 1910 for an orthotopic bladder replacement without achieving continence [13, 14]. The next descriptions of ileocaecal reservoirs followed in the 1950s by Gilchrist, who successfully developed the technique for a continent orthotopic reservoir. However, their approach was not reproducible by others [15].

In the 1970s, the first heterotopic continent ileocecal reservoir-based UDs were reported [16–18].

This period also marks the beginning of the "Lundiana pouch" with the use of a cecal reservoir and an ileal intussusception nipple as a continence mechanism [19]. After later modifications, the first clinical results were published in 1990 [20]. A recent publication with the largest cohort on the Lundiana pouch, including 64 women among 198 patients mostly operated for malignant indications, has reported continence rates of 91% and difficulties with catheterization in 5.3% of patients at a median follow-up of 13 years. Reoperations were performed at least once during follow-up in 54% of the patients, with 15% for uretero-intestinal stenoses, 14% for pouch stones, 8% for outlet revision, 8% for stomal stenosis, 5% for pouch perforation, and 2% for parastomal hernia. Overall, 25% of the patients had a major complication within 90 days of surgery [21].

The Mainz pouch I (mixed augmentation ileum and cecum) was first described in 1983, initially for bladder substitution in benign diseases, and, 3 years later, the first results of 11 bladder substitutions and 12 CCUDs were published [22]. Later publications included larger cohorts and different modifications [23–25]. The classical Mainz pouch I is created by antimesenteric opening and reconfiguration of the ileocecum (Fig. 15.1) and two ileal loops plus an additional 8–10-cm ileum left intact for the efferent segment. Subsequently, ureters are implanted with an anti-reflux technique using a submucosal tunnel or a serosa-lined extramural tunnel. The invaginated efferent segment fixated with staplers serves as the continence mechanism. Additional modifications in the following years included the appendix stoma, further developments of the ileum invagination nipple, and modifications of the efferent segment [23–26]. Moreover, antirefluxive techniques were abandoned over time based on the idea that in a low-pressure reservoir, reflux is less hazardous than implantation stenosis. The largest cohort on the Mainz pouch I was published in 2006 including 977 patients from Mainz and Würzburg who were treated with different techniques for ureter implantation and the continence mechanism

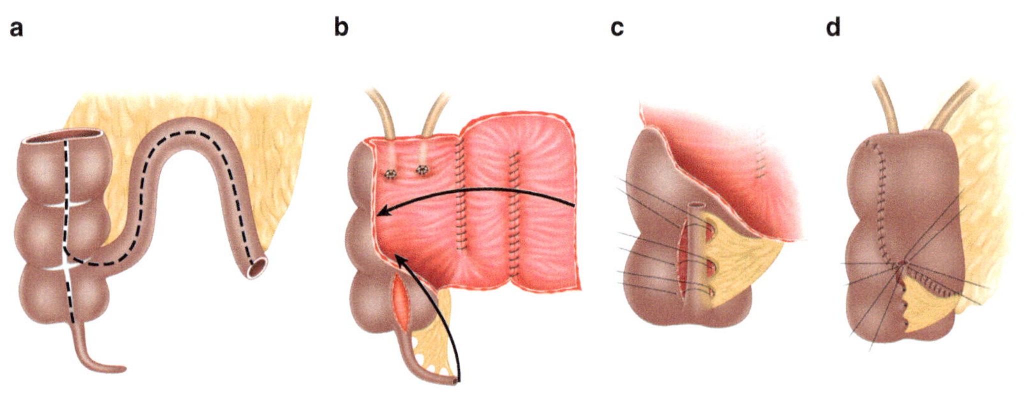

Fig. 15.1 Key steps of the Mainz pouch I with a Mitrofanoff nipple: (**a**) An antimesenteric longitudinal incision is made. (**b**) Detubularization and ureteral implantation are performed. (**c**) The appendix is folded cranially and sutures are placed. (**d**) After sutures are knotted, a segment of the appendix is placed submucosally

(mostly appendix stomas, $n = 419$, intussuscepted ileal nipple valves, $n = 491$, and 1470 renal units with uretero-intestinal anastomosis via the submucosal tunnel and 136 ureter implantations using a serosa-lined extramural tunnel). At a mean follow-up of 7.5 years, continence was reported by 96% of the patients with an appendix stoma and by 90% of the patients with an intussuscepted ileal nipple. Reoperations concerning the efferent segment occurred mainly due to stoma stenosis (24% of the patients with an appendix stoma and 15% with an intussuscepted ileal nipple) and calculus formation (5.6% of patients with an appendix stoma and 11% with an intussuscepted ileal nipple) as well as incontinence (1.5 vs. 5.2% for appendix stoma vs. intussuscepted ileal nipple, respectively). Overall, 6.5% of renal units undergoing uretero-intestinal reimplantation via the submucosal tunnel developed uretero-intestinal stenosis, compared to 5% of renal units with uretero-intestinal reimplantation via the serosa-lined extramural tunnel [26].

The Indiana pouch was developed and described in the 1980s by Rowland et al. [27] Herein, ureters are implanted along the tenia libera into an ileocecal reservoir using the ileocecal valve and the tapered terminal ileum as the continence mechanism (Fig. 15.2) [28]. The largest single-center Indiana pouch cohort was published in 2022 including 55 women among 137 patients, mostly undergoing radical cystectomy UD for bladder cancer. Herein, the authors report an overall complication rate of 39% within 1 year (Clavien–Dindo grades II–V only) and a major complication rate of 23% [29]. Continence rates for Indiana pouch vary from 72% at a mean follow-up of 41 months to 100% at a median follow-up of 21 months in smaller cohorts ($n < 100$) [30–32]. Reoperation rates vary from 7.3% within 90 days of surgery and 8% beyond 90 days, to 52% at a median follow-up of 41 months [29, 32–34].

The Florida pouch was developed in 1987 and comprises the ascending colon and the right flexure adjacent to the ileocecal segment. Ureters were first implanted directly and later according to Le Duc, and the continence mechanism was composed of the ileocecal valve and a double plication of the efferent segment [35]. In 2003, the largest Florida pouch cohort, which included 74 patients and 36 females, reported a continence rate of 93%. UD-related complications were grouped by etiology, resulting in 6.3% of ureteral obstruction, 5.5% of severe acidosis, 5.4% of reservoir stones, and 4% of parastomal hernia [36]. The initial series on the Florida pouch reports a reoperation rate of 5% (bowel obstruction, bilateral ureteral reimplantation, anti-incontinence segment replication, and abdominal wall closure) [35].

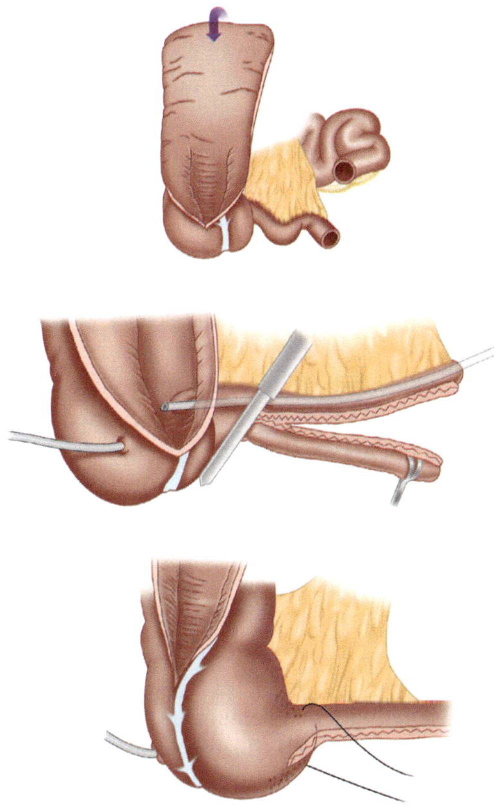

Fig. 15.2 Fundamental steps of the Indiana pouch procedure: After longitudinal detubularization, the colon segment is downfolded to form the pouch. For establishing the continence mechanism, the terminal ileum undergoes a reduction in diameter. Subsequently, a 12-Fr catheter is accurately positioned within the efferent segment. Concluding the procedure, imbricating seromuscular stitches are applied with nonabsorbable suture material, fortifying the ileocecal valve and thereby enabling continence

The Miami pouch was first described in 1988 and utilizes the same bowel components as the Florida pouch; ureters are implanted using a modified Le Duc technique, and the continence mechanism involves the terminal ileum, which is tapered and reinforced with three proximal sutures [37, 38]. The largest Miami pouch cohort consists of 90 patients from the Miami gynecology department, who underwent Miami pouch UD mostly due to pelvic malignancies with total pelvic exenteration in 79% of cases. Of note, 91% of these patients received prior pelvic radiotherapy. The continence rate was reported to be 92% at last follow-up after three open surgical revisions. Overall, 76% of the patients experienced non-UD-related complications within 60 days of surgery, including a mortality rate of 11% (mostly due to sepsis). UD-related complications during follow-up occurred in 53% of the patients, with ureteral obstruction in 20% and anastomotic leak in 14% of the patients [39]. Other series with small urological cohorts including women and using Clavien–Dindo grades for complication reporting show a 30-day overall complication rate of 93% with a 30-day major complication rate of 13% vs. 14% and continence rates ranging from 79% to 100% [37, 38, 40, 41].

The Rome pouch, a simplification of an ileocecal reservoir, was first described in 2006. Through transverse taeniamyotomies, detubularization of the colonic segment can be omitted [42]. This technique was previously described for orthotopic neobladders and showed sufficient capacity [43]. Ureteral implantation and the continence mechanism are based on the Miami pouch technique [42]. The Rome pouch series with the largest cohort size was published in 2011 and included 62 patients who underwent radical cystectomy mostly for bladder cancer but also for gynecological tumors. After the procedure, the continence rate for appendicostomies was 94% during the day and 88% during the night, while the continence rate for ileostomies was 90% during the day and 85% during the night. Forty-eight months after surgery, the Rome pouch appeared to have a median capacity of 607 ml [44]. In a gynecology-only cohort, late complications occurred in 32% and 24% of patients at 3 and 12 months, respectively, following surgery mostly due to stomal stenosis or ureteral stenosis [45]. These results match the reported complication rates for urological cohorts (30% long-term complications at a mean onset of 13 months postoperatively, mostly concerning the efferent limb) [46]. Notably, all publications on the Rome pouch originate from no more than three hospitals in Rome.

The most recently developed technique is the Turin pouch, which was first described in 2013 for patients with a prior appendectomy and consists of an ileocecal reservoir with 10 cm of the terminal ileum and 40 cm of the right colon, folded to obtain a U-shaped pouch via stapler detubularization, followed by the creation of an artificial efferent limb through stapler separation of a 5-cm tubularized flap of the colonic wall. Ureter implantation is performed according to the Nesbit technique into the preserved terminal ileum [47]. The largest and most recent cohort of Turin pouch, published in 2021, consisted primarily of females (79%) and bladder cancer patients and reported an approximate 90% daytime continence rate. In all, 24% of patients experienced stone formation within the pouch; 18% reported catheterization difficulties; 11% had efferent limb stenosis; and 10% observed ureteral stenosis and complicated urinary tract infection at their last follow-up. These numbers are roughly consistent with those of the initial series [47, 48].

In conclusion, ileocecal reservoirs provide good capacity with sufficient continence rates across all techniques and subtle differences regarding postoperative complications. However, due to mainly small cohorts as well as heterogeneous reporting of functional and objective outcomes, comparisons can often only be made with reservations.

Colonic Reservoirs

Irradiation of the pelvis compromises the use of ileocecal reservoirs; hence, a transverse colonic pouch using a transverse and upper ascending or descending colon was developed in 2000. The continence mechanism consisted of a narrowed colon segment that was incorporated into the anterior pouch wall [49]. In 2000, the largest cohort of Mainz pouch III patients was reported from Mainz, including 44 previously irradiated female patients. The continence rate was to be reported at 100% after two open revisions, with no early UD-related postoperative complications. However, 18% of patients developed late UD-related complications, mostly stoma stenosis. Each of the late complications required a reoperation. The median pouch capacity was found to be 480 ml [49]. A later publication described the use of Mainz pouch III also in non-irradiated patients and reported a continence rate of 83% for a small cohort of 24 patients, with 4% of them suffering from an early UD-related complication and late UD-related complications occurring in 8% of patients [50].

Ileal Reservoirs

The development of continent ileostomy and later the ileum reservoir for UD is attributed to Kock [51]. Nevertheless, other authors have also described the use of ileum reservoirs in the late 1940s and 1950s and also in the 1970s [52–56]. Kock worked intensively on how to create a low-pressure pouch that would enable continence, and he recognized the relevance of antimesenteric opening and reconfiguration of the bowel in a way that peristalsis would counteract itself and no increase in pressure would occur [51]. Kock presented the first clinical results on his pouch in 1982. The continence mechanism and the implantation site of the ureters were formed by two separate ileum intussusception nipples, which were reinforced by Marlex tapes and connected by the ileum reservoir [57]. The largest cohort of patients undergoing the Kock pouch dates back to 1989, when 489 patients received a continent cutaneous Kock pouch, predominantly for malignant causes. Due to several modifications over the years, late complication rates and incontinence rates decreased from above 40% and 20% to 22% and 15%, respectively. Early complications were reported in 16% of patients [58]. Several series reported significantly elevated reoperation rates for Kock pouch (38% and 53%) compared to other CCUDs [34, 59].

A few years later in 1998, Bochner, Stein, and Skinner published a novel antirefluxive valve mechanism and created the T-pouch [60]. Another modification was made by Abol-Enein, who implanted both ureters and the efferent segment into the W-shaped ileum reservoir using "serosa-lined extramural tunnels," also named the double T-pouch [11, 61]. This technique continues to be used in ileal reservoirs to date [62].

Outcomes, Complications, and Gender

To assess the functional and objective outcomes after establishing UD, authors have used a variety of study protocols, resulting in heterogeneous reporting over time. In addition, there is lack of evidence regarding the effect of gender on outcomes following CCUD, particularly as the overall rate of continent UDs decreases [7–9]. Few studies compared outcomes by gender for different types of UDs, including CCUD and/or ileal conduit and orthotopic neobladder and found that, in general, there were no significant differences. Yet, statistical power is consistently limited due to the small cohort sizes [63–67]. However, prior irradiation significantly increases the risk of both postoperative and UD-related complications [68, 69]. Unfortunately, pelvic irradiation is commonly indicated for gynecological malignancies.

Continence is an integral part of functional outcomes. However, authors have used different definitions of continence and reported data with varying levels of accuracy, making comparability impossible.

Postoperative complications are commonly divided into very early (≤30 days), early (≤90 days), and late complications. Overall, instruments for standardized reporting are rarely applied. In many cases, a rate of major complications is reported rather than an overall complication rate (major complications: grade IIIa and higher according to the Clavien–Dindo classification). Moreover, complications are sometimes divided into UD-related and UD-unrelated complications or into complications concerning the efferent or afferent limb.

The Efferent Segment

To ensure continence and feasible self-catheterization in CCUDs, many different techniques and modifications of the efferent segment have been described and published. Some of them can be applied to different reservoirs. In general, these techniques can be divided into different principles; the flap valve principle, the nipple valve principle, hydraulic valves, and artificial valves using tissue engineering [70].

The most common technique is probably the flap valve principle included in the Mitrofanoff procedure (Fig. 15.1), which uses the tunneled appendix to create the efferent segment. The largest published series for in situ appendix in the context of Mainz pouch I reports continence in 96% of patients and a stenosis rate of 24% [26]. If the appendix is not available, the Mitrofanoff principle can be applied according to Monti and Yang using a short section of the small intestine, which is antimesenterically detubularized and then transversally re-tubularized to create a narrower and longer tunnel [71, 72]. The largest series in children comparing Monti channels with appendicovesicostomy was published in 2015 and reported similar rates of stomal stenosis and incontinence (7.4% vs. 7.5% and 3.4% vs. 0.9%, respectively). However, the primary subfascial revision rate was significantly higher in Monti channels (16.6% vs. 6.5%, $p = 0.001$) [73]. Other techniques use a tapered ileum, stomach, ureter, fallopian tube, vas deferens, or skin as the efferent limb [74]. Serosa-lined extramural tunnels (Fig. 15.3), primarily described by Abol-Enein, also represent a common type of the flap valve principle. In 2004, Abol-Enein published a series featuring 93 patients, with a continence rate of 95%, stomal stenosis in 5%, and a failure to catheterize in 2% of patients over a mean follow-up period of 37 months [61].

The Kock pouch employs the nipple valve principle using an intussuscepted ileal nipple. The largest Kock pouch series reported an early complication rate of 17% and a late complication rate of 22%. Leakage was the leading cause of late complications in up to 15% of patients, whereas the stenosis rate was lower in 2.6% of patients compared to flap valves [70]. An intussuscepted ileal nipple is also described for Mainz pouch I (Fig. 15.4) and continues to be an

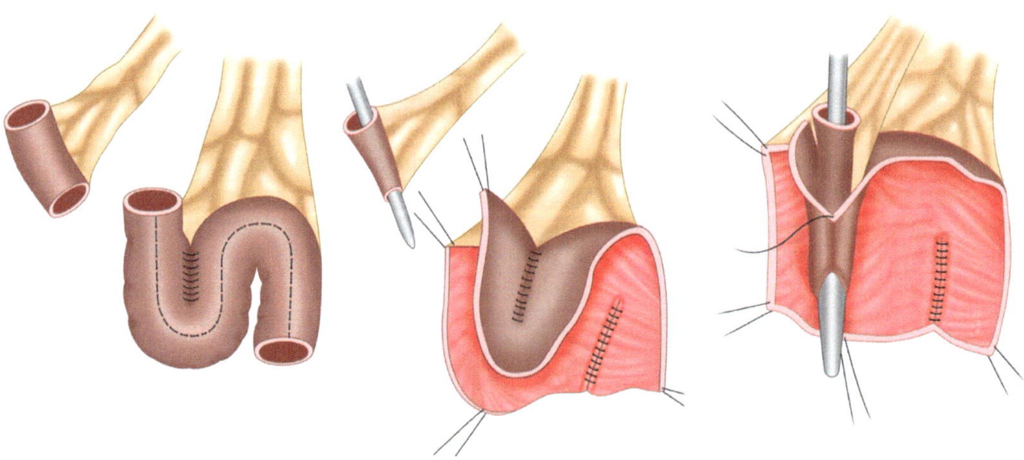

Fig. 15.3 Crafting a serous-lined extramural tunnel for ileal pouch continence. A 40-cm terminal ileum segment is partitioned into 30-cm oral and 10-cm caudal lengths. The oral segment is shaped into an "S," and its distal limbs is joined with a 4/0 seromuscular silk suture. The antimesenteric border is incised to form an ileal tunnel. The short caudal segment is adjusted around a 14-Fr catheter at its proximal two-thirds and is then implanted within the ileal tunnel

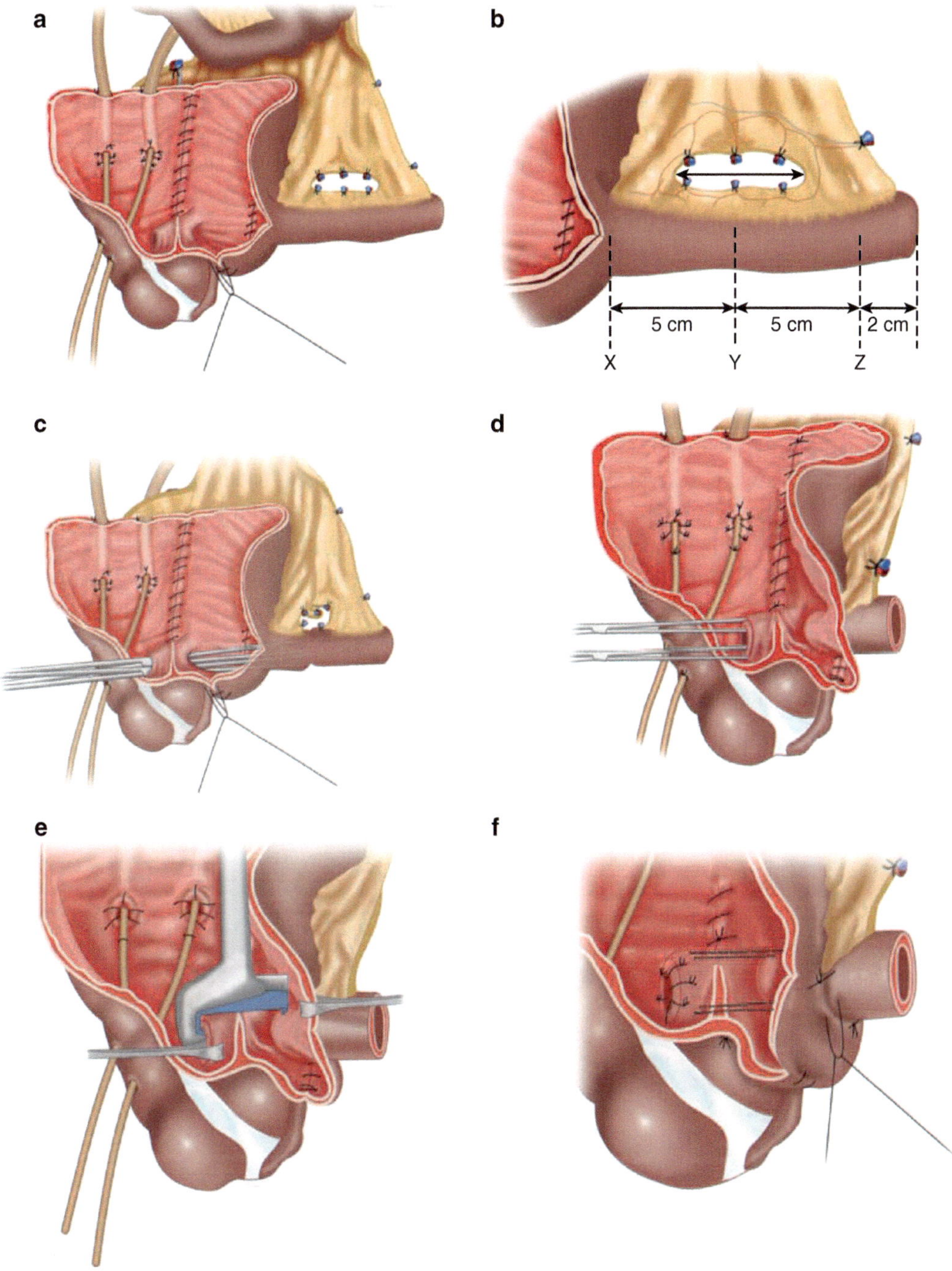

Fig. 15.4 Constructing an ileal intussusception nipple for a Mainz pouch 1 reservoir. (**a**) The intact proximal 12-cm ileum attached to the pouch is prepared for the nipple. The ileum's mesentery is separated 5 cm beyond the first arcade for easy intussusception. (**b**) Dimensions of the nipple segments are depicted: the mesenterial exclusion (5 cm over the nipple tip), the nipple tip (Y), the outer layer (X–Y), and the inner layer (Y–Z). The proximal 2 cm is reserved for umbilicus anastomosis. (**c**) Allis clamps grasp the ileal wall, inserted through the ileocecal valve, establishing the isoperistaltic nipple. (**d**) A completed 5-cm isoperistaltic nipple, pulled through the ileocecal valve with Allis clamps. (**e**) A nipple fixed to the ileocecal valve by three staple rows: two from inside the pouch and one from outside. (**f**) Closure of the nipple's mesenterial slit using several 3/0 polypropylene nonabsorbable sutures

option for patients without an appendix. The largest series of intussuscepted ileal nipple valves in Mainz pouch I included 491 patients, of whom 90% reported continence. The rate of stenosis was determined to be 15%, which was lower than the rate of stenosis for appendix stomas (24%) [26].

Benchekroun et al. described a hydraulic valve technique using a 14-cm ileal segment including its mesentery and creating a continence mechanism by folding the ileal segment inward so that the increase in pressure due to urine filling between the outer and inner parts of the folded ileum segment causes the inner canal to collapse and ensures continence [18]. The initial continence rates were described to be 75% at a median follow-up of 38 months [18] However, at 5 years' follow-up, 91% of patients had undergone surgical revision with stomal stenosis being the most common complication in 73% of patients [75].

To date, neither the artificial urinary sphincter system nor tissue engineering has been established in the context of CCUDs [70].

The Afferent Segment

Controversies regarding the use of antirefluxive or refluxive ureteral implantation techniques persist to date. While antirefluxive techniques are more likely to cause ureteral stenosis, refluxive techniques may cause reflux into the kidneys with subsequent upper urinary tract problems. However, higher rates of reflux with refluxive techniques do not appear to be associated with a reduction in renal function [76]. Given the context of a low-pressure reservoir and a higher risk of ureteral implantation stenosis with antirefluxive ureteral implantation techniques, some authors increased utilization of refluxive ureteral anastomoses in continent cutaneous urinary diversions over time [77, 78]. Well-known refluxive ureteral implantation techniques include Nesbit, Bricker, and Wallace (Fig. 15.5) [79–81]. The predominantly used antirefluxive implantation techniques include Leadbetter, Le Duc, the submucosal tunnel (Fig. 15.6), the serosa-lined extramural tunnel, the split-cuff nipple, and the intussuscepted ileal nipple [61, 82–85].

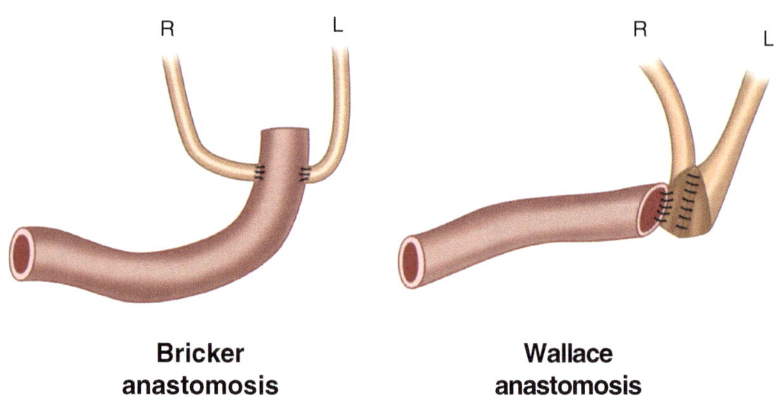

Fig. 15.5 Refluxive uretero-intestinal anastomosis techniques. In the Bricker method, spatulated ureters are individually anastomosed to the ileal segment. In the Wallace method, spatulated ureters are anastomosed along their medial walls, with the resultant conjoined ureters subsequently anastomosed to the ileal loop

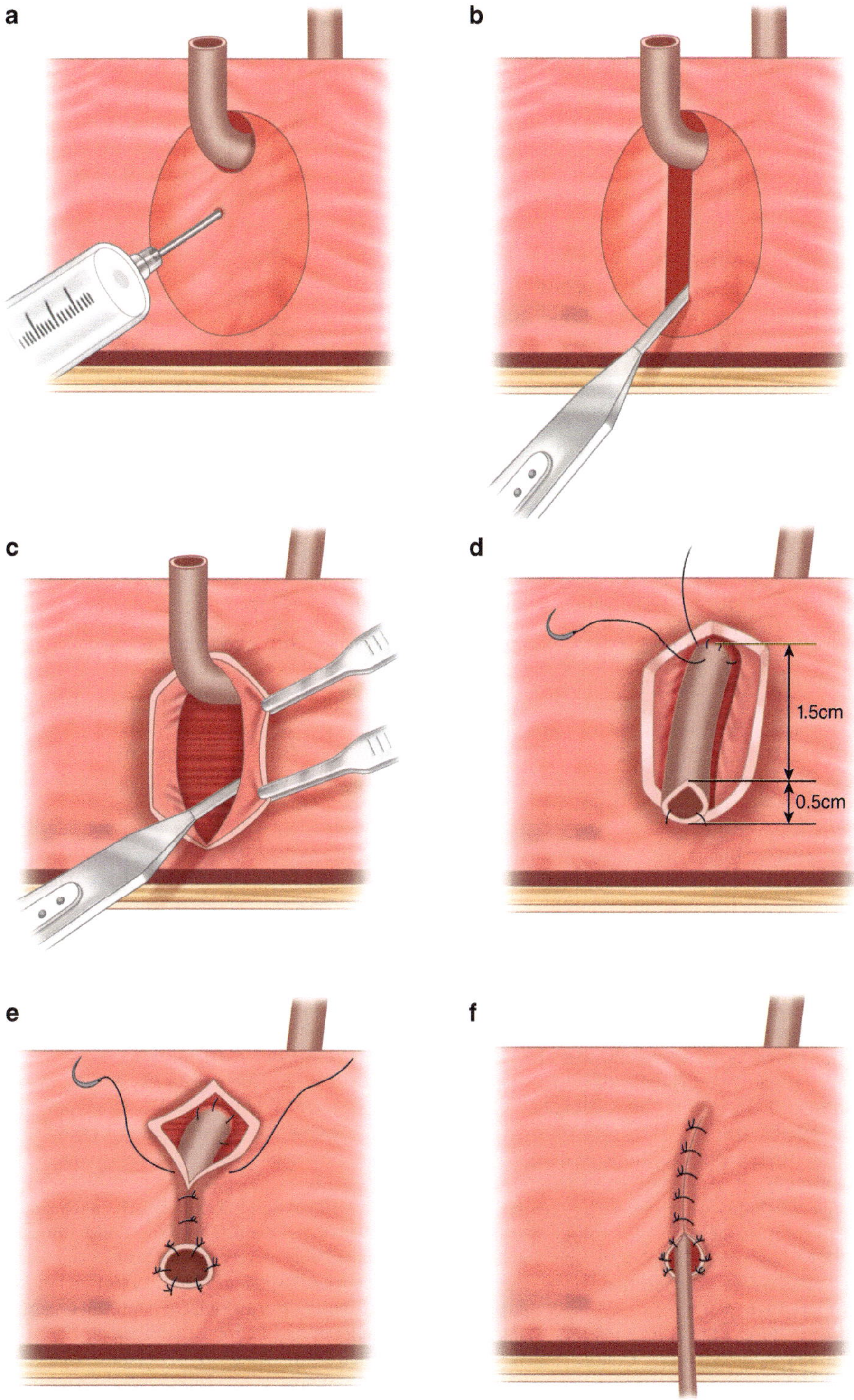

Fig. 15.6 A modified Le Duc submucosal tunnel. (**a**) The ureter is introduced 2 cm into the ileal lumen following saline injection. (**b**) A 2-cm full-thickness ileal mucosal sulcus is created. (**c**) The submucosal space is undermined, forming mucosal flaps. (**d**) The terminal ureter is spatulated for 5 mm, anchored, and the ureteral adventitia and ileal serosa are sutured. (**e**) A 1.5-cm non-spatulated ureter is concealed by mucosal flaps. (**f**) A ureteral stent is inserted

Conclusions

A variety of techniques exist for creating the reservoir, as well as the afferent and efferent segments, some of which can be combined in different ways. Mainz pouch I and Indiana pouch are among the most widely used CCUDs with excellent outcomes when performed by experienced surgeons and represent a valid alternative when an orthotopic neobladder is not feasible. However, careful patient selection is key to enable the best possible outcome.

Conflict of Interest None.

References

1. Sung H, Ferlay J, Siegel RL, Laversanne M, Soerjomataram I, Jemal A, et al. Global cancer statistics 2020: GLOBOCAN estimates of incidence and mortality worldwide for 36 cancers in 185 countries. CA Cancer J Clin. 2021;71(3):209–49.
2. Collaborative P. Minimum standards of pelvic exenterative practice: PelvEx Collaborative guideline. Br J Surg. 2022;109(12):1251–63.
3. Aftreth OP, Tenggardjaja CF, Reyblat P. Cystectomy for benign indications. Curr Urol Rep. 2022;23(9):195–201.
4. Vetterlein MW, Buhné MJ, Yu H, Klemm J, von Deimling M, Gild P, et al. Urinary diversion with or without concomitant cystectomy for benign conditions: a comparative morbidity assessment according to the updated European Association of Urology guidelines on reporting and grading of complications. Eur Urol Focus. 2022;8(6):1831–9.
5. European Association of Urology Guidelines on Muscle-invasive and Metastatic Bladder Cancer: Summary of the 2023 Guidelines European Urology. 2024;85(1):17–31. https://doi.org/10.1016/j.eururo.2023.08.016.
6. Vetterlein MW, Klemm J, Gild P, Bradtke M, Soave A, Dahlem R, et al. Improving estimates of perioperative morbidity after radical cystectomy using the European Association of Urology quality criteria for standardized reporting and introducing the comprehensive complication index. Eur Urol. 2020;77(1):55–65.
7. Klemm J, Fisch M, Laukhtina K, Dahlem R, Shariat SF, Vetterlein MW. Continent diversion is losing its momentum: a nationwide trend analysis from Germany 2005–2021. BJU International. 2024;133(2);154–157. https://doi.org/10.1111/bju.v133.210.1111/bju.16215.
8. Groeben C, Koch R, Baunacke M, Schmid M, Borkowetz A, Wirth MP, et al. Urinary diversion after radical cystectomy for bladder cancer: comparing trends in the US and Germany from 2006 to 2014. Ann Surg Oncol. 2018;25(12):3502–9.
9. Bachour K, Faiena I, Salmasi A, Lenis AT, Johnson DC, Pooli A, et al. Trends in urinary diversion after radical cystectomy for urothelial carcinoma. World J Urol. 2018;36(3):409–16.
10. von Deimling M, Laukhtina E, Pradere B, Pallauf M, Klemm J, Fisch M, et al. Radical cystectomy and urinary diversion in women: techniques, outcomes, and challenges-a narrative review. Transl Androl Urol. 2022;11(11):1598–610.
11. Fisch M, Thüroff JW. Continent cutaneous diversion. BJU Int. 2008;102(9 Pt B):1314–9.
12. Skinner EC. Continent cutaneous diversion. Curr Opin Urol. 2015;25(6):555–61.
13. Verhoogen J. Neostomie uretero-caecale: formation d'une nouvelle poche vesicale et d'un nouvel uretre. Assoc Franc Urol. 1908;12:362.
14. Makkas M. Zur behandlung der Blasenektopie. Umwandlung des ausgeschalteten Coecum zur Blase und der Appendix zur Urethra. Zentralbl Chir. 1910;37:1073–6.
15. Gilchrist RK, Merricks JW, Hamlin HH, Rieger IT. Construction of a substitute bladder and urethra. Surg Gynecol Obstet. 1950;90(6):752–60.
16. Zingg E, Tscholl R. Continent cecoileal conduit: preliminary report. J Urol. 1977;118(5):724–8.
17. Ashken MH. An appliance-free ileocaecal urinary diversion: preliminary communication. Br J Urol. 1974;46(6):631–7.
18. Benchekroun A. Continent caecal bladder. Eur Urol. 1977;3(4):248–50.
19. Mansson W, Sundin T. Experience with a continent cecal reservoir in urinary-diversion. Scand J Urol Nephrol. 1978; Scandinavian University Press Toyen, Journal Division Customer.
20. Månsson W, Davidsson T, Colleen S. The detubularized right colonic segment as urinary reservoir: evolution of technique for continent diversion. J Urol. 1990;144(6):1359–61.
21. Liedberg F, Gudjonsson S, Xu A, Bendahl PO, Davidsson T, Månsson W. Long-term third-party assessment of results after continent cutaneous diversion with Lundiana pouch. BJU Int. 2017;120(4):530–6.
22. Thüroff J, Alken P, Riedmiller H, Engelmann U, Jacobi G, Hohenfellner R. The Mainz pouch (mixed augmentation ileum and cecum) for bladder augmentation and continent diversion. J Urol. 1986;136(1):17–26.
23. Riedmiller H. Appendix as continent urinary reservoir outlet. Scand J Urol Nephrol Suppl. 1992;142:73–5.
24. Thüroff J, Alken P, Riedmiller H, Jacobi G, Hohenfellner R. 100 cases of Mainz pouch: continuing experience and evolution. J Urol. 1988;140(2):283–8.
25. Lampel A, Hohenfellner M, Schultz-Lampel D, Thuroff J. In situ tunneled bowel flap tubes: 2 new

techniques of a continent outlet for Mainz pouch cutaneous diversion. J Urol. 1995;153(2):308–15.
26. Wiesner C, Bonfig R, Stein R, Gerharz EW, Pahernik S, Riedmiller H, et al. Continent cutaneous urinary diversion: long-term follow-up of more than 800 patients with ileocecal reservoirs. World J Urol. 2006;24(3):315–8.
27. Rowland RG, Mitchell ME, Bihrle R. The cecoileal continent urinary reservoir. World J Urol. 1985;3:185–90.
28. Rowland RG, Mitchell ME, Bihrle R, Kahnoski RJ, Piser JE. Indiana continent urinary reservoir. J Urol. 1987;137(6):1136–9.
29. Burns R, Speir R, Kern SQ, Jarvis H, Schmidt J, Cary C, et al. Early and midterm complications of the continent Catheterizable Indiana pouch urinary diversion: a 7-year experience. Urology. 2022;167:229–33.
30. Al Hussein Al Awamlh B, Wang LC, Nguyen DP, Rieken M, Lee RK, Lee DJ, et al. Is continent cutaneous urinary diversion a suitable alternative to orthotopic bladder substitute and ileal conduit after cystectomy? BJU Int. 2015;116(5):805–14.
31. Cheng KW, Yip W, Shah A, Medina LG, Ghoreifi A, Miranda G, et al. Stoma complications and quality of life in patients with Indiana pouch versus appendico/neo-appendico-umbilicostomy urinary diversions. World J Urol. 2021;39(5):1521–9.
32. Holmes DG, Thrasher JB, Park GY, Kueker DC, Weigel JW. Long-term complications related to the modified Indiana pouch. Urology. 2002;60(4):603–6.
33. Bihrle R. The Indiana pouch continent urinary reservoir. Urol Clin North Am. 1997;24(4):773–9.
34. Okada Y, Shichiri Y, Terai A, Kakehi Y, Terachi T, Arai Y, et al. Management of late complications of continent urinary diversion using the Kock pouch and the Indiana pouch procedures. Int J Urol. 1996;3(5):334–9.
35. Lockhart JL, Pow-Sang JM, Persky L, Kahn P, Helal M, Sanford E. A continent colonic urinary reservoir: the Florida pouch. J Urol. 1990;144(4):864–7.
36. Webster C, Bukkapatnam R, Seigne JD, Pow-Sang J, Hoffman M, Helal M, et al. Continent colonic urinary reservoir (Florida pouch): long-term surgical complications (greater than 11 years). J Urol. 2003;169(1):174–6.
37. Bejany DE, Politano VA. Stapled and non-stapled tapered distal ileum for construction of a continent colonic urinary reservoir. J Urol. 1988;140(3):491–4.
38. Bloch WE, Bejany DE, Penalver MA, Politano VA. Complications of the Miami pouch. J Urol. 1992;147(4):1017–9.
39. Salom EM, Mendez LE, Schey D, Lambrou N, Kassira N, Gómez-Marn O, et al. Continent ileocolonic urinary reservoir (Miami pouch): the University of Miami experience over 15 years. Am J Obstet Gynecol. 2004;190(4):994–1003.
40. Baboudjian M, Gondran-Tellier B, Michel F, Abdallah R, Rouy M, Gaillet S, et al. Miami pouch: a simple technique for efficient continent cutaneous urinary diversion. Urology. 2021;152:178–83.
41. Pattou M, Baboudjian M, Pinar U, Parra J, Rouprêt M, Karsenty G, et al. Continent cutaneous urinary diversion with an ileal pouch with the Mitrofanoff principle versus a Miami pouch in patients undergoing cystectomy for bladder cancer: results of a comparative study. World J Urol. 2022;40(5):1159–65.
42. Panici PB, Angioli R, Plotti F, Muzii L, Zullo MA, Manci N, et al. Continent ileocolonic urinary diversion (Rome pouch) for gynecologic malignancies: technique and feasibility. Gynecol Oncol. 2007;107(2):194–9.
43. Alcini E, Racioppi M, D'Addessi A, Alcini A, Menchinelli P, Grassetti F, et al. The ileocaecourethrostomy with multiple transverse taeniamyotomies for bladder replacement: an alternative to detubularized neobladders. Morphological, functional and metabolic results after 9 years' experience. Br J Urol. 1997;79(3):333–8.
44. Ferriero M, Simone G, Papalia R, Guaglianone S, Forastiere E, Gallucci M. Early and late urodynamic assessment of simplified Indiana pouch with multiple taeniamyotomies. BJU Int. 2011;107(1):112–6.
45. Angioli R, Zullo MA, Plotti F, Bellati F, Basile S, Damiani P, et al. Urologic function and urodynamic evaluation of urinary diversion (Rome pouch) over time in gynecologic cancers patients. Gynecol Oncol. 2007;107(2):200–4.
46. Gallucci M, Leonardo C, Guaglianone S, Roccheggiani A, Alcini A, Flammia GP, et al. Simplified Indiana pouch with multiple teniamyotomies. Urology. 2006;67(1):93–6.
47. Muto G, Castelli E, D'Urso L, Leucci G, Collura D, Giacobbe A. The Turin pouch: a new technique of ileocecal cutaneous continent urinary diversion. Urology. 2013;81(3):663–8.
48. Muto G, Giacobbe A, Collura D, Germinale F, Kurti M, Papalia R, et al. A right colon pouch with a novel efferent channel concept: long-term results of the Turin pouch. World J Urol. 2021;39(6):1935–40.
49. Leissner J, Black P, Fisch M, Höckel M, Hohenfellner R. Colon pouch (Mainz pouch III) for continent urinary diversion after pelvic irradiation. Urology. 2000;56(5):798–802.
50. Stolzenburg JU, Schwalenberg T, Liatsikos EN, Sakelaropoulos G, Rödder K, Hohenfellner R, et al. Colon pouch (Mainz III) for continent urinary diversion. BJU Int. 2007;99(6):1473–7.
51. Kock NG. Intra-abdominal reservoir in patients with permanent ileostomy: preliminary observations on a procedure resulting in fecal continence in five ileostomy patients. Arch Surg. 1969;99(2):223–31.
52. Pearl JI. Intussuscepted conical valve formation in jejunostomies. Surgery. 1949;25(2):297–9.
53. Basso DE. The efficacy and applicability of an intussuscepted conical valve in preventing regurgitation and leakage of intestinal contents. Ann Surg. 1951;133(4):477.

54. Smith GI, Hinman F. The intussuscepted ileal cystostomy. J Urol. 1955;73(2):261–9.
55. Mayor G, Leisinger H, Säuberli H, Schauwecker H. Continent ileal bladder: first clinical experience. Eur Urol. 1976;2:8–12.
56. Madigan M. The continent ileostomy and the isolated ileal bladder. Ann R Coll Surg Engl. 1976;58(1):62.
57. Kock N, Nilson A, Nilsson L, Norlen L, Philipson B. Urinary diversion via a continent ileal reservoir: clinical results in 12 patients. J Urol. 1982;128(3):469–75.
58. Skinner DG, Lieskovsky G, Boyd S. Continent urinary diversion. J Urol. 1989;141(6):1323–7.
59. Carr LK, Webster GD. Kock versus right colon continent urinary diversion: comparison of outcome and reoperation rate. Urology. 1996;48(5):711–4.
60. Bochner BH, Stein JP, Ginsberg DA, Kurzrock E, Figueroa A, Skinner DG. A serous lined antireflux valve: in vivo fluorourodynamic evaluation of antireflux continence mechanism. J Urol. 1998;160(1):112–5.
61. Abol-Enein H, Salem M, Mesbah A, Abdel-Latif M, Kamal M, Shabaan A, et al. Continent cutaneous ileal pouch using the serous lined extramural valves. The Mansoura experience in more than 100 patients. J Urol. 2004;172(2):588–91.
62. Furrer MA, Noser L, Lyttwin B, Kiss B, Thomas BC, Bosshard P, et al. Functional results, complications associated with the serosa-lined tunnel, and quality of life with a cross-folded Ileal reservoir combined with an afferent tubular Isoperistaltic segment for heterotopic continent urinary diversion: an observational long-term cohort analysis. Eur Urol Focus. 2021;7(4):869–76.
63. Gellhaus PT, Cary C, Kaimakliotis HZ, Johnson CS, Weiner M, Koch MO, et al. Long-term health-related quality of life outcomes following radical cystectomy. Urology. 2017;106:82–6.
64. Myers JB, Martin C, Cheng PJ, Zhang C, Presson AP. Outcomes of right colon continent urinary pouch using standardized reporting methods. Neurourol Urodyn. 2019;38(5):1290–7.
65. Kern SQ, Speir RW, Tong Y, Kaimakliotis H, Masterson TA, Bihrle R, et al. Longitudinal health related quality of life after open radical cystectomy: comparison of Ileal conduit, Indiana pouch, and orthotopic neobladder. Urology. 2021;152:184–9.
66. Weijerman PC, Schurmans JR, Hop WC, Schröder FH, Bosch JL. Morbidity and quality of life in patients with orthotopic and heterotopic continent urinary diversion. Urology. 1998;51(1):51–6.
67. Large MC, Katz MH, Shikanov S, Eggener SE, Steinberg GD. Orthotopic neobladder versus Indiana pouch in women: a comparison of health related quality of life outcomes. J Urol. 2010;183(1):201–6.
68. Gontero P, Pisano F, Palou J, Joniau S, Albersen M, Colombo R, et al. Complication rate after cystectomy following pelvic radiotherapy: an international, multicenter, retrospective series of 682 cases. World J Urol. 2020;38(8):1959–68.
69. Eisenberg MS, Dorin RP, Bartsch G, Cai J, Miranda G, Skinner EC. Early complications of cystectomy after high dose pelvic radiation. J Urol. 2010;184(6):2264–9.
70. Ardelt PU, Woodhouse CR, Riedmiller H, Gerharz EW. The efferent segment in continent cutaneous urinary diversion: a comprehensive review of the literature. BJU Int. 2012;109(2):288–97.
71. Yang W-H. Yang needle tunneling technique in creating antireflux and continent mechanisms. J Urol. 1993;150(3):830–4.
72. Monti PR, Lara RC, Dutra MA, de Carvalho JR. New techniques for construction of efferent conduits based on the Mitrofanoff principle. Urology. 1997;49(1):112–5.
73. Szymanski KM, Whittam B, Misseri R, Flack CK, Hubert KC, Kaefer M, et al. Long-term outcomes of catheterizable continent urinary channels: what do you use, where you put it, and does it matter? J Pediatr Urol. 2015;11(4):210.e1–7.
74. Alsulihem A, Corcos J. Technical aspects and outcome review of continent catheterizable channels in the adult neurourologic population. Urol Ann. 2022;14(3):205–14.
75. Sanda MG, Jeffs RD, Gearhart JP. Evolution of outcomes with the ileal hydraulic valve continent diversion: reevaluation of the Benchekroun catheterizable stoma. World J Urol. 1996;14(2):108–11.
76. Zhang Y, Ding H, Zhang Y, Tian J, Yang L, Dong Z, et al. Is anti-reflux anastomosis an advantage in an Orthotopic Ileal Neobladder? A systematic review and meta-analysis. Urol Int. 2023;107(1):1–14.
77. von Knobloch R, Seybold M, Fischer HP, Kibele M, Samad WA. Modification of the Indiana pouch Ileo-Caecal cutaneous continent urinary diversion: tubular Ileal afferent limb for ureteral anastomosis has low stricture rate and allows Ileal ureter replacement. Urol Int. 2022;106(2):180–5.
78. Hohenfellner R, Black P, Leissner J, Allhoff EP. Refluxing ureterointestinal anastomosis for continent cutaneous urinary diversion. J Urol. 2002;168(3):1013–6. discussion 6–7
79. Nesbit RM. Ureterosigmoid anastomosis by direct elliptical connection. Univ Hosp Bull. 1948;14(6):45.
80. Wallace DM. Ureteric diversion using a conduit: a simplified technique. Br J Urol. 1966;38(5):522–7.
81. Bricker EM. Bladder substitution after pelvic evisceration. Surg Clin North Am. 1950;30(5):1511–21.
82. Politano VA, Leadbetter WF. An operative technique for the correction of vesicoureteral reflux. J Urol. 1958;79(6):932–41.
83. Le Duc A, Camey M, Teillac P. An original antireflux ureteroileal implantation technique: long-term followup. J Urol. 1987;137(6):1156–8.
84. Stone AR, MacDermott JP. The split-cuff ureteral nipple reimplantation technique: reliable reflux prevention from bowel segments. J Urol. 1989;142(3):707–9.
85. Janknegt RA. Construction of ileal nipples as antireflux valve technique. Eur Urol. 1988;14(1):46–9.

Complications of Ileal Conduit Urinary Diversion: A Comprehensive Review

16

Timothy Donahue and Charissa Chu

Introduction

Since the 1950s, the ileum has been the primary choice for urinary diversion after pelvic surgery to remove the bladder for conditions such as bladder cancer, severe neurogenic bladder, or other pelvic malignancies [1]. Despite seven decades of experience and technical advancements, ileal conduit urinary diversion remains associated with long- and short-term medical and surgical complications, with lasting effects on quality of life.

Complications with ileal conduit urinary diversion can be generally categorized into stoma and conduit-related, intestinal complications, infections, metabolic disturbances, and sexual health impacts. Although most of these complications affect both men and women, recent quality-of-life studies have highlighted the fact that female-specific changes after urinary diversion remain understudied. This chapter details the various complications associated with urinary diversion to better inform patient education and provide guidance on the management of various complications, as they may pertain to woman specifically.

T. Donahue (✉)
Department of Surgery, Memorial Sloan Kettering Cancer Center, New York, NY, USA
e-mail: donahuet@mskcc.org

C. Chu
Department of Urology, University of California, San Francisco, San Francisco, CA, USA
e-mail: carissa.chu@ucsf.edu

Stoma-Related Complications

Stoma-related complications can arise owing to poor stoma care, infection, or mechanical trauma. Common issues include peristomal skin irritation, stomal stenosis, prolapse, and retraction. Regular assessment, appropriate hygiene practices, and skilled stoma care education can minimize these complications and improve patients' quality of life.

Singh and colleagues reported complication rates after ileal conduit diversion for 93 patients, with an average follow-up of 5 years, and noted stoma-related complications were the most frequently encountered (31%), with reported rates in the literature varying from 27 to 50% [2].

Parastomal Hernia

The majority of parastomal hernias occur within the first 2 years after surgery. The most accurate clinical definition is any palpable defect or bulge adjacent to the stoma when the patient is supine with legs elevated or when straining in an upright position. If cross-sectional imaging is added to the clinical examination, a parastomal hernia can be defined as any intra-abdominal content protruding along the ostomy. Different types of parastomal hernias have been described. A type 1 parastomal hernia is defined as a hernia sac that contains prolapsed bowel forming the stoma.

M. Hoffman et al. (eds.), *Major Complications of Female Pelvic Surgery*,
https://doi.org/10.1007/978-3-031-66772-5_16

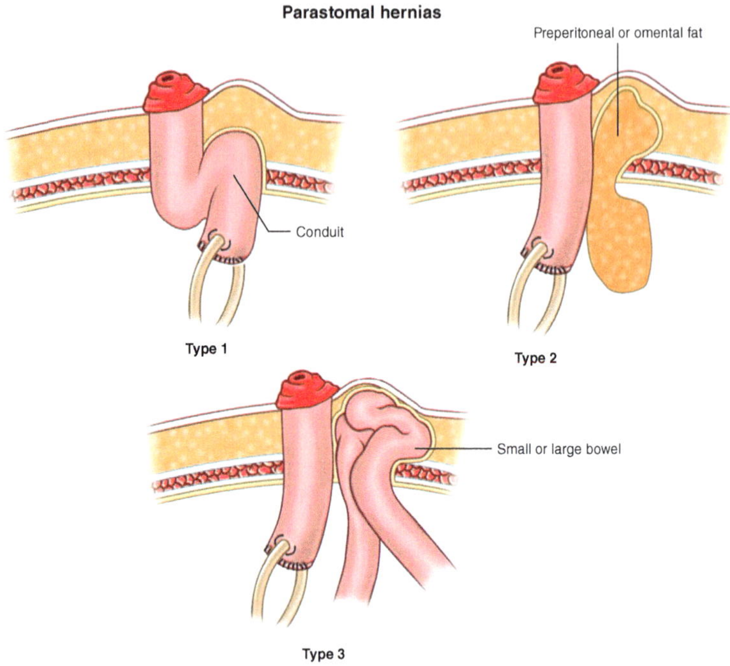

Fig. 16.1 Depiction of different types of parastomal hernias. Type 1, showing a hernia sac that contains prolapsed conduit. Type 2, showing abdominal fat or omentum hernia. Type 3 contains herniated loops of bowel other than that forming the stoma

Type 2 contains abdominal fat or omentum herniating through the abdominal wall defect created by the stoma. A type 3 hernia contains herniated loops of bowel other than that forming the stoma (Fig. 16.1).

The etiology of parastomal hernias is multifactorial and influenced by both technical and patient-related factors. In our published series of 386 patients undergoing open radical cystectomy and ileal conduit, risk of parastomal hernia formation was independently associated with female gender (HR 2.25; 95% CI 1.58, 3.21; $p < 0.0001$), higher body mass index (HR 1.08 per unit increase; 95% CI 1.05, 1.12; $p < 0.0001$) and lower preoperative albumin (HR 0.43 per g/dl; 95% CI 0.25, 0.75; $p = 0.003$) after adjusting for age, diabetes, smoking history, chronic obstructive pulmonary disorder, estimated blood loss, prior abdominal surgery, preoperative radiation therapy, neoadjuvant chemotherapy, and stoma type (end-stoma versus the Turnbull technique) [3].

Technical factors, such as the type of stoma created, the size and location of the stoma, the use of fascial anchoring sutures, and preoperative marking by a wound-ostomy nurse, may alter the risk of parastomal hernia development. Other patient-related factors believed to be associated with parastomal hernia development include obesity, age, prior abdominal surgery, smoking, poor nutrition, emergency surgery, postoperative sepsis, corticosteroid use, and history of malignancy [4–8].

Although most patients with parastomal hernias are asymptomatic, up to one third will undergo surgical repair on an elective basis for bothersome symptoms or occasionally under emergency circumstances owing to strangulation or bowel obstruction. Recurrences after hernia repair are frequent and often require reoperation [3, 9]. The benefit of prophylactic mesh placed at the time of conduit creation is currently being evaluated in a clinical trial.

Stomal Stenosis

Stomal stenosis may result from chronic ischemia, fascial narrowing, retraction of the stoma, or due to local skin changes from chronic irritation and dermatitis. Fluctuations in weight and body habitus can also affect the orientation of the stoma. When constructing the stoma, formation of a protrusion approximately 5 mm above the skin level allows for appropriate fit of the ostomy appliance and minimizes the local skin changes associated with leakage, skin irritation, and hyperkeratosis that can ultimately lead to stomal stenosis. Long-term sequelae of stomal stenosis may include urinary obstruction, recurrent infections, and upper tract deterioration. Historically, stomal stenosis rates have been reported to be as high as 25%. Historic series describe stomal stenosis rates as high as 25% for end-stomal ileal conduits and 10–20% for Turnbull loop stomas, although in more contemporary series stenosis rates are closer to 3% [22]. The role of gender in stomal stenosis remains undefined.

Turnbull loop stomas have been associated with significantly reduced rates of stomal stenosis [23] and should be considered in patients with a short mesentery and a thick abdominal wall, where an end-stoma approach may not be feasible. Surgical repair of stomal stenosis may be as simple as a circumferential releasing incision; however, more complex repairs such as a Y-V plasty or intra-abdominal release of the conduit may be necessary, depending on the severity and level of stenosis. Patients who are no longer surgical candidates may be managed with stomal catheters, which must be carefully irrigated and exchanged to maintain patency.

Ureterointestinal Stricture

Ureterointestinal strictures occur in 3–29% of patients, depending on the anastomotic technique used and the length of follow-up reported. Most strictures are felt to be due to ureteral ischemia and occur within the first 1–2 years after surgery irrespective of the type of anastomosis performed. Prior radiation, leak, or infection increase the risk of stricture development. These strictures are typically asymptomatic and only identified by changes in creatinine levels over time or on surveillance imaging studies. Minimizing mobilization and devascularization of ureters is paramount in reducing the risk of postoperative strictures. Care must be taken in routing the left ureter under the descending colon or through an avascular segment of its mesentery, which should be considered when passing the ureter beneath the colon might cause excessive angulation or place the anastomosis on tension. Controversy over interrupted and running sutures for anastomosis remains [10, 11]. In the open technique, our standard practice is to place interrupted simple sutures. Prior pelvic radiation is associated with an increased risk of stricture and leakage owing to delayed healing mechanisms and compromised blood supply [9, 12–14]. In clinical practice, we recommend higher excision of irradiated ureteral segments to mitigate the risk of stricture.

Antegrade and retrograde endoscopic as well as open surgical approaches have been described to address ureterointestinal strictures. Endoscopic management is recommended, with short (<2-cm) strictures. At 3 years' follow-up, endoscopic management of ureterointestinal strictures has a reported continued success rate of only 32% [15]. Open surgical approaches have success rates approaching 90%, but are the most invasive and technically challenging. It is important to evaluate the split function of the kidney and rule out recurrent malignancy prior to performing a repair.

Infection

Urinary tract infection and pyelonephritis are the most common infectious complications following ileal conduit urinary diversion and can occur both early and late. Bacterial colonization with the use of bowel substitution to skin is to be expected. Prompt diagnosis and effective antibiotic treatment are essential to prevent potential complications such as urosepsis.

Upper tract imaging should rule out nephrolithiasis or obstruction due to stricture, tumor, or stone as the possible underlying cause of recurrent pyelonephritis. Owing to reduced bile salt re-absorption, bacterial colonization, and chronic metabolic acidosis, patients with ileal conduits may be at increased risk of nephrolithiasis.

Patients with recurrent upper urinary tract infections should have workup for suspected strictures with cross-sectional and/or functional imaging, including CT, ultrasound, or renal scan. Fluoroscopic procedures, including antegrade nephrostogram or loopogram, can help to identify the underlying anatomical cause of recurrent infection as well. Last, the addition of prophylaxis may play a role in the prevention of recurrent infection, including cranberry extract, urinary alkalinization, or long-term antibiotics.

Ileus and Bowel Obstruction

Postoperative ileus remains one of the most common early complications (20–30%) after ileal conduit formation and typically occurs in the immediate postoperative setting, although readmissions for ileus do occur [16]. Although there is no standard definition, postoperative ileus is characterized by oral intake intolerance that persists beyond 5 days after surgery or by nausea and vomiting accompanied by abdominal distention that requires bowel rest, with or without a nasogastric tube [17, 18]. Ileus is associated with absent bowel sounds and delayed flatus.

Management of ileus is largely supportive care. Patients who are symptomatic may benefit from the use of a nasogastric tube for decompression. Imaging should be performed to differentiate ileus from early bowel obstruction. Although rare in the immediate postoperative period, bowel obstruction can be diagnosed by plain radiographs of the abdomen taken in the supine and upright positions, which may identify multiple air-fluid levels and lack of gas in the bowel distal to the point of obstruction. In contrast, patients with an ileus may also have air-fluid levels, but gas is typically seen throughout the entire gastrointestinal tract. Computed tomography with oral contrast medium has a sensitivity and specificity of over 90% in identifying small bowel obstruction [19]. Electrolyte abnormalities are common with nasogastric suction and ileus and should be monitored and corrected daily. Most patients regain bowel function with these supportive measures alone. Occasionally, parenteral nutrition may be required and should be carefully coordinated with inpatient nutrition and pharmacy teams.

The past decade has given rise to the development of enhanced recovery after surgery (ERAS) protocols for patients undergoing radical cystectomy to reduce rates of ileus and promote early return of gastrointestinal function. Although these protocols vary slightly by institution, ERAS emphasizes the avoidance of preoperative mechanical bowel preparation, reduction of opioid pain medication use, early ambulation, and addition of alvimopan, an oral μ-receptor antagonist [16, 20]. These measures have been associated with improved gastrointestinal recovery, shorter hospital stays, and reduced major adverse events [16, 20]. Liposomal or volume-expanded bupivacaine are other adjunctive measures for decreasing demand for postoperative opioid medications [21, 22].

Bowel obstruction is less common than ileus (0.7–11%) and refers to the absence of any passage of stool or flatus beyond an anatomically defined point of obstruction, as visualized on imaging [23]. Reoperation should be considered for lack of resolution by 10–14 days [24]. Partial bowel obstruction can also occur and is more likely to resolve with nasogastric tube decompression, fluid resuscitation, electrolyte replacement, and time. Upward of 90% of patients with a partial small bowel obstruction can be safely managed in this manner, with two thirds of these bowel obstructions resolving within 7 days and the remainder within 14 days [25].

Enterocutaneous Fistula

Fistulae are rare (<5%) after urinary diversion and refer to an anomalous communication between the bowel and adjacent organ, typically skin (enterocutaneous), but can include bowel–diversion (enterodiversion) and conduit–skin (diversion cutaneous) [26] Poor preoperative nutritional status is a major risk factor and is associated with an increased risk of anastomotic leak, wound infections, and poor healing. Patients with pre-existing conditions such as diabetes or renal insufficiency, prior chemotherapy use, and/or radiation exposure, or chronic steroid use, are at an increased risk of fistula formation.

The initial presentation for an enterocutaneous fistula often occurs between postoperative days 4 and 7 and is marked by signs and symptoms consistent with a wound infection: leukocytosis, fever, peri-incisional erythema, and edema, and drainage of either pus or feculent material from the wound. The initial management of a fistula is not operative but rather supportive, with attention directed toward managing the infection, ruling out leakage, and draining any intra-abdominal fluid collections, correcting electrolyte and fluid losses, and providing adequate nutrition. Patients may require parenteral antibiotics and bowel rest with total parenteral nutrition as well. Urostomy care is often compromised by the location of the fistula and complex management with a specialized urostomy nurse is recommended.

If the fistula does not resolve after 6 weeks of appropriate nutritional support and no evidence of infection, spontaneous resolution is unlikely, and further management is based upon the volume of enteric losses through the fistula and whether the patient is at risk of continued sepsis. Some small-volume enterocutaneous fistulas may be observed and managed non-operatively over the long term.

Anastomotic Leak

A rare but devastating complication is bowel leak at the ileo-ileal anastomosis, reported in 1–5% of patients after ileal conduit urinary diversion [27]. Factors that may contribute to the risk of bowel anastomotic leak include poor preoperative nutrition, ischemia at the site of the bowel anastomosis, prior intestinal surgery, chemotherapy exposure, history of radiation therapy, steroid use, excess tension on the anastomotic repair, and distal obstruction.

Anastomotic bowel is associated with sepsis, abscess formation, fistula formation, and wound breakdown. Exploratory laparotomy, segmental bowel resection, re-anastomosis, and proximal intestinal diversion are often required to address this severe complication.

Conduit Necrosis

Acute ischemia of the segment of bowel forming the conduit may be due to mesenteric compromise, inadequate preservation of the arterial arcades, or prior surgery to the bowel affecting collateral blood flow. Conduit necrosis must be distinguished from the typical edema that accompanies conduit construction immediately postoperatively. In contrast to stomal edema and venous congestion, conduit necrosis often manifests with a progressively darkening stoma, with retraction of the conduit away from the skin edges forming the border of the abdominal wall site. The conduit above and below the abdominal wall fascia demonstrates vascular compromise, which can be visualized during endoscopy of the conduit or gentle insertion of a test tube into the lumen of the conduit and illuminated to visualize the proximal bowel. Patients with a nonviable conduit may present clinically with sepsis, metabolic acidosis, hyperphosphatemia, and occasionally shock. Acute conduit necrosis is a surgical emergency and requires urgent abdominal exploration to inspect both the conduit and the entire small bowel to look for vascular compromise followed by excision and replacement of the ischemic conduit.

Metabolic Disturbances

The ileum is associated with the fewest electrolyte abnormalities compared to colon, stomach, or jejunal urinary substitution. Metabolic abnormalities occur because of the absorption of ammonium chloride in urine, resulting in hyperchloremic metabolic acidosis. Patients with impaired renal function can develop lethargy, anorexia, weight loss, and long-term risk of bone demineralization, leading to osteopenia. Symptomatic metabolic acidosis can be treated with alkalinizing agents such as sodium bicarbonate, maintaining good hydration, and optimizing urinary drainage.

The terminal ileum is also responsible for the absorption of bile salts, fat-soluble vitamins (K, A, D, and E), and the absorption of vitamin B-12. If excessive lengths of ileum are used for diversion, patients can develop steatorrhea, vitamin B-12 deficiency, and dehydration. These can be treated with cholestyramine and supplementation respectively. It is important to note that vitamin B-12 depletion occurs slowly, often taking 3–5 years to drop to a level sufficiently low enough to produce symptoms. Annual serum B-12 monitoring is recommended.

Chronic acidosis after urinary diversion occurs in 5.5–13.3% of patients at a mean follow-up of 51 months and can result long term in bone demineralization and osteomalacia. Decreased intestinal absorption of calcium can occur with resection of longer segments of ileum. Bone minerals, such as calcium and carbonate, act as buffers against hydrogen ions, leading to decreased skeletal calcium content. Chronic acidosis induces vitamin D deficiency, resulting in bone mineralization defects, and finally the acidic environment activates resorption of bone by osteoclasts. Laboratory values may show elevated alkaline phosphatase and reduced serum calcium and phosphate levels. Patients can present with a variety of issues related to bone demineralization ranging from being asymptomatic to pain in weight-bearing joints to having fractures [28].

Women appear to be at highest risk of the complications associated with bone demineralization and osteopenic fractures. Patients with impaired renal function are at a compounded risk of acidosis. Calcium and vitamin D supplementation is recommended for women and oral sodium bicarbonate should be considered for patients with a base deficit of −2.5 mmol/l to reduce the likelihood of developing bone sequelae from chronic acidosis [28]. Patients should undergo routine screening with metabolic panel for acidosis, with correction if needed with sodium bicarbonate and consultation with a nephrologist.

Sexual Side Effects and Quality of Life Impact

Ileal conduit urinary diversion can have a significant impact on a patient's sexual function and body image, leading to psychological distress. Addressing these concerns through counseling, support groups, and referral to appropriate specialists is crucial to help patients to cope with the psychological impact of the procedure.

One of the largest single-center series of 411 patients reporting comprehensive, 2-year longitudinal evaluation of contemporary patient-reported outcomes after cystectomy with urinary diversion (all types) found that there were no substantial detriments to patient-reported HRQOL within the first 2 years after surgery, other than worsened body image among patients receiving ileal conduit [29]. Although all patients (men and women) undergoing ileal conduits had lower baseline sexual function than all other patients undergoing continent diversion, no differences were detectable specifically among women when using the female-only Female Sexual Function Index surveys. Sexual function declined after surgery among all groups. A follow-up study among women showed that women may be more affected by body image perception after conduit (in publication).

Additional Thoughts

Women considering an ileal conduit procedure should undergo detailed discussions with their surgeon, as well as a specialized stoma nurse, who can provide personalized advice and guidance based on their individual needs and circumstances. Women may have unique considerations and providing gender-based support groups, counseling, and educational resources is critical in the short- and long-term recovery period.

Acknowledgement Catherine Tsai, MD, for contributing the illustration in Fig. 16.1.

References

1. Bricker EM. Bladder substitution after pelvic evisceration. Surg Clin North Am. 1950;30:1511–21.
2. Singh G, Wilkinson JM, Thomas DG. Supravesical diversion for incontinence: a long-term follow-up. Br J Urol. 1997;79:348–53.
3. Donahue TF, Bochner BH, Sfakianos JP, Kent M, Bernstein M, Hilton WM, et al. Risk factors for the development of parastomal hernia after radical cystectomy. J Urol. 2014;191:1708–13.
4. Nastro P, Knowles CH, McGrath A, Heyman B, Porrett TR, Lunniss PJ. Complications of intestinal stomas. Br J Surg. 2010;97:1885–9.
5. Arumugam PJ, Bevan L, Macdonald L, Watkins AJ, Morgan AR, Beynon J, et al. A prospective audit of stomas--analysis of risk factors and complications and their management. Color Dis. 2003;5:49–52.

6. Parmar KL, Zammit M, Smith A, Kenyon D, Lees NP. A prospective audit of early stoma complications in colorectal cancer treatment throughout the Greater Manchester and Cheshire colorectal cancer network. Color Dis. 2011;13:935–8.
7. De Raet J, Delvaux G, Haentjens P, Van Nieuwenhove Y. Waist circumference is an independent risk factor for the development of parastomal hernia after permanent colostomy. Dis Colon Rectum. 2008;51:1806–9.
8. Kouba E, Sands M, Lentz A, Wallen E, Pruthi RS. Incidence and risk factors of stomal complications in patients undergoing cystectomy with ileal conduit urinary diversion for bladder cancer. J Urol. 2007;178:950–4.
9. Liu NW, Hackney JT, Gellhaus PT, Monn MF, Masterson TA, Bihrle R, et al. Incidence and risk factors of parastomal hernia in patients undergoing radical cystectomy and ileal conduit diversion. J Urol. 2014;191:1313–8.
10. Large Michael C, Cohn Joshua A, Kiriluk Kyle J, Dangle P, Richards Kyle A, Smith Norm D, et al. The impact of running versus interrupted anastomosis on Ureterointestinal stricture rate after radical cystectomy. J Urol. 2013;190:923–7.
11. Reesink Daan J, Gerritsen Sarah L, Kelder H, van Melick Harm HE, Stijns Pascal EF. Evaluation of ureteroenteric anastomotic strictures after the introduction of robot-assisted radical cystectomy with Intracorporeal urinary diversion: results from a Large tertiary referral center. J Urol. 2021;205:1119–25.
12. Malgieri JJ, Persky L. Ileal loop in the treatment of radiation-treated pelvic malignancies: a comparative review. J Urol. 1978;120:32–4.
13. Alfert HJ, Gillenwater JY. The consequences of ureteral irradiation with special reference to subsequent ureteral injury. J Urol. 1972;107:369–71.
14. Ahlering TE, Kanellos A, Boyd SD, Lieskovsky G, Skinner DG, Bernstein L. A comparative study of perioperative complications with Kock pouch urinary diversion in highly irradiated versus nonirradiated patients. J Urol. 1988;139:1202–4.
15. Wolf JS Jr, Elashry OM, Clayman RV. Long-term results of endoureterotomy for benign ureteral and ureteroenteric strictures. J Urol. 1997;158:759–64.
16. Djaladat H, Daneshmand S. Gastrointestinal complications in patients who undergo radical cystectomy with enhanced recovery protocol. Curr Urol Rep. 2016;17:50.
17. Shabsigh A, Korets R, Vora KC, Brooks CM, Cronin AM, Savage C, et al. Defining early morbidity of radical cystectomy for patients with bladder cancer using a standardized reporting methodology. Eur Urol. 2009;55:164–74.
18. Ramirez JA, McIntosh AG, Strehlow R, Lawrence VA, Parekh DJ, Svatek RS. Definition, incidence, risk factors, and prevention of paralytic ileus following radical cystectomy: a systematic review. Eur Urol. 2013;64:588–97.
19. Donckier V, Closset J, Van Gansbeke D, Zalcman M, Sy M, Houben JJ, et al. Contribution of computed tomography to decision making in the management of adhesive small bowel obstruction. Br J Surg. 1998;85:1071–4.
20. Sultan S, Coles B, Dahm P. Alvimopan for recovery of bowel function after radical cystectomy. Cochrane Database Syst Rev. 2017;5:Cd012111.
21. Chu CE, Law L, Zuniga K, Lin TK, Tsourounis C, Rodriguez-Monguio R, et al. Liposomal bupivacaine decreases postoperative length of stay and opioid use in patients undergoing radical cystectomy. Urology. 2021;149:168–73.
22. Schmidt B, Bhambhvani HP, Greenberg DR, Prado K, Shafer S, Thong A, et al. Bupivacaine local anesthetic to decrease opioid requirements after radical cystectomy: does formulation matter? Urol Oncol. 2021;39:369.e1–8.
23. van Hemelrijck M, Thorstenson A, Smith P, Adolfsson J, Akre O. Risk of in-hospital complications after radical cystectomy for urinary bladder carcinoma: population-based follow-up study of 7608 patients. BJU Int. 2013;112:1113–20.
24. Ong AW, Myers SR. Early postoperative small bowel obstruction: a review. Am J Surg. 2020;219:535–9.
25. Pickleman J, Lee RM. The management of patients with suspected early postoperative small bowel obstruction. Ann Surg. 1989;210:216–9.
26. Smith ZL, Johnson SC, Golan S, McGinnis JR, Steinberg GD, Smith ND. Fistulous complications following radical cystectomy for bladder cancer: analysis of a large modern cohort. J Urol. 2018;199:663–8.
27. Taneja SS, Shah O. Complications of urologic surgery e-book: prevention and management. Elsevier Health Sciences; 2017.
28. Gupta A, Atoria CL, Ehdaie B, Shariat SF, Rabbani F, Herr HW, et al. Risk of fracture after radical cystectomy and urinary diversion for bladder cancer. J Clin Oncol. 2014;32:3291–8.
29. Clements MB, Atkinson TM, Dalbagni GM, Li Y, Vickers AJ, Herr HW, et al. Health-related quality of life for patients undergoing radical cystectomy: results of a Large prospective cohort. Eur Urol. 2022;81:294–304.

Part IV

Upper Urinary Tract

Injury Repair of Pelvic Ureter

17

Kyrollis Attalla and John P. Sfakianos

Background

Ureteral injury is a rare event, the most common cause being iatrogenic during open, minimally invasive, or endoscopic procedures. Penetrating trauma accounts for most non-iatrogenic ureteral injuries. The sequelae of unrecognized ureteral injuries range from urine leakage and abscess formation to severe complications, including ureteral stricture, loss of renal function, sepsis, urinary fistula, and even death. Often subtle in presentation, ureteral injuries require a high index of suspicion to obviate the potentially serious sequelae of unrecognized or mismanaged injuries.

Iatrogenic pelvic ureteral injuries are most common during hysterectomy and colorectal surgery; urological and vascular surgeries also account for a significant, albeit lower, incidence of pelvic ureteral injuries. Ureteral injury as a consequence of external trauma is rare, occurring in under 4% of penetrating trauma and less than 1% of cases of blunt trauma. In cases of penetrating trauma, the mechanism of injury is not only by direct transection but also indirectly subsequent to damage to the blood supply of the ureter. Concomitant abdominal or retroperitoneal organ injury is present in over 90% of patients with ureteral injuries, and mortality due to these injuries approaches 30% [1, 2].

The urological surgeon managing ureteral injuries requires a detailed understanding of the course and the associated anatomy of the ureters. The entirety of the ureter is divided into three distinct segments: (1) the proximal ureter, extending from the ureteropelvic junction to the upper border of the sacrum; (2) the middle ureter, coursing from the upper border of the sacrum to the iliac vessels; and (3) the distal ureter, extending from the iliac vessels to the urinary bladder. Likewise, an understanding of the proximity of the ureter to neighboring anatomy is critical in the prevention, identification, and subsequent management of a ureteral injury.

Descending from the upper retroperitoneum, the ureters lie atop the psoas muscle in the retroperitoneal space, taking a medial course of entry anteriorly over the common iliac arteries and posterior to the gonadal vessels prior to their entry at base of the bladder in the pelvis. In males, the ureter courses medial to the medial umbilical ligament and posteriorly under the vas deferens; in females, the proximity of the ureter to the uterine artery anteriorly at the ureterovesical junction brings a risk of injury to this segment of ureter during gynecological surgery.

K. Attalla · J. P. Sfakianos (✉)
Department of Urology, Icahn School of Medicine at Mount Sinai, New York, NY, USA
e-mail: john.sfakianos@mountsinai.org

M. Hoffman et al. (eds.), *Major Complications of Female Pelvic Surgery*,
https://doi.org/10.1007/978-3-031-66772-5_17

Prevention and Evaluation

Early recognition of a ureteral injury is critical to abate associated long-term sequelae. Thus, the earliest recognition of an iatrogenic ureteral injury is intraoperatively. Preventive measures include the use of intraoperatively placed ureteral stents to aid in identification of the ureters. Ureteral stents are often requested or placed by gynecological, colorectal, and vascular surgeons, given the relevant anatomy in close proximity to the ureters. Although prophylactic placement of ureteral stents may assist with identification of ureteral injuries, the ability to decrease the incidence of injury is unclear [3, 4]. Nevertheless, a recent review of the National Surgical Quality Improvement Program (NSQIP) demonstrated a lower rate of ureteral injury after colectomy with the use of ureteral stents [5]. In many situations there is anatomical distortion of the ureter secondary to mass effect, i.e. from gyn or colorectal tumors or fibrosis, i.e. from aortic aneurysms, that lead to difficulties in recognition or dissection of the ureter leading to increased risk of injury.

Postoperatively, a high index of suspicion is required to diagnose and localize a ureteral injury, which harbors several signs and symptoms. An even higher index of suspicion is required following laparoscopic or robotic cases; whereas one-third of ureteral injuries are recognized intraoperatively during open surgery, fewer injuries are recognized with minimally invasive approaches [6, 7]. Conditional upon the patient's clinical status, the recognition of ureteral injuries ranges from immediate to delayed. Fever, ileus, hematuria, leukocytosis, abdominal tenderness and/or distention, or a rise in serum creatinine secondary to peritoneal reabsorption of urine or secondary to an obstructed renal unit may be suggestive of ureteral injury with resultant peritoneal irritation, urinoma, or abscess formation. If a surgical drain was placed at the time of surgery, fluid may be sent for spot creatinine; it is positive for urine leakage if spot creatinine is greater than serum creatinine. If renal function permits the administration of intravenous (IV) contrast, computed tomography (CT) of the abdomen and pelvis with IV contrast medium and delayed urographic phase is an effective diagnostic tool in localizing ureteral injury. Retrograde pyelogram represents the most sensitive diagnostic tool to assess the location of injury and may also permit the simultaneous cystoscopic placement of a ureteral stent, depending on the extent of injury.

Management

Management of endoscopically induced ureteral injuries vary based on the extent of the injury. Perforation of the distal ureter is best managed with placement of a ureteral stent, typically removed approximately 4–6 weeks later. A urethral Foley catheter may or may not be placed temporarily to avoid reflux of urine from the bladder into the ureter to allow for maximal and optimal healing. Complete ureteral avulsions require surgical exploration and repair.

The evaluation of a suspected ureteral injury often occurs intraoperatively; as such, visualization of the pelvic ureter is limited by initial exposure achieved for the primary operation. The urological surgeon evaluating a possible pelvic ureteral injury may do so cystoscopically with a retrograde pyelogram if surgical exposure precludes direct access to the pelvic ureter. Intravenous administration of methylene blue may be a useful aid in localizing subtle injuries. Similarly, injection of methylene blue can be achieved cystoscopically in a retrograde fashion by ureteral catheterization. If on-table imaging is suggestive of injury, or if fluoroscopy is not readily available, the initial incision is extended or a counter-incision is created for adequate mobilization and direct visualization of the ureter. Inspection of the segment of ureter in question should note tissue viability, as evidenced by the appearance of the ureteral tissue, extravasation of urine, and size of the disruption or injury. Inquiry as to the mechanism of injury should be made, as thermal injuries requiring debridement beyond the readily apparent area of injury is required. Other common mechanisms of injury include sharp injury or transection, crush injuries, suture ligation, and the application of stapling or clip devices to the ureter. Prior to surgery proper inspection of patient imaging is important to understand anomalies of anatomy such as solitary kidneys or duplicated ureters.

Should the injury appear to be limited to a contusion with tissue viability, a ureteral stent may be cystoscopically placed as detailed previously. On the other hand the mechanism of injury such as thermal or high-powered projectile are important to recognize as the viability of the surrounding tissue maybe compromised requiring a larger resection area prior to reconstruction. Injuries recognized intraoperatively or within 1 week of surgery should be repaired immediately. In unstable trauma cases with concomitant ureteral injury, primary repair or reconstruction is delayed and the ureter is ligated proximal to the area of injury; a percutaneous nephrostomy tube is subsequently placed for drainage of the renal unit. Delayed recognition of a ureteral injury is managed with a ureteral stent, and/or percutaneous nephrostomy tube, or a percutaneous nephroureteral stent with a Foley catheter for complete drainage and maximal decompression of the urinary tract. Definitive repair is deferred until 6 weeks following the injury. Associated sequelae are additionally addressed; urinomas are optimally managed with the placement of a percutaneous drain, and abscesses are managed with percutaneous drain placement and culture-specific antibiotics.

The management and reconstruction of ureteral injuries are conditional upon the length of the defect and location of the injury. Primarily, short (3–4 cm) mid-ureteral defects can be repaired. Depending on the mechanism of injury, both ends of the ureter are debrided of all devascularized tissue accordingly. The proximal and distal ureter are both widely spatulated and an end-to-end anastomosis is completed using a 4-0 Vicryl suture in an interrupted fashion (Fig. 17.1). Careful handling of ureteral tissue with non-crushing forceps and the preservation of ureteral adventitia are critical to avoid disruption of the ureteral blood supply. A double-J ureteral stent is placed over a guidewire prior to completing the anastomosis (Fig. 17.1).

The preferred strategy for distal ureteral reconstruction is ureteral reimplant with or without a psoas hitch (Figs. 17.2 and 17.3). (insert the figure in this location; you have the figures at the end of the chapeter, please place them in the appropriate spot throughout the article: BB). The peritoneum overlying the ureter is incised proximally and distally to expose the injury and mobilize the ureter for a tension-free anastomosis. Dissection should be carried distally until the level of injury. The ovarian ligaments in females, may be retracted anteriorly to facilitate exposure. The ureter is transected just proximal to the injured segment of ureter; if already transected inadvertently, the ureteral tissue is carefully examined and debrided. If a refluxing extravesical reimplant is desired, an approximately 2-cm incision is made on the ipsilateral aspect of the bladder dome. The ureter is spatulated at the posterior, 6 o'clock aspect of the ureter and an anastomosis is performed in an interrupted fashion. Ureteral to bladder mucosal apposition is critical in maintaining optimal anastomotic principle. Prior to completing the anastomosis, a double-J ureteral stent is passed over a guidewire, with the proximal curl of the stent in the renal pelvis and the distal curl of the stent placed in the bladder. A second-layer closure of the bladder serosa to the ureteral adventitia may be performed. A leak test to assess the integrity of the anastomosis is completed by instilling 200–300 cc of normal saline into the bladder. In a similar fashion, a nonrefluxing anastomosis can be performed. To do this, a submucosal incision is made extravesically and a tunnel is formed. An incision is then made through into the bladder and the ureter is tunneled into the bladder. Similar to a refluxing procedure, the ureter is then spatulated and either in an interrupted or a running fashion anastomosed mucosa to mucosa.

A psoas hitch in addition to ureteroneocystomy is a highly effective approach to reconstructing the lower third of the ureter (Fig. 17.4). The ureteral gap is bridged by "hitching" the bladder to the ipsilateral psoas minor tendon using 2-0 Vicryl suture in a vertical manner to avoid entrapment of the genitofemoral nerve. For larger mid- to distal ureteral defects (Fig. 17.5), a

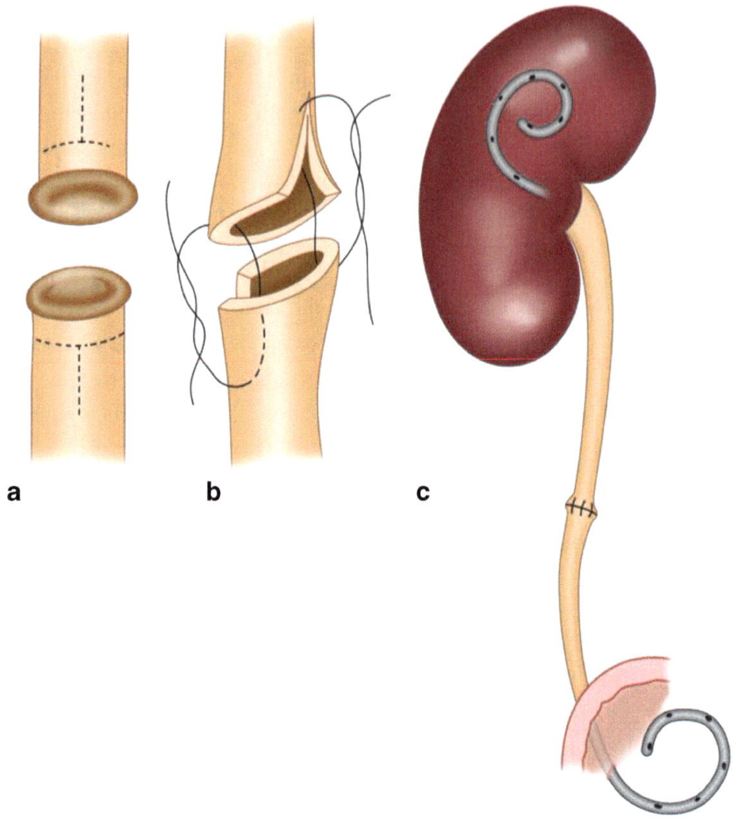

Fig. 17.1 (a–c) Double-spatulated ureteroureterostomy

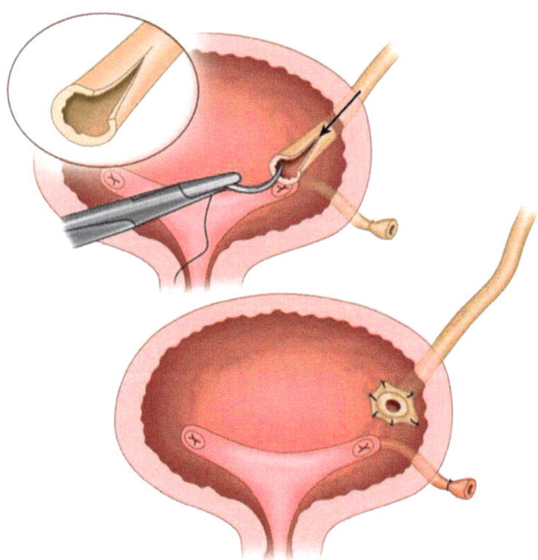

Fig. 17.2 Transvesical ureteroneocystostomy

Boari flap may be employed to create a tension-free anastomosis between the bladder and the ureter for larger areas requiring bridging (10–15 cm in length). Following assessment of the length of the defect and debridement of devitalized or injured ureteral tissue, the colon is mobilized medially by an incision along the white line of Toldt. An incision is made in the posterior peritoneum to dissect the proximal ureter; mobilizing the ureter at or above the level of the common iliac artery ensures adequate proximal mobilization. The contralateral aspect of the bladder is mobilized by dividing the superior vesicle pedicle. Division of the inferior vesicle pedicle is typically unnecessary, but may be performed if needed. Normal saline may be instilled through an indwelling urethral catheter to inflate the bladder and assist with dissecting the peritoneal lining off the bladder. Division of the ipsilateral medial umbilical ligament may help to further mobilize the bladder. A fine 4-0 or 5-0 stay suture is placed on the distal end of the proximal ureter.

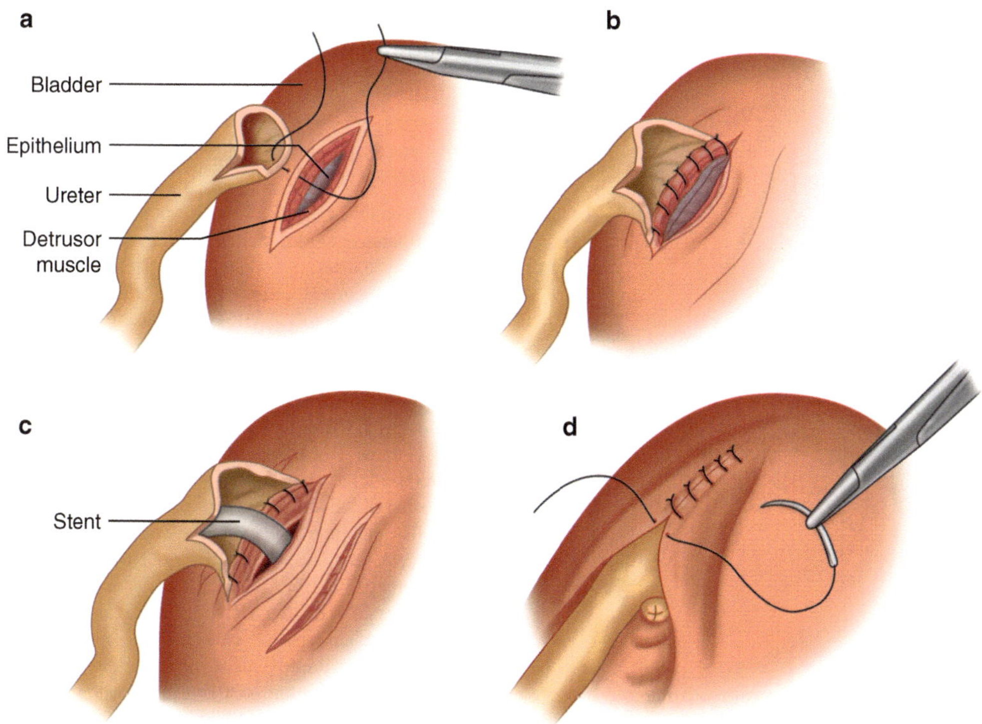

Fig. 17.3 (**a–d**) Direct ureteroneocystostomy

The bladder flap is prepared by instilling normal saline into the bladder, if not already performed. A surgical marking pen is used to outline the flap; the bladder flap should be no shorter than 4 cm at the base and 3 cm at the tip in order to avert distal ureteral constriction after tubularization. To ensure adequate blood supply to the flap, the ideal ratio of flap length to base width should be no greater than 3:1. The length of the flap should be equivalent to the length of the defect, plus an additional 3–4 cm to allow for a submucosal tunnel if a nonrefluxing anastomosis is desired. After the appropriate dimensions of the flap are outlined, four stay sutures are placed along the four corners of the flap.

An incision is made along the distal aspect of the flap. The posterior bladder wall is elevated toward the psoas muscle with insertion of an index finger into the bladder (if repair is being performed in an open fashion) and hitched to the psoas tendon. If concerns regarding tension on the anastomosis exist, the ipsilateral kidney may likewise be mobilized for an additional length of 5–8 cm. Likewise, a nonrefluxing anastomosis may be performed between a spatulated distal ureteral stump and the edge of the bladder flap.

If a nonrefluxing anastomosis is desired, an approximately 3-cm submucosal tunnel is created by hydrodistension beneath the mucosal layer with normal saline. The overlying mucosa is incised. The tagged end of the spatulated ureter is carefully brought through the tunnel and an anastomosis is performed using 4-0 Vicryl in an interrupted fashion. An initial stay stitch approximating the ureter to the bladder, incorporating the muscular layer of the bladder, may aid in stabilizing the anastomosis. A double-J ureteral stent is placed over a guidewire and the bladder is closed in a two-layer fashion, first by reapproximating the mucosal layer using a 4-0 Vicryl suture, followed by the muscularis and adventitial layers with a 3-0 Vicryl suture. The peritoneal lining of the bladder initially incised may be used as a third layer of reinforcement. An 18-French or

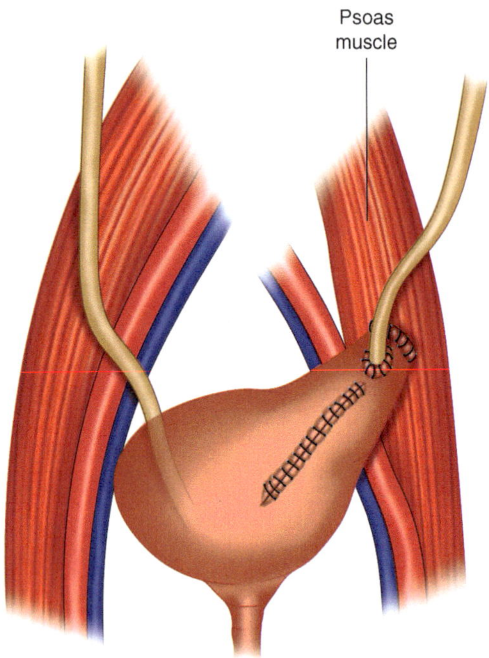

Fig. 17.4 Ureteroneocystostomy with bladder remodeling and psoas hitch

larger urethral catheter is left in place, and a closed-suction drain

may be placed at the discretion of the surgeon. A cystogram may be performed prior to catheter removal to confirm the integrity of the reconstruction and bladder closure.

References

1. Medina D, Lavery R, Ross SE, et al. Ureteral trauma: preoperative studies neither predict injury nor prevent missed injuries. J Am Coll Surg. 1998;186(6):641–4. https://doi.org/10.1016/s1072-7515(98)00108-2.
2. Pereira BM, Ogilvie MP, Gomez-Rodriguez JC, et al. A review of ureteral injuries after external trauma. Scand J Trauma Resusc Emerg Med. 2010;18(6) https://doi.org/10.1186/1757-7241-18-6.
3. Morrow J, Curry D, Dooher M, et al. Minimally invasive management of delayed recognition iatrogenic ureteric injury. Ulster Med J. 2017;86(3):181–4.
4. Norris BL, Everaerts W, Posma E, et al. The urologist's role in multidisciplinary management of placenta percreta. BJU Int. 2016;117(6):961–5. https://doi.org/10.1111/bju.13332.
5. Coakley KM, Kasten KR, Sims SM, et al. Prophylactic ureteral catheters for colectomy: a national surgical quality improvement program-based analysis. Dis Colon Rectum. 2018;61(1):84–8. https://doi.org/10.1097/DCR.0000000000000976.
6. Grainger DA, Soderstrom RM, Schiff SF, et al. Ureteral injuries at laparoscopy: insights into diagnosis, management, and prevention. Obstet Gynecol. 1990;75(5):839–43.
7. Parpala-Spårman T, Paananen I, Santala M, et al. Increasing numbers of ureteric injuries after the introduction of laparoscopic surgery. Scand J Urol Nephrol. 2008;42(5):422–7. https://doi.org/10.1080/00365590802025857.

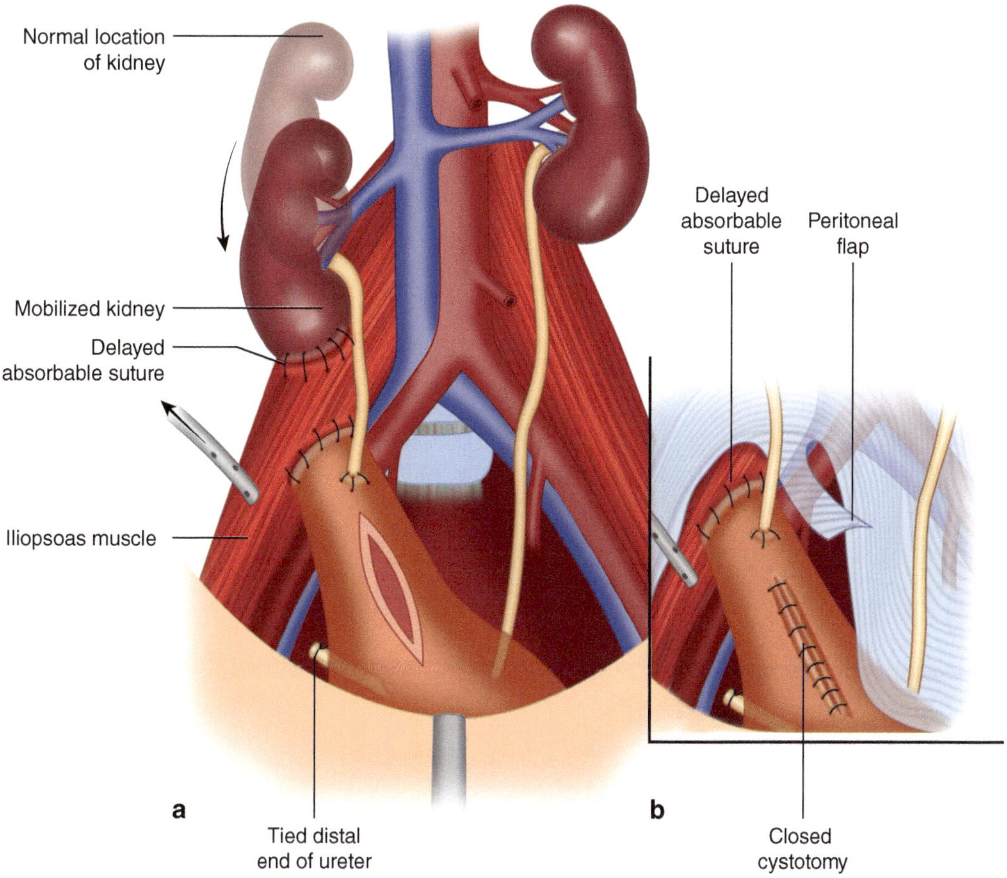

Fig. 17.5 (**a, b**) Loss of pelvic ureter. Ureteroneocystostomy to remodeled bladder with psoas hitch. Kidney mobilized caudad and secured in place with psoas hitch

Ureteroscopy

18

Jonathan Modai and Matthew D. Dunn

Introduction

Over the last several decades, technological advances in the fields of optics and camera design have led to the miniaturization of scopes, thus creating ureteroscopes, which allow access to all parts of the upper urinary tract. This has revolutionized the way urologists access, survey, and treat afflictions in the upper urinary tract, with renal stone disease being the most common. What used to require open surgery, which carried risks of relatively high morbidity and possible mortality, was suddenly possible through natural orifice surgery with a minimal risk of complications.

This is not to say that ureteroscopy is free of complications. Since it was first described in 1977 [1], reports of both minor and major complications have begun to surface, with modern data reporting an overall complication rate of 3.5% [2]. While most complications are minor and can be managed conservatively, some rare complications can have far-reaching consequences and, at times, can even be life-threatening. With modern reports showing a rise in the number of women suffering from upper urinary tract afflictions [3–5], their exposure to such complications has also increased. In this chapter, we will cover the known complications of ureteroscopy, dividing them into intraoperative, early postoperative, and late postoperative.

J. Modai · M. D. Dunn (✉)
Department of Urology, University of California Los Angeles, Los Angeles, CA, USA
e-mail: mddunn@mednet.ucla.edu

Intraoperative Complications

Ureteral Wall Injury

Background

Ureteroscopy involves many steps, including guidewire insertion to assist in the passage up to the ureter or access sheath placement if repeated entry to the upper tract is required. Wire and access sheath insertion, ureteral dilatation, ureteroscopic manipulation, stone extraction, and lithotripsy can all cause varying degrees of ureteral wall injury, ranging from superficial mucosal erosions to complete avulsion [6, 7]. Such complications are underreported, and their rates fluctuate wildly between different studies, ranging from 1.8% to 46.5% with severe injury reported in as high as 13.3% of patients [6, 8–25]. In rare cases, submucosal or extra-ureteral stone migration can further complicate the situation, making complete stone removal difficult and, at times, impossible [8, 10, 12].

Prevention

Prevention of injury requires using the smallest available instruments possible [21, 24, 26, 27] and respecting the ureteral anatomy by not

M. Hoffman et al. (eds.), *Major Complications of Female Pelvic Surgery*,
https://doi.org/10.1007/978-3-031-66772-5_18

forcing the tissues to accommodate instrumentation. Patience and using a gentle technique can assist in lowering the risk of ureteral damage. This is especially important in males, elderly patients, and patients who have not been prestented, as they were found to be at risk of access sheath insertion-related injury. If retrieval of a basketed stone fragment is difficult, force should not be applied, and the stone should be released and fragmented further before retrieval is attempted again. If the stone does not disengage from the basket, a laser fiber can be passed through the scope alongside the basket to fragment the stone within, or, if this is not possible, the basket can be disassembled and a ureteroscope with a laser fiber passed alongside it.

Recognition

An injury is usually recognized visually during the procedure or upon its conclusion when the ureter is surveyed along its length. In severe cases, extravasation of contrast can be seen on retrograde pyelography.

Management

When a minor ureteral injury is recognized during surgery, most clinicians recommend completing the procedure and leaving a ureteral stent in place. The stent is usually removed after 1–6 weeks, depending on the severity of the injury observed. If a major injury occurs, the procedure should be terminated and a stent, if possible, or a nephrostomy tube left in place.

Ureteral Avulsion and Intussusception

Background

Ureteral avulsion is one of the most feared complications of ureteroscopy, resulting in devastating damage to the ureter, requiring open or laparoscopic surgical repair, and, on some occasions, causing long-term patient morbidity. It is feared not only for its significant consequences but also for its preventable nature, as it is usually the result of a faulty surgical technique, where unduly force was applied during surgery. Fortunately, it is a rare complication, with a reported occurrence ranging from 0.04% to 1.3% [2, 8–14, 28]. Several mechanisms for avulsion have been described, the most common of which is a forceful attempt to retrieve a stone larger than the ureteral lumen [8–13]. Other less common scenarios include removal of an instrument from a tight ureter after ureteral injury has occurred [29, 30] or a trial to straighten and retrieve an ureteroscope with a broken deflection mechanism or a fractured distal section by forcefully withdrawing it [31, 32]. A variation on ureteral avulsion, ureteral intussusception, describes a partial-thickness circumferential mucosal sleeve that is withdrawn with the ureteroscope under the same circumstances that cause avulsion [33].

Prevention

Prevention of ureteral avulsion and intussusception follows the same principles as those for other ureteral injuries. Small instruments, a gentle technique, and patience are key. Surgeons should keep an eye out for ureteral injury during surgery and limit applying forces once an injury is recognized. If the injury is severe, surgery should be aborted and a ureteral stent left in place for several weeks. In case of a retained ureteroscope with a broken distal section or deflection mechanism, one can try to straighten the ureteroscope manually by passing a coaxial dilator alongside the ureteroscope, and, if that fails, one should cut the handle of the ureteroscope or its distal end using a percutaneous antegrade approach [31].

Recognition

Diagnosis of ureteral avulsion is straightforward, with the avulsed ureter seen within the bladder in men, outside the urethra in women, or over the ureteroscope itself. Diagnosis is confirmed by a retrograde pyelogram where extravasation of contrast to the retroperitoneum can be seen without any contrast reaching the renal cavities. Diagnosis of ureteral intussusception is less obvious and requires a high index of suspicion, as a retrograde pyelogram does not show contrast extravasation.

Management

Treatment of ureteral avulsion requires surgical repair ranging from a variety of ureteral reimplantation techniques, bowel transposition, kidney autotransplantation, and, at times, even nephrectomy. Even though ureteral intussusception preserves ureteral continuity and is thus theoretically less severe than ureteral avulsion, it requires the same treatment approach, for the intussuscepted segment is usually devascularized and destined to form a narrow stenotic and dysfunctional segment.

Bleeding

Background

Hematuria is a common occurrence after ureteroscopy, but significant bleeding is reported in 0.1–19% of cases [2, 8–11, 13–18, 25, 28, 34–36]. Most cases are classified as transient, meaning they resolve within 48 h [16, 34]. Bleeding occurs usually as the result of trauma to the urinary collecting system from instrumentation, excessive intrarenal pressures, or reckless application of energy, mostly laser, to the mucosa. In as many as 2.1% of cases, bleeding can result in poor visibility, requiring termination of the procedure [8–10, 18], and, in up to 1.6% of cases, it can be complicated by postoperative clot retention [34, 37]. The majority of intraoperative bleeding occurs mostly during endoscopic treatment of ureteropelvic junction stenosis by means of an endopyelotomy and is usually the result of injury to the nearby crossing vessels [29, 38].

Prevention

Because bleeding is a direct result of tissue injury, prevention mainly revolves around gentle instrumentation and careful application of energy modalities within the urinary system. Using smaller instruments [27] and gentle manipulation of instruments and wires can lower the risk of bleeding of an ureteral and renal origin. Using a ureteral access sheath and keeping the irrigation pressure low help keep the intrarenal pressures below 50 mmHg and prevents forniceal rupture and bleeding [39, 40]. When treating upper tract urothelial carcinoma, bleeding can be prevented by avoiding contact between the scope and laser fiber and the tumor and ablating it using a Tm:YAG laser or a Ho:YAG laser with a long pulse width and low energy and frequency settings [41]. To avoid major bleeding during endopyelotomy, ureteral incisions should be made in the posterolateral aspect of the proximal ureter, in the anterior aspect of the mid-ureter, and in the anteromedial aspect of the distal ureter. Preoperative CT angiography (CTA) is highly recommended as it allows for the localization of the vessels crossing the ureter near its narrowed section and for presurgical planning of the surgical incisions.

Management

Treatment of minor bleeding is mostly conservative, with cessation of bleeding without any intervention in the vast majority of cases and transfusion needed in only up to 0.7% of cases [2, 28, 34]. The majority of bleeding can be life-threatening [42], requiring immediate resuscitation maneuvers, insertion of a ureteral dilating balloon to tamponade the bleeding and embolization, and endovascular or open repair as needed.

Difficult Access

Access to the upper urinary tract without prior dilatation is unsuccessful in up to 37% of cases due to either a narrow ureteral orifice or an ureteral segment [43]. This narrowing can be due to a stricture or a ureteral wall spasm. In these cases, termination of the procedure, leaving a ureteral stent in place, allows for gradual dilatation of the ureter with subsequent ureteroscopy a week or more later. This is the preferred option, as attempts to dilate the ureter carry a 5% risk of ureteral perforation [44] and attempts to forcefully insert the ureteroscope can result in serious injury and future stricture formation [45].

Early Postoperative Complications

Vascular Anomalies

Background

Accidental or intentional application of energy to the renal parenchyma during ureteroscopy can, in rare occasions, result in the creation of either an arteriovenous fistula or a pseudoaneurysm [46–55]. These unstable vascular anomalies can rupture when subjected to high blood pressures and bleed into either the surrounding tissues or the urinary collecting system.

Recognition

Because these malformations take a few weeks to form, symptoms usually appear within weeks from the procedure and can include unexplained anemia, abdominal or flank pain, fever, and even life-threatening hemorrhage or hematuria. Once suspicion of a vascular anomaly arises, diagnosis is easily made with CTA or angiography.

Management

Treatment usually requires either embolization or surgical removal of the vascular anomaly, with unstable or feverish patients also requiring supportive treatment with fluid resuscitation, blood transfusions, or antibiotics if infection is present.

Urinoma, Perirenal Abscess, and Hematomas

High intrarenal pressures and instrument manipulation can cause damage to the pelvicalyceal system, resulting in urinoma, perirenal abscess, or subcapsular, perirenal, or retroperitoneal hematoma. These are uncommon, with a reported incidence of up to 2.2% [14, 18, 34, 46, 56–65]. Presenting symptoms include flank pain, hematuria, fever, sepsis, and even shock in the postoperative period, prompting CT scan or CTA where the lesion is identified. Depending on presentation and clinical course, treatment can be conservative or require antibiotic treatment, drain or stent placement, embolization, surgical repair and rarely nephrectomy.

Urinary Infection and Sepsis

Background

Urinary tract infection (UTI) after ureteroscopy is not uncommon, with up to 15% of patients developing a UTI after the procedure [2, 9, 14–19, 25, 28, 34–36, 58, 66, 67] and as many as 5% progressing to full-blown urosepsis [2, 8, 11, 14, 16, 18, 19, 28, 34, 35, 68–73]. Reported risk factors for postoperative UTI include preoperative UTI, history of recurrent UTIs, positive presurgical urine culture, high Charlson comorbidity or ASA scores, older age, female gender, smoking, diabetes, bowel surgery, coronary heart disease, anticoagulant therapy, chronic kidney disease, dyslipidemia, immunosuppression, presence and duration of indwelling ureteric stents, stone burden, presence of infectious stones, duration of surgery, presence of residual fragments, history of previous surgery for renal stones, long pre and post-operative hospital stay, deficient nutritional status, neurogenic bladder, and low and high body mass index [74].

Prevention

Prevention of postureteroscopy UTI relies on several factors. The procedure should be done in a sterile urinary system, and so preoperative urine cultures should be obtained, and if positive, appropriate antibiotic treatment given several days before the procedure. While single-dose preoperative antibiotic treatment failed to reduce the risk of postoperative UTI in multiple trials [75, 76], both the European and American urological associations recommend this practice. The addition of postoperative antibiotic treatment does not appear to decrease the risk of postoperative UTI any further [66]. Ureteral access sheath use might also reduce the risk of infectious complications due to the reduced intrapelvic pressures during the procedure [77]. Avoiding prolonged ureteroscopic procedures can also help lower the risk of infectious complications [73].

Recognition

A urinary tract infection can be difficult to diagnose in patients who have undergone ureteroscopy as most will report dysuria, urgency, and frequency in the postoperative period, especially if a ureteral stent was left in place. This difficulty is compounded by the fact that postoperative fever is nonspecific, with many possible alternative diagnoses, including atelectasis, phlebitis, and drug reactions. When a patient reports severe or prolonged lower urinary symptoms, especially when accompanied by fever, a UTI should be suspected and urine culture obtained before appropriate treatment is initiated, until the urine culture results come back. Physicians should keep an eye out for signs of sepsis, including severe malaise, pallor, perspiration, leukocytosis or leukopenia, and cardiovascular instability, and, if these occur, they should acquire blood culture and perform upper tract imaging before beginning aggressive treatment.

Management

If infection develops, most cases resolve with appropriate antibiotic treatment. If a ureteral stent was left in place, one should consider urethral catheter placement to prevent vesicoureteral reflux of infected urine and lower the risk of severe systemic infection. Nevertheless, physicians should stay alert for the development of urosepsis, as in these cases, immediate aggressive treatment can reduce mortality [46, 78]. Patients found to be at risk to develop post-surgical urosepsis are those with positive preoperative urine cultures, pre-stented patients, older patients, diabetic patients, those with ischemic heart disease, and those with longer procedural duration [73]. Common pathogens cultured in uroseptic patients include *Escherichia coli*, *Enterococcus*, *Proteus*, *Pseudomonas*, *Serratia*, group B *Streptococci*, *Staphylococcus aureus*, and *Candida* [79–81], with stone cultures more accurately identifying the culprit than preoperative urinary cultures [82]. Treatment includes broad spectrum antibiotic treatment, monitoring and supportive care, and urinary drainage as needed.

Pain and Ureteral Obstruction

Postoperative pain can plague 0.9–10.2% of patients undergoing ureteroscopy, affecting mostly the flank and lower abdominal regions [9, 17, 19, 28, 36, 83]. Most cases can be managed with analgesics, but, in up to 3.4% of patients, pain will be the result of ureteral obstruction caused by edema, blood clots, or residual fragments [2, 15, 18, 19, 28, 34, 58, 70]. These cases might require renal drainage by either a ureteral stent or nephrostomy tube placement or a repeat ureteroscopy.

Ureteral Stent Discomfort

Fear of postoperative pain and upper urinary tract obstruction is the foundation for the practice of ureteral stent placement at the end of ureteroscopy. However, studies have found that the presence of a ureteral stent is accompanied by complaints of dysuria, frequency, urgency, nocturia, flank discomfort, and hematuria in as many as 88% of patients, with more than 70% of them requiring analgesic support [84–86]. For this reason, both the European and American urological association guidelines recommend avoiding routine ureteral stent placement after an uncomplicated ureteroscopy, proposing that it should be considered only in patients with larger stone burden, requiring prolonged surgery, with obvious upper urinary tract damage or with a single functioning kidney.

Premature Labor

Possibly the only female-specific complication of ureteroscopy, premature labor, can occur in 4.3–8.7% of pregnant patients undergoing ureteroscopy [87, 88]. The most common indication is managing obstructing ureteral stones. The risk is higher during the third trimester, in patients with urinary tract infection at presentation, and when ureteroscopy is performed for stone removal and not for diagnostic purposes. Although conservative care in managing ureteral stones might seem prudent in light of these statistics, delayed intervention was also found to carry the risk of premature labor [87, 89]. No prospective studies have compared the obstetric complication profile of ureteroscopy to stent or nephrostomy placement, but, because of the higher encrustation rate seen during pregnancy [90] and the need for repeated exchanges, many believe that ureteroscopy is the better choice. In any case, a multidisciplinary approach to these patients is advised.

Ureteral Stent Migration

Background

Although designed to remain in a stable position, stent migration, either upward to the kidney or downward to the bladder, can occur in 0.7–3.6% of patients, caused by incorrect placement, incorrect stent size selection, or ureteral peristalsis [8, 14, 16, 18, 34, 35, 83, 70]. In some patients, the ureteral stent is left with a string attached to facilitate future removal, and, in these cases, unintentional tension can also cause the stent to dislodge from its position.

Prevention

Choosing the correct stent size and firmness to fit the patient's anatomy and using the correct technique are key to preventing ureteral stent migration after surgery. In patients for whom the ureteral stent was left with a string attached, positioning the string in a safe location, leaving it with some slack to accommodate movement, and informing the patient about the string and the importance of avoiding any tension on it can help prevent unintentional stent displacement.

Recognition

While some patients can be asymptomatic, others will present with flank pain, nausea, urine leakage, fever, and even full-blown sepsis. In some cases, mainly in women with complaints of urine leakage, especially if a string was left in place, the stent can be seen outside the urethral meatus on physical exam. In other cases, diagnosis can be easily made with either a ultrasound (US), abdominal X-ray, or CT showing the mispositioned ureteral stent.

Management

Treatment requires stent removal or repositioning, depending on the clinical scenario. In patients presenting with fever or sepsis, stent repositioning to ensure renal drainage, urethral catheter placement, urine and blood cultures, antibiotic treatment, and supportive care are suggested.

Intravascular Stent Misplacement

Unfortunately, the literature contains several accounts of stents being malpositioned into either the iliac veins or vena cava, resulting in postoperative hematuria, thromboembolic event, or obstruction of the upper urinary tract [91–100]. Most cases can be treated by endovascular extraction of the stent, with some requiring surgical removal.

Post-Obstructive Diuresis

In patients with a single functioning kidney or bilateral obstruction, ureteroscopy to relieve upper urinary tract obstruction can result in post-obstructive diuresis, putting the patient at risk of dehydration, serum electrolyte imbalances, arrhythmias, and death [16]. This complication is rarely reported on, and so its incidence is unknown. Patients developing post-obstructive diuresis will present with dramatically increased urine production with possible symptoms including malaise, fatigue, nausea, vomiting, confusion, and even stupor and coma. When a clinical suspicion arises, assessing hourly urine production and lab work showing hypernatremia and increased blood urea nitrogen and creatinine can establish the diagnosis. Careful monitoring, free access to water, and, at times, intravenous fluid support are required to avoid and treat this complication. If hyponatremia is present, careful fluid management is needed to avoid overzealous correction of serum sodium levels that can lead to cerebral edema.

Late Postoperative Complications

Ureteral Strictures

Background
According to the modern literature, 0.1–3% of patients will develop ureteral strictures after ureteroscopy [2, 8, 9, 12, 14, 18, 25, 28, 83, 101]. This is a significant complication, as it can result in prolonged discomfort, recurrent and complicated UTI, and loss of renal function, if not addressed in a timely manner. Moreover, treatment will frequently require surgical correction, with some amenable to endoscopic correction, while other more complicated cases may require laparoscopic, robotic, or open surgery [9, 12, 83, 102, 103].

Prevention
While the exact pathophysiology of ureteral stricture formation after ureteroscopy remains unknown, many believe it is the result of ureteral wall inflammation and fibrosis, caused by the presence of a stone or by insults suffered during the procedure itself [104, 105]. Because of that, suggested preventive measures include using a gentle surgical technique, using the smallest instruments possible, utilizing general and not regional or local anesthesia, complete removal of impacted stones to avoid formation of stone granulomas, and avoiding simultaneous performance of endopyelotomy and stone fragmentation and removal in the same session [9, 106–110].

Recognition
Ureteral strictures usually develop within weeks to months of the procedure. While some patients can be asymptomatic, others will present with flank or abdominal pain, fever, recurrent UTIs, or hematuria. Because some cases can be asymptomatic, and these silent cases can result in permanent renal damage, many suggest performing an imaging study a few weeks after ureteroscopy to rule out hydronephrosis as a sign of a possible stricture. The final diagnosis can be made with a CT urogram showing hydroureteronephrosis above the strictured area and a MAG3 (mercaptoacetyltriglycine) renal scan showing functional obstruction of the affected kidney. However, a more invasive, diagnostic ureteroscopy can also establish the diagnosis with the added benefit of enabling treatment of the stricture at the time of diagnosis.

Management
Possible treatments for ureteral stricture disease include endoscopic and open, laparoscopic, or robotic procedures. Endoscopic treatment is the least invasive and includes balloon dilatation and/or laser incision of the strictured section. These are mainly effective in the treatment of relatively short, non-obliterative strictures in well-vascularized tissue [111, 112]. If endoscopic treatment fails, the stricture is too long or tight, or the tissue is ischemic, then open, laparoscopic, or robotic surgical correction is required. This includes resection of the strictured section and re-anastomosis, buccal ureteroplasty, interposition of the interstitial graft, autotransplantation, and even nephrectomy [9, 12, 83, 102, 103].

Neglected Stents

Background
Ureteral stents placed at the end of ureteroscopy need to be removed in a timely manner. Failure to do so can result in stent encrustation, fragmentation, and obstruction [113, 114], subjecting the patient to prolonged stent-related discomfort, upper urinary tract obstruction, infectious complication risk [114, 115], and, in extreme scenarios, perinephric abscess formation, renocolic fistula formation, and death [116, 117].

Prevention
Stent neglection is mainly an issue of patient compliance. Physicians should make sure to educate patients with ureteral stents on the importance of removing the stents on time and staying under surveillance until their urological issues are resolved. Other key prevention measures include minimizing ureteral stent use and keeping close tabs on patients in whom a ureteral stent was placed. A patient registry is useful to keep track of patients who were stented in an emergent

setting or for those who require long-standing ureteral stents for chronic ureteral obstruction, such as those with a pelvic malignancy, and a complicated stricture disease.

Recognition

Patients with a neglected stent will present with either a stent-related complication, such as UTI, hematuria, or flank pain, or will incidentally be found when an imaging study performed for other reasons reveals the stent in the urinary system.

Management

Most neglected stents cannot be simply removed cystoscopically if they are heavily encrusted. Such stents require complex endoscopic, percutaneous, and even open surgical intervention to be removed [114, 115].

Conclusions

Although considered minimally invasive and generally safe, ureteroscopy is tied to a wide variety of complications, most of which are minor and self-limited, but some are serious with potential morbid and even fatal results. While an experienced, attentive clinician can lower the rate of these complications, all should keep alert, for delayed diagnosis of the complications can lead to devastating consequences.

References

1. Goodman TM. Ureteroscopy with pediatric cystoscope in adults. Urology. 1977;9(4):394.
2. de la Rosette J, Denstedt J, Geavlete P, Keeley F, Matsuda T, Pearle M, Preminger G, Traxer O, CROES URS Study Group. The clinical research office of the endourological society ureteroscopy global study: indications, complications, and outcomes in 11,885 patients. J Endourol. 2014;28(2):131–9.
3. Penniston KL, McLaren ID, Greenlee RT, Nakada SY. Urolithiasis in a rural Wisconsin population from 1992 to 2008: narrowing of the male-to-female ratio. J Urol. 2011;185(5):1731–6.
4. Scales CD Jr, Curtis LH, Norris RD, Springhart WP, Sur RL, Schulman KA, Preminger GM. Changing gender prevalence of stone disease. J Urol. 2007;177(3):979–82.
5. Lieske JC, Peña de la Vega LS, Slezak JM, Bergstralh EJ, Leibson CL, Ho KL, Gettman MT. Renal stone epidemiology in Rochester, Minnesota: an update. Kidney Int. 2006;69(4):760–4.
6. Traxer O, Thomas A. Prospective evaluation and classification of ureteral wall injuries resulting from insertion of a ureteral access sheath during retrograde intrarenal surgery. J Urol. 2013;189(2):580–4.
7. Schoenthaler M, Buchholz N, Farin E, Ather H, Bach C, Bach T, Denstedt JD, Fritsche HM, Grasso M, Hakenberg OW, Herwig R, Knoll T, Kuehhas FE, Liatsikos E, Liske P, Marberger M, Osther PJ, Santos JM, Sarica K, Seitz C, Straub M, Traxer O, Trinchieri A, Turney B, A, Miernik. The Post-Ureteroscopic Lesion Scale (PULS): a multicenter video-based evaluation of inter-rater reliability. World J Urol. 2014;32(4):1033–40.
8. Geavlete P, Georgescu D, Nita G, Mirciulescu V, Cauni V. Complications of 2735 retrograde semi-rigid ureteroscopy procedures: a single-center experience. J Endourol. 2006;20(3):179–85.
9. Elashry OM, Elgamasy AK, Sabaa MA, Abo-Elenien M, Omar MA, Eltatawy HH, El-Abd SA. Ureteroscopic management of lower ureteric calculi: a 15-year single-centre experience. BJU Int. 2008;102(8):1010–7.
10. Georgescu D, Multescu R, Geavlete B, Geavlete P. Intraoperative complications after 8150 semi-rigid ureteroscopies for ureteral lithiasis: risk analysis and management. Chirurgia (Bucur). 2014;109(3):369–74.
11. Taie K, Jasemi M, Khazaeli D, Fatholahi A. Prevalence and management of complications of ureteroscopy: a seven-year experience with introduction of a new maneuver to prevent ureteral avulsion. Urol J. 2012;9(1):356–60.
12. Fuganti PE, Pires S, Branco R, Porto J. Predictive factors for intraoperative complications in semirigid ureteroscopy: analysis of 1235 ballistic ureterolithotripsies. Urology. 2008;72(4):770–4.
13. Tanriverdi O, Silay MS, Kadihasanoglu M, Aydin M, Kendirci M, Miroglu C. Revisiting the predictive factors for intraoperative complications of rigid ureteroscopy: a 15-year experience. Urol J. 2012;9(2):457–64.
14. Öğreden E, Oğuz U, Demirelli E, Benli E, Sancak EB, Gülpinar MT, Akbaş A, Reşorlu B, Ayyildiz A, Yalçin O. Categorization of ureteroscopy complications and investigation of associated factors by using the modified Clavien classification system. Turk J Med Sci. 2016;46(3):686–94.
15. El-Nahas AR, El-Tabey NA, Eraky I, Shoma AM, El-Hefnawy AS, El-Assmy AM, Soliman S, Youssef RF, El-Kenawy MR, Shokeir AA, El-Kappany HA. Semirigid ureteroscopy for ureteral stones: a multivariate analysis of unfavorable results. J Urol. 2009;181(3):1158–62.

16. Ibrahim AK. Reporting ureteroscopy complications using the modified clavien classification system. Urol Ann. 2015;7(1):53–7.
17. Mursi K, Elsheemy MS, Morsi HA, Ali Ghaleb AK, Abdel-Razzak OM. Semi-rigid ureteroscopy for ureteric and renal pelvic calculi: predictive factors for complications and success. Arab J Urol. 2013;11(2):136–41.
18. Baş O, Tuygun C, Dede O, Sarı S, Çakıcı MÇ, Öztürk U, Göktuğ G, İmamoğlu A. Factors affecting complication rates of retrograde flexible ureterorenoscopy: analysis of 1571 procedures-a single-center experience. World J Urol. 2017;35:5.
19. Schuster TG, Hollenbeck BK, Faerber GJ, Wolf JS Jr. Complications of ureteroscopy: analysis of predictive factors. J Urol. 2001;166(2):538–40.
20. Abdel-Razzak OM, Bagley DH. Clinical experience with flexible ureteropyeloscopy. J Urol. 1992;148(6):1788–92.
21. Francesca F, Scattoni V, Nava L, Pompa P, Grasso M, Rigatti P. Failures and complications of transurethral ureteroscopy in 297 cases: conventional rigid instruments vs. small caliber semirigid ureteroscopes. Eur Urol. 1995;28(2):112–5.
22. Jeromin L, Sosnowski M. Ureteroscopy in the treatment of ureteral stones: over 10 years' experience. Eur Urol. 1998;34(4):344–9.
23. Blute ML, Segura JW, Patterson DE. Ureteroscopy. J Urol. 1988;139(3):510–2.
24. Aykanat C, Balci M, Senel C, Ozercan AY, Coser S, Aslan Y, Guzel O, Asfuroglu A, Karabulut E, Tuncel A. The impact of ureteral access sheath size on perioperative parameters and postoperative ureteral stricture in retrograde intrarenal surgery. J Endourol. 2022;36(8):1013–7.
25. Darwish AE, Gadelmoula MM, Abdelkawi IF, Abdellatif AM, Abdel-Moneim AM, Hammouda HM. Ureteral stricture after ureteroscopy for stones: A prospective study for the incidence and risk factors. Urol Ann. 2019;11(3):276–81.
26. Guzelburc V, Guven S, Boz MY, Erkurt B, Soytas M, Altay B, Albayrak S. Intraoperative evaluation of ureteral access sheath related injuries using post-ureteroscopic lesion scale. J Laparoendosc Adv Surg Tech A. 2016;26(1):23–6.
27. Atis G, Arikan O, Gurbuz C, Yildirim A, Erol B, Pelit S, Ulus I, Caskurlu T. Comparison of different ureteroscope sizes in treating ureteral calculi in adult patients. Urology. 2013;82(6):1231–5.
28. Perez Castro E, Osther PJ, Jinga V, Razvi H, Stravodimos KG, Parikh K, Kural AR, de la Rosette JJ, CROES Ureteroscopy Global Study Group. Differences in ureteroscopic stone treatment and outcomes for distal, mid-, proximal, or multiple ureteral locations: the Clinical Research Office of the Endourological Society ureteroscopy global study. Eur Urol. 2014;66(1):102–9.
29. Gerber GS, Lyon ES. Endopyelotomy: patient selection, results, and complications. Urology. 1994;43(1):2–10.
30. Badlani G, Karlin G, Smith AD. Complications of endopyelotomy: analysis in series of 64 patients. J Urol. 1988;140(3):473–5.
31. Hubosky SG, Raval AJ, Bagley DH. Locked deflection during flexible ureteroscopy: incidence and elucidation of the mechanism of an underreported complication. J Endourol. 2015;29(8):907–12.
32. Huynh M, Telfer S, Pautler S, Denstedt J, Razvi H. Retained digital flexible ureteroscopes. J Endo Urol Case Rep. 2017;3(1):24–7.
33. Bernhard PH, Reddy PK. Retrograde ureteral intussusception: a rare complication. J Endourol. 1996;10(4):349–51.
34. Mandal S, Goel A, Singh MK, Kathpalia R, Nagathan DS, Sankhwar SN, Singh V, Singh BP, Sinha RJ, Dalela D. Clavien classification of semirigid ureteroscopy complications: a prospective study. Urology. 2012;80(5):995–1001.
35. Somani BK, Giusti G, Sun Y, Osther PJ, Frank M, De Sio M, Turna B, de la Rosette J. Complications associated with ureterorenoscopy (URS) related to treatment of urolithiasis: the Clinical Research Office of Endourological Society URS Global study. World J Urol. 2017;35(4):675–81.
36. Salem HK. A prospective randomized study comparing shock wave lithotripsy and semirigid ureteroscopy for the management of proximal ureteral calculi. Urology. 2009;74(6):1216–21.
37. Cohen J, Cohen S, Grasso M. Ureteropyeloscopic treatment of large, complex intrarenal and proximal ureteral calculi. BJU Int. 2012;111:127–31.
38. Kim FJ, Herrell SD, Jahoda AE, Albala DM. Complications of acucise endopyelotomy. J Endourol. 1998;12(5):433–6.
39. Thomsen HS, Dorph S, Olsen S. Pyelorenal backflow in rabbits following clamping of the renal vein and artery: radiologic and microscopic investigation. Acta Radiol Diagn (Stockh). 1982;23(2):143–8.
40. Proietti S, Dragos L, Somani B, Butticè S, Talso M, Emiliani E, Baghdadi M, Giusti G, Traxer O. In vitro comparison of maximum pressure developed by irrigation systems in a kidney model. J Endourol. 2017;31(5):522–7.
41. Defidio L, De Dominicis M, Di Gianfrancesco L, Fuchs G, Patel A. First collaborative experience with thulium laser ablation of localized upper urinary tract urothelial tumors using retrograde intra-renal surgery. Arch Ital Urol Androl. 2011;83(3):147–53.
42. Lopes RI, Torricelli FC, Gomes CM, Carnevale F, Bruschini H, Srougi M. Endovascular repair of a nearly fatal iliac artery injury after endoureterotomy. Scand J Urol. 2013;47(5):437–9.
43. Hudson RG, Conlin MJ, Bagley DH. Ureteric access with flexible ureteroscopes: effect of the size of the ureteroscope. BJU Int. 2005;95(7):1043–4.
44. Kuntz NJ, Neisius A, Tsivian M, Ghaffar M, Patel N, Ferrandino MN, Sur RL, Preminger GM, Lipkin ME. Balloon dilation of the ureter: a contemporary review of outcomes and complications. J Urol. 2015;194(2):413–7.

45. Ambani SN, Faerber GJ, Roberts WW, Hollingsworth JM, Wolf JS Jr. Ureteral stents for impassable ureteroscopy. J Endourol. 2013;27(5):549–53.
46. Cindolo L, Castellan P, Primiceri G, Hoznek A, Cracco CM, Scoffone CM, Galfano A, Petralia G, Angelis MDE, Annino F, Malacasa E, Cormio L, Acquati P, Lorenzis EDE, Maugeri O, Arena G, Celia A, Giusti G, Schips L. Life-threatening complications after ureteroscopy for urinary stones: survey and systematic literature review. Minerva Urol Nefrol. 2017;69(5):421–31.
47. Jubber I, Patel PR, Hori S, Al-Hayek S. Renal pseudoaneurysm: a rare and potentially fatal complication following ureteroscopy and laser fragmentation of stones. rare and potentially fatal. Ann R Coll Surg Engl. 2018;100(3):51–2.
48. Aston W, Whiting R, Bultitude M, Challacombe B, Glass J, Dasgupta P. Pseudoaneurysm formation after flexible ureterorenoscopy and electrohydraulic lithotripsy. Int J Clin Pract. 2004;58(3):310–1.
49. Angelsen A, Talseth T, Mjones JG, Hedlund H. Hypertension and pseudoaneurism on the renal artery following retrograde endopyelotomy (Acucise). Scand J Urol Nephrol. 2000;34(1):79–80.
50. Durner L, El Howairis MEF, Buchholz N. Renal pseudoaneurysm after flexible ureterorenoscopy—an unusual complication. Urol Int. 2017;99(4):484–6.
51. Ngo TC, Lee JJ, Gonzalgo ML. Renal pseudoaneurysm: an overview. Nat Rev Urol. 2010;7(11):619–25.
52. Watanabe M, Padua HM, Nguyen HT, Alomari AI. Renal pseudoaneurysm following laser lithotripsy: endovascular treatment of a rare complication. J Pediatr Urol. 2010;6(4):420–2.
53. Rudnick DM, Dretler SP. Intrarenal pseudoaneurysm following ureterorenoscopy and electrohydraulic lithotripsy. J Urol. 1998;159(4):1290–1.
54. Tiplitsky SI, Milhoua PM, Patel MB, Minsky L, Hoenig DM. Case report: intrarenal arteriovenous fistula after ureteroscopic stone extraction with holmium laser lithotripsy. J Endourol. 2007;21(5):530–2.
55. Abogunrin FA. Renal arteriovenous fistula: a rare complication of electro-hydraulic lithotripsy. South Afr J Surg. 2012;50(4):134–5.
56. Bai J, Li C, Wang S, Liu J, Ye Z, Yu X, Xi Q, Ni M, He D. Subcapsular renal haematoma after holmium:yttrium-aluminum-garnet laser ureterolithotripsy. BJU Int. 2012;109(8):1230–4.
57. Chiu PK, Chan CK, Ma WK, To KC, Cheung FK, Yiu MK. Subcapsular hematoma after ureteroscopy and laser lithotripsy. J Endourol. 2013;27(9):1115–9.
58. Hyams ES, Munver R, Bird VG, Uberoi J, Shah O. Flexible ureterorenoscopy and holmium laser lithotripsy for the management of renal stone burdens that measure 2 to 3 cm: a multi-institutional experience. J Endourol. 2010;24(10):1583–8.
59. Paiva MM, da Silva RD, Jaworski P, Kim FJ, Molina WR. Subcapsular hematoma after ureteroscopy and laser lithotripsy. Can J Urol. 2016;23(4):8385–7.
60. Tao W, Cai CJ, Sun CY, Xue BX, Shan YX. Subcapsular renal hematoma after ureteroscopy with holmium:yttrium-aluminum-garnet laser lithotripsy. Lasers Med Sci. 2015;30(5):1527–32.
61. Vaidyanathan S, Samsudin A, Singh G, Hughes PL, Soni BM, Selmi F. Large subcapsular hematoma following ureteroscopic laser lithotripsy of renal calculi in a spina bifida patient: lessons we learn. Int Med Case Rep J. 2016;9:253–9.
62. Riley JM, Stearman L, Troxel S. Retrograde ureteroscopy for renal stones larger than 2.5 cm. J Endourol. 2009;23(9):1395–8.
63. Xu L, Li G. Life-threatening subcapsular renal hematoma after flexible ureteroscopic laser lithotripsy: treatment with superselective renal arterial embolization. Urolithiasis. 2013;41:5.
64. Meng HZ, Chen SW, Chen GM, Tan FQ, Wang CJ, Shen BH. Renal subcapsular hemorrhage complicating ureterolithotripsy: an unknown complication of a known day-to-day procedure. Urol Int. 2013;91(3):335–9.
65. Yahsi S, Tonyali S, Ceylan C, Yildiz KY, Ozdal L. Intraparenchymal hematoma as a late complication of retrograde intrarenal surgery. Int Braz J Urol. 2017;43(2):367–70.
66. Chew BH, Flannigan R, Kurtz M, Gershman B, Arsovska O, Paterson RF, Eisner BH, Lange D. A single dose of intraoperative antibiotics is sufficient to prevent urinary tract infection during ureteroscopy. J Endourol. 2016;30(1):63–8.
67. Sohn DW, Kim SW, Hong CG, Yoon BI, Ha US, Cho YH. Risk factors of infectious complication after ureteroscopic procedures of the upper urinary tract. J Infect Chemother. 2013;19(6):1102–8.
68. Berardinelli F, De Francesco P, Marchioni M, Cera N, Proietti S, Hennessey D, Dalpiaz O, Cracco C, Scoffone C, Schips L, Giusti G, Cindolo L. Infective complications after retrograde intrarenal surgery: a new standardized classification system. Int Urol Nephrol. 2016;48(11):1757–62.
69. Bloom J, Fox C, Fullerton S, Matthews G, Phillips J. Sepsis after elective ureteroscopy. Can J Urol. 2017;24(5):9017–23.
70. Giusti G, Proietti S, Villa L, Cloutier J, Rosso M, Gadda GM, Doizi S, Suardi N, Montorsi F, Gaboardi F, Traxer O. Current standard technique for modern flexible ureteroscopy: tips and tricks. Eur Urol. 2016;70(1):188–94.
71. Mitsuzuka K, Nakano O, Takahashi N, Satoh M. Identification of factors associated with postoperative febrile urinary tract infection after ureteroscopy for urinary stones. Urolithiasis. 2016;44(3):257–62.
72. Nevo A, Mano R, Baniel J, Lifshitz DA. Ureteric stent dwelling time: a risk factor for post-ureteroscopy sepsis. BJU Int. 2017;120(1):117–22.
73. Bhojani N, Miller LE, Bhattacharyya S, Cutone B, Chew BH. Risk factors for urosepsis after ureteroscopy for stone disease: a sys-

tematic review with meta-analysis. J Endourol. 2021;35(7):991–1000.
74. Chugh S, Pietropaolo A, Montanari E, Sarica K, Somani BK. Predictors of urinary infections and urosepsis after ureteroscopy for stone disease: a systematic review from EAU section of urolithiasis (EULIS). Curr Urol Rep. 2020;21:4.
75. Hsieh CH, Yang SS, Lin CD, Chang SJ. Are prophylactic antibiotics necessary in patients with preoperative sterile urine undergoing ureterorenoscopic lithotripsy? BJU Int. 2014;113(2):275–80.
76. Martov A, Gravas S, Etemadian M, Unsal A, Barusso G, D'Addessi A, Krambeck A, de la Rosette J, Clinical Research Office of the Endourological Society Ureteroscopy Study Group. Postoperative infection rates in patients with a negative baseline urine culture undergoing ureteroscopic stone removal: a matched case-control analysis on antibiotic prophyl. J Endourol. 2015;29(2):171–80.
77. Traxer O, Wendt-Nordahl G, Sodha H, Rassweiler J, Meretyk S, Tefekli A, Coz F, de la Rosette JJ. Differences in renal stone treatment and outcomes for patients treated either with or without the support of a ureteral access sheath: The Clinical Research Office of the Endourological Society Ureteroscopy Global Study. World J Urol. 2015;33(12):2137–44.
78. Ferrer R, Martin-Loeches I, Phillips G, Osborn TM, Townsend S, Dellinger RP, Artigas A, Schorr C, Levy MM. Empiric antibiotic treatment reduces mortality in severe sepsis and septic shock from the first hour: results from a guideline-based performance improvement program. Crit Care Med. 2014;42(8):1749–55.
79. Scotland KB, Lange D. Prevention and management of urosepsis triggered by ureteroscopy. Res Rep Urol. 2018;10:43–9.
80. Gautam G, Singh AK, Kumar R, Hemal AK, Kothari A. Beware! Fungal urosepsis may follow endoscopic intervention for prolonged indwelling ureteral stent. J Endourol. 2006;20(7):522–4.
81. Blackmur JP, Maitra NU, Marri RR, Housami F, Malki M, McIlhenny C. Analysis of factors' association with risk of postoperative urosepsis in patients undergoing ureteroscopy for treatment of stone disease. J Endourol. 2016;30(9):963–9.
82. Eswara JR, Shariftabrizi A, Sacco D. Positive stone culture is associated with a higher rate of sepsis after endourological procedures. Urolithiasis. 2013;41(5):411–4.
83. Cheung MC, Lee F, Leung YL, Wong BB, Chu SM, Tam PC. Outpatient ureteroscopy: predictive factors for postoperative events. Urology. 2001;58(6):914–8.
84. Joshi HB, Stainthorpe A, MacDonagh RP, Keeley FX Jr, Timoney AG, Barry MJ. Indwelling ureteral stents: evaluation of symptoms, quality of life and utility. J Urol. 2003;169(3):1065–9.
85. Al-Kandari AM, Al-Shaiji TF, Shaaban H, Ibrahim HM, Elshebiny YH, Shokeir AA. Effects of proximal and distal ends of double-J ureteral stent position on postprocedural symptoms and quality of life: a randomized clinical trial. J Endourol. 2007;21(7):698–702.
86. Giannarini G, Keeley FX Jr, Valent F, Manassero F, Mogorovich A, Autorino R, Selli C. Predictors of morbidity in patients with indwelling ureteric stents: results of a prospective study using the validated Ureteric Stent Symptoms Questionnaire. BJU Int. 2011;107(4):648–54.
87. Butticè S, Laganà AS, Vitale SG, Netsch C, Tanidir Y, Cantiello F, Dragos L, Talso M, Emiliani E, Pappalardo R, Sener TE. Ureteroscopy in pregnant women with complicated colic pain: Is there any risk of premature labor? Arch Ital Urol Androl. 2017;89(4):287–92.
88. Johnson EB, Krambeck AE, White WM, Hyams E, Beddies J, Marien T, Shah O, Matlaga B, Pais VM Jr. Obstetric complications of ureteroscopy during pregnancy. J Urol. 2012;188(1):151–4.
89. Zhang S, Liu G, Duo Y, Wang J, Li J, Li C. Application of ureteroscope in emergency treatment with persistent renal colic patients during pregnancy. PLos ONE. 2016;11:1.
90. Smith CL, Kristensen C, Davis M, Abraham PA. An evaluation of the physicochemical risk for renal stone disease during pregnancy. Clin Nephrol. 2001;55(3):205–11.
91. Michalopoulos AS, Tzoufl MJ, Theodorakis G, Mentzelopoulos SD. Acute postoperative pulmonary thromboembolism as a result of intravascular migration of a pigtail ureteral stent. Anesth Analg. 2002;95(5):1185–8.
92. Sabnis RB, Ganpule AP, Ganpule SA. Migration of double J stent into the inferior vena cava and the right atrium. Indian J Urol. 2013;29(4):353–4.
93. Farshi AR, Roshandel MR. Intracardiac migration of ureteral double-J stent: A case report and review. Can Urol Assoc J. 2015;9(10):661–4.
94. Ioannou CV, Velegrakis J, Kostas T, Georgakarakos E, Touloupakis E, Anezinis P, Katsamouris AN. Caval migration of a ureteral J-stent after simultaneous ureter and iliac vein perforation during its placement for obstructive pyelonephritis. Int Angiol. 2009;28(5):421–4.
95. Hajji M, Bennani MS, Bekkali S, Jroundi L. Intracaval migration of ureteral stent. J Belg. 2015;99(1):28–30.
96. Arab D, Ardestani Zadeh A, Eskandarian R, Asaadi M, Ghods K. An extremely rare complication of ureteral pigtail stent placement: a case report. Nephrourol Mon. 2016;8:3.
97. Falahatkar S, Hemmati H, Gholamjani MK. Intracaval migration: an uncommon complication of ureteral Double-J stent placement. J Endourol. 2012;26(2):119–21.
98. Hastaoglu IO, Tokoz H, Kavlak E, Bilgen F. Double J ureteral stent displaced through the right ventricle. Interact Cardiovasc Thorac Surg. 2014;18(6):853–4.
99. Marques V, Parada B, Rolo F, Figueiredo A. Intracaval misplacement of a double-J ureteral stent. BMJ Case Rep; 2018.

100. Li D, Xiao L, Tang Z, Qi L, Luo K, Huang L, Huang K, Zhou J, Tang Y, Li J. Management of intravenous migration of urologic catheter. Urology. 2013;82(1):248–52.
101. El-Abd AS, Suliman MG, Abo Farha MO, Ramadan AR, El-Tatawy HH, El-Gamal OM, El-Gamal SA, Figenshau R, El Abd SA. The development of ureteric strictures after ureteroscopic treatment for ureteric calculi: A long-term study at two academic centres. Arab J Urol. 2014;12(2):168–72.
102. Zhao LC, Weinberg AC, Lee Z, Ferretti MJ, Koo HP, Metro MJ, Eun DD, Stifelman MD. Robotic Ureteral Reconstruction Using Buccal Mucosa Grafts: A Multi-institutional Experience. Eur Urol. 2018;73(3):419–26.
103. Tran G, Ramaswamy K, Chi T, Meng M, Freise C, Stoller ML. Laparoscopic nephrectomy with autotransplantation: safety, efficacy and long-term durability. J Urol. 2015;194(3):738–43.
104. Roberts WW, Cadeddu JA, Micali S, Kavoussi LR, Moore RG. Ureteral stricture formation after removal of impacted calculi. J Urol. 1998;159(3):723–6.
105. Sener TE, Cloutier J, Audouin M, Villa L, Traxer O. A guidewire introducer as a ureteral foreign body: a case report. Can Urol Assoc J. 2015;9(5):384–6.
106. Harmon WJ, Sershon PD, Blute ML, Patterson DE, Segura JW. Ureteroscopy: current practice and long-term complications. J Urol. 1997;157(1):28–32.
107. Dretler SP, Young RH. Stone granuloma: a cause of ureteral. J Urol. 1993;150(6):1800–2.
108. Doddamani D, Kumar R, Hemal AK. Stone granuloma— not to be forgotten as a delayed complication of ureteroscopy. Uro Int. 2002;68(2):129–31.
109. Narcisi F, Castellani D, Di Marco G, Fileni A, Paradiso Galatioto G, Mancinotti A, Vicentini C. Uncommon complication of endoscopic ureterolithotripsy: the stone granuloma. Int J Urol. 2006;13(3):289–90.
110. Giddens JL, Grotas AB, Grasso M. Stone granuloma causes ureteropelvic junction obstruction after percutaneous nephrolithotomy and antegrade endopyelotomy. J Urol. 2000;164(1):118–9.
111. Richter F, Irwin RJ, Watson RA, Lang EK. Endourologic management of benign ureteral strictures with and without compromised vascular supply. Urology. 2000;55(5):652–7.
112. Wolf JS Jr, Elashry OM, Clayman RV. Long-term results of endoureterotomy for benign ureteral and ureteroenteric strictures. J Urol. 1997;158:759–64.
113. Fiuk J, Bao Y, Calleary JG, Schwartz BF, Denstedt JD. The use of internal stents in chronic ureteral obstruction. J Urol. 2015;193(4):1092–100.
114. Abdelaziz AY, Fouda WB, Mosharafa AA, Abelrasoul MA, Fayyad A, Fawzi K. Forgotten ureteral stents: risk factors, complications and management. Afr J Urol. 2018;24(1):28–33.
115. Thomas A, Cloutier J, Villa L, Letendre J, Ploumidis A, Traxer O. Prospective analysis of a complete retrograde ureteroscopic technique with holmium laser stent cutting for management of encrusted ureteral stents. J Endourol. 2017;31(5):476–81.
116. Singh V, Srinivastava A, Kapoor R, Kumar A. Can the complicated forgotten indwelling ureteric stents be lethal? Int Urol Nephrol. 2005;37(3):541–6.
117. Lee SW, Kim JH. Renocolic fistula secondary to a perinephric abscess: a late complication of a forgotten double J stent. J Korean Med Sci. 2009;24(5):960–2.

Part V

Anus and Rectum

Transanal Local Excisions and Endoluminal Approaches

19

Kamil Erozkan and Emre Gorgun

Introduction

As explained by the adenoma–carcinoma sequence, sporadic colorectal cancer begins with adenoma formation and progresses to cancer with recurrent driver mutations [1]. Screening colonoscopies aim to detect and destroy precancerous lesions before invasive carcinoma develops [2]. Early identification and removal of precancerous lesions during screening colonoscopies have led to a significant decrease in colorectal cancer incidence and mortality [3]. There are different methods to remove polyps of different sizes. Polyps smaller than 10 mm are typically excised with a cold snare, while larger polyps require historically segmental resections or, more recently, local excisions. Surgical organ resections can lead to a significant increase in mortality and morbidity, alongside increased postoperative pain, blood loss, and prolonged length of hospital stay. Histopathological analysis after major surgeries for premalignant lesions often reveals a high percentage of benign results [4], thus putting patients at an unnecessary risk. Surgeons have been adopting less invasive methods, such as transanal local excisions (TAEs) and endoluminal procedures, to remove premalignant lesions in order to reduce postoperative pain, permit shorter hospital stays, and enable a faster recovery process. These techniques can be applied to various benign diseases, but their growing appeal lies in their ability to serve as minimally invasive methods to remove early-stage malignant and premalignant lesions. Transanal local excision (TAE) is a commonly used surgical technique to remove certain types of benign or early-stage malignant lesions in the rectum using conventional retractors and sutures (Fig. 19.1). Another technique, transanal minimally invasive surgery (TAMIS), is the most popular transanal endoluminal approach among surgeons. TAMIS enables excision using conventional laparoscopic instruments or robotic surgical systems via transanal access platforms (e.g., the SILS™ Port (Medtronic, Minneapolis, MN, USA), the GelPOINT® Path transanal access platform (Applied Medical, Rancho Santa Margarita, CA, USA), the KeyPort Flex (Richard Wolf, Knittlingen, Germany), the SSL (Single Site Laparoscopy access system, Ethicon Endo-Surgery, Cincinnati, OH), and the Endorec® (Aspide Médical, La Talaudière, France)) placed in the anal canal. Full-thickness excision is possible through TAE and TAMIS procedures.

Supplementary Information The online version contains supplementary material available at https://doi.org/10.1007/978-3-031-66772-5_19.

K. Erozkan · E. Gorgun (✉)
Department of Colorectal Surgery, Digestive Disease and Surgery Institute, Cleveland Clinic, Cleveland, OH, USA
e-mail: gorgune@ccf.org

M. Hoffman et al. (eds.), *Major Complications of Female Pelvic Surgery*,
https://doi.org/10.1007/978-3-031-66772-5_19

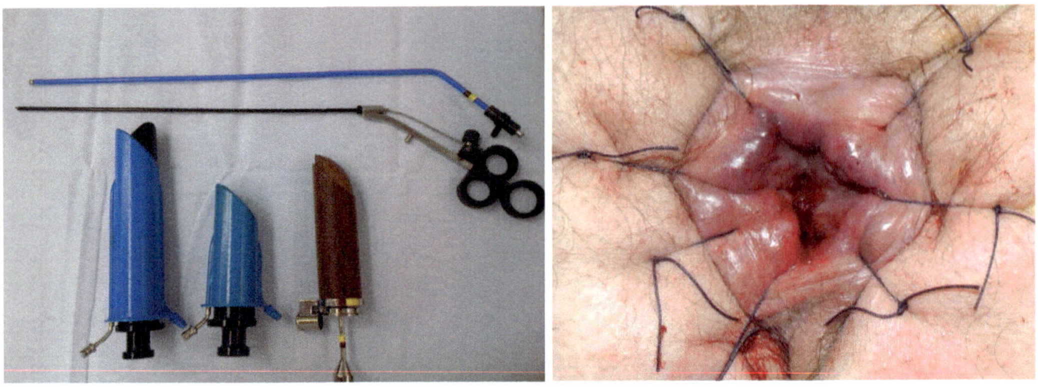

Fig. 19.1 Transanal local excision with conventional instruments

Nevertheless, dissection in the submucosal plane is sufficient for benign, premalignant, and superficial invasive cancers; however, intramuscular or full-thickness resection is recommended for the local management of rectal cancers >T1. Although access to proximal lesions is more efficient with TAMIS compared to TAE, the useability of both techniques is limited for distal colorectal lesions. For upper rectum and rectosigmoid lesions, advanced polypectomy techniques are preferred.

Endoscopic mucosal resection (EMR) and endoscopic submucosal dissection (ESD) are currently two of the most popular transanal endoscopic procedures for excising large premalignant lesions. EMR is a method that lifts, snares, and then excises lesions. The polyp is lifted using various solutions and snared by slowly closing a loop wire while simultaneously cauterizing it. Even though piecemeal excision is acceptable in the case of totally benign large lesions, the goal is to remove high-risk lesions in an en bloc manner. An increased number of snared pieces decreases the adequacy of the histopathological examination and can also lead to full-thickness defect as a result of entrapment of the muscle layer in the bite. On the other hand, ESD is a procedure in which the lesion is excised by dissecting within the submucosal plane. The ESD procedure begins by lifting the lesion using an injectate similar to the one used in the EMR technique. After the mucosal incision, dissection is carried out in the submucosal plane using an endoscopic cutting knife.

Although all the techniques mentioned above are minimally invasive, complications can be observed. The most common complications include perforation, bleeding, abscess, stricture, urinary retention, and fecal incontinence. This chapter provides an in-depth review of the common complications of transanal local excisions and endoluminal procedures, including their indications, background, and techniques for their prevention, recognition, and management..

Perforation

Background

The thickness of the colorectal wall, colonic folds, flexures, and peristalsis can lead to perforation during transanal local excisions and endoluminal approaches. Perforations are generally classified as either intraprocedural or delayed. Intraprocedural perforations should be examined separately as minor and major perforations (Fig. 19.2). Minor perforations are partial perforations generally characterized by defects in the muscularis propria, while major perforations describe full-thickness injuries in the colon and rectum wall. Intraprocedural perforations are commonly detected during the procedure, and appropriate treatments are performed. Major surgery is only required for a small number of patients. Delayed perforations occur after the procedure with a more severe clinical presentation and can lead to abscess formation or sepsis.

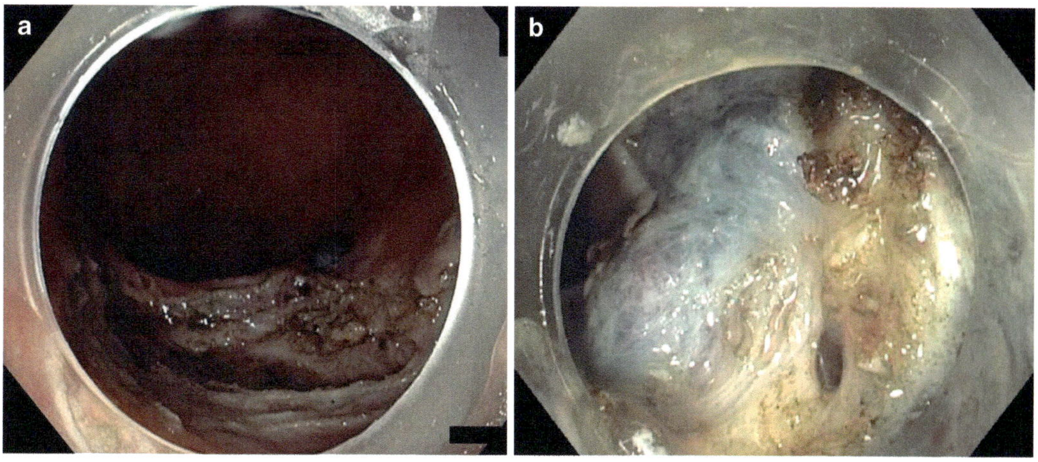

Fig. 19.2 Perforations. (**a**) Muscular defect. (**b**) Full-thickness perforation

Therefore, these should be quickly identified, evaluated, and treated. One common reason for delayed perforations is the overuse of electrocauterization during the procedure, leading to insufficient blood supply and eventual perforation. Even if any perforation is detected and closed during the procedure, delayed perforation can occur afterward. Another condition that can cause delayed perforation is the development of an abscess due to partial perforation of the colon wall. Fecal contamination causes inflammation and abscess in the muscular defect. Inflammation and abscess can lead to delayed perforations after the procedure.

Several perforation rates were previously reported after local excisions and endoluminal procedures, ranging from 2.5% to 18% [5–9]. Generally, ESD has a higher perforation rate than EMR [10]; however, with increasing experience and completion of the learning curve, perforation rates could be improved. A lesion's location, size, and histopathological morphology can all be risk factors for perforation. It is known that excision of rectum lesions leads to less perforation than that of colon lesions [11, 12]. Perforations are more common in lesions larger than 2 cm [12]. Submucosal fibrosis is also a risk factor for perforation in transanal and endoluminal approaches. A muscle-like structure in the submucosal plane, inadequate lifting, and a white web are all signs of submucosal fibrosis. Studies show that the perforation rate is higher in lesions with submucosal fibrosis [11, 13]. Submucosal fibrosis can occur in patients with recurrence, so they should be treated more carefully during procedures.

Post-polypectomy syndrome, first described in 1986, is another complication of conventional and advanced polypectomy techniques [14]. It may initially present as perforation and show fever, abdominal pain, and leukocytosis symptoms. However, peritonitis is generally localized in post-polypectomy, and there is no perforation in the bowel wall. Excessive electrocautery use, which is a significant risk factor for post-polypectomy syndrome, can cause burning in the muscular layer. Other risk factors include lesions larger than 3 cm, prolonged procedure time, and rectosigmoid lesions [15].

Prevention

Preoperative patient positioning is a factor that facilitates proper dissection. The position can be changed during procedures depending on the location of the lesion. In addition, the scope can be rotated 180° to position the target area at the 6 o'clock position during endoluminal procedures. TAMIS port placement and instrument choice should be made according to the location of the lesions.

Injection of the lifting solution into the submucosal area is the critical step for all transanal local excisions and endoluminal approaches. Submucosal injection is widely utilized in ESD and EMR. However, its application in TAMIS remains understudied and less commonly employed. As the authors of this chapter, we firmly believe that incorporating submucosal injection into TAMIS procedures not only facilitates dissection but also serves as a preventive measure for achieving superior outcomes. Nonetheless, challenges do exist when attempting a submucosal injection during TAMIS. To overcome these challenges, we employ through-the-scope (TTS) endoscopy injection needles. These needles are placed through the shaft of a laparoscopic instrument's metal sheet and subsequently directed into the target area (Fig. 19.3).

Sufficient injection into the submucosal area is essential to prevent perforations or other complications since injecting solutions under the muscle layer, or insufficient injections, can cause difficulties during dissection and excision. In case of unsuccessful injections, proper cushioning might not be created and the muscular layer can be trapped in the snare while snaring or dissection cannot be continued in a proper plane. If the patient is not under anesthesia, biting the muscular layer can result in abdominal pain. In the event of non-lifting, reapplication of the lifting solution should be preferred, even if it is time-consuming. If proper lifting cannot be achieved with reapplication, piecemeal removal might be considered to prevent perforation. Two types of solutions are available for lifting during transanal local excisions and endoluminal procedures. The Food and Drug Administration (FDA)-approved premixed solutions are LiftUp® (Ovesco Endoscopy AG, Tübingen, Germany), Blue Eye™ (The Standard Co., Ltd., Gunpo-si, Korea), Blue Beacon™ (Micro-Tech Co., Ltd., Nanjing, China), EverLift™ Submucosal Lifting Agent (Gi Supply, Inc.), Eleview® (SIC 8000) (Cosmo Technologies, Ltd., Dublin, Ireland), and EndoClot® solution (EndoClot Plus Co., Ltd., Santa Clara, CA, USA). These solutions remain in the submucosal plane for long durations, reducing the procedure time by eliminating preparation steps and repeat injections. In addition to premixed solutions, diluted adrenaline (1 mL of 0.1% adrenaline) and hydroxyethyl starch solution mixed with methylene blue or other dyes can also be used. Saline is not a preferred solution as it stays in the tissue only for a limited time and dissipates quickly.

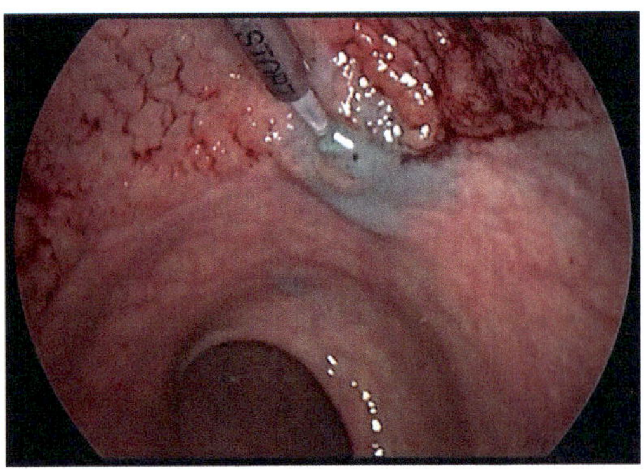

Fig. 19.3 Submucosal injection in TAMIS

Traction can also be applied to lesions for dissection and complication prevention. There are various traction techniques in anal procedures. Clips can be attached to the mucosa proximal or opposite to the lesion if a sufficient submucosal opening is not created during dissection. Alternatively, externally placed flexible endoscopic graspers can be used for distal lesions. Other traction methods, such as balloon-assisted overtube, thin-type endoscopy, or string clip traction devices, could improve the traction for colorectal ESD, especially in large lesions with submucosal fibrosis.

Special techniques can be considered to prevent perforation. Underwater EMR (UEMR), described by Binmoeller et al. [16], fills the bowel lumen with water so that the bowel maintains the circular shape of the muscle layer while the mucosa and submucosa float on water. This technique allows for proper excision without using an injection. Moreover, studies have shown that UEMR reduces complications such as perforation and delayed bleeding [16, 17]. Another technique is an adaptive customized approach, as shown in Video 19.1. In this video, we demonstrate how different approaches can be utilized if one technique does not work. For example, conversion to TAMIS to treat lesions that cannot be adequately accessed by transanal local excision or for which resection cannot be completed with techniques such as EMR and ESD is a customized approach. We believe that this can facilitate dissection and reduce the risk of complications.

In case of minor perforation or mucosal defect closure, endoscopic clips can close the defect area and prevent major perforation and later abscess development (Fig. 19.4). Through-the-scope (TTS) endoscopic clips are Resolution™ Clip (Boston Scientific, Marlborough, MA, USA), SureClip® (Micro-Tech Endoscopy, Ann Arbor, MI, USA), QuickClip Pro™ (Olympus America, Center Valley, PA, USA), EZ Clip™ (Olympus America, Center Valley, PA, USA), Tomel Clip™ (Century Medica, Inc., Tokyo, Japan), and ZEOCLIP™ (Zeon Medical Inc., Tokyo, Japan). These clips have higher rotation and repositioning ability [18]. Mucosal defect closure involves using a clip to grasp the edges of the defect. It is important to degas the intestinal lumen before clipping to grasp the mucosal defect edge. Several techniques have been described for closing large defects with clips. If the defect is wider than a clip, a mucosal incision method may be used, where a clip is hooked onto a small hole on one side of the mucosa [19]. Another method, the endoscopic mucosa–submucosa clip closure, uses a single clip to grasp the defect edge and the submucosa above the muscularis layer, reducing the size of the mucosal defect [20]. The clip-on-clip closure method involves placing one clip over another and using the gap between clips as an anchor (zipping technique) [21]. To close the defects in thin gastrointestinal sections such as the rectosigmoid colon, the mucosal and muscular layers can be softened by submerging them in water during clipping [22]. Various mucosal defect closure methods have been proposed using clips and special devices such as sutures, rings, endoloops, and double-channel endoscopes [23]. Additionally, TTS clips should not be used alone when inflamed or indurated tissue surrounds the defect or when anatomical variations prevent clip placement [24]. Clip-and-snare, clip-and-endoloop techniques, and band-assisted closure are more successful in such cases. Closed layer levels of these techniques are generally limited to the mucosa and submucosa. Endoscopic procedures such as over-the-scope clip (OTSC) or endoscopic suturing, described in the "Management" section, could be also an alternative option.

In TAMIS, flexible endoscopic clips or laparoscopic clips can be used via the transanal access platforms. Flexible endoscopic clips are suitable to pass along through trocars and placed with the assistance of TAMIS instruments. Primary suturing is an option for defect closure during

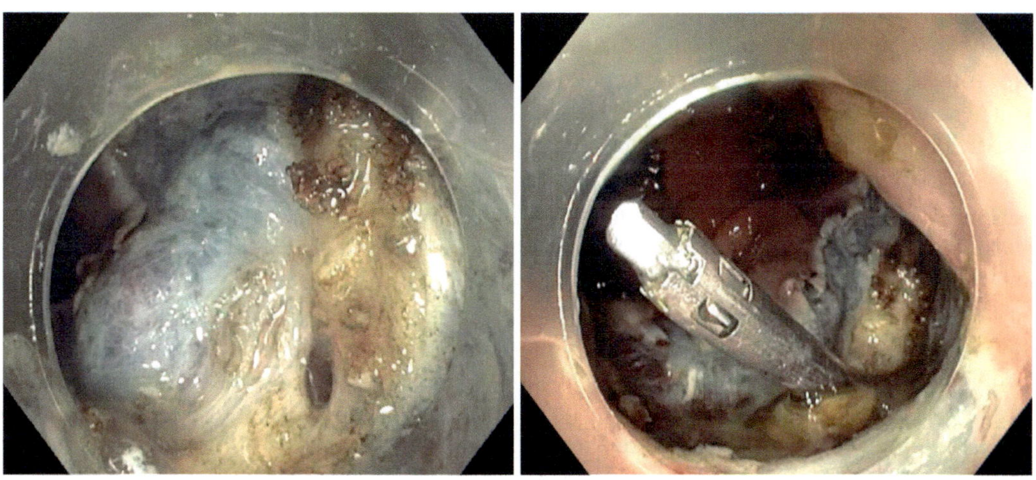

Fig. 19.4 Endoscopic clip placement for closure after a full-thickness perforation

TAMIS and TAE. Using flexible robotic platforms for transanal procedures facilitates the closure of defects with improved dexterity.

Endoscopic clips can be used to prevent post-polypectomy syndrome and bleeding. Prophylactic antibiotics can be administered to reduce the risk of post-polypectomy syndrome [25]. Endoscopic clips are also an option for preventing post-polypectomy syndrome.

Recognition

Early recognition and treatment of complications are crucial for reducing morbidity and mortality risks. Perforation and bleeding can be identified early by carefully observing the resection site during the procedure. Patients undergoing transanal local excisions and endoluminal approaches are typically observed for 3–4 h after the procedure, and those with complicated or larger lesions may stay overnight.

Perianal and pelvic abscesses can be seen in lower rectum lesions. Perforations after rectosigmoid and anteriorly located mid- and upper rectum lesion resections can be connected with the intraabdominal cavity. Surgeons should stay alert for perforation signs and symptoms, which include fever, leukocytosis, abdominal pain, distention, and rebound tenderness. Delayed complications can lead to more severe clinical presentations. In rare cases, the patient may develop pelvic sepsis and septic shock, which can be life-threatening. If perforation is suspected, the patient should undergo thorough physical examination, laboratory tests, or imaging studies. Laboratory tests such as a complete blood count (CBC) and C-reactive protein (CRP) can help identify the presence of inflammation and infection. Digital rectal examination and flexible sigmoidoscopy can help diagnose lesions at the distal level. Abdominal X-rays can verify free air's presence after suspicious procedures. In addition, computed tomography (CT) scanning, or in some cases magnetic resonance imaging (MRI), can provide more detailed information on the extent of the perforation and the presence of any associated abscess or bleeding.

Management

The management of perforation and bleeding depends on the timing of diagnosis and the patient's condition. Intraprocedural recognition and diagnosis of perforation are crucial for prompt management and to prevent further severe complications. Intraoperative detection and clipping can be performed to manage perforations and bleeding, preventing additional surgical procedures [26]. However, delayed complications may require more severe medical attention if perforation is detected later.

General strategies such as oral intake restriction, intravenous fluid resuscitation, and intravenous antibiotic therapy are commonly employed against perforation. Endoscopic and transanal methods are often the preferred initial treatment for early or delayed perforations in patients with stable vital signs and good overall health. Endoscopic procedures may be performed for delayed perforations, such as closure with TTS clips, OTSC, or endoscopic suturing. The OTSC® system (Ovesco Endoscopy AG, Tübingen, Germany) is generally used for tightly grasping large defects. It is recommended to create a slightly larger dissection area around the perforation and hook one side of the clip around the non-neoplastic mucosa to prevent the excision bed or muscle layer from tearing during clipping [27, 28]. Lumen occlusion is one of the worst and most unknown complications of OTSC application [29]. Endoscopists should check wall integrity and lumen patency each time after an OTSC clip placement. Closure of major perforations is feasible with an endoscopic suturing device. Overstitch™ (Apollo Endosurgerry Inc., Austin, TX, USA) is the only FDA-approved device for endoscopic suturing. This system comprises a cap attached to a scope, a hand lever-controlled needle driver, and an anchor exchange component. It enables the application of full-thickness sutures using different suturing patterns and comes with accessories such as scissors and grasping forceps that aid in targeting and tissue release.

Another defect closure technique can be applied using TAMIS. When a peritoneal breach occurs during TAMIS, immediate placement of a corner suture before completing the rectal mass removal provides control of the peritoneal defect site. Early suture placement can prevent losing control of the defect site and loss of pneumorectum. TAMIS can be a valuable option to repair the defect, especially for anteriorly located mid- and upper rectum lesions. A corner suture also prevents enlargement of the peritoneal breach, which could result in an uncontrollable pneumoperitoneum. After the dissection is completed, defect closure can be resumed (Video 19.2). This technical approach prompts successful TAMIS completion and reduces the risk of conversion to laparoscopy or laparotomy.

Sometimes in lesions with fibrosis, TAMIS can lead to full-thickness excision, which might lead to almost complete loss of the rectal domain. These challenging cases can be prone to potential complications, such as formation of mesorectal abscesses or the complete disruption of anatomy. To reinforce this issue, we believe that a sleeve advancement can be applied (Video 19.3).

In cases of diffuse peritonitis when endoscopic and transanal management is not feasible, alternative interventional options and abdominal surgical procedures can be considered. The choice of surgical approach depends on the extent and severity of the perforation as well as the surgeon's experience and preference. The management of delayed complications requires close monitoring and may require a multidisciplinary approach.

Bleeding

Background

Bleeding is one of the most common complications encountered during transanal local excisions and endoluminal approaches (Fig. 19.5). It develops as a result of vascular injury in the submucosal area. Studies have reported bleeding rates ranging from 2% to 13% [8, 9]. Delayed bleeding may also occur postoperatively, and it has been reported in 2% of colorectal ESD patients [30]. Although most bleeding is minor and managed conservatively, severe bleeding can sometimes occur. Risk factors for bleeding include using anticoagulant and antiplatelet drugs, previous ESD procedures, male gender, and lesions larger than 2 cm [8]. Hypertension and using hot biopsy forceps are additional risk factors for delayed bleeding [31]. Rectal lesions are specifically an independent risk factor for bleeding. Bleeding may occur due to injury to the hemorrhoidal venous plexus during lower rectal lesion excision. Hemorrhoidal bleeding comes from an easily accessible area and can be stopped with sutures.

Prevention

Before the procedure, it is crucial to evaluate the patient's risk of bleeding and discontinue any anticoagulant or antiplatelet therapy if possible.

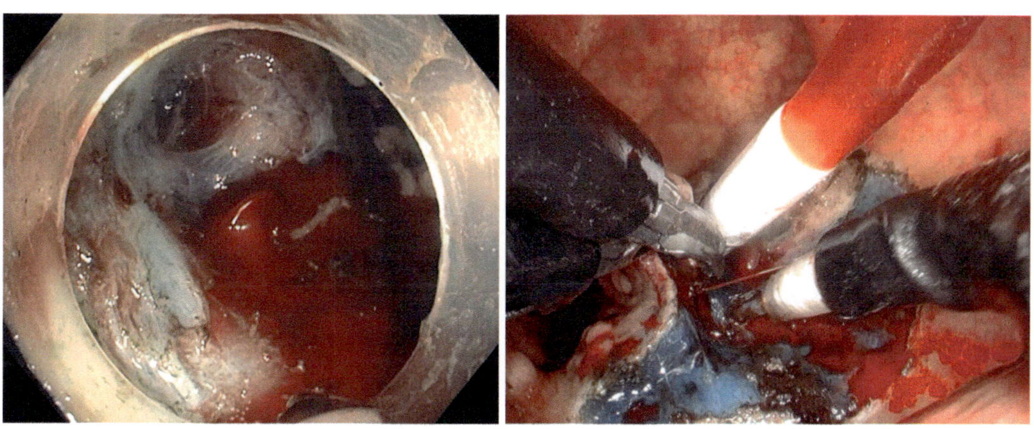

Fig. 19.5 Bleeding during ESD and endo-robotic submucosal dissection (ERSD)

Adequate submucosal injection, slow dissection pace, a stepwise approach, and preventive coagulation of visible blood vessels before the dissection are methods to prevent bleeding during the procedure [32]. Adding adrenaline to the injection solutions might also be considered in high-risk patients. Many methods and techniques for preventing and managing perforations can also be used for early or delayed bleeding. (Please refer to the perforation prevention and management section for submucosal injection, endoscopic clipping, UEMR, etc.). Endoscopic clips, cautery, or sutures can be used during the procedure to control bleeding, but, even if we use these techniques, delayed bleeding can occur. A multicentric study showed that prophylactic clipping could reduce the risk of delayed bleeding in high-risk groups with no complications such as perforation [33]; however, conflicting data also exist [34]. Using electrocautery for prophylactic coagulation is also a debated method to stop bleeding. A randomized controlled study showed that prophylactic coagulation of non-bleeding visible vessels is ineffective [35], but some studies claim the opposite [36]. We believe electrocautery use is a valuable option to prevent delayed bleeding with the proper device and technique (Please refer to the bleeding management section).

Recognition

Patients with bleeding may present with hematochezia, hypotension, tachycardia, low hemoglobin levels, or even hypovolemic shock. Melena is rarely seen after excisions at the pelvic level. Physical examination, CBC, and colonoscopy can be used for diagnosis. CT is the preferred imaging method for bleeding suspicions. Angiography can be used for both diagnosis and treatment in resilient patients with bleeding. Scintigraphy is theoretically an alternative option for the diagnosis of bleeding but is not common in practice.

Management

In case of minor bleeding, careful observation and cessation of anticoagulant therapy may be sufficient for management. If bleeding is continuous, endoscopic treatment methods, which are also options for managing perforation, such as clips or sutures, can be used to control bleeding. Conventional retractors can be used for identifying and managing bleeding. If it is not possible to identify a bleeding spot or continue dissection because of blood pooling, changing the patient's position by taking advantage of gravity can improve the view. Endoscopic coagulation of visible vessels can also be performed to stop bleeding, but excessive electrocautery should be avoided as it may lead to late perforation. Using proper coagulation devices and generators is essential, especially for endoluminal procedures. The most utilized energy towers are VIO®3 (Erbe USA, Inc., Marietta, GA, USA) and Geradores THUNDERBEAT (ESG-400 e USG-400) (Olympus America Inc., Center Valley, PA, USA). These generators are designed for endoluminal procedures providing different energy modalities, including swift, forced, and spray coagulation. In their cutting mode, blended energy can be applied that can be combined in the cutting mode with a blend of coagulation period. Additionally, incremental a coagulation modality can be added for patients with specific hematological issues to minimize bleeding even in the cutting or blend mode. The other advantage of these generators is that in the blend cutting mode, application of pulsatile energy is enabled, which allows physicians to make a clear cut at superficial levels that can expose deeper vessels more clearly. Subsequently, prophylactic coagulation can be performed in forced and spray coagulation modes. Additionally, topical agents, band ligation, and sclerosing agent injections can be preferred instead for bleeding treatment. Angiography or abdominal surgical approaches may be necessary in severe hypovolemic conditions unresponsive to intravenous resuscitation.

Abscesses

Background

Infections and abscesses are inflammatory complications of transanal local excisions and endoluminal approaches. Surgical site infections are the most common hospital-acquired infections after colorectal surgery, increasing morbidity, mortality, and hospital costs. However, these techniques are performed in the third space. Infections are generally related to perforation and usually result in abscesses. An abscess is a frequent complication of transanal local excisions and endoluminal approaches, often resulting from delayed perforations. However, minor perforations can also cause an abscess due to fecal obstruction of the muscularis propria defect and bacterial colonization. Insufficient blood supply, and inflammation secondary to bacterial colonization, may result in a full-thickness perforation. Abscesses can be localized within the abdominal cavity or cause diffuse peritonitis after rectosigmoid and anterior upper and mid-rectum procedures [37]. Lower rectum perforations generally result in perianal and pelvic abscesses, although delayed cases may develop Fournier's gangrene.

Prevention

Bowel preparation reduces contamination due to minor leakage and can effectively prevent abscess development [38]. Additionally, it provides a better operation view and facilitates dissection, which is important for preventing other complications. Position change can also reduce contamination in the peritoneal cavity in case of perforation [38].

Even though prophylactic antibiotics can reduce the incidence of clinical adverse events, including abdominal pain, diarrhea, hematochezia, and fever [39], their preoperative use is not recommended for preventing infections and abscess development [40, 41]. Antibiotic use can be considered in cases of perforation and large lesion resections [40]. Prophylactic antibiotics are not recommended for the excision of lesions smaller than 20 mm [41]. However, our prospective project, which is the implementation of the surgical site infection prevention bundle at our center, substantially declined surgical site infection rates in our department for all colorectal procedures [42]. We believe that prophylactic pre- and perioperative antibiotic use can reduce infections and abscess development after local anal operations and endoluminal approaches. In particular, we believe that it is effective in case of perforation and minimizes the contamination that may be caused by flow and blow.

Prevention and early management of perforations also prevent possible abscess development. The excision bed should be carefully evaluated for perforations at the end of the procedure. Endoscopic clips, sutures, and other techniques can be used as described in the "Perforation" section for early management of perforations (please refer to the perforation prevention and management section). Even within the mesorectum full-thickness defect, we prefer to close them using endoscopic clips or possibly suture closing. As discussed earlier, excessive use of electrocautery should be avoided to prevent disruption of blood flow, which might cause delayed perforations and abscesses.

Recognition

Abscess diagnosis is based on clinical symptoms and imaging methods. The diagnostic criteria for perianal abscesses include redness, warmth, tenderness, digital rectal fullness, and fluctuation. Digital rectal examination helps identify perianal and pelvic abscesses. Patients with a pelvic abscess, which is more common than an abdominal abscess after transanal excisions and endoluminal approaches, might present with sacral pain, pain when sitting, and tailbone pain. Patients may have abdominal abscesses in case of a peritoneal breach. These patients may have abdominal pain, tenderness, fever, nausea, and vomiting. CBC, possible emergency visits, and CT are recommended for these patients.

Management

The primary treatment of an abscess is surgical drainage. Once a perianal or perirectal abscess is diagnosed, it is crucial to promptly drain it, regardless of the presence of fluctuance. Delaying treatment can lead to the abscess expanding into nearby spaces and potentially causing a systemic infection. Depending on the localization, perianal abscesses can be drained via the endoluminal or perianal route. Perianal and ischiorectal abscesses can be drained by incision through the perineum. It is important to make the skin incisions as close to the anal verge as possible. This approach helps minimize the potential length of a fistula that may develop while still ensuring adequate drainage of the abscess. Following the incision and drainage procedure, wound packing is a common practice. However, it is worth stating that there is no proven benefit to this approach [43]. Although supra levator abscesses are generally rare, their incidence may increase after endoluminal approaches. They occur in case of perforation in the rectum wall. These abscesses should be drained into the rectum through an incision in the resection bed to avoid creating an extrasphincteric fistula.

If CT findings reveal presacral or abdominal fluid collections larger than 2 cm, possible drainage is highly recommended, especially for symptomatic patients. For collections smaller than 2 cm, a course of antibiotics might be trailed; however, even if the patients are symptomatic with smaller lesions, possible drainage and at least aspiration under CT guidance may be recommended. Typically, these drains are placed in the transgluteal area to collect a larger amount of liquids from the pelvis. This can be painful, and the access route should be explained to patients, as the insertion points for trans-gluteal drains can cause varying amounts of pain. These drains should be monitored daily until drainage is required. When using drains with negative pressure application, monitoring should continue until the amount of drainage becomes minimal. Especially in pelvic drains, daily irrigation is strongly advised to prevent clogging.

After the incision and drainage of an abscess, it is suggested to administer empiric antibiotics to all patients. This practice has been shown to potentially reduce the rate of fistula formation, according to available evidence. The duration of antibiotic coverage is based on extrapolating from studies focusing on intraabdominal infection following source control. A systematic review and meta-analysis of two randomized trials and one retrospective study provided the strongest evidence supporting the use of routine empiric antibiotics after drainage [44–46]. The analysis showed that the rate of fistula formation was lower in patients who received antibiotics compared to those who did not. The American Society of Colon and Rectal Surgeons (ASCRS) recommends empiric antibiotics after abscess drainage only for patients with extensive perianal/perineal cellulitis, signs of systemic infection, diabetes, valvular heart disease, or immunosuppression [47]. All these publications are based on perianal and pelvic abscesses and are not specific for abscesses after transanal local excisions and endoluminal procedures.

If interventional and antibiotic treatments are unsuccessful, abdominal surgical procedures can be an option for abscess treatment. Endoscopic ultrasound-guided (EUS-guided) drainage is feasible for localized abdominal and pelvic abscesses [48].

Strictures

Background

Strictures after colorectal local excisions are not as commonly seen as in esophageal and gastric antral lesions after tissue resections [49]. Preventive approaches enhance epithelialization and mucosal healing after colorectal lesions; however, strictures may occur, especially after circumferential resection, with reported rates of 50–70% [50–52]. We have found the rates to be lower in our practice, particularly if dissection is at a higher level in the rectum, farther from the anal canal. Rectal lesions with more than three-quarters of the luminal circumference carry a higher risk of post-ESD strictures, especially if they are large or have long longitudinal lengths or if mucosal defects cover more than 90% of the luminal circumference [51] (Fig. 19.6). Total circumferential resection possesses a high risk and requires close postoperative follow-up [38].

Prevention

Close monitoring of patients after circumferential excision is essential to prevent stricture formation. Prophylactic bougie or balloon dilation can be performed in the follow-up period. Steroid treatment to prevent stricture formation is controversial in colorectal lesions. Even though conflicting studies exist in the literature [50], prophylactic usage of steroids may be effective [51]. Steroid treatment has been reported to cause necrosis to prevent esophageal strictures, but there is no data for colorectal lesions [53]. Full-thickness resection and primary sleeve advancement with TAMIS can be an option to prevent strictures in cases of circumferential lesions [54].

Recognition

Strictures may present with constipation and develop over an extended period. The diagnosis is usually confirmed by flexible sigmoidoscopy and digital rectal examination. Imaging studies may show dilatation of the bowel loops.

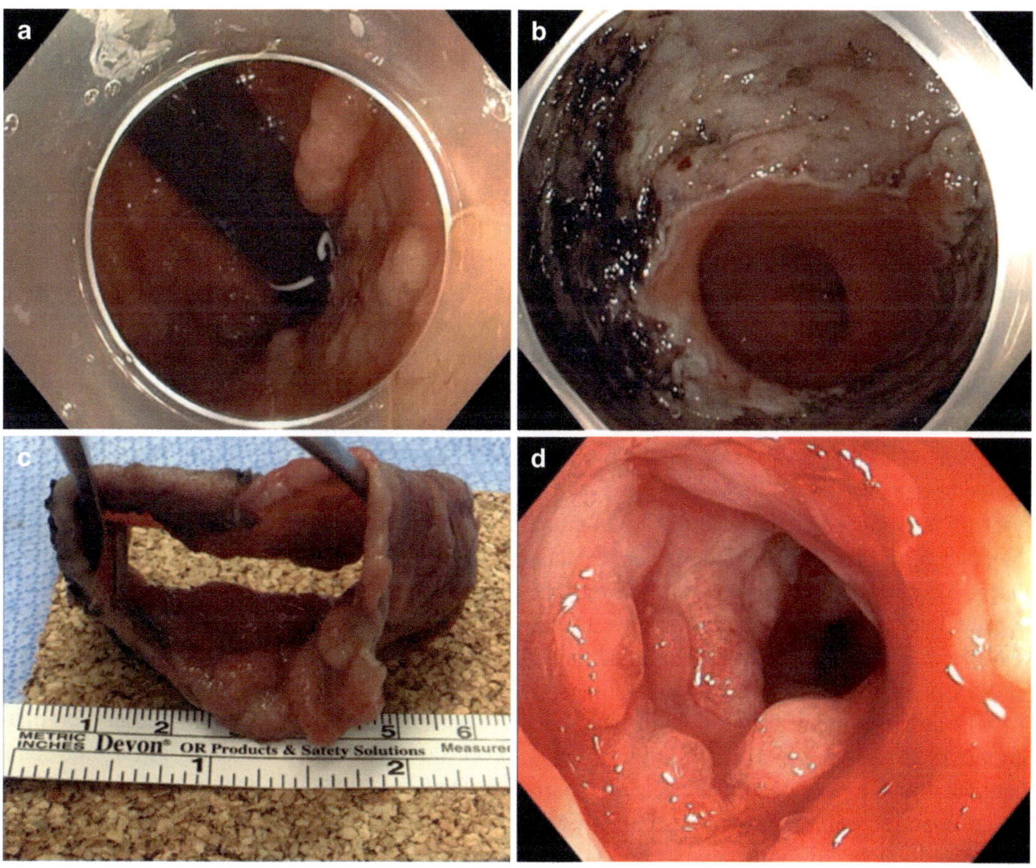

Fig. 19.6 Stricture development and treatment. (**a**) Circumferential lesion. (**b**) Resection bed. (**c**) Specimen. (**d**) Stricture

Management

Strictures that generally develop in distal lesions can be prevented and treated with bougie and balloon dilation [52]. In addition, dilation can be achieved by endoscopic knife escharotomy. Alternatively, a re-resection can be performed to manage strictures [49]. Triamcinolone–acetonide injection and rectal suppository hydrocortisone acetate may be adjuncts in healing and prevention [49, 50]. Fixing endoscopic stents with biomaterials, which can be used for esophageal lesions, are not preferred for colorectal lesions due to possible stent migration [55]. Close follow-up is essential to monitor the effectiveness of treatment and prevent recurrence of the stricture.

Fecal Incontinence

Background

Fecal incontinence is a distressing complication that can happen especially following transanal local excisions. The involuntary loss of fecal contents significantly impairs the quality of life of the affected patients. Postoperative fecal incontinence is observed in approximately 29% of patients who undergo transanal endoscopic microsurgery (TEM) with varying degrees of severity [56]. The TEM device's relatively large diameter and rigidity contribute to this higher incidence. Conventional retractors can cause sphincter damage during TAE procedures probably with the same pathophysiology. However, the diameter of the retractor in TAE is smaller than that in TEM and operation times are shorter. The expected fecal incontinence rate is lower than that of the TEM procedure. The introduction of TAMIS has helped mitigate fecal incontinence. TAMIS utilizes a more flexible platform, reducing the risk of sphincter damage and improving functional outcomes. Moreover, fecal incontinence is not an expected complication in EMR and ESD, which are more flexible approaches. Nevertheless, when these procedures are performed in the distal rectum, fecal incontinence can still arise from sphincter damage. Injuries that can occur during dissection or resection can cause a loss of anal sphincter pressure. Fecal incontinence may occur due to complications arising after the procedure. For example, a perforation or an abscess, which might occur after these procedures, can cause fecal incontinence. The severity of fecal incontinence symptoms gets worse after the procedure, especially in patients who have undergone TEM. However, most patients experience transient symptoms that improve over time [57]. The procedure-specific risk factors for the development of functional disorders after transanal excisions are the TEM procedure, prolonged operative time, tumor localization at <3 cm from the anal verge, and tumor size larger than 3 cm [56].

Prevention

Preventing fecal incontinence following transanal local excisions and endoluminal approaches requires a comprehensive approach. Surgeons should employ surgical techniques to minimize damage to the anal sphincter complex and surrounding structures. Careful dissection and preservation of the anal sphincter muscles, nerves, and blood supply are crucial for reducing the risk of fecal incontinence. Transitioning to more flexible platforms like EMR, ESD, and TAMIS has demonstrated a reduced incidence of sphincter damage and subsequent fecal incontinence. Flexible platforms should be considered for larger lesions, especially in older patients. Preoperative evaluation of anal sphincter function through anorectal manometry and endoanal ultrasonography can help identify patients at a higher risk. A trauma to the anal sphincters caused by inserting operating devices or platforms and prolonged stretching of the anal canal during surgery can impair continence [57]. Therefore, operative time should be kept to a minimum.

Recognition

Fecal incontinence can be detected through patient complaints. Associated symptoms may include altered bowel habits, such as increased frequency of bowel movements or urgency to defecate. Patients who complain about gas, solid or liquid stool incontinence, and frequent bathroom visits due to their inability to control their bowel movements might have fecal incontinence.

Management

Management of fecal incontinence should be individualized according to the underlying cause, type of operation, severity of symptoms, and patient preferences. It should be known that fecal incontinence is temporary in most cases. Initially, patients should be evaluated for sphincter damage and functions. Nonsurgical interventions such as dietary changes, bowel retraining, pelvic floor exercises (biofeedback therapy), and stool collection devices can be applied initially to improve symptoms and support continence in patients without sphincter injury.

Medical therapy aims to reduce stool frequency and improve stool consistency. While no specific medication has been proven to be universally effective, antidiarrheal drugs such as loperamide can be used to reduce fecal incontinence in patients with liquid stools. Dietary supplementation with bulking agents like psyllium or methylcellulose can improve stool consistency, especially in patients with low-volume, loose stools. In cases of fecal impaction, disimpaction and treatment of constipation are necessary.

If initial management fails, further evaluation with anorectal manometry and endorectal ultrasound/magnetic resonance imaging should be conducted to identify any functional or structural abnormalities causing fecal incontinence. Biofeedback therapy can be considered for patients with weakness of the external anal sphincter or decreased ability to perceive rectal distension. It aims to retrain the pelvic floor and abdominal wall muscles, improving coordination and sensation.

Injectable anal bulking agents, such as dextranomer stabilized in hyaluronic acid, may be used for passive fecal incontinence to enhance resting anal pressures. Anal sphincteroplasty, a surgical procedure, is reserved for patients who do not respond to initial management and have evidence of sphincter injury. Sacral nerve stimulation is an option for patients who do not respond to biofeedback or sphincteroplasty, involving electrical stimulation of the sacral nerve roots to improve fecal continence. For patients with intractable symptoms who have failed nonsurgical and surgical management, colostomy, sphincteroplasty, artificial anal sphincter, radio-frequency ablation, anal plugs can be an option.

Urinary Retention

Background

Urinary incontinence is a potential complication that might arise following transanal local excisions and endoluminal approaches. The surgical sites for these procedures are close to the urinary tract and often include the manipulation of pelvic tissues, which can disrupt normal voiding mechanisms and result in impaired bladder emptying. The incidence of urinary retention, a significant contributing factor to urinary incontinence, ranges from 4.1% to 9.4% [58, 59]. Notably, the utilization of spinal anesthesia during these procedures has been associated with a higher incidence of urinary retention. However, it is worth mentioning that endoscopic techniques, which can be performed under sedation, have demonstrated lower rates of urinary retention in colorectal lesions [60].

Prevention

Detail-oriented surgical techniques should be used to avoid injury to the urinary tract during procedures. Correct identification and careful dissection of anatomical landmarks can minimize injury. In addition, appropriate patient selection and comprehensive preoperative evaluation may help identify patients at a high risk of urinary retention, leading to appropriate surgical management. Sedation or general anesthesia may be preferred instead of spinal anesthesia to prevent urinary retention. Similarly, considering endoscopic techniques may be advantageous due to their lower rates of urinary retention. Enhanced recovery practices such as early mobilization, not using a urinary catheter, or removing the catheter in the early postoperative period can aid in preserving the urinary tract [61]. Conservative measures such as bladder training or pharmacological interventions to enhance bladder contractility may be attempted. Prophylactic alpha-adrenergic antagonists, such as tamsulosin, can also lower postoperative urinary retention [62].

Recognition

Patients may present with symptoms such as reduced urine output, difficulty initiating or maintaining urination, or a sense of incomplete bladder emptying. Patients' clinic examination and symptoms are important for diagnosis. Upon physical examination, the patient would demonstrate suprapubic tenderness and fullness.

Management

Prompt recognition and treatment of any underlying causes, such as urinary tract infection or medication-related factors, are essential. The surgical site should be controlled in case of hematoma, abscess, and perforation. More invasive interventions may be considered in the failure of conservative measures or in cases of persistent or recurrent urinary retention. These may include placement of a urethral catheter, suprapubic catheterization, or, in refractory cases, surgical procedures to relieve bladder outlet obstruction.

References

1. Fearon ER, Vogelstein B. A genetic model for colorectal tumorigenesis. Cell. 1990;61:759–67. https://doi.org/10.1016/0092-8674(90)90186-I.
2. Zauber AG, Winawer SJ, O'Brien MJ, et al. Colonoscopic polypectomy and long-term prevention of colorectal-cancer deaths. N Engl J Med. 2012;366:687–96. https://doi.org/10.1056/NEJMOA1100370.
3. US Preventive Services Task Force, Davidson KW, Barry MJ, et al. Screening for colorectal cancer: US preventive services task force recommendation statement. JAMA. 2021;325(19):1965–77. Published correction appears in JAMA. 2021 Aug 24;326(8):773.
4. Gorgun E, Benlice C, Abbas MA, Steele S. Experience in colon sparing surgery in North America: advanced endoscopic approaches for complex colorectal lesions. Surg Endosc. 2018;32:3114–21. https://doi.org/10.1007/S00464-018-6026-2.
5. Takamaru H, Saito Y, Yamada M, et al. Clinical impact of endoscopic clip closure of perforations during endoscopic submucosal dissection for colorectal tumors. Gastrointest Endosc. 2016;84:494–502.e1. https://doi.org/10.1016/J.GIE.2016.01.014.
6. Saito Y, Fukuzawa M, Matsuda T, et al. Clinical outcome of endoscopic submucosal dissection versus endoscopic mucosal resection of large colorectal tumors as determined by curative resection. Surg Endosc. 2010;24:343–52. https://doi.org/10.1007/S00464-009-0562-8.
7. Akintoye E, Kumar N, Aihara H, et al. Colorectal endoscopic submucosal dissection: a systematic review and meta-analysis. Endosc Int Open. 2016;4:E1030–44. https://doi.org/10.1055/S-0042-114774.
8. Sakamoto T, Mori G, Yamada M, et al. Endoscopic submucosal dissection for colorectal neoplasms: a review. WJG. 2014;20:16153. https://doi.org/10.3748/WJG.V20.I43.16153.
9. Rahmi G, Hotayt B, Chaussade S, et al. Endoscopic submucosal dissection for superficial rectal tumors: prospective evaluation in France. Endoscopy. 2014;46:670–6. https://doi.org/10.1055/S-0034-1365810.
10. Shahini E, Passera R, Lo Secco G, Arezzo A. A systematic review and meta-analysis of endoscopic mucosal resection vs endoscopic submucosal dissection for colorectal sessile/non-polypoid lesions. Minim Invasive Ther Allied Technol. 2022;31:835–47. https://doi.org/10.1080/13645706.2022.2032759.
11. Hong SN, Byeon JS, Lee BI, et al. Prediction model and risk score for perforation in patients undergoing colorectal endoscopic submucosal dissection. Gastrointest Endosc. 2016;84:98–108. https://doi.org/10.1016/J.GIE.2015.12.011.

12. Niikura R, Yasunaga H, Yamada A, et al. Factors predicting adverse events associated with therapeutic colonoscopy for colorectal neoplasia: a retrospective nationwide study in Japan. Gastrointest Endosc. 2016;84:971–982.e6. https://doi.org/10.1016/J.GIE.2016.05.013.
13. Mizushima T, Kato M, Iwanaga I, et al. Technical difficulty according to location, and risk factors for perforation, in endoscopic submucosal dissection of colorectal tumors. Surg Endosc. 2015;29:133–9. https://doi.org/10.1007/S00464-014-3665-9.
14. Nivatvongs S. Complications in colonoscopic polypectomy. An experience with 1,555 polypectomies. Dis Colon Rectum. 1986;29:825–30. https://doi.org/10.1007/BF02555356.
15. Jung D, Youn YH, Jahng J, et al. Risk of electrocoagulation syndrome after endoscopic submucosal dissection in the colon and rectum. Endoscopy. 2013;45:714–7. https://doi.org/10.1055/S-0033-1344555.
16. Binmoeller KF, Weilert F, Shah J, et al. "Underwater" EMR without submucosal injection for large sessile colorectal polyps (with video). Gastrointest Endosc. 2012;75:1086–91. https://doi.org/10.1016/J.GIE.2011.12.022.
17. Uedo N, Nemeth A, Johansson GW, et al. Underwater endoscopic mucosal resection of large colorectal lesions. Endoscopy. 2015;47:172–4. https://doi.org/10.1055/S-0034-1390749.
18. Daram SR, Tang SJ, Wu R, To SDF. Benchtop testing and comparisons among three types of through-the-scope endoscopic clipping devices. Surg Endosc. 2013;27:1521–9. https://doi.org/10.1007/S00464-012-2679-4.
19. Otake Y, Saito Y, Sakamoto T, et al. New closure technique for large mucosal defects after endoscopic submucosal dissection of colorectal tumors (with video). Gastrointest Endosc. 2012;75:663–7.
20. Banno S, Nishizawa T, Kinoshita S, Mori H, Uraoka T. Endoscopic mucosa-submucosal clip closure method. Endoscopy. 2017;49:E307–8.
21. Nomura T, Kamei A, Sugimoto S, Oyamada J. New closure method for a mucosal defect after endoscopic submucosal dissection—the clip-on-clip closure method. Endoscopy. 2018;50:547–8.
22. Yamasaki Y, Harada K, Oka S, et al. Feasibility of underwater clip closure for large mucosal defects after colorectal endoscopic submucosal dissection. Digestion. 2019;99:327–32.
23. Nomura T, Sugimoto S, Temma T, Oyamada J, Ito K, Kamei A. Suturing techniques with endoscopic clips and special devices after endoscopic resection. Dig Endosc. 2023;35(3):287–301. https://doi.org/10.1111/den.14427.
24. Kumar S, Youn YH, Lee JH. Life on a knife edge: the optimal approach to the management of perforations during endoscopic submucosal dissection (ESD). Expert Rev Gastroenterol Hepatol. 2020;14(10):965–73. https://doi.org/10.1080/17474124.2020.1791085.
25. Lee SP, Sung IK, Sung IK. A randomized controlled trial of prophylactic antibiotics in the prevention of electrocoagulation syndrome after colorectal endoscopic submucosal dissection. Gastrointest Endosc. 2017;86:349–357.e2.
26. Nakajima T, Saito Y, Tanaka S, et al. Current status of endoscopic resection strategy for large, early colorectal neoplasia in Japan. Surg Endosc. 2013;27:3262–70. https://doi.org/10.1007/S00464-013-2903-X.
27. Hu X, Xu QW, Liu WH. Endoscopic loop string-assisted clip suturing closure of large mucosal defects after endoscopic submucosal dissection in the sigmoid colon. Am J Gastroenterol. 2020;115:15. https://doi.org/10.14309/AJG.0000000000000505.
28. Yan B, Shi RH, Feng YD, Di ZH. Evaluating long-term attachment of a novel endoclip in porcine stomachs: a prospective study of initial deployment success and clip retention rates at different regions of the stomachs. Surg Endosc. 2016;30:1100–6. https://doi.org/10.1007/S00464-015-4305-8.
29. Dionigi B, Ozgur I, Sapci I, Church J, Gorgun E. Complete occlusion of lumen after over-the-scope-clip deployment during ESD: a lesson learned - a video vignette. Color Dis. 2022;24(5):664. https://doi.org/10.1111/codi.1605.
30. Repici A, Hassan C, De Paula PD, et al. Efficacy and safety of endoscopic submucosal dissection for colorectal neoplasia: a systematic review. Endoscopy. 2012;44:137–50. https://doi.org/10.1055/S-0031-1291448.
31. Li R, Cai S, Sun D, et al. Risk factors for delayed bleeding after endoscopic submucosal dissection of colorectal tumors. Surg Endosc. 2021;35:6583–90. https://doi.org/10.1007/S00464-020-08156-5.
32. Ahmed Y, Othman M. EMR/ESD: techniques, complications, and evidence. Curr Gastroenterol Rep. 2020;22(8):39. https://doi.org/10.1007/S11894-020-00777-Z.
33. Albéniz E, Enguita-Germán M, Gimeno-García AZ, et al. The answer to "when to clip" after colorectal endoscopic mucosal resection based on a cost-effectiveness analysis. Am J Gastroenterol. 2021;116:311–8. https://doi.org/10.14309/AJG.0000000000000943.
34. Spadaccini M, Albéniz E, Pohl H, et al. Prophylactic clipping after colorectal endoscopic resection prevents bleeding of large, proximal polyps: meta-analysis of randomized trials. Gastroenterology. 2020;159:148–158.e11. https://doi.org/10.1053/J.GASTRO.2020.03.051.
35. Lee HS, Jeon SW, Kwon YH, et al. Prophylactic endoscopic coagulation to prevent delayed post-EMR bleeding in the colorectum: a prospective randomized controlled trial (with videos). Gastrointest Endosc. 2019;90:813–22. https://doi.org/10.1016/J.GIE.2019.05.039.
36. Takizawa K, Oda I, Gotoda T, et al. Routine coagulation of visible vessels may prevent delayed bleeding after endoscopic submucosal dissection--an analysis

of risk factors. Endoscopy. 2008;40:179–83. https://doi.org/10.1055/S-2007-995530.
37. Kawashima K, Hikichi T, Fujiwara T, et al. Delayed perforation after endoscopic submucosal dissection for mucosal colon cancer: a conservatively treated case. Fukushima J Med Sci. 2018;64:157–62. https://doi.org/10.5387/FMS.2018-04.
38. Takamaru H, Goto R, Yamada M, et al. Predicting and managing complications following colonoscopy: risk factors and management of advanced interventional endoscopy with a focus on colorectal ESD. Expert Rev Med Devices. 2020;17:929–36. https://doi.org/10.1080/17434440.2020.1819788.
39. Zhang QS, Han B, Xu JH, Gao P, Shen YC. Antimicrobial prophylaxis in patients with colorectal lesions undergoing endoscopic resection. World J Gastroenterol. 2015;21(15):4715–21. https://doi.org/10.3748/wjg.v21.i15.4715. PMID: 25914483; PMCID: PMC4402321.
40. Muro T, Higuchi N, Imamura M, Nakagawa H, Honda M, Nakao K, Izumikawa K, Sasaki H, Kitahara T. Post-operative infection of endoscopic submucosal dissection of early colorectal neoplasms: a case-controlled study using a Japanese database. J Clin Pharm Ther. 2015;40(5):573–7. https://doi.org/10.1111/jcpt.12313. Epub 2015 Aug 6. PMID: 26249257.
41. Zheng L, Jiang L, Li D, Chen L, Jiang C, Xie L, Zhou L, Huang J, Liu M, Wang W. Antimicrobial prophylaxis in patients undergoing endoscopic mucosal resection for 10- to 20-mm colorectal polyps: a randomized prospective study. Medicine (Baltimore). 2022;101(50):e31440. https://doi.org/10.1097/MD.0000000000031440.
42. Gorgun E, Rencuzogullari A, Ozben V, et al. An effective bundled approach reduces surgical site infections in a high-outlier colorectal unit. Dis Colon Rectum. 2018;61(1):89–98. https://doi.org/10.1097/DCR.0000000000000929.
43. O'Malley GF, Dominici P, Giraldo P, et al. Routine packing of simple cutaneous abscesses is painful and probably unnecessary. Acad Emerg Med. 2009;16(5):470–3. https://doi.org/10.1111/j.1553-2712.2009.00409.x.
44. Mocanu V, Dang JT, Ladak F, et al. Antibiotic use in prevention of anal fistulas following incision and drainage of anorectal abscesses: a systematic review and meta-analysis. Am J Surg. 2019;217:910.
45. Sözener U, Gedik E, Kessaf Aslar A, et al. Does adjuvant antibiotic treatment after drainage of anorectal abscess prevent development of anal fistulas? A randomized, placebo-controlled, double-blind, multicenter study. Dis Colon Rectum. 2011;54:923.
46. Ghahramani L, Minaie MR, Arasteh P, et al. Antibiotic therapy for prevention of fistula in-ano after incision and drainage of simple perianal abscess: a randomized single blind clinical trial. Surgery. 2017;162:1017.
47. Gaertner WB, Burgess PL, Davids JS, et al. The American Society of Colon and Rectal Surgeons clinical practice guidelines for the Management of Anorectal Abscess, fistula-in-Ano, and Rectovaginal fistula. Dis Colon Rectum. 2022;65:964.
48. Liu S, Tian Z, Jiang Y, et al. Endoscopic ultrasound-guided drainage to abdominal abscess: a systematic review and meta-analysis. J Minim Access Surg. 2022;18:489–96. https://doi.org/10.4103/JMAS.JMAS_349_21.
49. Ozgur I, Lee GC, Gorgun E. Management of rectal stricture after en-bloc endoscopic submucosal dissection for a circumferential lateral spreading tumor. Dis Colon Rectum. 2023;66:E168. https://doi.org/10.1097/DCR.0000000000002611.
50. Abe S, Sakamoto T, Takamaru H, et al. Stenosis rates after endoscopic submucosal dissection of large rectal tumors involving greater than three quarters of the luminal circumference. Surg Endosc. 2016;30:5459–64. https://doi.org/10.1007/S00464-016-4906-X.
51. Ohara Y, Toyonaga T, Tanaka S, et al. Risk of stricture after endoscopic submucosal dissection for large rectal neoplasms. Endoscopy. 2016;48:62–70. https://doi.org/10.1055/S-0034-1392514.
52. Hayashi T, Kudo S, Miyachi H, et al. Management and risk factor of stenosis after endoscopic submucosal dissection for colorectal neoplasms. Gastrointest Endosc. 2017;86:358–69. https://doi.org/10.1016/J.GIE.2016.11.032.
53. Yamashita S, Kato M, Fujimoto A, et al. Inadequate steroid injection after esophageal ESD might cause mural necrosis. Endosc Int Open. 2019;7:E115. https://doi.org/10.1055/A-0781-2333.
54. Arezzo A, Arolfo S, Allaix ME, et al. Transanal endoscopic microsurgery for giant circumferential rectal adenomas. Color Dis. 2016;18:897–902. https://doi.org/10.1111/CODI.13279.
55. Dolezel R, Walterová B, Juhas S, et al. Fixation of biomaterial to metallic stent and fixation of stents after circular endoscopic dissection in the esophagus on an animal model. Rozhl Chir. 2018;97:208–13.
56. van Heinsbergen M, Leijtens JW, Slooter GD, Janssen-Heijnen ML, Konsten JL. Quality of life and bowel dysfunction after transanal endoscopic microsurgery for rectal cancer: one third of patients experience major low anterior resection syndrome. Dig Surg. 2020;37:39–46.
57. Khomyakov E, Chernyshov S, Fomenko O, Rybakov E. Does transanal endoscopic microsurgery affect reictal function? Ann Coloproctol. 2022;39(4):326–31. https://doi.org/10.3393/ac.2022.00220.0031. Published online ahead of print, 2022 Nov 14.
58. Altaf K, Slawik S, Sochorova D, et al. Long-term outcomes of open versus closed rectal defect after transanal endoscopic microscopic surgery. Color Dis. 2021;23(11):2904–10. https://doi.org/10.1111/codi.15830.
59. Mehraj A, Saqib N, Wani R, Chowdri N, Parray F, Khan M. Transanal minimal invasive surgery (TAMIS): safety and feasibility for the resection of

benign and malignant lesions of the rectum. Turk J Surg. 2021;37(1):6–12. Published 2021 Mar 22. https://doi.org/10.47717/turkjsurg.2021.5057.
60. Naughton AP, Ryan ÉJ, Bardon CT, et al. Endoscopic management versus transanal surgery for early primary or early locally recurrent rectal neoplasms-a systematic review and meta-analysis. Int J Color Dis. 2020;35(12):2347–59. https://doi.org/10.1007/s00384-020-03715-7.
61. Hung LY, Benlice C, Jia X, et al. Outcomes after early versus delayed urinary bladder catheter removal after Proctectomy for benign and malignant disease in 2,429 patients: an observational cohort study. Surg Infect. 2021;22(3):310–7. https://doi.org/10.1089/sur.2020.159.
62. Gao B, Zhang D, Wang Y, Wang Z, Wang Z. The effect of tamsulosin in post-operative urinary retention: a meta-analysis of randomized controlled trials. Naunyn Schmiedeberg's Arch Pharmacol. 2023;396(3):441–51. https://doi.org/10.1007/s00210-022-02343-y.

Perianal Abscess and Fistula

20

Valery Vilchez and Amy L. Lightner

Cryptoglandular Pathophysiology—Abscess

Cryptoglandular abscess and fistula-in-ano arise from glands at the dentate line, between the anal papilla and the columns of Morgagni. These glands extend into the submucosal space, internal sphincter, intersphincteric space, and external sphincter. When bacteria and debris are entrapped in these glands, infection begins and subsequently tracks along the course of the gland and/or path of least resistance from its origin (most likely the perianal skin) [1].

Anorectal abscesses may originate from multiple anatomical locations of the pelvis and are then classified on the basis of these locations into perianal, ischiorectal, intersphincteric, and supralevator (Fig. 20.1). A horseshoe abscess is an abscess that courses posteriorly through the deep postanal space to involve the bilateral ischiorectal spaces.

Perianal and ischiorectal abscesses represent the most common anorectal abscesses. Ramanujam et al. described in their series that perianal abscesses accounted for 42.7%, ischiorectal for 22.7%, intersphincteric for 21.4%, and supralevator for 7.3% of all anorectal abscesses [2]. Perianal and ischiorectal abscesses typically present with perianal pain, swelling, fluctuance, and potential spontaneous drainage of purulent liquid. Intersphincteric abscesses are characterized by intense pain but typically do not have external manifestations. Supralevator abscesses may arise from the superior extension of a cryptoglandular origin but may also be associated with an intra-abdominal process, including diverticular disease, Crohn's disease, or malignancy.

History and physical examination are typically sufficient to diagnose perianal and ischiorectal abscesses. Imaging adjuncts including CT scanning, magnetic resonance imaging (MRI), endoanal ultrasound, and fistulogram are not generally indicated for uncomplicated disease or for patients without significant comorbidities with an easily recognizable diagnosis. Imaging would be valuable in some instances in patients with an isolated intersphincteric abscess or in those who have a complicated history, including malignancy, radiation, Crohn's disease, prior anorectal operations, trauma, or a complex disease (horseshoe and/or a supralevator component).

Primary treatment for an anorectal abscess is timely incision and drainage. Perianal and ischiorectal abscesses should be drained through the skin overlying the area of fluctuance. If the abscess cavity is large, the incision should be made in the area closest to the anal

V. Vilchez
Division of Colon and Rectal Surgery, University of California at Irvine, Irvine, CA, USA

A. L. Lightner (✉)
Department of General Surgery, Scripps Clinic Medical Group, San Diego, CA, USA
e-mail: lightner.amy@scrippshealth.org

M. Hoffman et al. (eds.), *Major Complications of Female Pelvic Surgery*,
https://doi.org/10.1007/978-3-031-66772-5_20

Fig. 20.1 Schematic representation of a cross-sectional image showing potential spaces of abscess formation

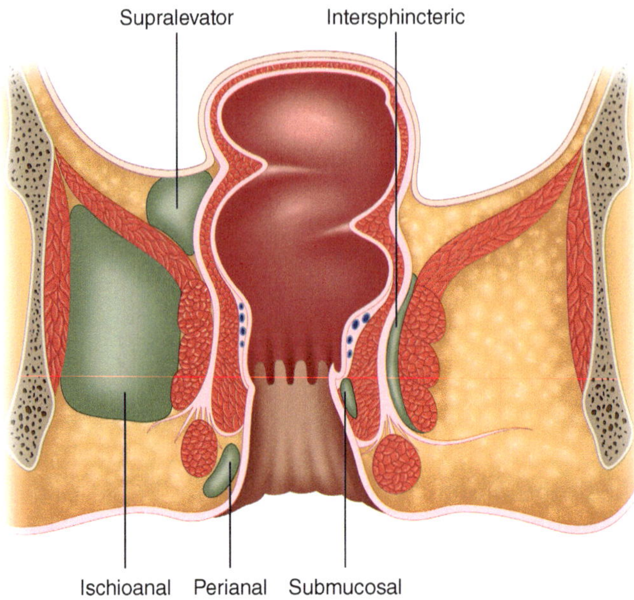

verge. If a fistula-in-ano develops post-abscess drainage, the fistula tract will be as short as feasible [3]. Intersphincteric abscesses typically require internal drainage at the dentate line via sphincterotomy if there is no external area of fluctuance.

The route of drainage is particularly important for supralevator abscesses to avoid iatrogenic creation of a suprasphincteric fistula. Those that arise from an intra-abdominal source should be drained transabdominally or transrectally. Those that arise from superior extension via the intersphincteric space should be drained transrectally. Those that arise from a superior extension of an ischiorectal abscess should be drained transcutaneously (Fig. 20.2).

Horseshoe abscess drainage requires a thorough understanding of the anatomy. To adequately drain these abscesses, there must be both bilateral transcutaneous ischiorectal drainage and posterior drainage after division of the anococcygeal ligament to access the deep postanal space (Hanley procedure) (Fig. 20.3). For those arising from a perianal abscess extending through the postanal space, posterior fistulotomy with seton

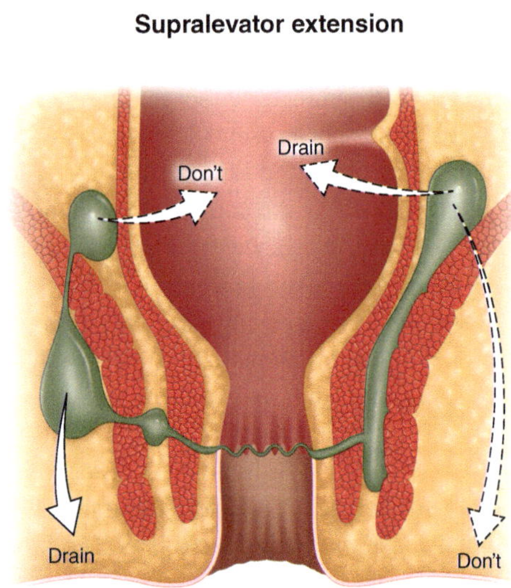

Fig. 20.2 Schematic representation of an appropriate drainage route for a supralevator abscess

placement has also been described for adequate drainage (modified Hanley procedure).

Of those undergoing abscess drainage, 30–70% of patients have a non-identifiable fistula tract at the time of drainage and 30–35% will develop a mature fistula tract [4]. In the setting of

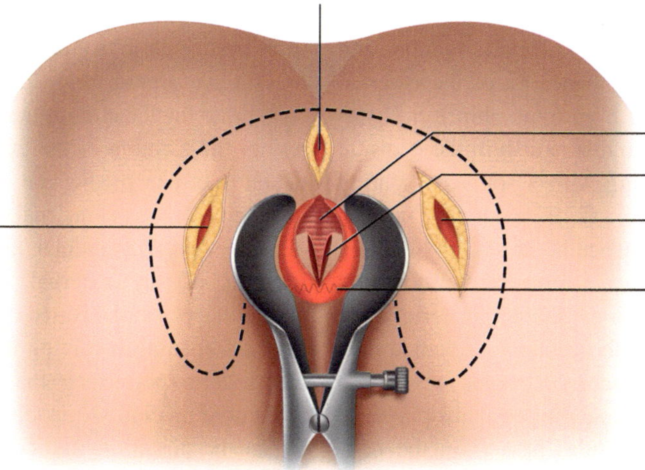

Fig. 20.3 Schematic representation of horseshoe fistula drainage via the Hanley procedure

acute inflammation, there is a risk of creating a false passage and/or unnecessary sphincter division (increasing the risk of incontinence post-procedure) while attempting to identify a fistula tract. Thus, given the potential risks, it is not generally recommended to manage this tract at the time of abscess drainage.

Incision and drainage of an abscess is preferred when the patient is first evaluated in the clinic. This reduces any unnecessary delay in time to controlling sepsis. If performed in the clinic, one must ensure that there is an adequate setup and that the patient is amenable to proceed under local anesthesia. Complex abscesses or those associated with tissue necrosis and/or patients who are intolerant of a bedside procedure should be managed in the operating room. Packing is not recommended as wounds left unpacked are associated with less pain and faster healing [5]. For large or deep abscess cavities, a catheter (such as a mushroom-type catheter) can be placed in the cavity to promote drainage and minimize the size of the external incision. Antibiotics are recommended for those with extensive cellulitis or signs of sepsis or in immunocompromised patients, but routine antibiotics are not recommended [6].

Fistula-in-Ano

Patients with fistula-in-ano present with a wide range of complaints, including hemorrhoids, a history of anorectal abscess with spontaneous drainage or prior surgical drainage, intermittent perianal bleeding from an external opening, and cyclical perianal pain and swelling that is relieved with expression of fluid. Given the wide variety of presenting symptoms, a good physical examination is critical for appropriately diagnosing and guiding medical decision-making.

The most common etiology of fistula-in-ano is cryptoglandular progression. Fistulas are categorized based on the degree of sphincter involvement with varying incidences, including subcutaneous/submucosal (2–3%), intersphincteric (24–45%), transsphincteric (30–60%), and suprasphincteric (2–20%) [7].

Subcutaneous or submucosal fistulas begin at the dentate line and course deep into the anoderm without sphincter involvement. Intersphincteric fistulas cross the internal sphincter and then have a tract to the perianal skin and do not involve any external anal sphincter muscles. Transsphincteric fistulas track from the internal opening at the dentate line via the internal and external anal sphincters to the perianal skin or perineum. Those involving 30% or less of the external sphincter are considered low transsphincteric fistulas, and those involving more than 30% of the external sphincter are named high transsphincteric fistulas. It is important to distinguish in the decision making of proceeding with a sphincter-sparing technique due to the risk of developing postoperative fecal incontinence in the setting of a high transsphincteric fistula. Suprasphincteric fistulas course superiorly into the intersphincteric space over the top of the puborectalis muscle and then descend through the ischiococcygeus muscle into the ischiorectal fossa and the perianal skin.

Extrasphincteric fistulas pass from the perineal skin through the ischiorectal fossa and levator muscles and then into the rectum and reside completely outside of the external sphincter complex. These fistulas arise from intra-abdominal sources such as diverticular disease and/or malignancy, are associated with different underlying etiologies such as Crohn's disease, or may arise from iatrogenic injury or inappropriate drainage of a supralevator abscess (Fig. 20.4).

Neither the location of the initial abscess cavity nor the location of the external opening of a fistula tract can predict the degree of sphincter involvement, but the internal opening can be predicted for cryptoglandular fistulas based on the location of the external opening following Goodsall's principle. Based on this principle, any external opening involving the posterior half of the anoderm (posterior to the transverse anal line) will curve medially to involve an internal opening in the posterior midline. External openings involving the anterior half of the anal verge (anterior to the transverse anal line) will correspond to a radially located internal opening. This is most accurate for posterior and intersphincteric fistulas, 91% and 93%, respectively, compared to

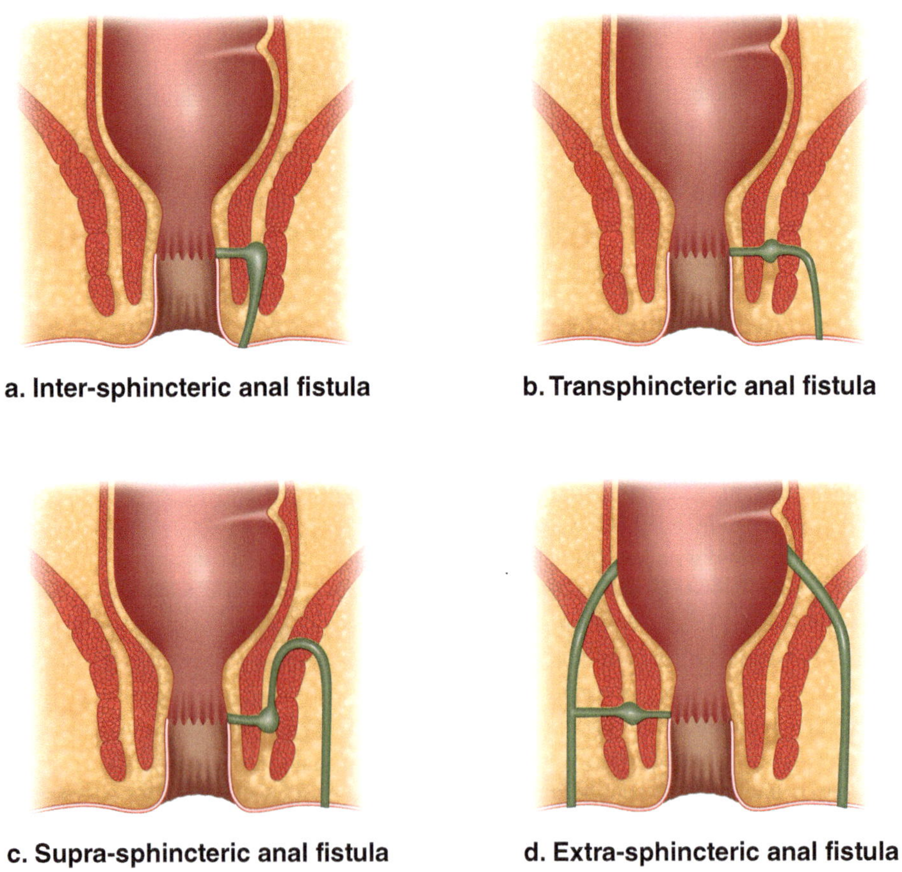

Fig. 20.4 Schematic representation of the anatomy of a fistula-in-ano

anterior and transsphincteric fistulas, 69% and 68%, respectively [8].

Routine use of diagnostic imaging is not typically necessary for patients with an anorectal fistula. However, imaging may be considered in selected patients with an occult anorectal abscess, a recurrent or complex anal fistula, immunosuppression, or anorectal Crohn's disease [6]. The imaging modality selected is highly dependent on surgeon preference, access of care to certain imaging modalities, and, in case of ultrasound, surgeon experience. Overall, pelvic magnetic resonance imaging (MRI) is the preferred imaging modality to characterize anal fistulas given its accuracy, reproducibility, non-instrumentation of the fistula tract, and ability to localize abscesses and fistula anatomy considering the surrounding anatomy.

Treatment Strategies for Fistula-in-Ano

Management of a fistula-in-ano entails a fine balance between the control of sepsis, definitive repair of the fistula without disease recurrence, and preservation of continence. The first step is an anorectal examination under anesthesia to ensure that *all* sepsis has been drained and evaluate the fistula, delineate the anatomy, and characterize the degree of sphincter involvement. Consideration to avoid any advanced repair beyond fistulotomy should be given if there is evidence of any sepsis.

Anorectal examination under anesthesia should begin with a digital rectal exam using a circumferential anoscope both to identify the internal opening and rule out concurrent or alternative anal canal pathologies. The external opening is gently probed with a fistula probe, and the probe is passed along the tract until it communicates with the internal opening with care to avoid creation of a false passage. Intraoperative hydrogen peroxide or methylene blue may be injected into the external fistula opening to aid in identification of the exact site of the internal opening [9]. Alternatively, intraoperative ultrasound with and without hydrogen peroxide contrast enhancement may be used. However, as with any ultrasound modality, endoanal ultrasound is highly user-dependent. Occasionally, the surgeon should abandon the examination under anesthesia with fistula repair if an internal opening is not identified. This preserves a future opportunity to identify the fistula tract without injury to the anal canal or sphincter complex.

Fistulas are classified as simple or complex based on the risk of incontinence after a sphincter-dividing procedure. Complex fistulas are described as involving more than 30% of the external sphincter, anterior location in a female, multiple tracts, recurrent fistula, preexisting baseline incontinence, history of radiation, and Crohn's disease [6]. Simple fistulas can be treated with sphincter-dividing surgery at the time of initial presentation, while all others should undergo a sphincter-preserving procedure, typically starting with placement of a seton.

Fistulotomy

A fistulotomy is generally safe in appropriately selected simple fistulas with recurrence rates less than 10% and incontinence rates between 0 and 37% [10, 11]. At the time of exam under anesthesia, a fistulotomy is performed by laying open the fistula tract to allow complete and adequate drainage. The tract is debrided with electrocautery or curetting. Marsupialization of the wound edges has been shown to decrease the overall wound size, shorten the time to healing, and reduce postoperative bleeding [12]. Concomitant fistulectomy is not recommended due to the risk of increased wound size, postoperative sphincter defect, and increased healing time.

Seton Placement

Setons are characterized as either draining setons or cutting setons. A draining seton is secured loosely to itself such that there is no significant tension on the involved tissues. Setons are used in cases of complex fistulas or significant inflammation. The two main goals of seton placement include sepsis control and maturation of the fistula tract.

A cutting seton is placed similarly to a draining seton, but it is secured tightly to itself with tension and compression on the involved tissues.

Division of the anoderm overlying the fistula is required. Then, the seton is serially tightened in clinic and slowly cuts through the involved tissue layers, leaving an intact scar once all tissues have been cut at the seton fall out. The duration for the seton to fall out and mature scar to develop depends on the amount of tissue to be divided. There is a large variability in the incontinence rate observed with this technique ranging up to 60% on follow-up and surveillance after the procedure [13, 14]. A cutting seton may be used selectively in the management of complex cryptoglandular anal fistula if other options have been exhausted. While this treatment was considered more readily in the past, it has largely been abandoned in routine clinical practice due to its high rates of incontinence [6]. However, it still holds a place in selected circumstances, which involve dividing more muscle than the surgeon is comfortable dividing for a fistulotomy, but other more advanced treatments are not feasible.

Fistula Plugs/Fibrin Glue

Anal fistula plugs and fibrin glue are relatively ineffective treatments for fistula-in-ano [6].

A bioprosthetic anal fistula plug, an acellular collagen matrix used to close the internal fistula opening, provides a scaffold for native tissue ingrowth to obliterate a fistula tract. Although early data demonstrated 70%–100% clinical healing with the plug, more recently published outcomes have been less encouraging with healing rates of 50% or less [15–17]. Plug failure is reported to be more common in patients with Crohn's disease, anovaginal fistula, or recurrent fistula and in active smokers.

Fibrin glue injection for treating anal fistulas has decreased in popularity because of disappointing contemporary data. In a 2019 randomized controlled double-blind trial, only 10 of 24 patients (41%) in the fibrin glue treatment arm had complete fistula healing [18]. In a retrospective review of 462 patients who underwent sphincter-preserving surgery for cryptoglandular anal fistula between 2005 and 2015, the use of an anal fistula plug (healing rate of 24%) and fibrin glue (healing rate of 18%) decreased significantly over the interval and the overall fistula healing rate increased significantly from 32% to 64% [19]. This decreased success has been attributed to multiple variables, including inadequate tract debridement, excessive tract debridement, an inadequately secured plug, and the presence or lack of a preoperative seton. The sphincter-preserving nature, even coupled with a remote chance of success, has allowed for the continued selective use of these approaches [6].

Ligation of Intersphincteric Fistula Tract (LIFT)

LIFT was developed as a sphincter-preserving technique in 2007 by Rojanasakul et al. [20] and entails dissection of the intersphincteric space until the mature fistula is encountered and subsequently divided and double ligated. The internal and external openings are debrided and left open to drain. In the initial description, the authors reported a 94.4% healing rate with a 0% rate of incontinence [20] (Fig. 20.5).

Overall, the rates of success range from 61% to 94% with rare instances of change in continence. Recurrence is associated with a shorter fistula tract. When the LIFT procedure fails, it may result in drainage via the intersphincteric incision as a persistent intersphincteric fistula, which can be subsequently managed by fistulotomy [21, 22]. A draining seton may be used before the LIFT procedure to allow for fibrosis of the tract that may facilitate the procedure, but this has not been shown to affect the success rate of the LIFT procedure.

Modifications of the LIFT procedure, including excising the lateral aspect of the tract, incorporating a fistula plug or biologic mesh interposition, or using video-assisted techniques, have been described and, in some studies, are

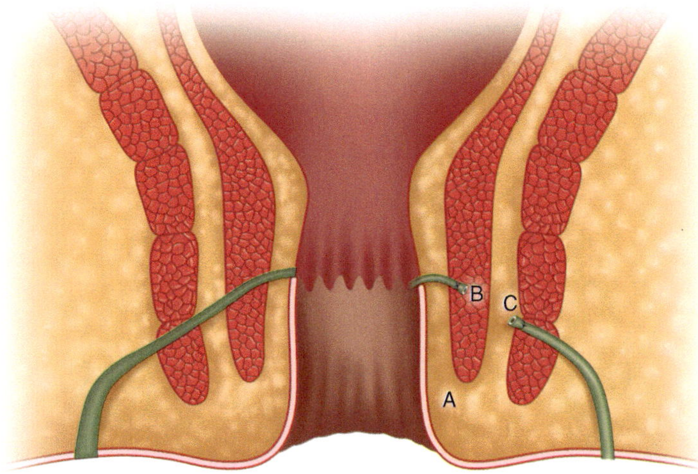

Fig. 20.5 Schematic representation of the LIFT procedure. Fistula tract is divided at points B and C, and a suture is placed at both points

associated with improved healing rates compared to the standard LIFT. However, the evidence evaluating these techniques is limited to small studies, and such modifications to the standard LIFT technique are typically not recommended [23–25].

Endorectal Advancement Flap (ERAF)

The technique of an endorectal advancement flap (ERAF) entails debridement or excision of the fistula tract and mobilization of a wide-based mucosal/submucosal rectal flap, followed by coverage of the internal opening after removal of the overlying tissues and suture closure of the internal opening. (Fig. 20.6). Given its reproducible success rate of 60–100%, ERAF is recommended as a treatment option for complex anal fistulas [6, 26–28].

Successful flaps require adequate blood supply (wide-based submucosal plexus) and lack of tension (adequate mobilization/length). Recurrence has been associated with smoking, Crohn's disease, a prior horseshoe abscess, and a high body mass index (BMI). Contraindications to ERAF include undrained sepsis, persistent secondary tracts, a fistula with a diameter greater than 3 cm, a malignancy or radiation-related etiology, and an anorectal stricture [29]. Flap configuration does not make a significant difference in the recurrence rate. Repeat ERAF is feasible and carries an acceptable success rate; however, it is also associated with a higher rate of recurrence than initial ERAF repair [30]. The technique does not divide the sphincter muscle but the incorporation of the sphincter fibers into the flap to varying degrees can lead to worsening continence in up to 35% of patients [6]. It can be a balance between having some of the fibers of the sphincter incorporated into the body of the flap (which provides the flap with thickness) and the concern for incontinence.

An alternative flap design has been described using a dermal advancement flap instead of a mucosal flap. These flaps can be in a house, diamond, or V-Y advancement of the skin. Studies evaluating this type of flap are heterogeneous, but, overall, the procedure is safe and has low-to-moderate rates of incontinence of up to 20% and moderate rates of success between 50 and 70% [29].

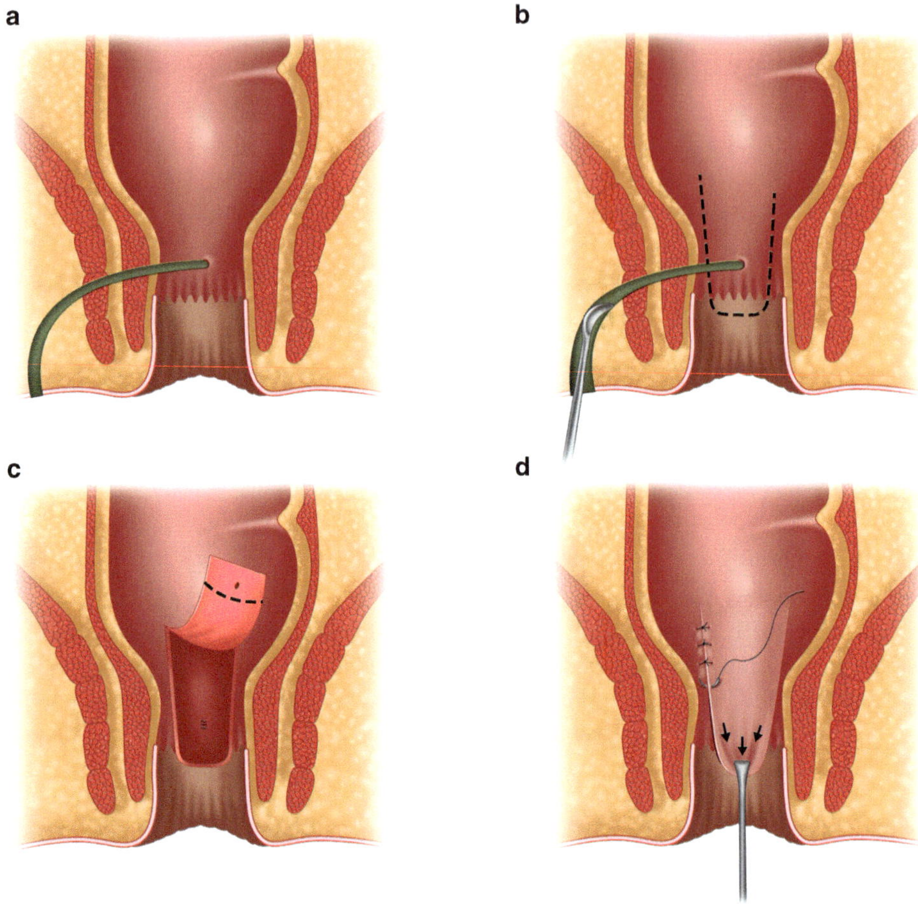

Fig. 20.6 Schematic representation of the ERAF procedure. (**a**) Fistula tract. (**b**) Curettage of the fistula tract. Dotted line represents the outline of the intended tissue flap harvest. (**c**) Flap raised with appropriate dimensions. (**d**) Flap being stretched into place after closure of the internal opening at the muscular level

Minimally Invasive Approaches

Minimally invasive techniques to treat anal fistulas have been studied over the past two decades to develop approaches with improved outcomes compared to more conventional fistula operations. Endoscopic or laser closure techniques have reasonable short-term healing rates but unknown long-term fistula healing and recurrence rates [6]. These techniques, described in small, single-institution series with limited follow-up and with various degrees of industry support, include video-assisted anal fistula treatment (VAAFT), fistula-tract laser closure (FiLaC), and endoscopic clipping using an over-the-scope clip (OTSC) device.

Most institutional experiences with VAAFT have been preliminary. This technique involves fistuloscopy through the external opening to identify the internal opening, closure of the internal orifice with sutures, clips, or a stapling device, and selective debridement or closure of the fistula tract. Reported healing rates after VAAFT range from 71% to 85% with no reported incontinence at a follow-up of less than 12 months [31–34].

FiLaC uses a radially emitting laser probe that, when passed along the tract, traumatizes the epithelium and, in this way, closes the fistula tract. In a recent meta-analysis, Elfeki et al. have reviewed 7 case series and comparative studies involving 454 patients who underwent FiLaC. At a median follow-up of 24 months, 65% of patients were healed, 4% experienced a complication, and the mean rate of incontinence was 1% [35].

Closure of the internal opening of a fistula tract has also been described using an OTSC device. This approach, frequently combined with a fistuloscopy, places a superelastic nitinol clip over the internal fistula opening with the aid of a transanal applicator. Outcomes of this technique have been reported in small, single-institution reviews showing primary healing rates of 79%–90% with limited follow-up [36]. Clip removal to relieve pain has been required in a minority of patients.

Anorectal Fistula Associated with Crohn's Disease

The management of fistulizing anorectal Crohn's disease typically involves a multidisciplinary approach to control infection and optimize the medical management used to treat the underlying Crohn's disease [6]. The mainstay of medical management of anorectal Crohn's disease is biological therapy [37–39]. Randomized controlled trials have shown initial fistula healing rates of 38%–55% in patients treated with infliximab, with long-term healing occurring in 39% of patients [39]. In many instances, medical therapy is combined, at least initially, with a draining seton [37, 38].

The decision to perform definitive fistula surgery in selected patients with anorectal Crohn's must be individualized and should take into consideration the severity of symptoms, the presence of infection, the fistula tract's anatomy, the presence of a stricture, and the status of Crohn's disease (especially the presence of proctitis). Following fistula surgery, patients with Crohn's disease may require additional interventions for nonhealing wounds or recurrent fistula more often than patients with cryptoglandular fistula [6].

In patients who do not require drainage, antibiotic therapy alone has been shown to be effective in fistulizing Crohn's disease; treatment with metronidazole and fluoroquinolones has demonstrated improvement in symptoms (at least temporarily) in more than 90% of patients [6, 40]. Despite medical and surgical management, patients with Crohn's disease with severe refractory anorectal fistulizing disease may ultimately require proctectomy and permanent fecal diversion [41–43].

Patients with Crohn's disease who present with an asymptomatic fistula secondary to Crohn's disease or a cryptoglandular infection without signs of local sepsis do not require surgical intervention as these tracts may remain quiescent for extended periods of time. Draining setons are typically useful in the multimodality therapy of fistulizing anorectal Crohn's disease and may be used for long-term disease control [6]. However, setons can be associated with persistent seepage, a chronic and bothersome symptom for patients, and recurrent sepsis can occur in more than 20% of patients.

In a retrospective study of 32 consecutive patients treated with infliximab for anorectal Crohn's disease, patients who also underwent seton placement ($n = 9$) had a lower fistula recurrence rate (44% vs. 79%; $p < 0.001$) at 3 months and longer time to recurrence (13.5 vs. 3.6 months; $p < 0.001$) [44]. A systematic review and meta-analysis of 10 studies, including 4 randomized controlled trials, concluded that anti-tumor necrosis factor (anti-TNF) therapy in combination with temporary seton placement was likely beneficial for fistula healing [45]. Multimodal treatment with biological agents and seton drainage has also been associated with improved fistula healing rates [46, 47]. The time to continue with a seton in place and/or removal has not been well-elucidated.

Fistulotomy may be safely performed in appropriately selected patients with Crohn's disease with an uncomplicated low fistula in the absence of proctitis. Healing rates after fistulotomy range from 62% to 100%, and 6% to 12% of patients report mild incontinence. However, some studies report higher rates of postoperative incontinence (up to 50%), especially in patients with active proctitis, underscoring the importance of appropriate patient selection [6].

Fistula patients with Crohn's disease may be considered for definitive operative repair if the fistula has a single dominant tract without associated sepsis, anal stenosis, proctitis, or interfering scarring from previous anorectal disease or procedures. In patients without signs of sepsis and with otherwise well-controlled disease, the most commonly performed repairs are ERAF and LIFT. A systematic review including 91 patients with Crohn's disease who underwent endorectal advancement flap reported overall fistula healing in 64% of patients at a median follow-up of 29 months. Incontinence was reported in 9.4% of patients after flap procedures and was associated with having had previous surgical repairs [48].

The LIFT procedure was evaluated in a prospective study of 15 patients with Crohn's disease with transsphincteric fistulas. In this study, 10 patients (67%) remained healed 12 months after surgery, no patients reported incontinence, and quality of life was significantly improved postoperatively [49]. A subsequent retrospective study of 23 consecutive patients with Crohn's disease with transsphincteric fistulas who underwent LIFT found that 11 patients (48%) healed after a median follow-up of 23 months; in patients who failed LIFT, the median time to failure was 9 months [50].

In patients with severe anorectal fistulizing Crohn's disease who do not respond adequately to medical therapy, local surgical intervention or long-term seton drainage fecal diversion with or without proctectomy to control anorectal sepsis and improve incontinence symptoms and overall quality of life may be considered [6].

Mesenchymal Stem Cell (MSC) Therapy

The local administration of mesenchymal stem cells (MSCs) appears safe and effective in selected patients with refractory anorectal fistulas in the setting of Crohn's disease [6]. Several phase I, II, and III clinical trials recently conducted have consistently demonstrated the safety and efficacy of the direct injection of MSCs in the treatment of medically and surgically refractory fistulizing anorectal Crohn's disease [51–54]. There are multiple varied study protocols. Some of the variations include using allogeneic or autologous MSCs derived from the bone marrow or adipose tissue. Other variations are on the delivery of the product—with or without scaffolding at varying doses ranging from 20 million to 120 million cells. Despite the heterogenicity of all published studies, the only reported adverse events have been anorectal pain and abscesses. The efficacy of MSCs ranges from 50% to 83% at follow-up intervals ranging from 6 months to 1 year with no reported rates of incontinence. ADMIRE was a randomized controlled double-blind phase III trial, including 212 patients receiving either placebo or 120 million MSCs. The reported results were equivalent rates of anorectal pain and abscess in the two arms of the study (13% vs. 11% and 12% vs. 13%, respectively). In this trial, study patients had significantly improved fistula healing rates compared to placebo control patients (50% vs. 34%; $p = 0.02$) at 6 and 12 months of follow-up [52]. This led to approval of the adipose-derived MSC product Alofisel in Europe for the treatment of perianal fistulizing Crohn's disease [55]. Further clinical trials investigating MSCs in the setting of Crohn's disease are underway including the completion of ADMIRE II and clinical trials evaluating MSCs in rectovaginal fistula, pouch fistula, and pediatric patients.

Complex Advanced Fistula Therapy

Fistulas that develop in the setting of pelvic radiation and recurrent and complex rectovaginal fistulas may be repaired with a muscle flap interposition or proctectomy with a primary or staged coloanal anastomosis.

In patients with severe, complex fistulizing disease secondary to Crohn's disease for whom proctectomy is considered, Marchesa et al. described the advancement rectal sleeve procedure. This involves circumferential excision, lifting the anal canal mucosa from the dentate line to the anorectal ring, mobilization of a full-thickness rectal flap, and anastomosis of the rectal sleeve to the dentate line [56].

In the setting of proctectomy, a primary or staged coloanal anastomosis may be used to restore continuity of the bowel. The Turnbull–Cutait technique is reserved for situations in which there are multiple fistulous tracts or an internal opening close to the suture line. Circumferential sutures are placed at the neo-dentate line. The proximal bowel is prolapsed out of the anus and wrapped in gauze for 5–7 days at which point the patient returns to the operating room for amputation of the prolapsed rectum and suture fixation to the neo-dentate line. Temporary fecal diversion is recommended in the setting of abdominal procedures and history of radiation [57, 58]. Karakayali et al. reported outcomes on 10 patients with rectovaginal fistula secondary to pelvic radiation who underwent pull-through and straight coloanal anastomosis with proximal diversion, and all patients healed without a leak and without significant changes in reported continence and improved quality of life [59].

Conclusions

At least one-third of cryptoglandular abscesses will progress to fistulas. Anorectal abscess should be treated with surgical drainage. Antibiotics are reserved for special circumstances when cellulitis, sepsis, or immunosuppression is present. Anal fistulas should be evaluated with examination under anesthesia prior to determining subsequent management. With any surgical management, control of sepsis and maintenance of continence are imperative. It important the surgeon takes into consideration and guides the decision-making process by the patient's presenting symptoms, the underlying etiology of the problem, the anatomy of the fistula tract, the quality of the surrounding tissues, and prior attempts at fistula repair. It is important to learn and take into consideration the different techniques that can be used to treat anal fistulas. When one method fails or is not adequate for the occasion, another approach should be considered. Patient expectations should be set at the initial visit, and failure rates as well as recurrence and potential need of further interventions should be discussed with the patients during the informed consent process.

Perianal Crohn's disease can be a source of significant morbidity for the affected patients. Combined medical and surgical therapy is essential for optimal outcomes, especially in complex disease. Sepsis control, adequate symptom control, continence preservation and function, and optimizing quality of life should be the goals of any attempt at treatment.

Conflict of Interest ALL: CMO at Direct Biologics; consultant CMO at Boomerang Medical.

References

1. Eisenhammer S. The internal anal sphincter and the anorectal abscess. Surg Gynecol Obstet. 1956;103(4):501–6.
2. Ramanujam PS, Prasad ML, Abcarian H, et al. Perianal abscesses and fistulas. A study of 1023 patients. Dis Colon Rectum. 1984;27(9):593–7.
3. Lohsiriwat V, Yodying H, Lohsiriwat D. Incidence and factors influencing the development of fistula-in-ano after incision and drainage of perianal abscesses. J Med Assoc Thail. 2010;93(1):61–5.
4. Cox SW, Senagore AK, Luchtefeld MA, et al. Outcome after incision and drainage with fistulotomy for ischiorectal abscess. Am Surg. 1997;63(8):686–9.
5. Perera AP, Howell AM, Sodergren MH, et al. A pilot randomized controlled trial evaluating postoperative packing of the perianal abscess. Langebecks Arch Surg. 2015;400(2):267–71.
6. Wolfgang B, Burgess P, Davids J, et al. Management of anorectal abscess, fistula-in-ano, and rectovaginal fistula. Dis Colon Rectum. 2022;65:964–85.
7. Parks AG, Gordon PH, Hardcastle JD. A classification of fistula-in-ano. Br J Surg. 1976;63(1):1–12.
8. Barwood N, Clarke G, Levitt S, et al. Fistula-in-ano: a prospective study of 107 patients. Aust N Z J Surg. 1997;67(2–3):98–102.
9. Gonzalez-Ruiz C, Kaiser AM, Vukasin P, et al. Intraoperative physical diagnosis in the management of anal fistula. Am Surg. 2006;72(1):11–5.
10. Garcia-Aguilar J, Belmote C, Wong WD, et al. Anal fistula surgery. Factors associated with recurrence and incontinence. Dis Colon Rectum. 1996;39(7):723–9.
11. Van Tets WF, Kuipers HC. Continence disorders after anal fistulotomy. Dis Colon Rectum. 1994;37(12):1194–7.
12. Pescatori M, Ayabaca SM, Cafaro D, et al. Marsupialization of fistulotomy and fistulectomy wounds improves healing and decreases bleeding: a randomized controlled trial. Color Dis. 2006;8(1):11–4.

13. Ritchie RD, Sackier JM, Hodde JP. Incontinence rates after cutting seton treatment for anal fistula. Color Dis. 2009;11(6):564–71.
14. Vial M, Pares D, Pera M, et al. Faecal incontinence after seton treatment for anal fistulae with and without surgical division of internal anal sphincter: a systematic review. Color Dis. 2010;12(3):172–8.
15. Herold A, Ommer A, Fürst A, et al. Results of the Gore bio-a fistula plug implantation in the treatment of anal fistula: a multicentre study. Tech Coloproctol. 2016;20:585–90.
16. Bondi J, Avdagic J, Karlbom U, et al. Randomized clinical trial comparing collagen plug and advancement flap for transsphincteric anal fistula. Br J Surg. 2017;104:1160–6.
17. Kontovounisios C, Tekkis P, Tan E, Rasheed S, Darzi A, Wexner SD. Adoption and success rates of perineal procedures for fistula-in-ano: a systematic review. Color Dis. 2016;18:441–58.
18. de la Portilla F, Muñoz-Cruzado MVD, Maestre MV, et al. Platelet-rich plasma (PRP) versus fibrin glue in cryptogenic fistula-in-ano: a phase III single-center, randomized, doubleblind trial. Int J Color Dis. 2019;34:1113–9.
19. Sugrue J, Mantilla N, Abcarian A, et al. Sphincter-sparing anal fistula repair: are we getting better? Dis Colon Rectum. 2017;60:1071–7.
20. Rojanasakul A, Pattanaarun J, Sahakitrungruang C, et al. Total anal sphincter preserving technique for fistula-in-ano; the ligation of intersphincteric fistula tract. J Med Assoc Thail. 2007;90(3):581–6.
21. Liu WY, Aboulian A, Kaji AH, et al. Long-term results of ligation of intersphincteric fistula tract (LIFT) for fistula-in-ano. Dis Colon Rectum. 2013;56(3):343–7.
22. Tan KK, Tan IJ, Lim FS, et al. The anatomy of failures following the ligation of intersphincteric tract technique for anal fistula: a review of 93 patients over 4 years. Dis Colon Rectum. 2011;54(11):1368–72.
23. Han JG, Wang ZJ, Zheng Y, et al. Ligation of intersphincteric fistula tract vs ligation of the intersphincteric fistula tract plus a bioprosthetic anal fistula plug procedure in patients with transsphincteric anal fistula: early results of a multicenter prospective randomized trial. Ann Surg. 2016;264:917–22.
24. Wanitsuwan W, Junmitsakul K, Jearanai S, Lohsiriwat V. Video-assisted ligation of intersphincteric fistula tract for complex anal fistula: technique and preliminary outcomes. Dis Colon Rectum. 2020;63:1534–40.
25. Zwiep TM, Gilbert R, Boushey RP, et al. Comparison of ligation of the intersphincteric fistula tract and BioLIFT for the treatment of transsphincteric anal fistula: a retrospective analysis. Dis Colon Rectum. 2020;63:365–70.
26. Jones IT, Fazio WW, Jagelman DG. The use of transanal rectal advancement flaps in the management of fistulas involving the anorectum. Dis Colon Rectum. 1987;30(12):919–23.
27. Jarrar A, Church J. Advancement flap repair: a good option for complex anorectal fistulas. Dis Colon Rectum. 2011;54(12):1537–41.
28. Hall JF, Bordeainou L, Hyman N, et al. Outcomes after operations for anal fistula: results of a prospective, multicenter, regional study. Dis Colon Rectum. 2014;57(11):1304–8.
29. Ozuner G, Hull TL, Cartmill J, et al. Long-term analysis of the use of transanal rectal advancement flaps for complicated anorectal/vaginal fistulas. Dis Colon Rectum. 1996;39(1):10–4.
30. Stremitzer S, Riss S, Swoboda P, et al. Repeat endorectal advancement flap after flap breakdown and recurrence of fistula-in-ano: is it an option? Color Dis. 2012;14(11):1389–93.
31. Jiang HH, Liu HL, Li Z, et al. Video-assisted anal fistula treatment (VAAFT) for complex anal fistula: a preliminary evaluation in China. Med Sci Monit. 2017;23:2065–71.
32. Seow-En I, Seow-Choen F, Koh PK. An experience with video-assisted anal fistula treatment (VAAFT) with new insights into the treatment of anal fistulae. Tech Coloproctol. 2016;20:389–93.
33. Schwandner O. Video-assisted anal fistula treatment (VAAFT) combined with advancement flap repair in Crohn's disease. Tech Coloproctol. 2013;17:221–5.
34. Meinero P, Mori L. Video-assisted anal fistula treatment (VAAFT): a novel sphincter-saving procedure for treating complex anal fistulas. Tech Coloproctol. 2011;15:417–22.
35. Elfeki H, Shalaby M, Emile SH, Sakr A, Mikael M, Lundby L. A systematic review and meta-analysis of the safety and efficacy of fistula laser closure. Tech Coloproctol. 2020;24:265–74.
36. Prosst RL, Joos AK, Ehni W, Bussen D, Herold A. Prospective pilot study of anorectal fistula closure with the OTSC proctology. Color Dis. 2015;17:81–6.
37. Guidi L, Ratto C, Semeraro S, et al. Combined therapy with infliximab and seton drainage for perianal fistulizing Crohn's disease with anal endosonographic monitoring: a single-Centre experience. Tech Coloproctol. 2008;12:111–7.
38. Topstad DR, Panaccione R, Heine JA, Johnson DR, MacLean AR, Buie WD. Combined seton placement, infliximab infusion, and maintenance immunosuppressives improve healing rate in fistulizing anorectal Crohn's disease: a single center experience. Dis Colon Rectum. 2003;46:577–83.
39. Sands BE, Anderson FH, Bernstein CN, et al. Infliximab maintenance therapy for fistulizing Crohn's disease. N Engl J Med. 2004;350:876–85.
40. Gecse KB, Bemelman W, Kamm MA, et al. World gastroenterology organization, international organisation for inflammatory bowel diseases IOIBD, European Society of Coloproctology and Robarts Clinical Trials; world gastroenterology organization international organisation for inflammatory bowel diseases IOIBD European Society of Coloproctology and Robarts Clinical Trials. A global consensus on the classification, diagnosis and multidisciplinary treatment of perianal fistulising Crohn's disease. Gut. 2014;63:1381–92.

41. Gu J, Valente MA, Remzi FH, et al. Factors affecting the fate of faecal diversion in patients with perianal Crohn's disease. Color Dis. 2015;17:66–72.
42. Löffler T, Welsch T, Mühl S, et al. Long-term success rate after surgical treatment of anorectal and recto-vaginal fistulas in Crohn's disease. Int J Color Dis. 2009;24:521–6.
43. Sauk J, Nguyen D, Yajnik V, et al. Natural history of perianal Crohn's disease after fecal diversion. Inflamm Bowel Dis. 2014;20:2260–5.
44. Regueiro M, Mardini H. Treatment of perianal fistulizing Crohn's disease with infliximab alone or as an adjunct to exam under anesthesia with seton placement. Inflamm Bowel Dis. 2003;9:98–103.
45. de Groof EJ, Sahami S, Lucas C, Ponsioen CY, Bemelman WA, Buskens CJ. Treatment of perianal fistula in Crohn's disease: a systematic review and meta-analysis comparing seton drainage and anti-tumour necrosis factor treatment. Color Dis. 2016;18:667–75.
46. Yang BL, Chen YG, Gu YF, et al. Long-term outcome of infliximab combined with surgery for perianal fistulizing Crohn's disease. World J Gastroenterol. 2015;21:2475–82.
47. Sebastian S, Black C, Pugliese D, et al. The role of multimodal treatment in Crohn's disease patients with perianal fistula: a multicentre retrospective cohort study. Aliment Pharmacol Ther. 2018;48:941–50.
48. Soltani A, Kaiser AM. Endorectal advancement flap for cryptoglandular or Crohn's fistula-in-ano. Dis Colon Rectum. 2010;53:486–95.
49. Gingold DS, Murrell ZA, Fleshner PR. A prospective evaluation of the ligation of the intersphincteric tract procedure for complex anal fistula in patients with Crohn's disease. Ann Surg. 2014;260:1057–61.
50. Kamiński JP, Zaghiyan K, Fleshner P. Increasing experience of ligation of the intersphincteric fistula tract for patients with Crohn's disease: what have we learned? Color Dis. 2017;19:750–5.
51. de la Portilla F, Alba F, García-Olmo D, Herrerías JM, González FX, Galindo A. Expanded allogeneic adipose-derived stem cells (eASCs) for the treatment of complex perianal fistula in Crohn's disease: results from a multicenter phase I/IIa clinical trial. Int J Color Dis. 2013;28:313–23.
52. Panés J, García-Olmo D, Van Assche G, ADMIRE CD Study Group Collaborators, et al. Expanded allogeneic adipose-derived mesenchymal stem cells (Cx601) for complex perianal fistulas in Crohn's disease: a phase 3 randomised, double-blind controlled trial. Lancet. 2016;388:1281–90.
53. Ciccocioppo R, Bernardo ME, Sgarella A, et al. Autologous bone marrow-derived mesenchymal stromal cells in the treatment of fistulising Crohn's disease. Gut. 2011;60:788–98.
54. Panés J, García-Olmo D, Van Assche G, et al. ADMIRE CD Study Group Collaborators. Long-term efficacy and safety of stem cell therapy (Cx601) for complex perianal fistulas in patients with Crohn's disease. Gastroenterology. 2018;154:1334–1342.e4.
55. Scott LJ. Darvadstrocel: a review in treatment-refractory complex perianal fistulas in Crohn's disease. BioDrugs. 2018;32(6):627–34.
56. Marchesa P, Hull TL, Fazio WW. Advancement sleeve flaps for treatment of severe perianal Crohn's disease. Br J Surg. 1998;85(12):1695–8.
57. Cutait DE, Figliolini FJ. A new method of colorectal anastomosis in abdominoperineal resection. Dis Colon Rectum. 1961;4:335–42.
58. De C, Cutait R, Ioshimoto M, et al. Abdominoperineal endoanal pull-through resection. A comparative study between immediate and delayed colorectal anastomosis. Dis Colon Rectum. 1985;28(5):294–9.
59. Karakayali FY, Tezcaner T, Ozcelik U, et al. The outcomes of ultralow anterior resection or and abdominoperineal pull-through resection and coloanal anastomosis for radiation-induced recto-vaginal fistula patients. J Gastrointest Surg. 2016;20(5):994–1001.

Fecal Incontinence

21

Anna R. Spivak

Fecal incontinence (FI) is defined as uncontrolled passage of stool lasting for the duration of 3 months in a patient who previously had control [1]. Severity and frequency of FI can be debilitating and have a great impact on one's quality of life.

Fecal continence is one of the most important early acquired social habits and depends on the function of multiple variables such as sphincter anatomy and function, rectal compliance, neurologic state, sensorimotor function, pelvic floor muscle coordination, stool consistency, colonic transit and motility, mental cognition, as well as psychological state. Any alterations to the abovementioned anatomy, function, innervation, or mentation can become a factor leading to fecal incontinence.

Fecal incontinence has been well-documented as a consequence of obstetrical trauma, pelvic surgery, and pelvic radiation. Sideris et al. reviewed 103 studies involving 16,110 women. Obstetric anal sphincter injuries (OASIS) were diagnosed on ultrasound in 26% of women and 19% experienced FI. [2] Obstetric-related occult sphincter injury can occur and not be recognized at the time of delivery. This is reported to occur in 21–35% of women after vaginal delivery. Therefore, occult anal sphincter injuries are not uncommon and may result in FI later in life. [2]

FI has also been documented to occur after pelvic surgery. Al-Mehaisen et al. followed 59 women for 10 years after an abdominal hysterectomy and found an increased risk of mild-to-moderate FI postoperatively with the risk being increased by simultaneous bilateral salpingo-oopherectomy. An increased risk of FI symptoms was not identified in patients who underwent vaginal hysterectomy [3].

Bowel function can be altered by pelvic surgery and can affect FI. Women who underwent surgery for deep pelvic endometriosis and segmental resection were compared to those who only underwent a shaving technique to excise their endometriosis. Patients who underwent segmental resection had higher scores on a standardized questionnaire (low anterior resection syndrome (LARS) score, which measures some elements of FI), and this correlated with a lower sexual quality of life. In the group that underwent the shaving technique, one-third presented with FI-type symptoms (when LARS scores were measured), which was surprising as no bowel was resected. [4] Another study looked at urinary and fecal incontinence in patients with ovarian cancer who were treated with debulking surgery and hyperthermic intraperitoneal chemotherapy. The results showed an increased rate of fecal and urinary incontinence [5].

A. R. Spivak (✉)
Cleveland Clinic Foundation, Cleveland, OH, USA
e-mail: spivaka2@ccf.org

M. Hoffman et al. (eds.), *Major Complications of Female Pelvic Surgery*,
https://doi.org/10.1007/978-3-031-66772-5_21

Problems with FI, loose stools, and defecation urgency has been reported in patients after pelvic radiotherapy. [6] Radiation can affect many areas that maintain continence. These include damage to the sphincter complex, leading to weakness and reduced compliance of the rectal wall. The reduced compliance is associated with heightened rectal sensitivity. All these changes can result in altered continence. The dose of radiation therapy to the pelvis has been found to affect FI symptoms. In patients who required radiation therapy to the pelvis for a gynecological malignancy, a mean dose of >50 Gy was associated with the occurrence of FI symptoms. Twelve percent of patients reported having FI symptoms post-treatment [7].

Surgery for a gynecological malignancy has been associated with FI and defecation alteration. Ribas et al. utilized a questionnaire to access bowel function in patients who were treated for endometrial (71.8%) and cervical cancers (28.2%). Of the 109 patients who responded, FI was reported in 10% of the endometrial group and in 15% of the cervical cancer group. [8] Dunberger et al. evaluated 616 gynecological cancer survivors and compared them to 344 controls to assess FI. Loose stools leading to fecal urgency and FI symptoms were 7.7 times higher in cancer survivors than in the controls. [9] Damage to the sphincter can occur during vulvar cancer excision. Hoffman et al. reviewed patients undergoing resection for carcinoma of the vulva involving perianal tissue. They found that in most cases, the external anal sphincter could be spared when resecting the cancer. If the sphincter required resection for adequate cancer removal, the patient was then at a significant risk of subsequent FI. [10] When extensive resection involving the sphincter is required, anal reconstruction consisting of plication of both the external anal sphincter and the puborectalis muscles leads to significant improvement in bowel function and FI in the postoperative period. [11] Overall, fecal incontinence can be a sequala of pelvic surgery for benign condition, malignancy, pelvic radiation, and perineum.

Diagnosis and Evaluation of FI

Diagnosis of FI involves a thorough history and physical exam focusing on the time at the onset of symptoms, duration of symptoms, character of the stool, assessment of bowel habits and bowel regiment, and review of new medications. Delineation of the exact symptoms is crucial as some patients report FI and really have diarrhea. Relevant details of FI symptoms include frequency, severity, urgency, character of the stool, continence to flatus, usage of pads, nocturnal accidents, and the presence of sensations to defecate prior to having an accident. A history of chronic conditions that can affect continence, such as diabetes, stroke, neurological conditions, previous pelvic radiation, irritable bowel syndrome, and inflammatory bowel disease, is recorded.

Surgical history, including obstetrical history, episiotomy and tears, usage of forceps during delivery, a prolonged second stage of labor, history of pelvic and abdominal surgery, history of radiation, anorectal procedures, sphincter repairs, and prior hemorrhoidectomy and fistula repair, is reviewed.

The physical exam begins with evaluation of the perianal skin to look for skin irritation, scars, trauma, fistulas, hemorrhoids, an open or patulous anus, full-thickness or mucosal rectal prolapse, and length of the perineal body. Sensations can be assessed by stoking the perianal skin with a Q-tip. This stimulation leads to contraction of the anal sphincter and is called anocutaneous reflex. Seeing the reflex signals an intact sacral reflex arch and pudendal nerve innervation of the anal sphincter.

A digital rectal exam is performed in order to determine anal sphincter tone while at rest and then asking the patient to squeeze. It is important to rule out a distal rectal mass, a stricture, or fecal impaction. Other findings to note during a digital exam include the presence of a rectocele, rectal intussusception, or tenderness, particularly of the levator muscles. If rectal prolapse is suspected, the patient is asked to bear down while sitting on the commode with or without giving an enema. The goal is to check whether the rectum is protruding out of the anus.

Anorectal manometry can help in evaluating pelvic floor function. Quantification of anal muscle strength during rest and squeeze can provide valuable information. The capacitance of the rectum, the presence of a recto-anal inhibitory reflex, and electromyography (EMG) can also be obtained as part of the anorectal manometry test. Along with the physical exam, anorectal manometry aids in assessing pelvic floor muscle coordination. Sphincter pressures on manometry are expected to be low in FI; however, high pressures can be seen in patients with FI and should alert the caregiver to rule out problems like animus or overflow incontinence. Patients with chronic constipation and urgency may also have high anal rest and squeeze pressures as a result of the sequela of constant squeezing out of fear of having an accident.

Rectal hyposensitivity (a stretched-out rectum) may be seen in chronically constipated patients with overflow incontinence where the rectum has reduced sensation and enlarges to a point that it is filled with stool that can uncontrollably run out the anus. Rectal hypersensitivity which can be thought of as similar to a stiff walled rectum, more typically is noted in patients with some forms of irritable bowel syndrome, low anterior resection syndrome, inflammatory bowel disease, scleroderma and after pelvic radiation. The absence of a recto-anal inhibitory reflex is seen in patients with Hirschsprung disease and after some anorectal surgery. Pudendal nerve terminal motor latency (PNTML) testing is no longer recommended or performed as it adds little to the evaluation and treatment plan. [1]

Ultrasound is a useful tool to assess sphincter morphology in the setting of FI. In experienced hands, ultrasound can also be used to diagnose rectal intussusception and pelvic organ prolapse (Fig. 21.1).

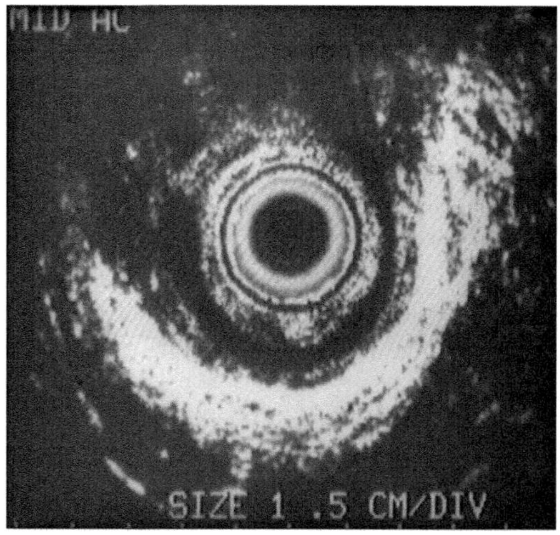

Fig. 21.1 Endoanal ultrasound: sphincter defect

Defecography can be performed dynamically with fluoroscopy or during an MRI. This allows visualization of the pelvic structures during the simulated act of squeezing and then defecation. For patients with FI, there is limited utility as most patients will not be able to retain contrast to complete the study. For patients who can retain contrast, evaluation for rectal intussusception may be useful as, if present, it may be associated with a suboptimal response to treatments like sacral nerve neuromodulation (SNM).

When to consider a colonoscopy is individualized for patients based on age, symptoms, and family history of colon cancer. Colonoscopy is recommended for anyone over 45 who has never had a colonoscopy or for patients with a change in their bowel habits. If there is a strong family history, typically, a colonoscopy is recommended when the patient is 10 years younger than the youngest person in their family who had colorectal cancer. A colonoscopy is performed to exclude pathology such as a malignancy or inflammatory bowel disease. For patients with diarrhea, random biopsies are performed to rule out microscopic colitis.

Survey tools to assess FI can be helpful. We prefer the Cleveland Clinic Fecal Incontinence Score (CCF FI 0–20 with 20 being totally incontinent) which is a validated tool that is helpful in objective documentation of symptoms of fecal incontinence and can be used to evaluate and follow FI after treatment.

Treatment

The goals of treatment include decreasing episodes of FI and improving quality of life. Conservative treatment is the first line of therapy and involves optimizing bowel function with dietary modifications, fluid management, correcting loose stools with bulking agents, antidiarrheal medications, and pelvic floor exercises, and incorporating behavioral changes.

Dietary modifications include eliminating caffeine, artificial sweeteners, lactose, gluten, and dietary supplements. The goal is to optimize stool consistency and eliminate foods that contribute to loose stools and urgency. Maintaining a diary, which documents food intake, bowel movement frequency, and consistency, as well as episodes of urgency and FI, can be extremely helpful to pinpoint dietary agents that contribute to bowel dysfunction.

Medical management utilizing medications designed to slow colonic motility and optimize stool consistency is also frequently started at this stage. Figure 21.2 lists the commonly recommended medications.

Regiments designed to facilitate emptying the rectum and left colon using scheduled enemas or

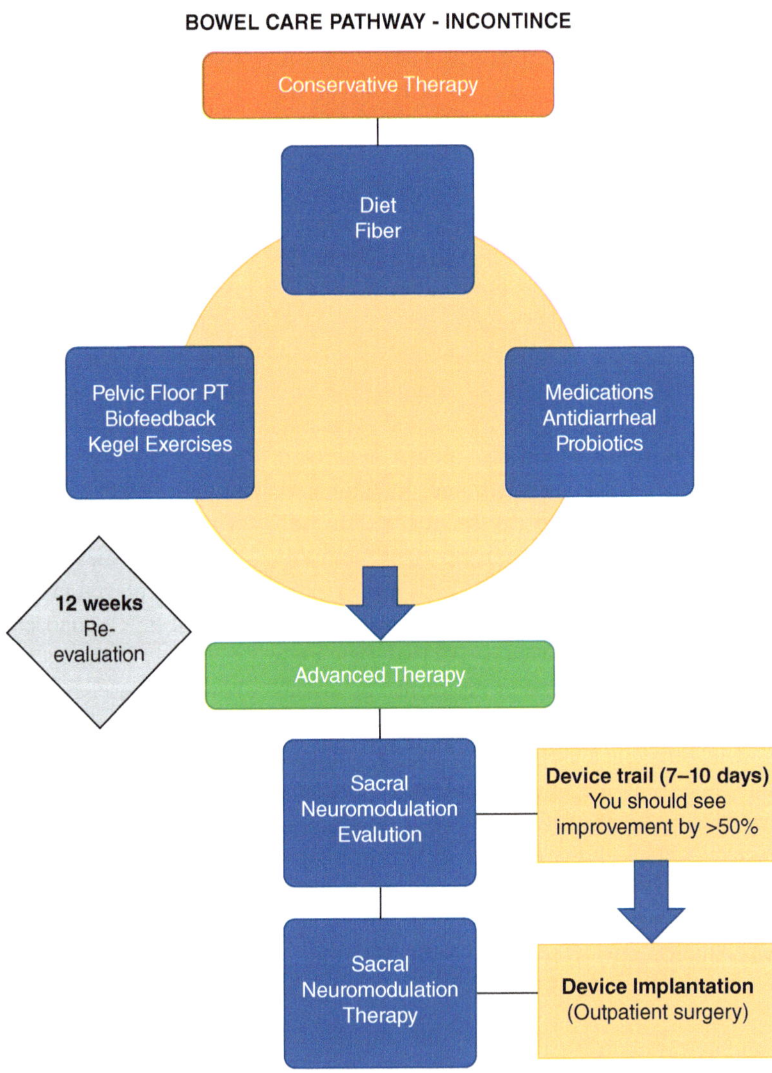

Fig. 21.2 Clinic bowel care pathway

suppositories can aid in the management of FI. There are some commercial products available to assist in this process. The Peristeen® anal irrigation system can be purchased online and is used in adults to improve quality of life symptoms. This device consists of a catheter with a balloon, a pump, and a water container. Patients are taught to insert the balloon via their anus into their rectum and inflate the balloon. They then irrigate their rectum and colon with water. Expelling the water with stool cleans out the left colon. When the left colon is cleansed of stool, FI cannot occur. Typically, this is performed several times a week [12].

Pelvic floor physical therapy is used to rehabilitate pelvic floor in order to improve sensation, muscle coordination, and anal strength. Ragadas et al. found in 124 patients treated with physical therapy, 50% demonstrated reduction in FI scores. They noted that patients who were less likely to respond had a CCF-FI score >10, a previous vaginal delivery, an anorectal or colon surgery, and were not able to maintain a squeezing effort [13].

Anal skin care is a forgotten need in patients with FI. It is important to counsel patients on correct use of barrier ointments (e.g., zinc oxide), gentle soaps, avoiding over wiping, and use of a bidet which all can improve irritated anal skin. Patients are also cautioned that deodorants can irritate the skin and that rubbing with perineal pads can further lead to perineal skin breakdown and irritation.

When conservative management does not sufficiently improve the patient's quality of life, more advanced therapy is considered and will be discussed next.

Anal Insertion Devices

Anal plugs can be used as an adjunct to conservative therapy. A plug is inserted into the distal part of the rectum to provide mechanical obstruction and prevent stool leakage. Plugs are no longer recommended in the guidelines published by the American Society of Colon and Rectal Surgeons [1] (ASCRS) due to variable results. Previous studies have demonstrated a 50% improvement in FI symptoms in 62% of patients over a 12-week observation period [12] (Fig. 21.3). There is little drawback to trying an anal plug, and some patients with limited FI may find it extremely helpful.

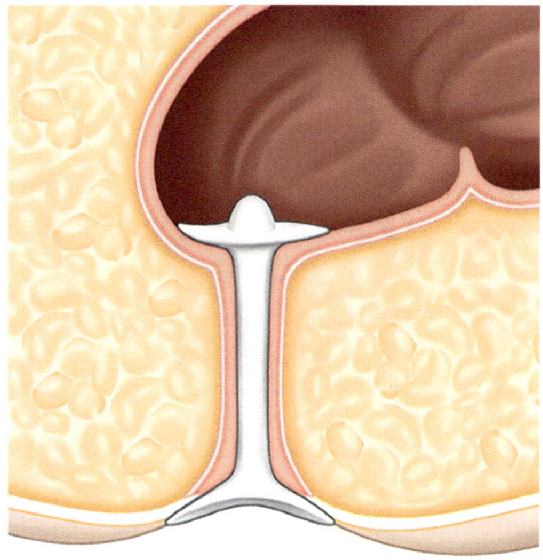

Fig. 21.3 An anal plug

Vaginal Bowel Control Systems

Vaginal bowel control systems can also be used as an adjunct to conservative therapy. A pessary-like device is introduced into the vagina. This has an attached balloon. When the balloon around the pessary is inflated, there is impingement on the rectovaginal septum, pushing the rectum toward the sacrum and mechanically occluding the rectum temporarily. This prevents stool from passing beyond this point. The balloon needs to be deflated for defecation. In a multicenter study of 137 patients, 62% were able to be fitted with and tolerate such a device. Of those, 94% had a reduction of their FI symptoms over a 12-month period [14] (Fig. 21.4).

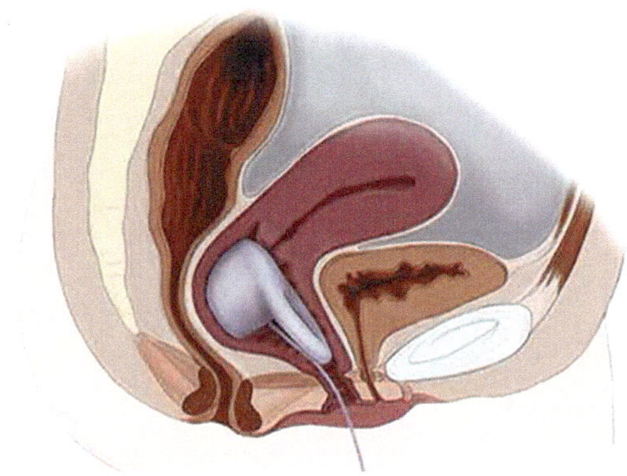

Fig. 21.4 A vaginal insertion device

Bulking Agents

Multiple types of bulking agents have been injected into the anal region in an attempt to increase the bulk of the anal sphincter with the goal of improving FI.

Dextranomer/hyaluronic acid (Solesta®), which is available in the United States, is a biocompatible bulking agent administered by submucosal injection. It is hypothesized to expand the submucosal layer of the proximal anal canal, thereby augmenting bowel control. Limited studies comparing injections to patients injected with a sham control demonstrated >25% reduction in FI symptoms over a 12-month period [15]. Bulking agent injections are not routinely recommended as treatment for FI in the updated ASCRS practice guidelines [1] due to lack of significant FI improvement in most studies (Fig. 21.5).

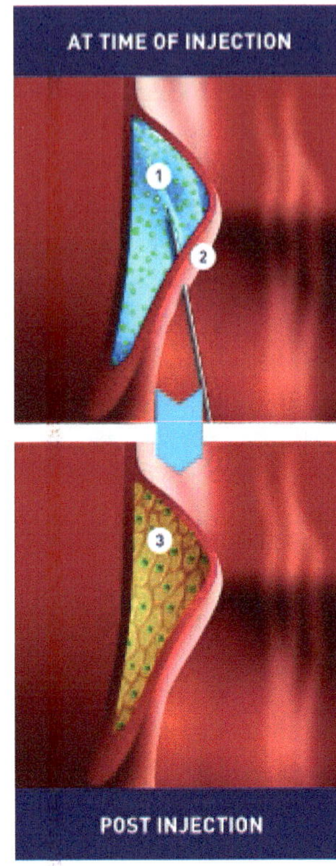

Fig. 21.5 Solesta® injection

Radio-Frequency Tissue Remodeling (SECCA®)

Radio-frequency tissue remodeling involves delivery of radio-frequency energy into the internal anal sphincter. This stimulates collagen deposition and thickening of the muscularis propria, which leads to an increased bulk and outlet resistance of the anal canal. Frascio et al. reviewed the published outcomes from several studies and found a 55–80% symptom improvement in patients with mild-to-moderate FI [17]. Long-term date is limited, and this treatment has not been recommended for treatment of FI in the most recent ASCRS practice guidelines [1] again due to concerns of limited significant improvement.

Percutaneous Tibial Nerve Stimulation (PTNS)

Percutaneous tibial nerve stimulation (PTNS) indirectly stimulates nerves supplying the pelvis by electrically stimulating the tibial nerve. It involves sitting with the stimulator over the tibial nerve for about 30 min several times per week for up to 3 months. If there is improvement, then occasional treatments will be needed to sustain the response. An advantage of PTNS is that no surgical procedure is required as the stimulator is external. In a randomized double-blind trial performed in the United Kingdom, 115 patients received PTNS and 112 sham stimulation. There was no significant difference between the two groups after 12 weeks of treatment [16].

Sacral Nerve Neuromodulation (SNM)

Sacral nerve neuromodulation is currently the recommended first-line surgical option for patients with FI—even in those with sphincter defects. The SNM procedure is performed in two stages. The first stage is called peripheral nerve evaluation (PNE) and involves inserting a wire into the S3 sacral foramen. This is usually performed in the office. This wire is a temporary lead and is attached to an external stimulator. The patient tracks their episodes of FI. After about a week, the wire is removed. If there has been a 50% improvement in symptoms, at a later date in the operating room, a permanent lead is placed in S3 and the stimulator implanted in the buttock. For some patients, stage one is performed in the operating room, and the permanent lead is inserted during this phase. The stimulator is still external during this modified phase one. If there is 50% improvement, the stimulator is implanted approximately a week later in the operating room (Fig. 21.6). The United States multicenter trial that led to Food and Drug Administration (FDA) approval involved 120 patients. In all, 83% had more than a 50% improvement in symptoms at 1 year and 41% achieved 100% continence. This stimulator is powered by a battery in the implanted device. In the past, the stimulator was not MRI-compatible. The most recent update to the device has made it MRI-compatible and prolonged the battery life to 10 years [18].

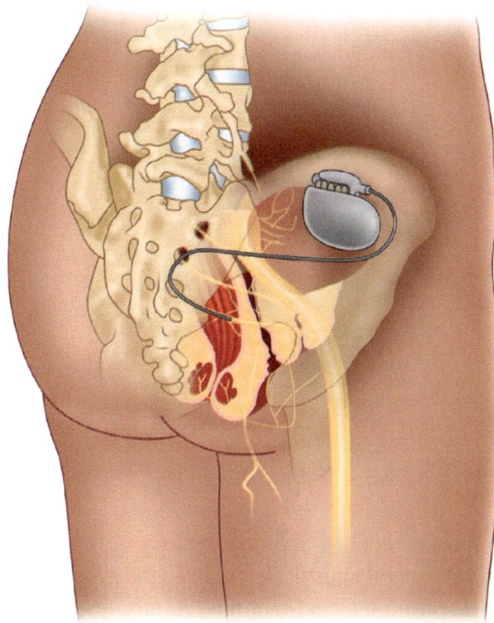

Fig. 21.6 Sacral nerve neuromodulation

Surgical Sphincter Repair (Sphincteroplasty)

Damage to the anal sphincter most commonly occurs during childbirth. Sphincter disruption may be undiagnosed at the time. As a women ages, weakening of the pelvic floor and a reduction in anal muscle bulk can occur. All these factors, combined with a remote obstetric anal sphincter injury, may lead to FI decades after childbirth. Sphincter disruption is typically diagnosed with anal ultrasound. When the disruption is diagnosed within a year after childbirth, repair of the sphincter may be an acceptable surgical treatment of FI. Sphincter repair can also be considered as a treatment option for FI when SNM is

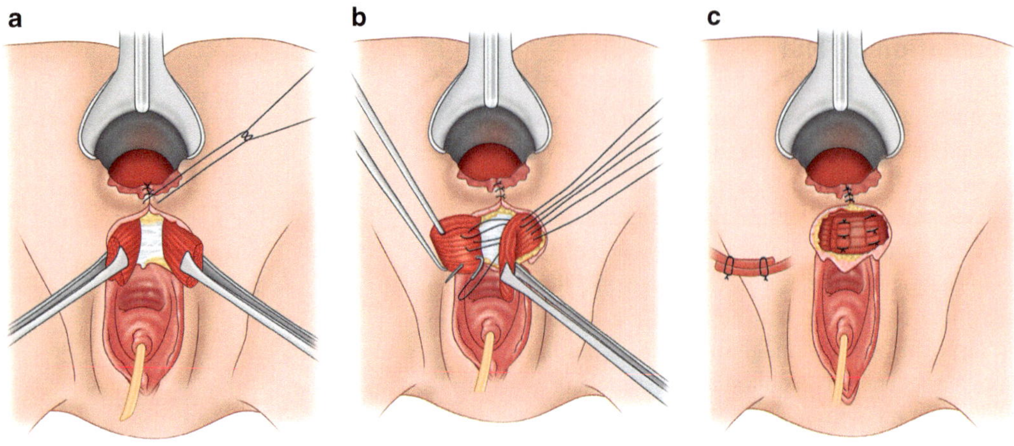

Fig. 21.7 (**a**) A dissected sphincter. (**b**) Overlapping sphincter repair. (**c**) Completed sphincteroplasty

not available [19]. Sphincteroplasty is performed under general anesthesia either in the prone jackknife position or in lithotomy. A curvilinear incision is made in the perineum, the dissection is carried laterally, and the ends of the anal sphincter are identified. Retaining the scar on the ends for tissue integrity, the internal and external sphincters are overlapped together in a vest-over-pants-type configuration and secured with absorbable sutures. This recreates the sphincter complex (Fig. 21.7).

Short-term published outcomes (<5 years) after sphincteroplasty demonstrate improvement of FI symptoms in 50–86% of patients. However, repair deteriorates over time. In patients reassessed at 10 years, none were totally continent. Redo repair has limited success and is rarely recommended [20].

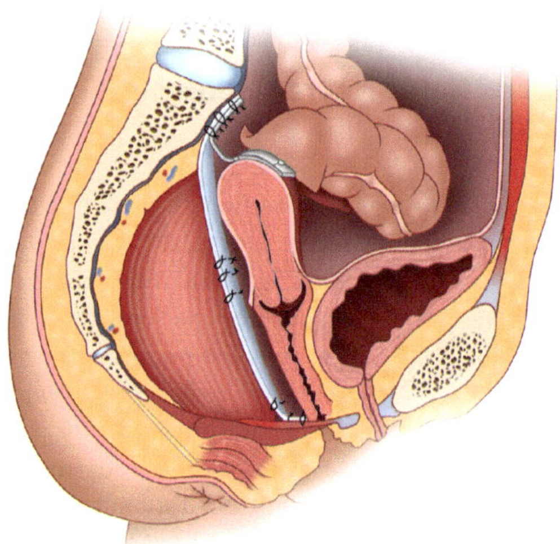

Fig. 21.8 Ventral mesh rectopexy

Ventral Mesh Rectopexy (VMR)

External rectal prolapse or significant rectal internal intussusception can add to FI. If present, response to any other FI therapy will be limited and the anatomic abnormality needs to be surgically corrected. In VMR, the space between the rectum and vagina is developed down to the pelvic floor. Mesh is sutured to the rectum, and then the other end is fixed to the sacral promontory. This lifts the posterior and middle compartments and stabilizes the rectum. Multiple studies document FI improvement after VMR correction of intussusception or external prolapse [21] (Fig. 21.8).

Other Treatments

Other treatments have been performed in the past for FI such as gracilis muscle transposition, magnetic anal sphincter augmentation, and artificial bowel sphincter. None of these are currently available or recommended in the United States [1].

Antegrade colonic enemas can be an option for a motivated patient who wants to avoid colostomy. This involves creation of appendicostomy and daily high-volume irrigations through the appendicostomy to cleanse the stool from the colon.

In patients who still suffer from a poor quality of life despite trying multiple FI therapies, a colostomy is an option. This can provide patients with the ability to leave their home without the worry of FI.

References

1. Bordeianou LG, Thorsen AJ, Keller DS, et al. The American Society of Colon and Rectal Surgeons clinical practice guidelines for the Management of Fecal Incontinence. Dis Colon Rectum. 2023;66(5):647–61. https://doi.org/10.1097/DCR.0000000000002776.
2. Sideris M, McCaughey T, Hanrahan JG, et al. Risk of obstetric anal sphincter injuries (OASIS) and anal incontinence: a meta-analysis. Eur J Obstet Gynecol Reprod Biol. 2020;252:303–12. https://doi.org/10.1016/j.ejogrb.2020.06.048.
3. Al-Mehaisen LM, Al-Kuran O, Lataifeh I, Ramsay I. Effect of abdominal hysterectomy on developing urinary and faecal incontinence later in life. J Obstet Gynaecol. 2009;29(8):742–8. https://doi.org/10.3109/01443610903207701.
4. Scheepers WFW, Maas JWM, Van De Kar MMA. Bowel function and quality of life following surgery for deep endometriosis. J Psychosom Obstet Gynecol. 2022;43(3):334–9. https://doi.org/10.1080/0167482X.2021.1952570.
5. Cascales-Campos PA, González-Gil A, Fernández-Luna E, et al. Urinary and fecal incontinence in patients with advanced ovarian cancer treated with CRS + HIPEC. Surg Oncol. 2021;36:115–9. https://doi.org/10.1016/j.suronc.2020.12.001.
6. Jadon R, Hanna L, Parsons P, Staffurth J. Dose–volume predictors for patient-reported Late diarrhoea, faecal incontinence and urgency after pelvic radiotherapy. Clin Oncol. 2021;33(8):536–45. https://doi.org/10.1016/j.clon.2021.03.011.
7. Lind H, Alevronta E, Steineck G, et al. Defecation into clothing without forewarning and mean radiation dose to bowel and anal-sphincter among gynecological cancer survivors. Acta Oncol. 2016;55(11):1285–93. https://doi.org/10.1080/0284186X.2016.1176247.
8. Ribas Y, Bonet M, Torres L, et al. Bowel dysfunction in survivors of gynaecologic malignancies. Support Care Cancer. 2020;28(11):5501–10. https://doi.org/10.1007/s00520-020-05402-3.
9. Dunberger G, Lind H, Steineck G, Waldenström AC, Onelöv E, Åvall-Lundqvist E. Loose stools lead to fecal incontinence among gynecological cancer survivors. Acta Oncol. 2011;50(2):233–42. https://doi.org/10.3109/0284186X.2010.535013.
10. Huffman MS, Roberts WS, LaPolla JP, Fiorica JV, Cavanagh D. Carcinoma of the vulva involving the perianal or anal skin. Gynecol Oncol. 1989;35(2):215–8. https://doi.org/10.1016/0090-8258(89)90046-2.
11. Hoffman MS, LaPolla JP, Roberts WS, Fiorica JV, Cavanagh D. Use of local flaps for primary anal reconstruction following perianal resection for neoplasia. Gynecol Oncol. 1990;36(3):348–52. https://doi.org/10.1016/0090-8258(90)90140-G.
12. Chew MH, Quah HM, Ooi BS, et al. A prospective study assessing anal plug for containment of faecal soilage and incontinence: assessing anal plug for containment of faecal soilage and incontinence. Color Dis. 2008;10(7):677–80. https://doi.org/10.1111/j.1463-1318.2007.01422.x.
13. Murad-Regadas SM, Regadas FSP, Regadas Filho FSP, Mendonça Filho JJD, Andrade Filho RS, Vilarinho ADS. Predictors of unsuccessful of treatment for fecal incontinence biofeedback for fecal incontinence in female. Arq Gastroenterol. 2019;56(1):61–5. https://doi.org/10.1590/s0004-2803.201900000-17.
14. Richter HE, Matthews CA, Muir T, et al. A vaginal bowel-control system for the treatment of fecal incontinence. Obstet Gynecol. 2015;125(3):540–7. https://doi.org/10.1097/AOG.0000000000000639.
15. Hoy SM. Dextranomer in stabilized sodium hyaluronate (Solesta®): in adults with faecal incontinence. Drugs. 2012;72(12):1671–8. https://doi.org/10.2165/11209030-000000000-00000.
16. Zyczynski HM, Richter HE, Sung VW, et al. Percutaneous Tibial nerve stimulation vs sham stimulation for fecal incontinence in women: NeurOmodulaTion for accidental bowel leakage randomized clinical trial. Am J Gastroenterol. 2022;117(4):654–67. https://doi.org/10.14309/ajg.0000000000001605.
17. Frascio M, Mandolfino F, Imperatore M, et al. The SECCA procedure for faecal incontinence: a review. Color Dis. 2014;16(3):167–72. https://doi.org/10.1111/codi.12403.
18. Mellgren A, Wexner SD, Coller JA, et al. Long-term efficacy and safety of sacral nerve stimulation for fecal incontinence. Dis Colon Rectum. 2011;54(9):1065–75. https://doi.org/10.1097/DCR.0b013e31822155e9.
19. Spivak AR, Hull TL. The role of sphincter repair for fecal incontinence. Ann Laparosc Endosc Surg. 2022;7:11.
20. Halverson AL, Hull TL. Long-term outcome of overlapping anal sphincter repair. Dis Colon Rectum. 2002;45(3):345–8. https://doi.org/10.1007/s10350-004-6180-6.
21. Portier G, Kirzin S, Cabarrot P, Queralto M, Lazorthes F. The effect of abdominal ventral rectopexy on faecal incontinence and constipation in patients with internal intra-anal rectal intussusception: ventral rectopexy and faecal incontinence. Color Dis. 2011;13(8):914–7. https://doi.org/10.1111/j.1463-1318.2010.02327.x.

Operations for Rectal Prolapse

22

Jennifer Shearer, Brooke Gurland,
and Caitlin Bungo

General Background

Rectal prolapse or procidentia is defined as a circumferential full-thickness protrusion of the rectal wall through the anus. Rectal prolapse is estimated to affect 1% of adults over the age of 65, and 3% of women in the United States have some form of pelvic organ prolapse—rectal prolapse, cystocele, uterine prolapse, or multi-organ prolapse [1, 2]. Females over the age of 50 are six times more likely to develop rectal prolapse compared to their male counterparts [3, 4]. Risk factors for rectal prolapse include laxity of the pelvic floor muscles, aberrant fixation of the rectum, increased depth of the pouch of Douglas, a redundant sigmoid, pudendal neuropathy, and weakness of the internal or external sphincters [4–6].

Rectal prolapse commonly presents as a rectal bulge, mucus discharge from the rectum, tenesmus, rectal bleeding, fecal incontinence, or constipation [1, 7]. Rectal prolapse can be internal and/or external. A solitary rectal ulcer may also suggest mucosal trauma secondary to the strain of the prolapsed rectal tissue against the anterior wall of the anal canal [5]. On physical exam, external prolapsed tissues appear as concentric folds protruding from the anal canal, and internal rectal prolapse can be visualized on anoscopy. Diagnosis is made by a clinical exam or a photograph, and colonoscopy may be recommended for cancer screening or to identify proximal colonic inflammation that may require treatment. If prolapse is suspected but not visualized on exam, dynamic defecography may aid in its characterization and diagnosis [2].

External rectal prolapse can occur during defecation or Valsalva activities (walking, exercising, or urination). However, in individuals with weak pelvic floor supports, the rectum can prolapse with standing and will remain out. Pain and pressure from the prolapse can limit mobility and further debilitate our most vulnerable elderly population. Unlike pelvic organ prolapse in which a pessary can be inserted vaginally to reduce uterine or bladder prolapse, no similar device exists for rectal prolapse. Surgical repair is the fundamental treatment for symptomatic external rectal prolapse with the goal of restoring the pelvic anatomy and correcting functional abnormalities without creating new bowel dysfunction [4]. Preoperative evaluation should include screening for anterior compartment prolapse, including symptoms of urinary incontinence or vaginal/uterine prolapse. A multidisciplinary surgical approach is preferred for multi-organ prolapse [4]. In this chapter, we will share with the reader our own unpublished surgical complications and management strategies in addition to the complication profiles of

J. Shearer · B. Gurland (✉) · C. Bungo
Department of Surgery, Division of Colorectal Surgery, Stanford University, Palo Alto, CA, USA
e-mail: jlsheare@stanford.edu; bgurland@stanford.edu; cbungo@stanford.edu

M. Hoffman et al. (eds.), *Major Complications of Female Pelvic Surgery*,
https://doi.org/10.1007/978-3-031-66772-5_22

rectopexy reported in the literature. All of patients in these data are prospectively entered into an IRB-approved prolapse registry.

Preoperative Procedural Considerations

Decision-making regarding which surgical approach and technique depends on a combination of patient, surgeon and prolapse features [8]. A body mass index (BMI) >30, inactivity or limited mobility, smoking, poor nutrition, and substance abuse are associated with higher complication profiles [9]. We advocate lifestyle modification programs with weight loss, exercise, and smoking and substance abuse cessation, which should be initiated prior to surgery. For women with multicompartment prolapse undergoing rectal and vaginal or anti-incontinence procedures, the operative time can be substantially longer than that of rectal prolapse alone and this should also be considered during operative planning. Reoperative abdominal or pelvic surgery and prior rectal prolapse repairs can influence which type of repair can be offered to avoid bowel ischemic complications and a perineal approach may be chosen to avoid entering a hostile abdomen. Individuals on blood thinners or antiplatelet agents may have a higher bleeding risk, and medications should be stopped at least 3 days prior to surgery. Precautions such as type and screen should be available at the time of surgery in the event of intraoperative or postoperative hemorrhage. Finally, if either synthetic mesh or biological graft is being considered, this decision should be discussed and consented with the patient preoperatively.

Abdominal Procedures for Rectal Prolapse

For non-frail individuals, abdominal approaches to rectal prolapse repair are recommended since they are considered more durable with lower prolapse recurrence rates (ranging from 8% to 15%) as compared to perineal repairs (recurrence rates ranging from 20% to 40%) [4]. Rectopexy involves variable degrees of mobilization of the rectum and can include dissection along the posterior, anterior, or lateral rectal attachments and fixation to the anterior lateral ligament along the sacrum. The rectal mesentery or lateral rectal attachments can be used for fixation, such as in a suture rectopexy (SR), or mesh can be incorporated either posteriorly (Well's rectopexy) or anteriorly (ventral mesh rectopexy (VR)) for additional support [4]. In selected cases such as the setting of diverticulitis or uncontrolled constipation, sigmoid resection with primary anastomosis is performed in addition to the rectopexy [4]. Our preference is an abdominal robotic ventral mesh rectopexy with biological graft. For patients who would like to avoid mesh, suture rectopexy is performed, and, for patients with uncontrolled constipation or diverticulitis, resection rectopexy is offered. Table 22.1 lists our break down of procedure and common abdominal rectopexy complication.

Table 22.1 Common complications of abdominal rectopexy by procedure type

Complication	Ventral mesh rectopexy; N = 128	Suture rectopexy; N = 26	Resection rectopexy; N = 15
Cardiac morbidity	0 (0%)	0 (0%)	0 (0%)
Pneumonia	1 (1%)	1(4%)	0 (0%)
Abscess	4 (3%)	0 (0%)	0 (0%)
Hemorrhage	2 (2%)	0 (0%)	0 (0%)
Ileus/bowel obstruction	1(1%)	1 (4%)	0 (0%)
Anastomotic leak	NA	NA	0 (0%)
Thromboembolic Events/Deep Vein Thrombosis/ Pulmonary Embolism (DVT/PE)	1 (1%)	0 (0%)	0 (0%)

(continued)

Table 22.1 (continued)

Complication	Ventral mesh rectopexy; N = 128	Suture rectopexy; N = 26	Resection rectopexy; N = 15
Wound hematoma	2 (2%)	1 (4%)	1 (1%)
Wound infection	1 (1%)	2 (8%)	2 (1%)
Port site hernia	2 (2%)	0 (0%)	0 (0%)
Discitis	0 (0)	0 (0%)	0 (0%)
Mesh complication	0 (0%)	NA	0 (0%)
Readmission	7 (5%)	1 (4%)	1 (1%)
Return to the OR	4 (3%)	0 (0%)	0 (0%)
Urinary retention	10 (8%)	1 (4%)	0 (0%)
Urinary tract infection	9 (7%)	0 (0%)	0 (0%)
Missed enterotomy	0 (0%)	0 (0%)	0 (0%)

Note: Data from the Stanford Rectal Prolapse Registry between 2017 and May 2023

General Abdominal Surgery Complications

For abdominal rectal prolapse procedures, minimally invasive techniques are preferred over open laparotomy. Laparoscopic repairs are associated with fewer overall complications, shorter length of stay, improved pain control, and earlier return of bowel function [10, 11]. Robotic surgery has also been associated with less blood loss, better visualization, and decreased morbidity [12, 13]. The robot's ability to dissect and suture in the narrow spaces of the pelvis, to enhance visualizations of the hypogastric region and to avoid injury makes robotic techniques ideal for rectopexy techniques. However, minimally invasive surgery does carry the risks of port site hematoma, hernia, wound infection, and possible inadvertent enterotomy [14, 15].

The most common minor complications of rectopexy are nonspecific and, like those of any general surgery procedure, include ileus, wound infection, hospital-acquired pneumonia, respiratory failure, small bowel obstruction (SBO), or incisional hernia. The likelihood of developing any of these complications after rectopexy is reported to be between 0.5 and 6% [14, 16]. Postoperative monitoring of bowel function, tolerance of oral intake, cardiopulmonary stability, and fever is essential for expediting the diagnosis of these common postoperative complications.

Port site complications such as hernias and hematomas account for 0.5–2% of postoperative complications after laparoscopic and robotic repair [16, 17]. Recognition is often made by physical exam of the abdominal wall to evaluate for mass, palpation of fascial defect, or bowel obstruction. Imaging provides further characterization of the size and structures involved in hernias or hematomas. Early recognition of a patient with a partial obstructive symptoms and a bulge or mass on abdominal exam is key as a port site hernia may warrant return to the OR and will avoid delay in care that could lead to bowel ischemia, gangrene and possible bowel resection. In our series, we report two cases of incarcerated hernia identified with 1 week of robotic rectopexy at the 8-mm robotic port site. Previously, we were not closing the fascia on these ports, but we are more liberal in closing them in octogenarians and a patients with poor tissue quality.

For patients with prior abdominal surgeries, abdominal access may be challenging and the risk of enterotomy or colotomy is higher such that entry under direct vision is recommended. If not appropriately recognized and repaired, a missed enterotomy can be fatal.

In the setting of prior pelvic surgery, ureteral visualization and risk of inadvertent injury should be considered and urinary lighted stents or retrograde injection of ICG into the urethral opening or stents can help with visualization of course of the ureter at the pelvic brim and during left lateral dissection (Fig. 22.1) [18].

Reoperation for abdominal rectopexy is reported in approximately 4% of cases, which is similar to our finding of 3% for reoperation and 5% for hospital readmission [14]. In our series, a

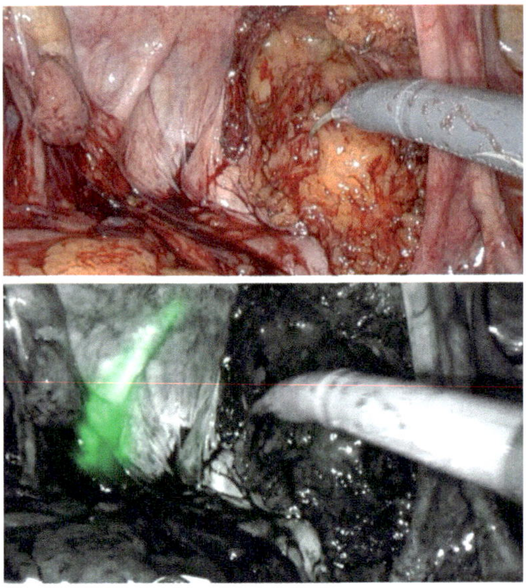

Fig. 22.1 Visualization of the ureteral course at the pelvic brim utilizing ICG

return to the OR within 30 days was secondary to bowel obstruction, incarcerated hernia, and one negative exam under anesthesia.

Hemorrhagic Complications During Rectopexy

Hemorrhagic complications during dissection of the presacral space can be devastating, and knowledge of the sacral anatomy is critical. The anatomy depicted in Fig. 22.2 highlights the vulnerability of the left common iliac vein crossing the sacral promontory and the middle sacral vessels while clearing the sacral promontory for suture fixation or during shearing for posterior rectal dissection of the small presacral veins [19–21]. Presacral venous bleeding after posterior rectal dissection is reported with an inci-

Fig. 22.2 The presacral veins, common iliac vein, and middle sacral veins are vulnerable to injury while clearing the sacral promontory

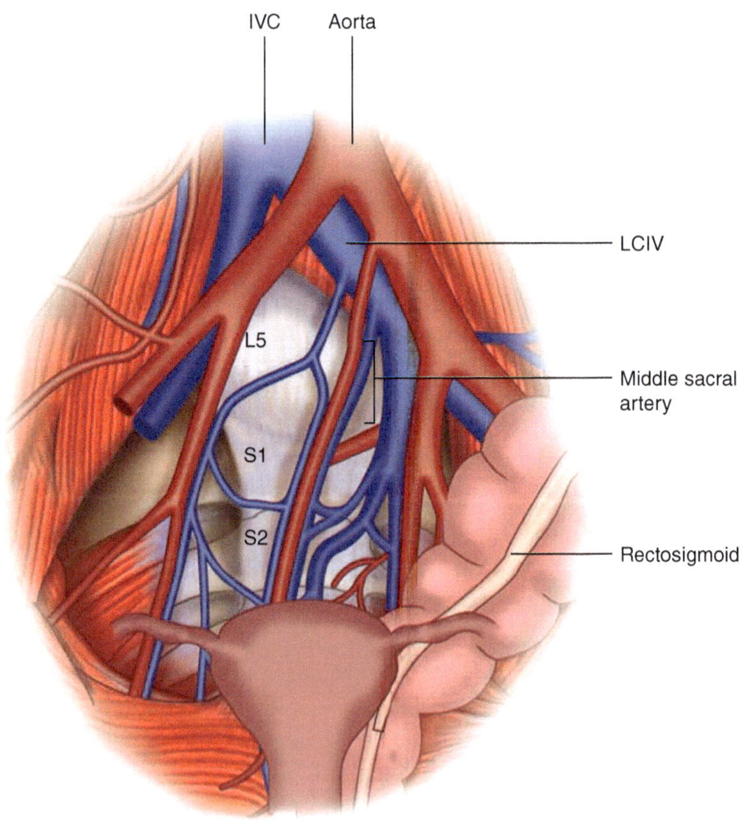

dence of 3–9% [19]. Rapid control is important and holding steady pressure is a critical first step. In our experience, most bleeding can be controlled with pressure alone but communication with the anesthesia and nursing team to be prepared for in the event that blood products are required or conversion to an open technique is warranted. If bleeding persists despite pressure, there are a variety of packing techniques, topical hemostatic agents, tacks, or coagulation devices that can be utilized to control bleeding. In an unstable patient, packing, ICU resuscitation, and hemodynamic stabilization are appropriate with a planned return to the OR within 48 h to remove packing and complete the procedure.

We report two cases of postoperative hemorrhage after ventral mesh robotic rectopexy. One patient responded to transfusions, and the bleeding ultimately stopped. The other patient underwent interventional radiology (IR) embolization. There were no long-term sequelae for either patient and no evidence of prolapse recurrence at 24 months.

Mesh Complications

Augmenting rectal prolapse repair with mesh varies with regard to the location of mesh placement (anterior or posterior) and the range of materials used (fascia lata, nonabsorbable synthetic mesh, and biological grafts) [5]. In this chapter, we will focus on ventral mesh rectopexy (VR), which has gained acceptance worldwide as a preferred abdominal mesh procedure [5]. VR involves dissection along the anterior rectum below the peritoneal reflection, suturing of mesh to the ventral rectum, and suspension by fixation of the mesh to the anterior ligament along the sacrum (Fig. 22.3). Adverse events related to mesh use include infection, erosion (into the rectum or vagina), rectal vaginal fistula, or chronic pelvic pain [12, 17, 22, 23]. The type of mesh, the sutures used to secure the mesh to the rectum, the depth of the suture into the rectal wall, and ischemia secondary to excessive tension around the rectum have all been implicated as risk factors for

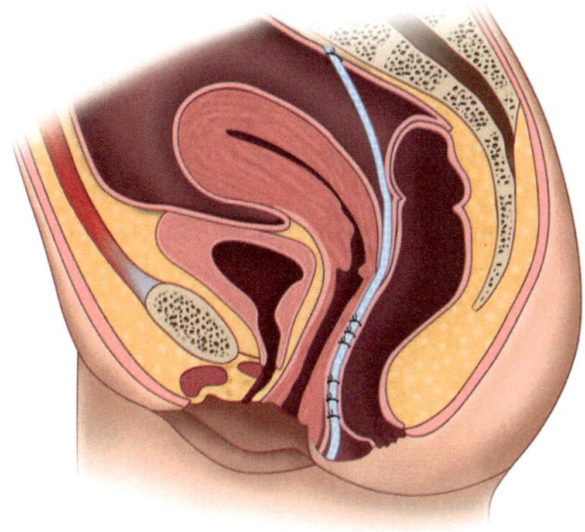

Fig. 22.3 Ventral mesh rectopexy includes mobilizing the anterior rectum down to below peritoneal reflection and securing mesh to the ventral rectum and the anterior ligament along the sacrum

mesh complications. Polyester material has been associated with higher erosion rates and is contraindicated, while titanium-coated light-weight polypropylene is preferred [17]. Looking at 11 studies with 4001 patients, the incidence of synthetic mesh related complications ranges from 0–2.4% as compared to 762 patients implanted with biological material with mesh complications ranging from 0–0.7% [23]. With biologics, the risk of mesh-related infection is assumed to be lower due to degradation and resorption of the graft and regeneration of the host tissue. There are concerns that biologic repairs may not be as durable, but short-term recurrence rates are similar between synthetic and biologic mesh and long-term recurrence rates require further evaluation [22, 24, 25]. Currently, there is no consensus on the preferred type of mesh [26].

Surgical technique and suture material may also impact complication rates. Seromuscular bites along the rectum are recommended to secure the mesh. Full-thickness suture placement into the rectal lumen is avoided, but if this misplacement does occur, the suture is cut and removed. The suture material used for mesh fixation to the rectum has also been implicated as a risk factor for erosion. Tejedor et al. revealed a decrease in erosion rates when changing from permanent to absorbable sutures [27]. There is a current recommendation that permanent, braided sutures be avoided in favor of absorbable monofilament for mesh to rectal or vaginal fixation [27, 28].

Patients with mesh erosion can present with symptoms of pain, dyspareunia, discharge, or fecal complaints immediately following surgery or years later [28–33]. Asymptomatic mesh erosions noted on vaginal or rectal examinations have also been reported. Mesh erosion and migration may or may not require surgical excision. Rectovaginal erosions less than 1 cm^2 can be managed with topical estrogen cream. If no response is seen within 3 months or if the erosion enlarges, as is the most common outcome, surgical management may be required [33, 34].

Indications for mesh excision include pain, perforation, and fistula formation [30]. Transvaginal, transanal, laparoscopic, and open en bloc resection may be used for mesh excision [6, 28]. For cases with large areas of dissection needed, en bloc resections may also require left anterior colonic resections with proximal diversion. Local stich or mesh excision is also possible with a microsurgical technique such as transanal endoscopic microsurgery (TEMS) or transanal minimally invasive surgery (TAMIS) [35]. These microsurgical techniques may require multiple procedures for complete resolution. One study found that vaginal erosions required a median number of two procedures and that rectal erosions required five procedures for adequate resolution of erosion, fistula takedown, and repair [28]. As removal of mesh likely occurs after postoperative scarring has taken place, removal of mesh does not fully equate with recurrence of rectal prolapse [28].

In our series, we report 128 cases of ventral rectopexy with 108 using (Cook BioTech® Rectopexy Graft) with 3.0 PDS used to suture to the mesh to the rectum and avoiding excessive tension on the rectum. There were no mesh-related complications.

Discitis

Infection of the disc space is an uncommon complication after sacrocolpopexy or rectopexy procedures [36]. Clinical presentation of discitis is variable, including severe back pain, tenderness of the paraspinal muscles or spasm, pain when walking or standing, and fever [37]. Symptoms may occur several weeks after surgery. If infection spreads to the epidural space, neurologic deficits may also be present [37]. Leukocytosis and an elevated erythrocyte sedimentation rate are common lab findings. Imaging, including CT scanning and magnetic resonance imaging (MRI), may reveal disc space narrowing, end plate irregularities, loss of psoas shadow, or loss of lordosis [37]. MRI is the imaging of choice with a sensitivity and a specificity greater than 90% [38].

In most cases, vertebral discitis is caused by hematogenous spread of pathogens. Although the exact pathophysiology of discitis after rectopexy is unknown, it is theorized that direct inoculation of the disc space can occur after deep suture placement. The mesh acts as a scaffold, which facilitates bacterial translocation from the distal rectum to the sacrum. The following techniques are recommended to avoid this dreaded complication:

1. Appropriate placement of sutures into the seromuscular layer of the rectum rather than penetration into the bowel wall to minimize contamination of the suture, fistula formation, and/or potential bacterial spread to the spinal discs [39].
2. Careful placement of the sacral sutures by avoiding deep penetration of the needle into the disc space.
3. Avoiding tight tensioning of the mesh, which could lead to bacterial translocation.
4. If findings are concerning for discitis, biopsy and blood cultures should be obtained.

Discitis requires broad spectrum antibiotics with coverage of cologenic flora and which are then narrowed given biopsy and cultures sensitivities. The initial course of antibiotics is 6–12 weeks [36, 37]. The majority of patients will respond to nonoperative management. Operative treatment is indicated for patients with neurologic symptoms concerning cord compression, instability of the spine, or a large epidural abscess requiring drainage. An anterior or posterior approach can be used to relieve spinal compression, drain the abscess, or stabilize the spine [37].

Intra-Abdominal Collections/Seromas/Abscesses

Seromas, hematomas, or abscesses can be identified on imaging after rectopexy. Incidental findings with minimal symptoms require no treatment. Findings can also be associated with abdominal, pelvic, or rectal pain, fevers, and/or leukocytosis. In a current meta-analysis comparing 616 patients following suture rectopexy (SR) to 1232 patients following VR, intra-abdominal collections and abscesses were reported in 0.5% of SR compared to 0 in VR [16]. Evans et al. retrospectively reviewed 2203 patients with VR and reported pelvic hematoma in 0.5% of them [17]. We advocate for antibiotics and, if needed, interventional radiology (IR) drainage. In our series, we readmitted three patients after VR (N = 128) with pelvic pain and collections on CT scan. Symptoms resolved with intravenous (IV) antibiotics, followed by an outpatient course of oral antibiotics. Repeat imaging revealed resolution of the fluid. None of the patients required IR drainage, and there were no long-term infectious mesh sequelae, but one patient had rectal prolapse recurrence 1 year after surgery.

Ureteral Injury

Closure of the peritoneum at completion of the rectopexy can cause tenting or obstruction of the ureter. Care should be taken to visualize the ureter and to only suture the edge of the peritoneum. For discussion of ureteral injury after rectal prolapse repair, please refer the other chapters in this text for recognition and management of this complication in the setting of pelvic surgery.

Bowel Obstruction

Small bowel obstruction (SBO) after rectopexy can occur if the small bowel adheres to the rectopexy sutures or to the mesh. Closing the peritoneum covers the mesh and is thought to prevent small bowel fixation in the pelvis. Rarely, a closed-loop obstruction may also develop despite peritoneal closure if a loop passes through a peritoneal defect or dehiscent suture in the right side of the pelvis and herniates medially and inferiorly between the rectum and uterus. This malposition typically results in inverted C-shaped loops that open toward the right and can be visualized on CT [38]. Barbed sutures for peritoneal closure have been associated with SBO requiring reoperation [40]. Our preference is to avoid using barbed sutures for peritoneal closure.

Anastomotic Leaks

In selected cases, sigmoid resection is added to rectopexy. This addition has a risk of anastomotic leak, abscess formation, and pelvic sepsis. However, the leak rates following resection rectopexy are very low, generally less than 1% [41–43]. The morbidity of pelvic sepsis after anastomotic leaks is approximately 2–16% [5].

For patients with anastomotic leaks, hemodynamic stability is the priority. Patients may require drain placement or taken back to the operative room for abdominal washouts of the infected cavity and repair of the leak. Broad-spectrum antibiotics should be initiated including anaerobic coverage for cologenic flora. For poorly contained leaks, a loop ileostomy or end colostomy may be needed for diversion [5]. However, this patient population is unlikely to need a permanent stoma and most leaks can be diverted.

Postoperative Pain

Pelvic pain is a common presenting symptom of rectal prolapse preoperatively, which improves for over two-thirds of patients postoperatively [44]. However, 12–19% of patients may experience pelvic pain postoperatively, including those showing no improvement, worsening, or de novo pelvic pain [23, 44]. Pelvic pain may also be a symptom of another complication such a mesh erosion, requiring reoperation [23]. For patients with preexisting pain syndromes, we consider avoiding mesh in favor of suture rectopexy or using biological grafts, which will reabsorb over time.

Perineal Surgery

The perineal approaches are transitionally preferred for high-risk operative candidates as the procedure generally has shorter operative times [8], avoids hemodynamic impact of laparoscopic insufflation, and can be performed under local or spinal anesthesia. Across surgical interventions, frail patients have almost four times the rate of wound complications, reoperation, readmission, and morality [9]. Risk calculators like the Frailty Index offer a multivariable evaluation of frailty compared to the traditional but limited basis of chronological age [45]. Therefore, a preoperative assessment of frailty may aid in determining the best candidates for a perineal repair.

When considering a perineal repair, there are two predominant perineal approaches: the Delorme and the Altemeier. The Delorme includes a short mucosal sleeve resection and imbrication of the muscularis layer of the rectum. The Altemeier is a transanal full-thickness resection of the prolapsed rectum with coloanal anastomosis, which can be sutured or stapled [5]. The Delorme avoids anastomotic complications but has the highest rate of prolapse recurrence.

The Delorme's procedure has a rate of early complication ranging from 4% to 12%, including infection, urinary retention, bleeding, and fecal impaction [1]. The low coloanal anastomosis performed during an Altemeier poses a risk of anastomotic leak, stricture, or stenosis as well as rectal perforation [1]. Anastomotic leaks and hematomas predispose patients to pelvic abscess formation postoperatively [5]. Alwahid et al. found that during the initial hospital stay, reoperation was required in approximately 7% of Altemeier cases [1]. Reoperation was most commonly secondary to anastomotic leak, and the authors report three patients with leaks: two underwent anastomotic takedown and end colostomy and one underwent a washout. Since Altemeier anastomosis remains extraperitoneal some cases, it is possible for anastomotic leaks to drain through the anus. This physiology may explain why the perineal approach is associated with a lower operative morbidity and faster postoperative recovery for patients with postoperative anastomotic leaks after rectal prolapse repair [1].

Anastomotic leaks typically present in the first week postoperatively [46]. Intraoperative technical considerations include minimizing disruption of peri-anastomotic blood supply and anastomotic tension to reduce the incidence of early anastomotic leak within the immediate postoperative period [31, 46]. Resection of too much bowel or mesentery should also be avoided to prevent ischemia at the anastomosis, which may also result in stenosis [31]. Late anastomotic leaks, greater than 30-days postoperatively, are associated with poor nutrition, immunosuppression, and obesity. Anastomotic leaks and pelvic abscesses typically present clinically with high-grade fever, tachypnea, lower abdominal pain, prolonged ileus, and possibly peritonitis. Labs are likely to reflect leukocytosis and elevated C-reactive protein levels. For patients with non-specific symptoms, diagnostic imaging will aid in diagnosis.

In Table 22.2, we report complication profile for our patients and common reports in the literature for perineal procedures.

We had no anastomotic leaks, but we did report five patients with postoperative bleeding. Four patients responded to blood transfusions. One patient developed an infected hematoma requiring sacral IR drainage. One patient required IR embolization, and, 6 months later, she presented with an anastomotic stricture requiring dilatation under anesthesia.

Table 22.2 Common complications of perineal rectal prolapse repair

Complication	Altemeier; N = 46	Delorme; N = 18
Cardiac morbidity	2 (4%)	0 (0%)
Pneumonia	1(2%)	0 (0%)
Abscess	2 (4%)	0 (0%)
Hemorrhage	5 (11%)	0 (0%)
Ileus/bowel obstruction	1 (2%)	0 (0%)
Anastomotic leak	0 (0%)	0 (0%)
DVT/PE	0 (0%)	0 (0%)
Wound hematoma	0 (0%)	0 (0%)
Wound infection	0 (0%)	0 (0%)
Readmission	3(7%)	1 (6%)
Return to the OR	3 (7%)	1 (6%)
Urinary retention	3 (7%)	3 (17%)
Urinary tract infection	1(2%)	0 (0%)

Note: Data from the Stanford Rectal Prolapse Registry between 2017 and May 2023

Multicompartment Prolapse Repairs

Mulitcompartment repairs can safely be performed for patients with cystocele or vaginal prolapse in addition to rectal prolapse [9, 47, 48]. These repairs involve dissection into the anterior and middle pelvic compartments. Due to the involved anatomy, these repairs have a higher rate of urinary complications, including leak, voiding dysfunction, or retention secondary to injury to the urethra, bladder, or ureters [49]. Additional sites of potential bleeding in the anterior compartment also include the iliac vessels and the vascular pedicle of the bladder [49]. From the Stanford database, 95 (41%) patients underwent multicompartment repairs.

Postoperative Constipation/Fecal Impaction

Bowel frequency and coordination should be evaluated and addressed prior to surgery with education and laxatives as needed. Managing bowel function after prolapse surgery with diet, fibers, and laxatives is imperative to avoid excessive straining. Prescription promotility agents can be prescribed to optimize stool consistency and frequency. Suppositories and enemas are not recommended in the first few weeks after repair. Patients with stenosis or anastomotic stricture may complain of worsening constipation, and digital examination or sigmoidoscopy is necessary. An exam under anesthesia and fecal disimpaction may be warranted in patients with hard stools, and anastomotic dilatation can be performed if a stricture or stenosis is present.

Conclusions

Morbidity after rectal prolapse repair is low. Patient selection for abdominal or perineal procedures and perioperative optimization are key to successful outcomes. Avoiding technical errors such as injuring the sacral vessels, deep suture bites along the rectum, or excessive tension can prevent postoperative bleeding, anastomotic issues, or mesh complications. Bleeding complications are primarily managed with transfusion, but IR embolization may be necessary. Urinary retention and infections are common and expected, especially if concomitant vaginal prolapse or anti-incontinence procedures are performed.

References

1. Alwahid M, Knight SR, Wadhawan H, Campbell KL, Ziyaie D, Koch SMP. Perineal rectosigmoidectomy for rectal prolapse—the preferred procedure for the unfit elderly patient? 10 years experience from a UK tertiary centre. Tech Coloproctol. 2019;23(11):1065–72. https://doi.org/10.1007/s10151-019-02100-z.
2. Bordeianou L, Hicks CW, Kaiser AM, Alavi K, Sudan R, Wise PE. Rectal prolapse: an overview of clinical features, diagnosis, and patient-specific management strategies. J Gastrointest Surg. 2014;18(5):1059–69. https://doi.org/10.1007/s11605-013-2427-7.
3. Vogel JD, de Campos-Lobato LF, Chapman BC, Bronsert MR, Birnbaum EH, Meguid RA. Rectal prolapse surgery in males and females: an ACS NSQIP-based comparative analysis of over 12,000 patients. Am J Surg. 2020;220(3):697–705. https://doi.org/10.1016/j.amjsurg.2020.01.017.
4. Bordeianou L, Paquette I, Johnson E, et al. Clinical practice guidelines for the treatment of rectal prolapse. Dis Colon Rectum. 2017;60(11):1121–31. https://doi.org/10.1097/DCR.0000000000000889.

5. Madiba TE, Baig MK, Wexner SD. Surgical management of rectal prolapse. Arch Surg. 2005;140(1):63–73.
6. Balla A, Quaresima S, Smolarek S, Shalaby M, Missori G, Sileri P. Synthetic versus biological mesh-related erosion after laparoscopic ventral mesh rectopexy: a systematic review. Ann Coloproctol. 2017;33(2):46–51. https://doi.org/10.3393/ac.2017.33.2.46.
7. Yasukawa D, Hori T, Machimoto T, et al. Outcome of a modified laparoscopic suture rectopexy for rectal prolapse with the use of a single or double suture: a case series of 15 patients. Am J Case Rep. 2017;18:599–604. https://doi.org/10.12659/AJCR.905118.
8. Lee A, Kin C, Syan R, Morris A, Gurland B. Surgical decision-making for rectal prolapse: one size does not fit all. Postgrad Med. 2020;132(3):256–62. https://doi.org/10.1080/00325481.2019.1669330.
9. Geltzeiler CB, Birnbaum EH, Silviera ML, et al. Combined rectopexy and sacrocolpopexy is safe for correction of pelvic organ prolapse. Int J Color Dis. 2018;33(10):1453–9. https://doi.org/10.1007/s00384-018-3140-5.
10. Bao X, Wang H, Song W, Chen Y, Luo Y. Meta-analysis on current status, efficacy, and safety of laparoscopic and robotic ventral mesh rectopexy for rectal prolapse treatment: can robotic surgery become the gold standard? Int J Color Dis. 2021;36(8):1685–94.
11. Clark CE, Jupiter DC, Thomas SJ, Papaconstantinou HT. Rectal prolapse in the elderly: trends in surgical management and outcomes from the American College of Surgeons National Surgical Quality Improvement Program Database. J Am Coll Surg. 2012;215(5):709–14.
12. van Iersel JJ, Paulides TJC, Verheijen PM, Lumley JW, Broeders IAMJ, Consten ECJ. Current status of laparoscopic and robotic ventral mesh rectopexy for external and internal rectal prolapse. WJG. 2016;22(21):4977.
13. Rondelli F, Bugiantella W, Villa F, et al. Robot-assisted or conventional laparoscoic rectopexy for rectal prolapse? Systematic review and meta-analysis. Int J Surg. 2014;12:S153–9.
14. de Bruijn H, Maeda Y, Tan KN, Jenkins JT, Kennedy RH. Long-term outcome of laparoscopic rectopexy for full-thickness rectal prolapse. Tech Coloproctol. 2019;23(1):25–31. https://doi.org/10.1007/s10151-018-1913-z.
15. Hajibandeh S, Hajibandeh S, Arun C, Adeyemo A, McIlroy B, Peravali R. Meta-analysis of laparoscopic mesh rectopexy versus posterior sutured rectopexy for management of complete rectal prolapse. Int J Color Dis. 2021;36(7):1357–66. https://doi.org/10.1007/s00384-021-03883-0.
16. Lobb HS, Kearsey CC, Ahmed S, Rajaganeshan R. Suture rectopexy versus ventral mesh rectopexy for complete full-thickness rectal prolapse and intussusception: systematic review and meta-analysis. BJS Open. 2021;5(1):zraa037. https://doi.org/10.1093/bjsopen/zraa037.
17. Evans C, Stevenson ARL, Sileri P, et al. A multicenter collaboration to assess the safety of laparoscopic ventral rectopexy. Dis Colon Rectum. 2015;58(8):799–807. https://doi.org/10.1097/DCR.0000000000000402.
18. Kimura C, Dawes A, Gurland B. Avoiding ureteral injury in reoperative ventral rectopexy. Presented at: Annual scientific meeting of the American Society of Colon and Rectal Surgeons; May 2022; Tampa, FL. https://doi.org/10.1097/DCR.000000000000245.
19. Lazarou G, Rahimi S, Cui N, Zormpa M. Variant iliocaval confluence discovered during sacrocolpopexy. Obstet Gynecol. 2011;117(2 Pt 2):436–7. https://doi.org/10.1097/AOG.0b013e3182062053.
20. Florian-Rodriguez ME, Hamner JJ, Corton MM. First sacral nerve and anterior longitudinal ligament anatomy: clinical applications during sacrocolpopexy. Am J Obstet Gynecol. 2017;217(5):607.e1–4. https://doi.org/10.1016/j.ajog.2017.07.008.
21. Good MM, Abele TA, Balgobin S, et al. Preventing L5-S1 discitis associated with sacrocolpopexy. Obstet Gynecol. 2013;121(2 Pt 1):285–90. https://doi.org/10.1097/AOG.0b013e31827c61de.
22. Smart NJ, Pathak S, Boorman P, Daniels IR. Synthetic or biological mesh use in laparoscopic ventral mesh rectopexy—a systematic review. Colorectal Dis. 2013;15(6):650–4. https://doi.org/10.1111/codi.12219.
23. van der Schans EM, Verheijen PM, Broeders IAMJ, Consten ECJ. Ninety-day morbidity of robot-assisted redo surgery for recurrent rectal prolapse, mesh erosion and pelvic pain: lessons learned from 9 years' experience in a tertiary referral centre. Colorectal Dis. 2021;23(12):3205–12. https://doi.org/10.1111/codi.15979.
24. Ogilvie JWJ, Stevenson ARL, Powar M. Case-matched series of a non-cross-linked biologic versus non-absorbable mesh in laparoscopic ventral rectopexy. Int J Color Dis. 2014;29(12):1477–83. https://doi.org/10.1007/s00384-014-2016-6.
25. Stevenson ARL. Erosion versus recurrence: is there a compromise using biologics for ventral rectopexy? Tech Coloproctol. 2015;19(4):199–200. https://doi.org/10.1007/s10151-015-1291-8.
26. Mercer-Jones MA, Brown SR, Knowles CH, Williams AB. Position statement by the pelvic floor society on behalf of the Association of Coloproctology of Great Britain and Ireland on the use of mesh in ventral mesh rectopexy. Colorectal Dis. 2020;22(10):1429–35. https://doi.org/10.1111/codi.13893.
27. Tejedor P, Lindsey I, Jones OM, et al. Impact of suture type on erosion rate after laparoscopic ventral mesh Rectopexy: a case-matched study. Dis Colon Rectum. 2019;62(12):1512–7. https://doi.org/10.1097/DCR.0000000000001510.
28. Ratnatunga K, Singh S, Bolckmans R, et al. Minimally invasive organ-preserving approaches in the management of mesh erosion after laparoscopic ventral mesh rectopexy. Color Dis. 2020;22(11):1642–8. https://doi.org/10.1111/codi.15257.

29. Borie F, Coste T, Bigourdan JM, Guillon F. Incidence and surgical treatment of synthetic mesh-related infectious complications after laparoscopic ventral rectopexy. Tech Coloproctol. 2016;20(11):759–65. https://doi.org/10.1007/s10151-016-1538-z.
30. Badrek-Al Amoudi AH, Greenslade GL, Dixon AR. How to deal with complications after laparoscopic ventral mesh rectopexy: lessons learnt from a tertiary referral centre. Colorectal Dis. 2013;15(6):707–12. https://doi.org/10.1111/codi.12164.
31. Goldstein S, Maxwell P. Rectal Prolapse. Clin Colon Rectal Surg. 2011;24(01):039–45. https://doi.org/10.1055/s-0031-1272822.
32. Ratneswaren A, Laskaratos FM, Kumar A, Hepworth C. Rectal bleeding due to rectal erosion of vaginal mesh. Ann Gastroenterol. 2015;28(4):498.
33. Mathew MJ, Parmar AK, Reddy PK. Mesh erosion after laparoscopic posterior rectopexy: a rare complication. J Minim Access Surg. 2014;10(1):40–1. https://doi.org/10.4103/0972-9941.124473.
34. Tuma F, McKeown DG, Al-Wahab Z. Rectovaginal Fistula. In: StatPearls. StatPearls Publishing; 2023.
35. Patil NS, Saluja SS, Mishra PK, Solanki N, Parasar K. Intrarectal migration of mesh following Rectopexy: case series and review of literature. Int J Surg. 2015;20:145–8.
36. Draaisma WA, van Eijck MM, Vos J, Consten ECJ. Lumbar discitis after laparoscopic ventral rectopexy for rectal prolapse. Int J Color Dis. 2011;26(2):255–6.
37. Shenoy K, Singla A, Krystal JD, Razi AE, Kim YH, Sharan AD. Discitis in adults. JBJS Rev. 2018;6(6):e6. https://doi.org/10.2106/JBJS.RVW.17.00104.
38. Haouari MA, Boulay-Coletta I, Khatri G, et al. Complications of mesh Sacrocolpopexy and Rectopexy: imaging review. Radiographics. 2023;43(2):e220137. https://doi.org/10.1148/rg.220137.
39. Hyun K, Yang SJ, Lim KY, Lee JK, Yoon SG. Laparoscopic Posterolateral Rectopexy for the treatment of patients with a full thickness rectal prolapse: experience with 63 patients and short-term outcomes. Ann Coloproctol. 2018;34(3):119–24.
40. Salminen HJ, Tan WS, Jayne DG. Three cases of small bowel obstruction after laparoscopic ventral rectopexy using the V-Loc(®) suture. Tech Coloproctol. 2014;18(6):601–2. https://doi.org/10.1007/s10151-013-1074-z.
41. Ashari LHS, Lumley JW, Stevenson ARL, Stitz RW. Laparoscopically-assisted resection rectopexy for rectal prolapse: ten years' experience. Dis Colon Rectum. 2005;48(5):982–7. https://doi.org/10.1007/s10350-004-0886-3.
42. Carvalho E, Carvalho ME, Hull T, Zutshi M, Gurland BH. Resection Rectopexy is still an acceptable operation for rectal prolapse. Am Surg. 2018;84(9):1470–5.
43. Laubert T, Bader FG, Kleemann M, et al. Outcome analysis of elderly patients undergoing laparoscopic resection rectopexy for rectal prolapse. Int J Color Dis. 2012;27(6):789–95. https://doi.org/10.1007/s00384-011-1395-1.
44. Singh S, Bolckmans R, Ratnatunga K, et al. Pelvic pain is a common prolapse symptom and improvement after ventral mesh rectopexy is more frequent than deterioration or de novo pain. Colorectal Dis. 2023;25(1):118–27. https://doi.org/10.1111/codi.16321.
45. Rockwood K, Song X, MacKnight C, Bergman H, Hogan DB, McDowell I, Mitnitski A. A global clinical measure of fitness and frailty in elderly people. CMAJ. 2005 Aug 30;173(5):489–95. https://doi.org/10.1503/cmaj.050051.
46. Chiarello MM, Fransvea P, Cariati M, Adams NJ, Bianchi V, Brisinda G. Anastomotic leakage in colorectal cancer surgery. Surg Oncol. 2022;40:101708.
47. Weinberg D, Qeadan F, McKee R, Rogers RG, Komesu YM. Safety of laparoscopic sacrocolpopexy with concurrent rectopexy: peri-operative morbidity in a nationwide cohort. Int Urogynecol J. 2019;30(3):385–92. https://doi.org/10.1007/s00192-018-3699-y.
48. Wallace SL, Syan R, Enemchukwu EA, Mishra K, Sokol ER, Gurland B. Surgical approach, complications, and reoperation rates of combined rectal and pelvic organ prolapse surgery. Int Urogynecol J. 2020;31(10):2101–8. https://doi.org/10.1007/s00192-020-04394-2.
49. Rovner ES. Complications of anterior compartment vaginal surgery. Curr Urol Rep. 2007;8(5):405–12. https://doi.org/10.1007/s11934-007-0039-z.

Part VI

Miscellaneous

Complications of Minimally Invasive Surgery

23

Dandi Huang and Kenneth H. Kim

Trocar Injury: Vascular and Bowel Injuries

Background

Abdominal entry is often the most dangerous step of minimally invasive surgery and accounts for approximately 50% of serious laparoscopic complications such as visceral and vascular injuries as well as medico-legal litigations [1–3]. Even though the rate of complication with the first trocar entry is only about 1%, laparoscopic trocars are still the most common device named in these litigations, making up one-third of all claims [3]. Multiple methods of entry exist, such as direct entry, Veress needle (VN) entry, and Hassan (open) entry.

This section will focus on trocar-related injuries. It is important to note that a Cochrane review showed no difference in safety of one technique over another [3]. The 2023 Cochrane review also compared blind VN and direct trocar insertion (DTI) and found no difference in the rate of bowel or major vascular injury. DTI was associated with a lower risk of omental bleeding, omental emphysema, subcutaneous emphysema, and extraperitoneal insufflation. Additionally, no single study has compared the different trocar types (i.e., radially expanding, conical blunt-shaped, single-bladed, cutting trocar, etc.). The existing data comparing visceral injury, vascular injury, trocar site herniation, trocar site bleeding, and postoperative pain of different trocar types have low quality of evidence [4]. We will focus on two of the most serious complications here, which are vascular and bowel injuries.

Prevention

Entry sites should be carefully chosen based on the patient's surgical history and likelihood of abdominal adhesions. The left upper quadrant (Palmer's point) should be considered if lower abdominal adhesions are anticipated. A nasogastric tube should be placed with left upper quadrant entry to decompress the stomach, decreasing the risk of gastric injury. The risk of major vascular injury can be decreased in most cases by introducing instruments at an approximately 45° angle from the plane of the patient's spine in the supine position (Figure 23.1a,b), as Trendelenburg can distort this angle [5]. For secondary ports, placement about 8 cm laterally from the midline can help avoid injury to the abdominal wall vessels. Once the initial trocar is placed, it is prudent to place the remaining trocars under direct visualization with a laparoscopic camera.

D. Huang · K. H. Kim (✉)
Department of Obstetrics and Gynecology, Division of Gynecologic Oncology, Cedars-Sinai Medical Center, West Hollywood, CA, USA
e-mail: dandi.huang@cshs.org; kenneth.kim3@cshs.org

M. Hoffman et al. (eds.), *Major Complications of Female Pelvic Surgery*,
https://doi.org/10.1007/978-3-031-66772-5_23

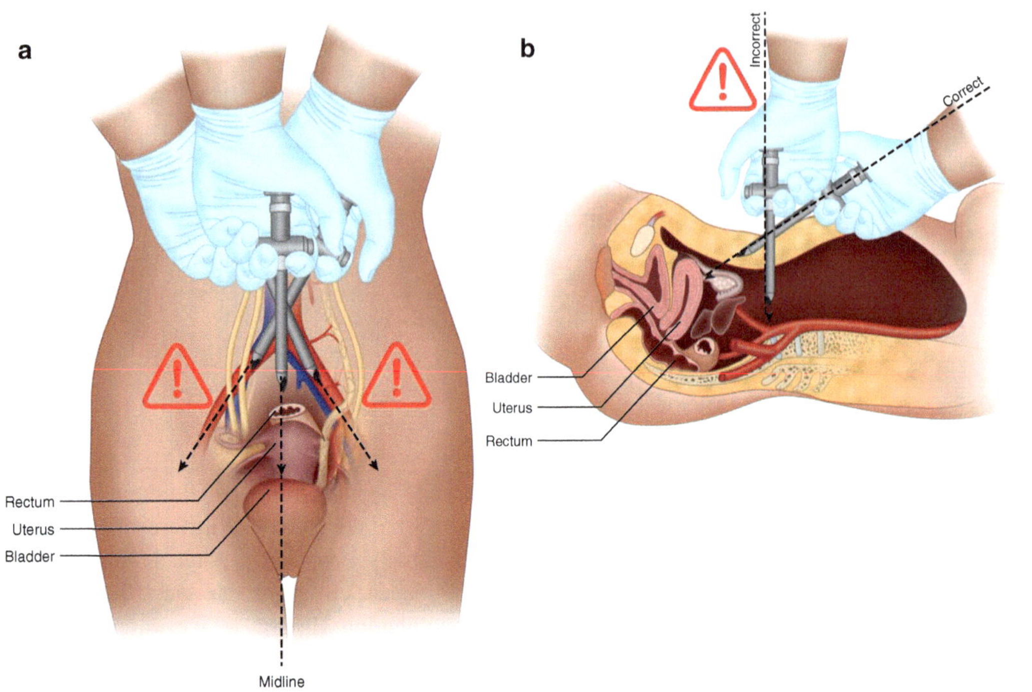

Fig. 23.1 (**a, b**) Incorrect and correct angels of midline trocar placement

Recognition

Early recognition of vascular and bowel injuries is of critical importance due to the high morbidity and mortality associated with such injuries.

Injuries to the abdominal wall vessels occur in 0.3–2.5% of procedures, and about half of these injuries affect the inferior epigastric vessels. More seriously, vascular injury to a major retroperitoneal vessel occurs in 0.3–1.0% of all procedures and accounts for 74–82% of all laparoscopy-related deaths [5–12]. The rate of major vascular injury during initial entry is 0.05–0.5%, and trocars account for 54–83% of these. The sites of vascular injury in decreasing frequency are the iliac vein, greater omental vessels, inferior vena cava, aorta, pelvic, and superior mesenteric veins, and lumbar veins.

The incidence of bowel injury ranges from 0.03 to 0.18% and accounts for 19% of deaths from trocar-related injury. Bowel injury occurs most frequently during entry (41.8%), and the sites of bowel injury in decreasing frequency are the small bowel (55.8%), large intestine (38.6%), and stomach (3.9%) [13–15].

Vascular Injury

Trocar injury to a major vessel will almost always result in brisk bleeding, regardless of whether the bleeding is arterial or venous. Signs of injury include rapidly increasing hemoperitoneum and changes to the patient's pulse and blood pressure. Intravascular insufflation is rare but can be fatal as massive venous gas embolism can lead to rapid cardiopulmonary collapse. Early signs may present as decreased end-tidal carbon dioxide (CO_2), decreased oxygen saturation, or a "mill wheel" murmur audible with a stethoscope. Tachyarrhythmias and right-sided heart strain with ST-T wave changes may also be seen. Later findings include increased central venous pressure and jugular venous distension. Fortunately, a lethal dose of intravascular CO_2 is much higher than air (i.e., air embolism) as CO_2 is rapidly absorbed and has higher solubility in blood.

Bowel Injury

Unlike thermal injury, trocar-related bowel injuries are typically recognizable at the time of surgery, but up to 50% can still be missed and about 10% are diagnosed after 48 h. An unrecognized bowel injury carries a mortality rate of up to 30%. Common intraoperative findings include foul smelling gas, visible bowel contents, asymmetric distention, and high insufflation pressure. If injury is not identified at the time of surgery, these traumatic perforations will typically present with symptoms within 48 h [13].

Management

Major Vascular Injury

It is important to ensure adequate vascular access and cardiovascular resuscitation. Anesthesia and the operating staff should also be promptly notified to help obtain ancillary equipment and ensure that blood products are available. A vascular or trauma surgeon should be called if needed and available. It is important to check the hospital protocol for these complications ahead of time as intravascular insufflation and major vascular injury with laparoscopy are rare, and some institutions may not have a standard protocol in place.

The abdominal wall vessels are smaller, and bleeding may be stopped with cautery or tamponade with a trocar (i.e., a balloon trocar) or a Foley catheter passed into the port site. Direct ligation may also be performed with a fascial closure device. Transmural suturing has also been done; these sutures may need to be removed at around 24 h to prevent abdominal wall necrosis. If abdominal wall swelling or bruising is noted postoperatively, it can often be managed conservatively while also monitoring hemoglobin levels. If this area is expanding or if the patient is hemodynamically unstable, exploration should be performed.

For a major retroperitoneal vascular injury, the following basic principles of management as summarized by Suarez should be followed [11]:

- Immediate conversion to an open procedure must be considered.
- Direct compression of the bleeding site is the quickest and safest way to gain initial control of blood loss, especially for a venous injury.
- If the patient exhibits unstable vital signs, adequate volume replacement, while controlling the blood loss, must take place prior to attempting repair of the injury.
- If the bleeding site is difficult to see, early and wide exposure of the site and the surrounding structures must be obtained.
- The vessel wall must be repaired with precise intima-to-intima apposition without tension.
- Venous injuries may be best handled by ligation rather than suture repair if the patient is unstable.
- If ligation of a vessel does not lead to ischemia, definitive repair may be postponed until the patient is stable and/or when the appropriate vascular surgeon is available.
- In some circumstances of minor venous bleeding, hemostasis can be obtained by applying pressure, increasing the insufflation pressure, and placing a clip or suture.

Carbon Dioxide Embolism

Key initial steps include discontinuing insufflation, releasing the pneumoperitoneum, and ventilating the patient with 100% oxygen. Clear communication with the anesthesia team is necessary. Aggressive fluid resuscitation can help elevate the central venous pressure and decrease further CO_2 entry. The patient should also be placed in steep Trendelenburg and left lateral decubitus position to allow the gas bubbles to rise into the right atrium and prevent gas entry into the pulmonary artery. Management of this serious and potentially fatal condition relies heavily on collaboration with the anesthesia team, which is beyond the scope of this text [16].

Bowel Injury

Bowel injury, if recognized during surgery, can typically be repaired laparoscopically by an experienced laparoscopic surgeon. If there is any concern, one should err toward converting to laparotomy to maximize repair and minimize any further complication. Veress needle injury can potentially be managed conservatively with observation due to the small diameter of the needle, as the muscular layer will close the defect. If the injury is limited to a serosal abrasion, then this may be left unrepaired. For deeper injuries less than 1 cm, primary closure is employed. With a trocar injury, leaving the trocar in situ can help identify the site of injury and a one- or two-layer closure is performed. Injury to the muscularis is repaired with a single layer of interrupted imbricating (Lembert) stitches using 3-0 absorbable or permanent silk sutures on a tapered needle. The sutures should be placed perpendicular to the longitudinal axis of the bowel at 2–3-mm intervals to prevent stenosis. For a full-thickness injury, a two-layer closure is typically performed. The mucosa should be closed with running or interrupted 3-0 absorbable sutures, and the seromuscular layer is closed with interrupted Lembert stitches of 3-0 absorbable or silk sutures. If the injury is larger than 1 cm or otherwise complicated, resection and re-anastomosis may be required.

In the large colon, serosal defects and small lacerations can be managed in a similar manner to the small bowel with the addition of prophylactic broad-spectrum antibiotics for 24 h. Colonic injuries that are delayed in recognition may require open repair, washout, and proximal diversion. For both small bowel and large bowel injuries, nasogastric tube placement is not always warranted post repair and early feeding is acceptable.

If gastric injury is discovered, a nasogastric tube should be placed and broad-spectrum antibiotics are initiated. A proton pump inhibitor is also considered. The appropriate surgeon should be notified for primary repair, and most patients may be fed in 1 or 2 days, depending on the nature and degree of injury [14].

Surgical Energy and Thermal Injury

Background

Electrosurgery is widely used in minimally invasive surgery. Electrical energy is converted into heat as the tissue resists the flow of the current, resulting in cutting, desiccation, or fulguration. Thermal injury from these instruments can result from direct contact, direct coupling, capacitive coupling, and/or insulation failure. The incidence of inadvertent electrothermal injuries ranges between 1 and 5 per 1000 surgeries and most commonly affects the bowel [17, 18]. In one study, roughly 26% of bowel injuries during laparoscopic surgery were related to thermal injury [19].

The risk of thermal injury differs by the energy modality due to the difference in thermal spread as summarized below [20–28]:

Energy modality (ESD type)	Working temperature range [°C]	Thermal spread within tissue [mm]
Monopolar	100–400	2–22
Bipolar (conventional)	80–120	2–6
Bipolar (advanced)	60–100	1–7
Ultrasonic	60–200	1–4
Hybrid (bipolar-ultrasonic)	100–220	2–3

The risk of thermal injury also varies by the electrical waveform and the intended tissue effect.

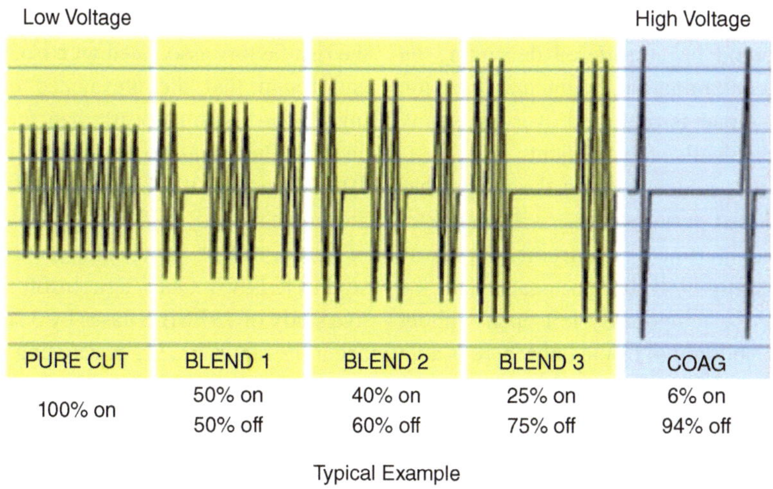

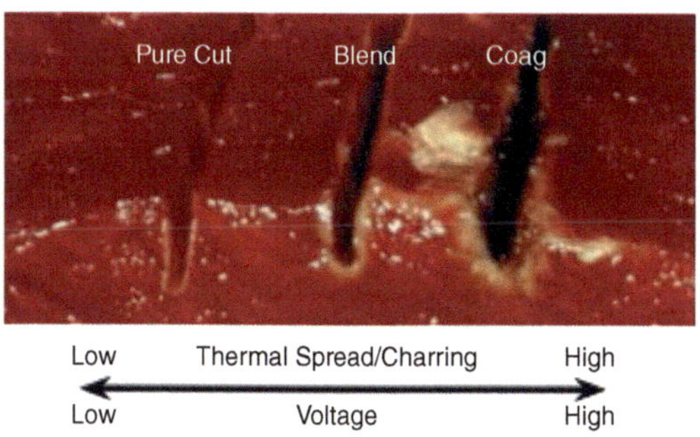

Recognition

Unfortunately, most thermal injuries to the bowel are unrecognized at the time of occurrence. The ileum is most frequently involved. Thermal injury to the bowel typically presents 4–10 days after surgery as compared to direct traumatic perforation, which will typically present within 12–36 h of surgery. A high clinical suspicion is necessary for early diagnosis; delayed diagnosis can result in a fatal outcome.

Common clinical findings include abdominal pain, inability to tolerate oral intake, fever, and even septic shock with altered mental status. Exam findings may include signs of peritonitis such as abdominal distension, guarding, and rebound tenderness.

Management and Prevention

If thermal bowel injury is recognized early, repair may be performed by laparoscopy or mini-laparotomy. Thermal injury from bipolar energy is easier to identify than that resulting from monopolar energy. Superficial, small thermal injuries may be oversewn with one layer of 3-0 absorbable or permanent silk sutures. For significant thermal damage, it is recommended to excise the injured area with at least a 1-cm margin followed by re-anastomosis to prevent subsequent perforation from coagulation necrosis due to thermal spread.

Additionally, delayed and extensive colonic injury may require a diverting colostomy depending on the clinical circumstance. Broad-spectrum antibiotics should also be administered, and drain placement should be considered depending on the extent of contamination. Segmental resection with primary repair is preferred over colostomy in a hemodynamically stable patient.

If recognition is delayed and the patient has already developed peritonitis, there is the risk of abdominal compartment syndrome. In these cases, laparotomy will be necessary and the abdomen may be temporarily left open without closure of the abdominal fascia until there is adequate source control of the infection. Loss of the peritoneal cavity domain is a concern.

Steps to prevent thermal injury have been outlined by Alkatout et al. as below:

1. Inspect insulation carefully.
2. Use the lowest possible power setting.
3. Use a low-voltage waveform (cut).
4. Use brief intermittent activation.
5. Do not activate in open circuit.
6. Do not activate in close proximity or direct contact with another instrument.
7. Use bipolar electrosurgery when appropriate.
8. Select an all-metal cannula system as the safest choice.
9. Utilize available technology (tissue response generator, active electrode monitoring) to eliminate concerns about insulation failure and capacitive coupling.

Incision Site Hernia

Background

The incidence of trocar site hernia ranges from 0.65 to 2.80% and can have early or late onset [29]. Risk factors include an elevated body mass index (BMI), preexisting hernia, wound infection, age, and gender. Early onset occurs within 2 weeks of surgery, involves dehiscence of the fascia and peritoneum, and commonly involves small bowel or omental herniation. Late onset occurs after 2 weeks with dehiscence of the fascial plane and a sac consisting of the peritoneum [29]. The umbilicus is also the most common site for trocar site hernia due to inherent anatomical weakness. A 2011 systematic review evaluated the risk factors associated with trocar site hernias and found that the prevalence of hernia was higher for 12-mm trocars than for 10-mm ones and that there was no difference between 5- and 10-mm trocars [30]. Data for single-incision laparoscopic surgery (SILS) are limited, and the rate of hernia ranges from 2.9% to 8.4% in various studies [31–35]. One single-institution retrospective study of 787 SILS cases by 3 surgeons found a hernia rate of 6.35; preexisting insertion site hernia, age and BMI ≥40 were risk factors, increasing incisional hernia rate to 12.64% and 18.18% respectively.

Recognition

There are more cases of incidentally found trocar site hernias on imaging than symptomatic cases. Symptomatic trocar site hernias will require repair. When there is bowel herniation, patients will often present with nausea, vomiting, and abdominal pain, and timely diagnosis is important to preserve bowel viability. Physical exam may show a nonreducible bulge at the prior trocar site and imaging such as abdominal X-ray or CT can help in the diagnosis.

Management and Prevention

A trocar-related hernia may be repaired laparoscopically or with an open approach by primary anatomical repair or mesh repair. In early-onset hernias, where bowel strangulation can occur, the bowel must be carefully evaluated and resection may be needed if gangrenous segments are present [36–38].

Trocar site herniation is multifactorial, and there are multiple preventative measures. There is a general consensus that the fascia of a 15-mm port should be closed to prevent a trocar site hernia. The closure of 10- and 12-mm port sites is more variable. In bariatric surgery, a prospective observational study and a retrospective study showed that closure of 12-mm epigastric port sites can decrease the trocar site hernia rate by half. Multiple closure techniques have been described, including single stitch, figure-of-eight stitch, and even mesh incorporation, although some of the previously studied mesh materials have now been withdrawn from the market. Unfortunately, midline trocar placement through the avascular linea alba carries a higher hernia rate even if the defect is closed. Trocar type may also contribute to hernia risk as there is some evidence that cutting blades are associated with a higher risk of postoperative hernia.

Considerations for Obesity

Obesity has been increasing worldwide and has tripled since 1975 [39]. In the United States, the obesity prevalence was 41.9% between 2017 and 2020 [40]. Previously, obesity was viewed as a relative contraindication to laparoscopy, especially due to the higher risk of associated comorbidities. However, recent studies have shown that minimally invasive surgery is safe and effective in obese patients and has advantages of shorter hospital stay, less postoperative pain, and fewer wound infections compared to traditional laparotomy [41]. A Swedish prospective study of more than 12,000 women undergoing hysterectomy found that in those with a BMI ≥30, abdominal hysterectomy had a higher overall complication rate compared to robot-assisted laparoscopic hysterectomy. Robot-assisted laparoscopic surgery had a lower rate of conversion to laparotomy compared to traditional laparoscopy as well as lower blood loss compared to abdominal, vaginal, and traditional laparoscopic hysterectomy in women with a BMI ≥30 [42].

Below are the key considerations to ensure safety in performing laparoscopy or robot-assisted laparoscopic surgery in obese patients.

Respiratory Mechanics

Obesity, especially class 3 (BMI ≥40), can lead to reduced functional residual capacity (FRC), lower chest wall compliance, and increased carbon dioxide production in the supine position as well as change in oropharyngeal anatomy [42, 43]. Pneumoperitoneum can also further reduce compliance in obese patients. Therefore, close communication with the anesthesia team will be important to ensure patient safety. Interestingly, pulmonary artery oxygen levels are adversely affected by increasing body weight, but this is not affected by Trendelenburg positioning. Thus, patients who tolerate supine positioning and anesthesia induction will likely tolerate pneumoperitoneum and Trendelenburg positioning [42].

Preoperative Evaluation

Preoperative evaluation should include a thorough history to evaluate for any cardiovascular or respiratory disease, including hypertension, sleep apnea, obstructive pulmonary disease, and peripheral vascular disease. Blood pressure should also be obtained with an appropriately sized blood pressure cuff. Baseline laboratory screening should include complete blood count and basic metabolic panel including creatine and glucose concentration. Preoperative anesthesia consultation is also beneficial to ensure safe surgical planning. An electrocardiogram and chest X-ray may also be recommended in the assessment of cardiopulmonary status.

Positioning

It is important to ensure that the operating table supports the patient's weight and that the table is wide enough to safely tuck the patient's arms by their sides. Table extenders may be used when needed. Appropriately sized stirrups and sequential calf compression devices should be used. To prevent patients from slipping cephalad in the Trendelenburg position, a nonslip mattress or bean bag may be used [44]. It is also important to remember that the umbilicus is not a reliable landmark in obese patients.[7] The panniculus can also be repositioned caudally with tape, clamps, or orthopedic weights to move it out of the way and thin the abdominal wall for placement of trocars.[7]

Trendelenburg Complications

Cardiopulmonary

A steep Trendelenburg position can increase mean arterial pressure due to increased venous return from gravity [45]. This also causes increased cardiac output. However, in a healthy patient, this is not sustained and the cardiac output will return to normal within 10 min. Although Trendelenburg displaces the diaphragm and mediastinal structures caudally, leading to decreased functional residual capacity and lung compliance, changes in lung physiology are affected more by pneumoperitoneum than by Trendelenburg [45].

Ocular Complications

Although no cases of postoperative vision loss have been reported in gynecological surgery, a steep Trendelenburg position can cause vision loss from ischemic optic neuropathy secondary to high venous pressure and interstitial edema that results in decreased blood flow [45].

Peripheral Nerve Injury

A recent meta-analysis has reported an overall peripheral nerve injury rate of 0.16–10.0% from being positioned in lithotomy with steep Trendelenburg [46]. The incidence of upper extremity peripheral nerve injury was 0.1–3.6% and that of lower extremity injury was 0.2–10%. The most commonly affected upper extremity nerves are the brachial plexus, ulnar nerve, median nerve, radial nerve, and humeral nerve. The most at-risk nerves in the lower extremity are the sciatic, femoral, obturator, and femoral cutaneous nerves. One study also found that operations lasting for more than 2 h in lithotomy and steep Trendelenburg position were associated with an increased risk of peripheral nerve injury. Multiple studies have also shown that a higher American Society of Anesthesiologists (ASA) score is also associated with an increased risk of peripheral nerve injury, and only one study showed that a higher BMI was a risk factor [46–49].

References

1. Taskforce for Abdominal Entry. Principles of safe laparoscopic entry. Eur J Obstet Gynecol Reprod Biol. 2016;201:179–88. https://doi.org/10.1016/j.ejogrb.2016.03.040.
2. Jansen FW, Kolkman W, Bakkum EA, de Kroon CD, Trimbos-Kemper TC, Trimbos JB. Complications of laparoscopy: an inquiry about closed- versus open-entry technique. Am J Obstet Gynecol. 2004;190(3):634–8. https://doi.org/10.1016/j.ajog.2003.09.035.
3. Ahmad G, Baker J, Finnerty J, et al. Laparoscopic entry techniques (Review). Cochrane Database Syst Rev. 2019;1(1):CD006583. https://doi.org/10.1002/14651858.CD006583.pub5.
4. la Chapelle CF, Swank HA, Wessels ME, Mol BWJ, Rubinstein SM, Jansen FW. Trocar types in laparoscopy. Cochrane Database Syst Rev. 2015;2015(12):CD009814. https://doi.org/10.1002/14651858.CD009814.pub2.
5. Sandadi S, Johannigman JA, Wong VL, et al. Recognition and Management of Major Vessel Injury during laparoscopy. J Minim Invasive Gynecol. 2010;17(6):692–702. https://doi.org/10.1016/j.jmig.2010.06.005.
6. Ahmed SA, Ali M. Fecal contamination of the peritoneum from laparoscopic trocar injury: a routine operation goes wrong. PSNet. October, 2022. https://psnet.ahrq.gov/web-mm/fecal-contamination-peritoneum-laparoscopic-trocar-injury-routine-operation-goes-wrong.
7. https://www.acog.org/education-and-events/creog/curriculum-resources/-/media/1b0feca92c284445ae1a16ddceda1ec9.ashx.
8. https://wchh.onlinelibrary.wiley.com/doi/pdf/10.1002/tre.188.
9. https://journals.lww.com/journalacs/Abstract/2001/06000/Trocar_Injuries_in_Laparoscopic_Surgery.1.aspx.
10. https://www.sciencedirect.com/science/article/pii/S1553465005002979.
11. Suarez CA. Chapter 12: Vascular complications in laparoscopy. Internet. http://laparoscopy.blogs.com/prevention_management/chapter_12_vascular_surgery. Aug 15, 2009.
12. Watrowski R, Kostov S, Alkatout I. Complications in laparoscopic and robotic-assisted surgery: definitions, classifications, incidence and risk factors - an up-to-date review. Wideochir Inne Tech Maloinwazyjne. 2021;16(3):501–25. https://doi.org/10.5114/wiitm.2021.108800. Epub 2021 Aug 28. PMID: 34691301; PMCID: PMC8512506.

13. van der Voort M, et al. Bowel injury as a complication of laparoscopy. Br J Surg. 2004;91(10):1253–8. https://doi.org/10.1002/bjs.4716.
14. Sigmon DF, Tuma F, Kamel BG, et al. Gastric Perforation. [Updated 2022 Jun 27]. StatPearls [Internet]. Treasure Island, FL: StatPearls Publishing; 2023 Jan. Available from: https://www.ncbi.nlm.nih.gov/books/NBK519554/.
15. https://www.pm360online.com/approaching-intraoperative-bowel-injury/.
16. Park EY, Kwon JY, Kim KJ. Carbon dioxide embolism during laparoscopic surgery. Yonsei Med J. 2012;53(3):459–66. https://doi.org/10.3349/ymj.2012.53.3.459. PMID: 22476987; PMCID: PMC3343430.
17. Alkatout I, Schollmeyer T, Hawaldar N, et al. Principles and safety measures of electosurgery in laparoscopy. J Soc Laparoscop Rob Surg. 2012;16(1):130–9. https://doi.org/10.4293/108680812X13291597716348.
18. Druzijanic N, Pogorelic Z, Perko Z, et al. Comparison of lateral thermal damage of the human peritoneum using monopolar diathermy, harmonic scalpel and LigaSure. Can J Surg. 2012;55(5):317–21.
19. Elbiss H, Abu-Zidian F. Bowel injury following gynecological laparoscopic surgery. Afr Health Sci. 2017;17(4):1237–45. https://www.ncbi.nlm.nih.gov/pmc/articles/PMC5870274/.
20. Kirby R, Arnold F, Challacombe B, et al. Diagnosis and management of bowel injury during laparoscopic surgery. Trend Urol Men Heal. 2011. https://wchh.onlinelibrary.wiley.com/doi/pdf/10.1002/tre.188.
21. https://journals.lww.com/greenjournal/Fulltext/2015/06000/Bowel_Injury_in_Gynecologic_Laparoscopy__A.20.aspx.
22. Brecht L, Wallwiener M, Schott S, Domschke C, Dinkic C, Golatta M, Schuetz F, Fluhr H, Stenzinger A, Kirchner M, Sohn C. Implementation of a novel efficacy score to compare sealing and cutting devices in a porcine model. Surg Endosc. 2018;32(2):1002–11.
23. Hefermehl LJ, Largo RA, Hermanns T, Poyet C, Sulser T, Eberli D. Lateral temperature spread of monopolar, bipolar and ultrasonic instruments for robot-assisted laparoscopic surgery. BJU Int. 2014;114(2):245–52.
24. Carus T, Rackebrandt K. Collateral tissue damage by several types of coagulation (monopolar, bipolar, cold plasma and ultrasonic) in a minimally invasive, perfused liver model. ISRN Surg. 2011;2011:518924.
25. Sutton PA, Awad S, Perkins AC, Lobo DN. Comparison of lateral thermal spread using monopolar and bipolar diathermy, the Harmonic Scalpel™ and the Ligasure™. J Br Surg. 2010;97(3):428–33.
26. https://www.asit.org/assets/documents/Prinicpals_in_electrosurgery.pdf.
27. Kobylianskii A, Zakhari A, Bougie O, et al. Bowel complications in laparoscopic gynecologic surgery. J Obstet Gynaecol Can. 2021;5(43):673. https://doi.org/10.1016/j.jogc.2021.02.082.
28. Karadag M, Cecen K, Demir A, Bagcioglu M, Kocaaslan R, Kadioglu T. Gastrointestinal complications of laparoscopic/robot-assisted urologic surgery and a review of the literature. J Clin Med Res NA. 2015;7(4):203–10. Available at: https://www.jocmr.org/index.php/JOCMR/article/view/2090/1015.
29. Rao P, Ghosh K, Sudhan D. Port site hernia: a rare complication of laparoscopy. Med J Armed Forces India. 2008;64(2):187–8. https://doi.org/10.1016/S0377-1237(08)80081-0. Epub 2011 Jul 21. PMID: 27408134; PMCID: PMC4921558. https://www.ncbi.nlm.nih.gov/pmc/articles/PMC4921558/.
30. Swank HA, et al. Systematic review of trocar-site hernia. Br J Surg. 2012;99(3):315–23. https://doi.org/10.1002/bjs.7836.
31. Tonouchi H, Ohmori Y, Kobayashi M, Kusunoki M. Trocar site hernia. Arch Surg. 2004;139(11):1248–56. https://doi.org/10.1001/archsurg.139.11.1248. https://jamanetwork.com/journals/jamasurgery/fullarticle/397584.
32. den Hartog FPJ, van Egmond S, Poelman MM, Menon AG, Kleinrensink G-J, Lange JF, et al. The incidence of extraction site incisional hernia after minimally invasive colorectal surgery: a systematic review and meta-analysis. Color Dis. 2023;25:586–99. https://doi.org/10.1111/codi.16455. https://onlinelibrary.wiley.com/doi/10.1111/codi.16455.
33. Yamamoto M, Minikel L, Zaritsky E. Laparoscopic 5-mm trocar site herniation and literature review. JSLS. 2011;15(1):122–6. https://doi.org/10.4293/108680811X13022985131697. PMID: 21902958; PMCID: PMC3134687.
34. Buckley FP, Vassaur HE, Jupiter DC, et al. Influencing factors for port-site hernias after single-incision laparoscopy. Hernia. 2016;20:729–33. https://doi.org/10.1007/s10029-016-1512-8.
35. Antoniou SA, García-Alamino JM, Hajibandeh S, et al. Single-incision surgery trocar-site hernia: an updated systematic review meta-analysis with trial sequential analysis by the minimally invasive surgery synthesis of interventions outcomes network (MISSION). Surg Endosc. 2018;32:14–23. https://doi.org/10.1007/s00464-017-5717-4.
36. https://www.frontierspartnerships.org/articles/10.3389/jaws.2022.11034/full.
37. Pulle MH, Siddartha R, Dey A, et al. Port site hernia in laparoscopic surgery: mechanism, prevention and management. Curr Med Res Prac. 2010;5(3):130–7. https://doi.org/10.1016/j.cmrp.2015.05.008.
38. Sıkar HE, Çetin K. Laparoscopic repair of lateral sided trocar site hernias. Turk J Surg. 2020;36(3):278–83. https://doi.org/10.47717/turkjsurg.2020.4447. PMID: 33778383; PMCID: PMC7963324.
39. https://www.who.int/news-room/fact-sheets/detail/obesity-and-overweight.
40. https://www.cdc.gov/obesity/data/adult.html.
41. Afors K, Centini G, Murtada R, et al. Obesity in laparoscopic surgery. Best Pract Res Clin Obstet Gynaecol. 2015;29(4):554–64. https://doi.org/10.1016/j.bpobgyn.2015.02.001.
42. https://www-clinicalkey-com.mlprox.csmc.edu/#!/content/playContent/1-s2.0-S1553465020302272?returnurl=null&referrer=null.

43. https://doi.org/10.1016/j.ajog.2004.05.077.
44. https://link-springer-com.mlprox.csmc.edu/article/10.1007/s00404-014-3600-2.
45. Arvizo C, Mehta ST, Yunker A. Adverse events related to Trendelenburg position during laparoscopic surgery: recommendations and review of the literature. Curr Opin Obstetr Gynecol. 2018;30(4):272–8. https://doi.org/10.1097/GCO.0000000000000471.
46. Bjøro B, Mykkeltveit I, Rustøen T, Candas Altinbas B, Røise O, Bentsen SB. Intraoperative peripheral nerve injury related to lithotomy positioning with steep Trendelenburg in patients undergoing robotic-assisted laparoscopic surgery—a systematic review. J Adv Nurs. 2020;76:490–503. https://doi.org/10.1111/jan.14271.
47. Souki FG, Rodriguez-Blanco YF, Polu SR, Eber S, Candiotti KA. Survey of anesthesiologists' practices related to steep Trendelenburg positioning in the USA. BMC Anesthesiol. 2018;18(1):117. https://doi.org/10.1186/s12871-018-0578-5. PMID: 30131061; PMCID: PMC6104011
48. Katayama S, Mori K, Pradere B, et al. Influence of steep Trendelenburg position on postoperative complications: a systematic review and meta-analysis. J Robotic Surg. 2022;16:1233–47. https://doi.org/10.1007/s11701-021-01361-x.
49. https://ales.amegroups.com/article/view/5380/pdf.

24 Composite Pelvic Resection for Deeply Infiltrating Endometriosis

Aparna R. Ramanathan, Rebecca E. Thompson, Elissa Trieu, and Vadim Morozov

Background

Endometriosis is a chronic gynecologic condition associated with chronic pelvic pain and infertility and affects approximately 6–10% of women of reproductive age [1]. It is characterized by endometrial tissue outside the uterus, which can invade various organs and structures. Its pathophysiology is still under investigation but is likely a combination of retrograde menstruation, immune dysfunction, and coelomic metaplasia, amongst other contributing factors. Endometriosis may be difficult to diagnose as symptoms vary per individual. Common clinical presentations include pelvic pain, dysmenorrhea, dyspareunia, and infertility. Endometrial implants trigger an inflammatory response, which can cause pain, adhesions, dyspareunia, and infertility. Symptoms often depend on the location of the endometrial implants.

Deep infiltrating endometriosis (DIE) is a form of endometriosis that involves the infiltration of endometrial tissue more than 5 mm below the peritoneum [2]. The lesions can range in size from small nodules to large masses that can distort the shape and function of the affected organ. In severe cases, DIE can lead to the formation of adhesions and scarring and retroperitoneal fibrosis, which can further impact organ function.

Diagnosis

The diagnosis of endometriosis can be challenging and often requires a combination of clinical evaluation, imaging studies, and surgical confirmation. There is no unique laboratory finding. Initial evaluation via a thorough history and physical examination may suggest endometriosis. Imaging via ultrasonography, magnetic resonance imaging (MRI), and computed tomography (CT) can help detect pelvic masses such as endometriomas. On ultrasound, endometriotic lesions appear hypoechoic and an endometrioma appears as a unilocular cyst with internal low-level echoes and a homogeneous "ground-glass" appearance [3]. Endometriotic lesions may be difficult to see and generally require specialized review [4]. On MRI, endometriosis is associated with DIE T2 hypointensity [5]. Intraoperatively, superficial

A. R. Ramanathan · R. E. Thompson
Obstetrics and Gynecology, Division of Minimally Invasive Gynecologic Surgery, MedStar Washington Hospital Center, Washington, DC, USA
e-mail: Aparna.R.Ramanathan@medstar.net; Rebecca.E.Thompson@medstar.net

E. Trieu
Obstetrics & Gynecology, Washington Hospital Center, Washington, DC, USA

V. Morozov (✉)
Obstetrics and Gynecology, MedStar Washington Hospital Center/Georgetown University School of Medicine, Washington, DC, USA
e-mail: Vadim.morozov@medsatr.net

M. Hoffman et al. (eds.), *Major Complications of Female Pelvic Surgery*,
https://doi.org/10.1007/978-3-031-66772-5_24

implants can have a wide range of characteristics, including "powder burn" lesions, white opacifications, and translucent blebs. The definitive diagnosis of endometriosis can only be made surgically via visualization or biopsy.

Treatment

Initial treatment depends on the patients' symptoms and goals. Patients can opt for expectant management if asymptomatic. Nonsurgical options include a combination of nonsteroidal anti-inflammatory drugs and hormonal suppression via progestins, gonadotropin-releasing hormone agonists, or gonadotropin-releasing hormone antagonists. If ineffective, further treatment involves surgical resection. The risk of endometriosis recurrence after surgery based on symptoms is up to 21.5% at 2 years and 40–50% at 5 years [6].

Goals of Treatment

Surgical excision of endometriosis has traditionally had three main goals: improvement in sexual function, pain, and infertility. It is widely known that DIE reduces quality of life and sexual function [8]. Improvement after surgical resection has been shown in several studies. Prospective studies showed improvement in sexual function after resection of DIE comparable to women without endometriosis at 6 and 36 months postoperatively [8–10]. These data were also supported in a systematic review [11]. Surgical excision itself can worsen sexual function if care is not taken when performing nerve-sparing techniques [7].

Pain is the central symptom of endometriosis [12, 13]. Although defining the best surgical treatment of endometriosis-related pain remains controversial, pain relief after surgery has been reported to be excellent [14]. In a prospective study of 981 women, improvement in pain after laparoscopic excision of endometriosis was shown to be significant over 36 months after surgery [13].

DIE does impact fertility, although the data are poor with regard to determining whether surgical excision of DIE improves fertility rates [15]. A systematic review which examined 29 studies reporting outcomes in 2730 women suggested that spontaneous fertility rates were high after DIE excision that did not involve the bowel and low spontaneous overall fertility rates after DIE excision with bowel involvement, suggesting a role for assisted reproductive technology in these patients [16].

The General Surgical Approach

In general, fertility-sparing surgery can be performed for excision of endometriosis. In those with significant symptoms and not desiring fertility, the risks and benefits of total laparoscopic hysterectomy and bilateral salpingectomy should be discussed. Postoperative hormonal suppression to prevent recurrence of symptoms should also be addressed [13].

Laparoscopic excision with or without robotic assistance is the preferred surgical approach. In our practice, we place higher and more medial ports (one-third of the distance between the anterior superior iliac spine (ASIS) and umbilicus) to facilitate excision of endometriosis along the pelvic sidewall. A 30-degree laparoscope can be used for improved visualization of these lateral lesions. The ovaries and uterus must be lifted from the surgical field for clear visualization of potential lesions in the posterior compartment. Ovariopexy to the round ligament or pelvic sidewall is routinely performed, and we use a uterine manipulator to elevate the uterus from the surgical field. Uteropexy to the anterior wall has also been described [17].

Nerve-Sparing Surgery

The nerves of the pelvic plexus run in close proximity to the uterosacral ligament and ureter and are at risk of injury during dissection for excision of endometriosis. Iatrogenic injury to these nerves can cause lifelong debilitating injury to the urinary or gastrointestinal systems, which cannot be repaired. Care must be taken when performing nerve-sparing techniques during endometriosis excision, with dissection of the connective tissue and separation of the nerves and surrounding fascia from the underlying peritoneum and endometriotic lesions [18, 19].

Approach to Urologic Endometriosis

Urinary tract involvement by endometriosis is a rare occurrence, affecting only 1–2% of women with endometriosis [20]. This number may be underreported. The symptomatology of urinary tract endometriosis varies based on the location of the endometriotic lesions, and diagnosis is often challenging due to the complexity of symptoms and difficulty in identifying lesions through imaging studies. The distribution of bladder to ureteral to urethral endometriosis follows a ratio of 40:5:1 [21].

Bladder Endometriosis

Diagnosis

Bladder involvement by endometriosis typically presents with urinary frequency, hematuria, and dysuria (symptoms similar to urinary tract infection). A high level of suspicion is prudent. MRI and ultrasound can be useful for visualizing lesions above 3 cm [22]. Cystoscopy and intravenous pyelogram (IVP) are good adjuvant studies.

Treatment

The treatment of bladder endometriosis involves both medical and surgical evaluation. In cases where lesions are situated near the trigone, medical management is typically indicated to avoid postoperative morbidity related to bladder neck surgery [23]. If the detrusor muscle is affected, the condition is more likely to be an endometrioma of the bladder [23] and resection is the preferred surgical treatment option.

Resection of bladder endometriosis can be performed via a combination of laparoscopic and cystoscopic techniques to excise deep bladder endometriosis without removal of the normal bladder tissue. The lesion can be visualized cystoscopically to better define its margins. Via laparoscopy, the medial and lateral paravesical spaces can be taken down and the vesicouterine space should be dissected to allow for adequate bladder visualization [24]. Dissection should then be carried out through the layers of the bladder [25]. Closure of the resection site can be achieved with one or two layers of either barbed or monofilament sutures [23]. The healing process is typically uncomplicated due to the vascularity of the area. Complications include leakage, fistula formation, and bleeding. Complications of bladder resection are covered in detail in Chap. 12. Rates of bladder recurrence are low: 2% at 12 months and 4% at 24 months [24].

Ureteral Endometriosis (UE)

Diagnosis

Ureteral endometriosis (UE) often affects the distal portion of the ureter, more commonly the left side [26]. It can be either extrinsic or intrinsic, with a ratio of 1:4 [27]. Extrinsic disease is caused by endometriosis that compresses the ureter, whether it is from peritoneal adhesions overlying the ureter or a large endometrioma. Intrinsic endometriosis involves invasion of the ureteral muscular or uroepithelial layer. Diagnosis of ureteral endometriosis is frequently delayed, and most women do not present until they experience silent renal failure [20]. Some patients have cyclic hematuria or cyclic colicky flank pain [28].

Imaging studies can be useful in assisting to visualize any obstruction or narrowing caused by an endometriotic lesion. Ultrasound has difficulty visualizing endometriosis in the ureter, but it can identify hydronephrosis. Magnetic resonance imaging (MRI) and computed tomography (CT) scans can also be helpful in identifying ureteral endometriosis. Retrograde pyelography or intravenous pyelogram are useful to identify the degree and level of ureteral involvement [23]. In some cases, ureteroscopy may be necessary to confirm the diagnosis and obtain a tissue sample for histological analysis.

Treatment

Treatment is focused on relieving the obstruction, improving symptoms, and addressing any renal dysfunction. Similar to endometriosis in other locations, UE can be treated via hormonal suppression or surgical resection. Hormonal suppression is risky as endometriosis is a progressive disease. If there are signs of obstruction, surgical treatment is the most appropriate management.

The goal of surgery is to remove any ureteral obstruction. Laparoscopy is the recommended approach. Ureteral stents are not necessary prior to starting the procedure and have not been shown to improve outcomes [29]. Resection of extrinsic endometriosis involves ureterolysis. Ureterolysis alone is useful to treat approximately 90% of cases of hydroureter [30]. There are multiple techniques for ureterolysis, with the overlying goal being to free the intact ureter from any fibrotic tissue and restore normal anatomy.

Intrinsic ureteral disease can impact all layers of the ureter, including the muscularis, lamina propria, and ureteral lumen. Intrinsic disease is more likely with deep infiltrating endometriosis. Treatment necessitates resecting the involved segment and, then, depending on the location of the resection, performing a primary ureteroureterostomy or ureteroneocystostomy with or without a psoas hitch [21]. This often requires a multidisciplinary approach.

While there is a risk of recurrence, a conservative ureter-sparing approach is preferred. Half of patients who presented with hydronephrosis preoperatively showed improvement after ureterolysis and ureteral preservation [30]. Untreated UE can lead to ureteral compression, hydroureter, hydronephrosis, and, ultimately, loss of kidney function.

The overall complication rates are low, occurring in 1–5% of patients [30]. Major postoperative complications include ureteral fistula or stenosis, hemorrhage, anastomotic bowel leakage, bowel perforation, bowel atony, and vesicovaginal fistula. Ureteral and bladder complications are covered in detail in Chaps. 17 and 12. Approximately 4% needed reoperation for endometriosis recurrence or persistence [30].

Ureteral Complications

Complications can occur from deep endometriosis resection in the genitourinary (GU) system. Endometriosis is a risk factor for ureteral injury. DIE is a benign but infiltrating pelvic disease. The ureters are frequently densely adherent to the affected endometriotic tissues and are occasionally encased or even infiltrated themselves. Surgical expiration of DIE therefore commonly requires extensive ureterolysis and, occasionally, purposeful ureteral resection. Expected ureteral complications include leak, fistulas, or strictures. Other risk factors include prior surgery, history of pelvic inflammatory disease, history of pelvic radiation, and ureteral duplication [35]. It is important to diagnose ureteral and bladder injuries intraoperatively as this leads to improved outcomes [35]. Overall, intraoperative complications are rare [30]. Complications include hemorrhage requiring conversion, visceral injury, and ureteral injury. Postoperative injuries occur in as many as 16% of women treated for ureteral endometriosis, significantly less in women treated for bladder endometriosis [20]. Injuries include ureteral injury, ureteral strictures, ureteral fistulas, and bladder dysfunction [20]. There is also the risk of endometriosis recurrence: the need for reoperation is 3.9%.

In order to avoid complications, a multidisciplinary team is crucial in respect to management of GU endometriosis. This includes a gynecologist, a urologist, and a gastrointestinal surgeon when the digestive tract is involved. Careful dissection must be undertaken near the ureters and bladder to avoid excessive denervation or thermal injury. Careful technique with surgical exposure of the pelvic retroperitoneum is important toward preventing ureteral injury [35]. Knowledge regarding the ureteral course and measures such as adequate mobilization, ureteral tracing, and avoidance of blind clamping for hemostasis can assist in avoiding injury [36]. After resection, a cystoscopy can be performed to evaluate the bladder and ureteral jets. If ureteral jets are not visualized, an intraoperative intravenous pyelogram or retrograde pyelogram with possible ureteral stent placement is indicated next. A cystoscopy can detect most bladder injuries and up to 80–90% of ureteral injuries. It is important to recog-

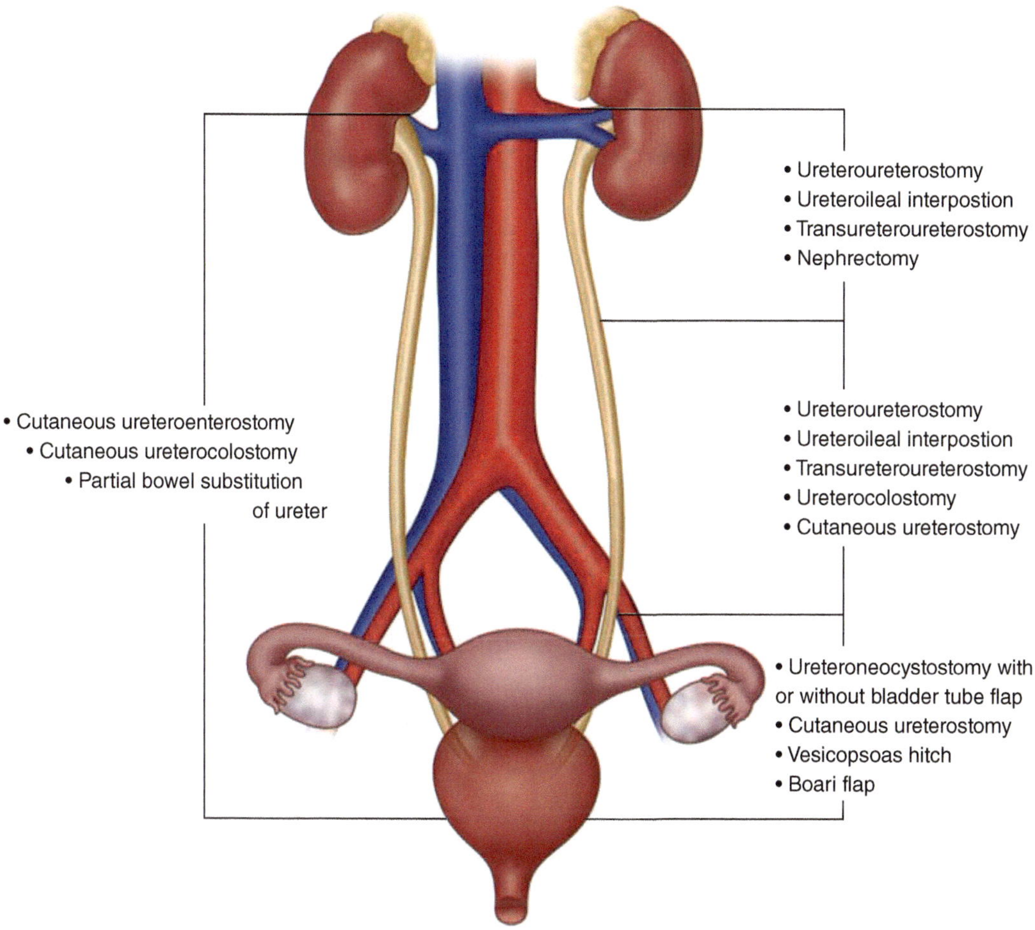

Fig. 24.1 Ureteral injury

nize injury of the ureter intraoperatively. The surgeon must maintain a high level of vigilance during any steps of an operation that are in close proximity to the ureter, as injury can be most easily recognized the moment it happens. Upon completion of the case, inspection of the operative field includes examination for possible ureteral injury. This may be facilitated by an intravenous injection of fluorescein dye to look for a leak, an intravenous injection of ICG to evaluate the integrity of the blood supply, and cystoscopy. Ureteral injuries caused by a postoperative swelling of nonocclusive suture ligatures and thermal injuries can be missed [34].

The surgeon operating on DIE must have thorough knowledge of the normal course of the ureters as well as the effect of DIE on the ureteral anatomy. Resection of DIE must often begin with extensive ureterolysis, which must be meticulous and gentle in order to avoid direct injury, loss of adventitia, and occult thermal damage. Ureteral stents have a controversial role and may even be detrimental as they stiffen the ureter which may predispose to stripping of adventitia. Use of indocyanine green (ICG) dye with a near infrared camera is a good alternative. When ureteral resection is necessary for the management of DIE, prevention of complications is based on an appropriately selected and performed ureteral reconstruction (see Chap. 17). For a ureteral injury, repair depends on the location (Fig. 24.1). This can include ureteroureterostomy, primary closure, or ureteroneocystostomy. Generally, ureteral injuries at the pelvic brim can be managed with an end-to-end anastomosis around a ureteric stent. The principle involves ureteral mobilization, resection of the nonviable tissue, and then a tension-free anastomosis [38]. Depending on the length and integrity of the distal segment, the injury can be repaired with either an end-to-end anastomosis or a Boari flap for ureteric reimplantation [36]. Management of ureteral injury is covered in detail in Chap. 17.

For bladder injury, repair depends on the grade of the injury. Surgical management includes repair with Polyglactin 910 in one or two layers, depending on the size of the defect [37], followed by an indwelling catheter.

Endometriosis is a risk factor for ureteral and bladder injury. Careful dissection is important to help avoid injury. Intraoperative diagnosis of injury leads to improved outcomes.

Approach to Gastrointestinal Endometriosis

Diagnosis

Endometriosis of the bowel affects 3.8–37% of patients and can be a superficial disease on the bowel serosa or a deeply infiltrative disease within the muscularis or mucosa. Common symptoms include dysmenorrhea, deep dyspareunia, chronic pain, and/or dyschezia [31]. Physical exam can be helpful with typical findings including palpable nodules or thickened areas along the uterosacral ligaments on rectovaginal exam. If the exam is performed during menstruation, lesions may be more inflamed, tender, and palpable. A speculum exam may reveal a blackish-blue lesion [32].

Several imaging modalities may be used to visualize endometriosis of the bowel, including transvaginal ultrasonography, rectal water contrast transvaginal ultrasonography, rectal endoscopic sonography, MRI, and double barium contrast enema. In our practice, MRI is typically used which has the benefit of being easily accessible by patients and providing information about lesions above the sigmoid colon. It can lack sensitivity in determining the depth of invasion of lesions [23]. In our practice, such images are often reviewed at a multidisciplinary conference involving radiologists and minimally invasive gynecologic surgeons to discuss lesion characteristics and the treatment plan.

Surgical Treatment

Surgical resection of these bowel lesions also benefits from a multidisciplinary approach. Typically, a minimally invasive trained gynecologic surgeon and a colorectal surgeon experienced in endometriosis should be involved. We recommend laparoscopic excision with or without robotic assistance for its superior outcomes when compared with an open approach.

There are three surgical options with regard to excision of bowel endometriosis (Fig. 24.2): superficial shaving, disc resection, and segmental resection of the rectosigmoid colon. The choice of technique has been the subject of extensive debate. Considerations should include the location of the bowel lesion, depth of infiltration, number of nodules, and the presence or absence of strictures. Some would argue that a more extensive excision with segmental resection translates to less residual disease and a lower risk of recurrence; however, even with radical excision, occult endometriosis has been shown to be present in the resection margins in up to 15% of patients [33]. We opt for a more conservative approach to minimize the risks of neurologic injury and long-term morbidity.

Shaving Excision

Shaving excision is the most conservative form of surgical management. With shaving excision, diseased tissue is removed layer by layer until healthy underlying tissue is reached. The aim is to remove the majority of endometriosis while preserving bowel integrity. Complication rates with this technique are low with good long-term outcomes reported [23].

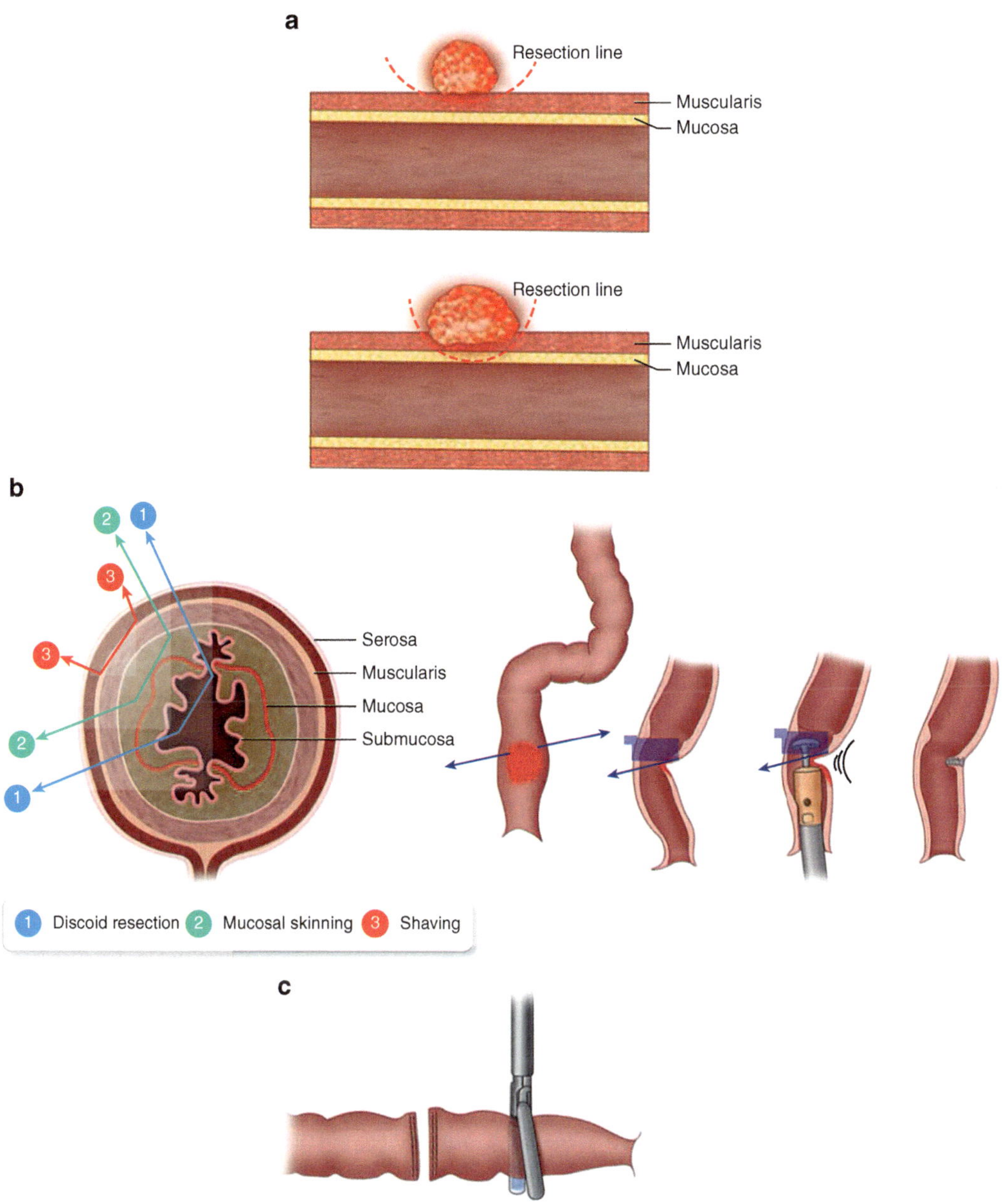

Fig. 24.2 Superficial shaving, disc resection, and segmental resection of the recto-sigmoid colon

Laparoscopic Disk Excision

Laparoscopic disk excision can be used to excise full-thickness bowel lesions that are limited to less than 50% of the circumference of the bowel. The resultant defect is stapled or sutured. Outcomes are good, and complication rates are lower than those of segmental resection [23].

Segmental Resection

Segmental resection involves complete resection of the segment of bowel containing endometriotic disease. Primary or end-to-end anastomosis of the bowel can be performed following excision. It is generally avoided when possible due to higher rates of serious complications, including anastomotic leak and anastomotic stricture [23]. Complications of bowel resection are covered in multiple other chapters.

Bowel Complications

The estimated rate of bowel injury during surgery for endometriosis is 3–5/1000 cases [19]. When resection of DIE nodules is undertaken, bowel complication rates range from 2 to 3%. Laparoscopic excision of bowel endometriosis has been associated with multiple intestinal complications, including bowel anastomotic dehiscence, rectovaginal fistula, anastomotic bleeding, intra-abdominal and wound infection, bowel stricture, intestinal obstruction, chronic constipation, and diarrhea. These complications may happen in the immediate postoperative period or later. Early recognition is fundamental to decreasing morbidity and mortality [39].

Contributing factors to bowel injury include laparoscopic entry, electrosurgery, and injury from grasping forceps or scissors. Approximately 40% of injuries are not recognized at the time of surgery [40].

Preoperatively, nutritional deficiencies should be corrected as patients with low albumin and low total protein are at a higher risk of anastomotic leaks. The evidence for or against mechanical bowel preparation is unclear. Prophylactic antibiotics prior to elective gastrointestinal surgery have been shown to decrease the rate of wound infection. Most bowel injuries can be repaired primarily in one or two layers. Intraoperatively, rectosigmoid integrity testing with air ("bubble" or "flat tire" test) in a fluid-filled abdomen can help in the early diagnosis of a leak [39].

Conclusions

Endometriosis is a complex disease that can be difficult to diagnose and causes significant morbidity. It can affect multiple organ systems, and surgical excision requires careful planning with consideration of a multidisciplinary approach. With knowledge of the pelvic anatomy and the distortions caused by DIE, as well as sound surgical judgment and technique, the likelihood of major complications can be reduced.

References

1. Practice bulletin no. 114: management of endometriosis. 2010;116:223–36. https://doi.org/10.1097/aog.0b013e3181e8b073.
2. De Cicco C, Corona R, Schonman R, et al. Bowel resection for deep endometriosis: a systematic review. BJOG. 2011;118:285–91. https://doi.org/10.1111/j.1471-0528.2010.02744.x.
3. Van Holsbeke C, Van Calster B, Guerriero S, et al. Endometriomas: their ultrasound characteristics. Ultrasound Obstet Gynecol. 2010;35(6):730–40. https://doi.org/10.1002/uog.7668.
4. Quesada J, Härmä K, Reid S, et al. Endometriosis: a multimodal imaging review. Eur J Radiol. 2023;158:110610. https://doi.org/10.1016/j.ejrad.2022.110610.
5. Bazot M, Daraï E. Diagnosis of deep endometriosis: clinical examination, ultrasonography, magnetic resonance imaging, and other techniques. Fertil Steril. 2017;108:886–94. https://doi.org/10.1016/j.fertnstert.2017.10.026.
6. Guo S-W. Recurrence of endometriosis and its control. Hum Reprod Update. 2009;15:441–61. https://doi.org/10.1093/humupd/dmp007.
7. Ianieri MM, Raimondo D, Rosati A, et al. Impact of nerve-sparing posterolateral parametrial excision for deep infiltrating endometriosis on postoperative bowel, urinary, and sexual function. Intl J Gynecol Obstet. 2022;159:152–9. https://doi.org/10.1002/ijgo.14089.
8. Di Donato N, Montanari G, Benfenati A, et al. Sexual function in women undergoing surgery for deep infiltrating endometriosis: a comparison with healthy women. J Fam Plann Reprod Health Care. 2015;41:278–83. https://doi.org/10.1136/jfprhc-2014-100993.
9. Pluchino N, Wenger J-M, Petignat P, et al. Sexual function in endometriosis patients and their partners: effect of the disease and consequences of treatment. Hum Reprod Update. 2016;22:762–74. https://doi.org/10.1093/humupd/dmw031.
10. Martínez-Zamora M-A, Coloma JL, Gracia M, et al. Long-term follow-up of sexual quality of life after laparoscopic surgery in patients with deep infiltrating endometriosis. J Minim Invasive Gynecol. 2021;28:1912–9. https://doi.org/10.1016/j.jmig.2021.04.023.
11. Franck C, Poulsen MH, Karampas G, et al. Questionnaire-based evaluation of sexual life after laparoscopic surgery for endometriosis: a systematic

review of prospective studies. Acta Obstet Gynecol Scand. 2018;97:1091–104. https://doi.org/10.1111/aogs.13369.
12. Morotti M, Vincent K, Becker CM. Mechanisms of pain in endometriosis. Eur J Obstet Gynecol Reprod Biol. 2017;209:8–13. https://doi.org/10.1016/j.ejogrb.2016.07.497.
13. Nezhat C, Vang N, Tanaka PP, Nezhat C. Optimal Management of Endometriosis and Pain. Obstet Gynecol. 2019;134:834–9. https://doi.org/10.1097/aog.0000000000003461.
14. Koninckx PR, Ussia A, Adamyan L, et al. Deep endometriosis: definition, diagnosis, and treatment. Fertil Steril. 2012;98:564–71. https://doi.org/10.1016/j.fertnstert.2012.07.1061.
15. Bafort C, Beebeejaun Y, Tomassetti C, et al. Laparoscopic surgery for endometriosis. 2020;2020(10):CD011031. https://doi.org/10.1002/14651858.cd011031.pub3.
16. Cohen J, Thomin A, Mathieu D'Argent E, et al. Fertility before and after surgery for deep infiltrating endometriosis with and without bowel involvement: a literature review. Minerva Ginecol. 2014;66:575–87.
17. Delara R, Wasson M. Temporary oophoropexy and uteropexy during gynecologic surgery. Am J Obstet Gynecol. 2020;223:279–80. https://doi.org/10.1016/j.ajog.2020.04.027.
18. Kahno K, Andou M, Aiko K, et al. Fertility- and nerve-sparing laparoscopic eradication of deep endometriosis with total posterior compartment peritonectomy: the Kurashiki method. J Minim Invasive Gynecol. 2021;28:170–1. https://doi.org/10.1016/j.jmig.2020.05.028.
19. Nezhat C, Li A, Falik R, et al. Bowel endometriosis: diagnosis and management. Am J Obstet Gynecol. 2018;218:549–62. https://doi.org/10.1016/j.ajog.2017.09.023.
20. Darwish B, Stochino-Loi E, Pasquier G, et al. Surgical outcomes of urinary tract deep infiltrating endometriosis. J Minim Invasive Gynecol. 2017;24:998–1006. https://doi.org/10.1016/j.jmig.2017.06.005.
21. Yohannes P. Ureteral Endometriosis. J Urol. 2003;170:20–5. https://doi.org/10.1097/01.ju.0000054836.32660.9e.
22. Kołodziej A, Krajewski W, Dołowy L, et al. Urinary tract endometriosis. Urol J. 2015;12:2213–7. https://doi.org/10.22037/uj.v12i4.2838.
23. Nezhat C, Falik R, McKinney S, King LP. Pathophysiology and management of urinary tract endometriosis. Nat Rev Urol. 2017;14:359–72. https://doi.org/10.1038/nrurol.2017.58.
24. Ceccaroni M, Clarizia R, Ceccarello M, et al. Total laparoscopic bladder resection in the management of deep endometriosis: "take it or leave it." Radicality versus persistence. Int Urogynecol J. 2020;31:1683–90. https://doi.org/10.1007/s00192-019-04107-4.
25. Guan Z, Soni SD, Zhou J, et al. Cystoscopic-guided robotic resection of bladder trigone endometriosis nodule with ureteral preservation. J Minim Invasive Gynecol. 2022;29:930–1. https://doi.org/10.1016/j.jmig.2022.05.012.
26. Cunha FLD, Arcoverde FVL, Andres MP, et al. Laparoscopic treatment of ureteral endometriosis: a systematic review. J Minim Invasive Gynecol. 2021;28:779–87. https://doi.org/10.1016/j.jmig.2020.11.022.
27. Bosev D, Nicoll LM, Bhagan L, et al. Laparoscopic management of ureteral endometriosis: the Stanford University Hospital experience with 96 consecutive cases. J Urol. 2009;182:2748–52. https://doi.org/10.1016/j.juro.2009.08.019.
28. Gustilo-Ashby AM, Paraiso MFR. Treatment of urinary tract endometriosis. J Minim Invasive Gynecol. 2006;13:559–65. https://doi.org/10.1016/j.jmig.2006.07.012.
29. Piriyev E, Schiermeier S, Römer T. Are double-J stents in surgery for deep infiltrating endometriosis always necessary? A retrospective analysis. Wideochir Inne Tech Maloinwazyjne. 2022;17:533–9. https://doi.org/10.5114/wiitm.2022.116325.
30. Cavaco-Gomes J, Martinho M, Gilabert-Aguilar J, Gilabert-Estélles J. Laparoscopic management of ureteral endometriosis: a systematic review. Eur J Obstet Gynecol Reprod Biol. 2017;210:94–101. https://doi.org/10.1016/j.ejogrb.2016.12.011.
31. Stratton P, Berkley KJ. Chronic pelvic pain and endometriosis: translational evidence of the relationship and implications. Hum Reprod Update. 2011;17:327–46. https://doi.org/10.1093/humupd/dmq050.
32. Alabiso G, Alio L, Arena S, et al. How to manage bowel endometriosis: the ETIC approach. J Minim Invasive Gynecol. 2015;22:517–29. https://doi.org/10.1016/j.jmig.2015.01.021.
33. Roman H, Hennetier C, Darwish B, et al. Bowel occult microscopic endometriosis in resection margins in deep colorectal endometriosis specimens has no impact on short-term postoperative outcomes. Fertil Steril. 2016;105:423–429.e7. https://doi.org/10.1016/j.fertnstert.2015.09.030.
34. AAGL Advancing Minimally Invasive Gynecology Worldwide. AAGL practice report: practice guidelines for intraoperative cystoscopy in laparoscopic hysterectomy. J Minim Invasive Gynecol. 2012;19(4):407–11. https://doi.org/10.1016/j.jmig.2012.05.001. PMID: 22748947.
35. Park JH, Park JW, Song K, Jo MK. Ureteral injury in gynecologic surgery: a 5-year review in a community hospital. Korean. J Urol. 2012;53(2):120–5. https://doi.org/10.4111/kju.2012.53.2.120. Epub 2012 Feb 20. PMID: 22379592; PMCID: PMC3285707.
36. Sakellariou P, Protopapas AG, Voulgaris Z, Kyritsis N, Rodolakis A, Vlachos G, Diakomanolis E, Michalas S. Management of ureteric injuries during gynecological operations: 10 years experience. Eur J Obstet Gynecol Reprod Biol. 2002;101(2):179–84. https://doi.org/10.1016/s0301-2115(01)00521-8. PMID: 11858895.

37. Zelivianskaia AS, Bradley SE, Morozov VV. Best practices for repair of iatrogenic bladder injury. AJOG Glob Rep. 2022;2(3):100062. https://doi.org/10.1016/j.xagr.2022.100062. PMID: 36276798; PMCID: PMC9563547.
38. Elliott SP, McAninch JW. Ureteral injuries: external and iatrogenic. Urol Clin North Am. 2006;33(1):55–66, vi. https://doi.org/10.1016/j.ucl.2005.11.005. PMID: 16488280.
39. Oliveira MAP, Pereira TRD, Gilbert A, Tulandi T, De Oliveira HC, De Wilde RL. Bowel complications in endometriosis surgery. Best Pract Res Clin Obstet Gynaecol. 2016;35:51–62. https://pubmed.ncbi.nlm.nih.gov/26694586/.
40. Llarena NC, Shah AB, Milad MP. Bowel injury in gynecologic laparoscopy: a systematic review. Obstet Gynecol. 2015;125(6):1407e17. https://pubmed.ncbi.nlm.nih.gov/26000512/.

Inflammatory Bowel Disease

25

Scott A. Strong

Introduction

Women afflicted with inflammatory bowel disease (IBD), including Crohn's disease and ulcerative colitis, often require resection of the rectum when their disease is refractory to appropriate medical therapy, or they develop a complication that cannot be resolved with medications. These procedures can be plagued by intraoperative and postoperative complications that can be occasionally avoided but more commonly require management based on patient-related factors, disease-specific variables, and complication-associated features.

Intraoperative Complications

Injuries to other pelvic structures can occur during surgery for IBD, especially if inflammatory or reoperative conditions distort the normal anatomy. Careful review of preoperative cross-sectional imaging studies can help identify individuals in whom lateral structures have been drawn more medially or were previously mobilized to lie in an abnormal position.

S. A. Strong (✉)
Department of Surgery, Feinberg School of Medicine, Northwestern University, Chicago, IL, USA
e-mail: scott.strong@nm.org

Injury to the Ureter and Bladder

Injury to a ureter or the bladder uncommonly occurs and is best managed by recognition at the time of the index operation as opposed to discovery during the postoperative period. The prevention, recognition, and management of this type of injury are discussed in Chap. 17.

Injury to the Reproductive Organs

An injury to a fallopian tube or an ovary is rare but occurs more often during pelvic surgery for Crohn's disease than for ulcerative colitis because extensive inflammation or fistulas complicating Crohn's disease can cause the diseased bowel to be densely adherent to the fallopian tubes and ovaries. If a fallopian tube is injured, it might be repaired to restore its function depending on the type and extent of the injury and the woman's desire for future conception. The approach largely depends on the location and severity of the damage [1]. A salpingostomy or fimbrioplasty is performed for distal tubal occlusions, especially if the fimbrial portion of the tube is involved. A salpingo-salpingostomy is used for more extensive injuries where a portion of the fallopian tube has been damaged or resected, and tubal implantation is recommended when the proximal aspect of the tube has been injured and the distal, healthy segment can be implanted

M. Hoffman et al. (eds.), *Major Complications of Female Pelvic Surgery*,
https://doi.org/10.1007/978-3-031-66772-5_25

directly into the uterus. An accidentally resected ovary can be grafted to a pelvic site with a good blood supply (e.g., a broad ligament, peritoneal surface). Following such transplantation, the ovarian tissue can begin to function, producing hormones and potentially allowing for natural conception. However, the duration of function varies, with some grafts functioning for a few months and others for several years. Successful pregnancies have been reported following ovarian tissue transplantation, both through natural conception and assisted reproductive technologies [2].

An injury to the vagina can occur when its posterior aspect is being mobilized off the anterior wall of the rectum. These injuries are usually readily identified and primarily suture repaired in a transverse manner, but closure can be challenging if the injury occurs near the apex of the vagina because the cervix must be accommodated. If the repair is going to lie close to a bowel anastomosis, it is advisable to interpose a tissue such as the omentum between the two suture lines to avoid breakdown at either site, leading to the development of a fistula. Alternatively, the mesentery of the bowel used for an ileal pouch or a neo-rectum can be oriented to lie anterior rather than posterior to separate the suture lines.

Injury to the Vessels

Major vascular injuries are rare but can be catastrophic and most commonly involve the internal iliac vein, internal iliac artery, or branches of these vessels. Proper management of a vascular injury entails control of hemorrhage through direct pressure, clamp application, or temporary packing to halt or tamponade the bleeding and stabilize the patient while appropriate blood products are made available, the team is readied, and repair is planned. The extent and type of injury should be assessed, and the surrounding structures must be examined to exclude concomitant damage. Small lacerations can be directly sutured, but larger injuries or transections may require more complex repair, such as end-to-end anastomosis, placement of patches or interposition grafts, or ligation. Ligation is a last resort option because ligating the internal iliac vein or artery can have consequences depending on other factors such as the level of injury, integrity of the collateral vessels, and remaining pelvic structures. Consultation with a vascular surgeon is sometimes warranted, especially if the responsible surgeon does not have sufficient experience with vascular repairs.

Pelvic bleeding can also arise from the veins of the vertebral venous system located both outside and inside the vertebral canal that communicate via the sacral basivertebral veins that penetrate the boney surface of the anterior sacrum within the foramina located in the bodies of S3–S5 [3]. The adventitia of these sacral basivertebral veins is blended with the sacral periosteum at the margin of the opening of the foramina. When the presacral fascia tissue is lifted during dissection, the basivertebral vein is potentially lacerated near the opening of the foramen and the transected end retracts into the foramen causing massive hemorrhage (Fig. 25.1). Massive presacral bleeding is best avoided by deliberate incision of the rectosacral fascia, and sharp dissection

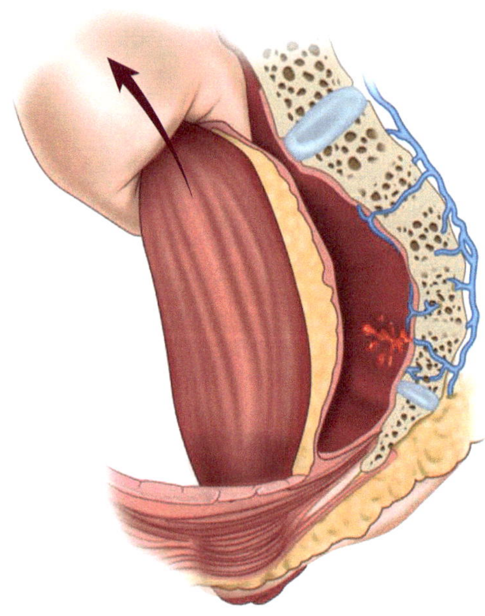

Fig. 25.1 Presacral bleeding from the basivertebral vein secondary to blunt dissection of the posterior mesorectum

distal to the fascia recalling the dissection continues in a more anterior direction toward the levator hiatus following the curve of the distal sacrum. Whenever massive presacral bleeding is encountered, the initial step is to achieve direct pressure control of the bleeding site as well as notifying the anesthesiologist and surgical team to prepare for the possibility of profound bleeding. If the bleeding site cannot be controlled in this manner, the posterior pelvis is packed to halt the hemorrhage. Once the patient is stabilized, blood products are made available, and all personnel are adequately readied, the pressure or pelvic packing is removed. Bleeding from the veins of the presacral venous plexus can be suture ligated, but hemorrhage originating from a sacral basivertebral vein retracted into a sacral foramen requires obliteration using a variety of techniques used individually or in combination, such as biologic tissue (e.g., the epiploic appendix, omental scrap, rectus muscle) welding, directed coagulation (e.g., an argon beam coagulator, electrocautery), focal tamponade (e.g., bone wax, a hemostatic sponge, a matrix hemostatic agent, rectus muscle/fascia), and occlusive pin (e.g., a thumb tack) placement (Fig. 25.2).

If sidewall or presacral bleeding cannot be controlled after the above-outlined approaches or the patient becomes unstable or coagulopathic, the pelvis is packed to achieve hemostasis and the abdomen is closed with plans to return to the operating room in 2–3 days after the patient is optimized. It is important to arrest all bleeding prior to constructing any anastomosis because efforts to control bleeding after an ileal pouch or neo-rectum is in place can be more difficult and pelvic packing potentially threatens future problems affecting the bowel or low-lying anastomosis.

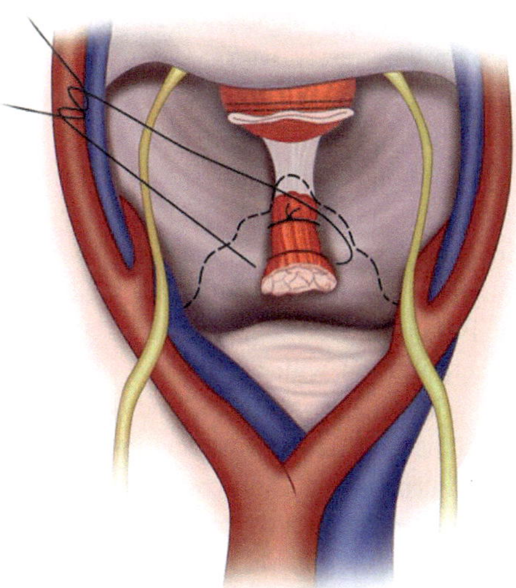

Fig. 25.2 Rectus muscle/fascia sutured into position to tamponade presacral bleeding from the basivertebral vein

Early Postoperative Complications

Surgical Site Infections

Surgical site infections (SSIs) are one of the potential complications associated with any surgical procedure, and their incidence after pelvic surgery for IBD can vary based on several factors, including the patient's overall health, the type of procedure performed, the surgical technique used, and the hospital's infection control practices. Many of these variables have been discussed in other chapters, but a few aspects unique to IBD-related surgery warrant mention. IBD is an inflammatory condition that can be complicated by malnutrition, fistulas, and abscesses, and these factors increase the incidence of postoperative SSIs. Moreover, many women with IBD are being treated with corticosteroids, immunomodulators, biologic agents, and/or small molecule medications prior to surgery, but only high-dose corticosteroids—prednisone (at least 20 mg daily) for at least 6 weeks—have been consistently shown to increase the risk of incisional and organ/space infections, including anastomotic leaks [4, 5].

Anastomotic/Pouch Leaks and Pelvic Abscesses

Women with IBD requiring pelvic surgery commonly wish to avoid a permanent stoma. Individuals suffering from Crohn's disease of the large intestine are sometimes candidates for segmental resection and creation of a low colorectal anastomosis or proctocolectomy and ileal pouch-anal anastomosis (IPAA) while many patients requiring surgery for ulcerative colitis elect to undergo proctocolectomy and IPAA. A leak from an anastomosis or the ileal pouch can be one of the more devastating complications (Fig. 25.3). Construction of a diverting loop ileostomy at the time of the initial operation does not necessarily decrease the risk of anastomotic leak but does minimize its consequences. Another technique used to potentially reduce the risk of leak associated with an IPAA employs close rectal dissection instead of total mesorectal excision. In the former technique, the superior rectal artery and mesorectum are left intact and the dissection is performed close to the muscular tube of the rectum. This close dissection is technically more challenging but tends to be associated with fewer anastomotic leaks, improved short-term quality of life, and better fecal continence compared to the total mesorectal excision approach [6, 7]. Lastly, long-term follow-up suggests that close dissection might also lessen the risk of chronic pelvic sepsis [8].

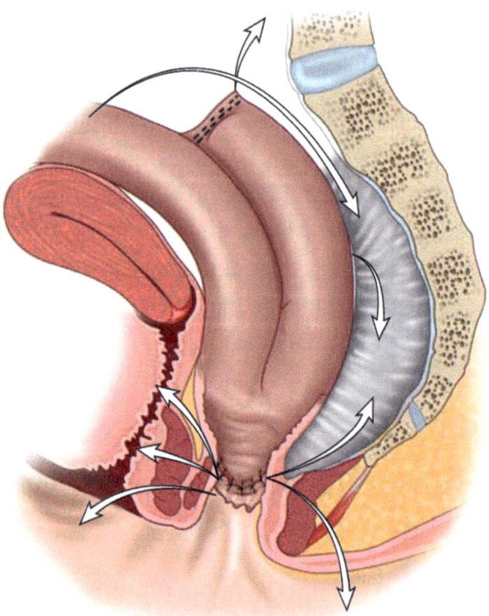

Fig. 25.3 Potential sites of leak from ileal pouch and ileal pouch-anal anastomosis

Other locations prone to leak include the tip of the J-pouch and the pouch body staple/suture line. Both locations are relatively risk-free staple/suture lines, but a leak can develop due to a technical error or insufficient blood supply, especially at the tip of the J-pouch. Leaks from a low coloproctostomy, IPAA, or ileal pouch can manifest themselves through a variety of symptoms (e.g., fever, ileus, pain, rigors) and signs (e.g., elevated C-reactive protein, leukocytosis, tachycardia). These leaks are generally diagnosed with cross-sectional imaging that includes delivery of intravenous, oral, and transanal contrast and/or lower endoscopy. Some are only identified on routine transanal contrast imaging performed prior to ileostomy closure in a patient that had an uneventful postoperative recovery.

Treatment of a pelvic abscess or leak will depend on the clinical status of the patient, preexisting diversion, and the location of the abscess and/or leak. Patients should receive broad-spectrum antibiotics directed against anaerobic and Gram-negative bacilli bacteria, and an undiverted anastomotic leak causing pelvic sepsis is likely to require fecal diversion, abdominopelvic washout, and extensive drainage. An isolated pelvic abscess can usually be managed by percutaneous transgluteal drainage, but sometimes they are too small or not accessible; most abscesses less than 4–5 cm in size can be sterilized with antibiotic therapy alone. Repeat laparoscopy/laparotomy is rarely warranted in the diverted patient, except for a large inaccessible abscess that is causing significant sepsis.

Anastomotic leaks with or without an associated abscess are best managed in the operating room by placing a suitably sized Pezzer catheter through the anastomotic defect via the anus. The drain is passed to the height of the associated cavity/tract, secured with a suture to the proximal bowel at the site of the defect, and trimmed 5 cm beyond the anal verge. Most cavities will quickly collapse around the drain catheter as evidenced by a drain injection study performed 4–6 weeks later. The catheter can be replaced by a smaller-caliber drain that is passed only halfway along the tract every 4–6 weeks after imaging to confirm shortening of the tract. The drain is ultimately discontinued, and the defect is saucerized when the residual tract measures only 2–3 cm in length. If the tract does not shorten as anticipated, a septotomy can be performed if the tract is less than 4–5 cm in length using an energy device or mechanical stapler. Longer tracts or selected short tracts may require advancement of the proximal bowel and construction of a neo-anastomosis. Vacuum-assisted devices like those commercially available outside the United States can be pieced together, placed through an endoscopically reachable anastomotic defect, used to expedite the collapse of a cavity, and may be linked to improved pouch function and a lower risk of pouch loss compared to more conventional management [9].

Percutaneous drainage of an abscess arising from an anastomotic leak has the potential to cause an extrasphincteric fistula, but this rarely materializes [10]. This approach can be coupled with efforts at endoscopic or transanal suture closure of the anastomotic defect prior to discontinuation of the percutaneous drain. Abscesses caused by leaks from the tip of the J-pouch or body of the ileal pouch commonly require percutaneous drainage for source control and fecal diversion if not already in place. Endoscopic closure of the defect can be subsequently attempted but the success rate is low, especially with leaks from the tip of the J-pouch, which typically require mobilization of the upper pouch and amputation of the culprit segment or ileal pouch excision and construction of a neo-ileal pouch [11]. That operation is usually scheduled to occur no sooner than 6 months after the last abdominal operation.

Late Postoperative Complications

Anastomotic/Pouch Fistulas

Although most women undergoing a proctocolectomy and creation of an IPAA experience acceptable functional outcomes and satisfactory quality of life, complications such as ileal pouch-related fistulas (e.g., pouch-perineal fistula, pouch-vaginal fistula) occur in 1.5–12% of cases [12]. They usually occur several months after IPAA and are commonly predated by early postoperative sepsis. Other risk factors include preoperative high-dose corticosteroid usage, technical problems encountered during proctectomy or ileal pouch creation, and a postoperative diagnosis of Crohn's disease. These fistulas are typically diagnosed with contrast-enhanced imaging studies and lower endoscopy studies and their management can range from observation for simple asymptomatic fistulas to pouch excision and creation of a permanent ileostomy for unsalvageable situations with debilitating symptoms. Patients with fistulas linked to Crohn's disease complicated by inflammation of the ileal pouch or anal canal are best treated with medical therapy and are generally not operative candidates. Most other cases suitable for operative repair will begin with fecal diversion and drainage of the fistula when possible. An ileostomy is created using a segment of the bowel located more proximally than usual in case construction of a neo-ileal pouch is required during the next operation.

Fistulas arising from a stapled IPAA extending to the perineum can be treated with transanal or transabdominal ileal pouch advancement and construction of a neo-IPAA (Figs. 25.4 and 25.5). Similar fistulas involving the vagina may resolve with observation if they are diagnosed in the early postoperative period but will require surgi-

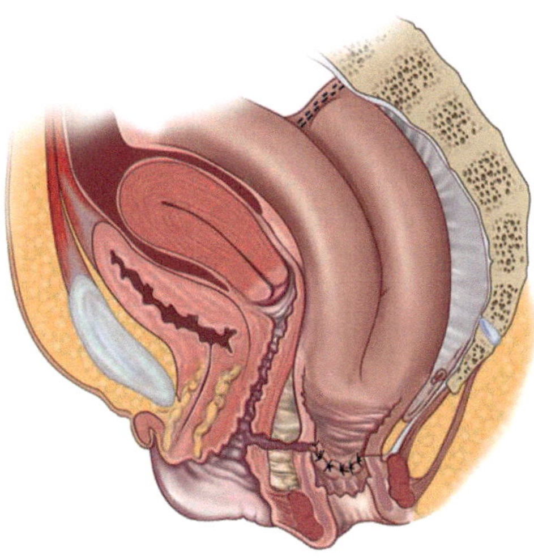

Fig. 25.4 A fistula extending from ileal pouch-anal anastomosis to the posterior vagina

cal repair if they persist or develop later, although the underlying Crohn's disease must always be excluded. In women who are candidates for repair, the integrity of the anal sphincter must be assessed and concomitant sphincteroplasty is generally indicated if a sphincter defect is noted in addition to the fistula (Fig. 25.6). The repair can be performed as described for a fistula to the perineum, but a transvaginal approach can also be considered. Pouch-vaginal fistula repair can be further buttressed using an interposed tissue such as a Martius flap or the gracilis muscle, but this is often reserved for a repeated attempt at repair (Fig. 25.7).

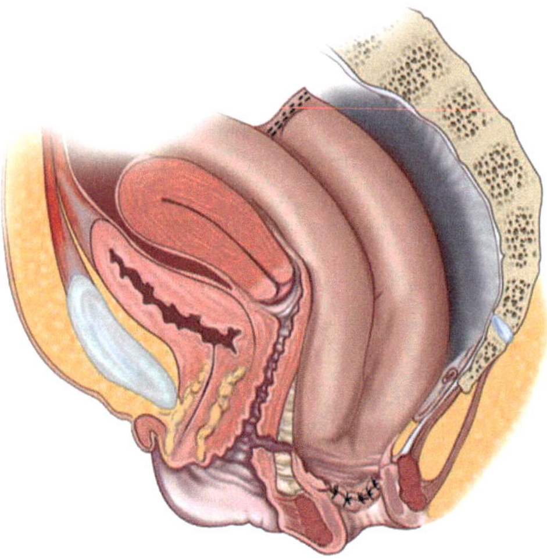

Fig. 25.5 A fistula from ileal pouch-anal anastomosis to the vagina repaired by mucosectomy, ileal pouch advancement, and creation of neo-ileal pouch-anal anastomosis

Enterocutaneous fistulas caused by leaks from the tip of the J-pouch were discussed earlier. Similar fistulas from the body of the ileal pouch require mobilization of the ileal pouch and usually disconnection of the IPAA, repair of the defect or creation of a neo-ileal pouch depending upon the condition of the affected pouch, and creation of a handsewn neo-IPAA.

Transabdominal redo ileal pouch surgery is warranted for several other indications such as obstruction, dysfunction, pouchitis, prolapse, and neoplasm, and the conduct of that operation is predicated upon the underlying problem, condition of the existing ileal pouch, and integrity of the existing anastomosis [13].

A recent systematic literature search of women with ileal pouch-vaginal fistulas has identified 34 relevant studies and suggested that a repeat IPAA

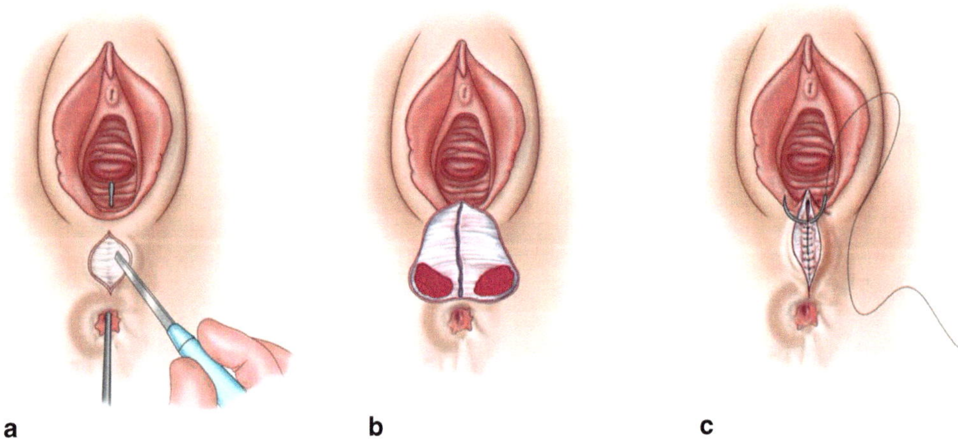

Fig. 25.6 Repair of fistula from ileal pouch-anal anastomosis to the vagina with concomitant anal sphincteroplasty

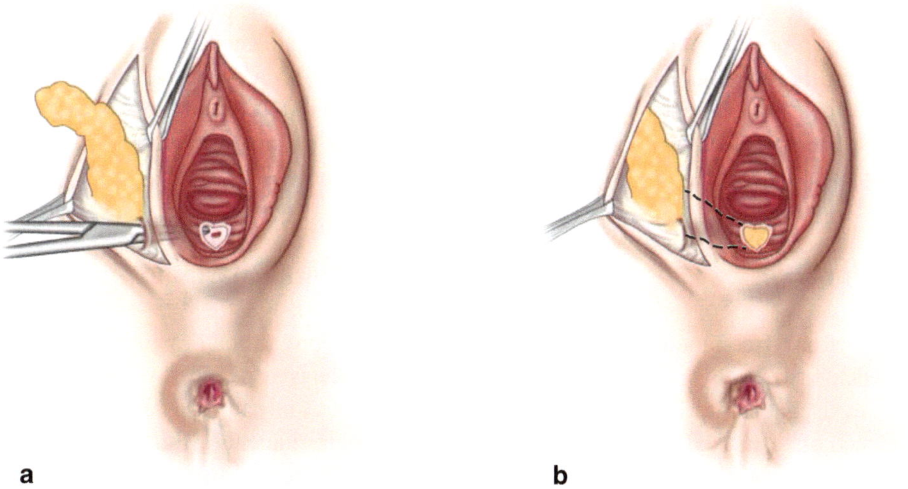

Fig. 25.7 Repair of fistula from ileal pouch-anal anastomosis to the vagina with a Martius flap

procedure is associated with the lowest recurrence rate (42%), while the transanal ileal pouch advancement operation had the highest risk of recurrence (57%) [12]. It was also noted that Crohn's disease is responsible for one in four pouch-vaginal fistulas. When considering redo ileal pouch surgery for all indications, a new pouch is created in 41% of patients, the short-term anastomotic leak rate is 8%, and 20% of individuals are expected to experience redo IPAA failure after a median follow-up of 7 years with pelvic sepsis developing after redo ileal pouch surgery as the primary predictor of pouch failure [13]. Overall functional outcomes and quality of life scores are acceptable following a redo operation.

Infertility

The effect of surgery on infertility and pregnancy outcomes was assessed in a recent Cochran review [14]. Nine studies compared patients with and without a history of prior IBD-related surgery, and another study contrasted women undergoing open versus laparoscopic IPAA. Unfortunately, all the studies showed a high risk of bias in at least two domains. They reported that IBD surgery may increase the likelihood of infertility at 24 months [(relative risk (RR) 3.59, 95% confidence interval (95% CI) 1.32–9.73; 190 participants; 1 study)] while the incidence of infertility seems comparable in women who undergo open compared to laparoscopic restorative proctocolectomy at 12 months (RR 0.70, 95% CI 0.38–1.27; 37 participants; 1 study). IBD surgery may also adversely affect pregnancy-related outcomes including miscarriage (odds ratio (OR) 2.03, 95% CI 1.14–3.60; 776 pregnancies; 5 studies) and usage of assisted reproductive technology (RR 25.09, 95% CI 1.56–403.76; 106 participants; 1 study) but not the incidence of stillbirth (RR 1.96, 95% CI 0.42–9.18; 246 pregnancies; 3 studies), preterm birth (RR 1.91, 95% CI 0.67–5.48; 194 pregnancies; 3 studies), low-birth-weight babies (RR 0.61, 95% CI 0.08–4.83), or small-for-gestational-age infants (RR 2.54, 95% CI 0.80–8.01; 65 pregnancies; 1 study). While assisted reproductive technology is safe and effective in patients with IBD, that efficacy is reduced in women who had previously undergone Crohn's disease-related surgery and others experiencing pouch failure [15].

Sexual Dysfunction

Sexual dysfunction is common among women with IBD as demonstrated by a systematic review and meta-analysis that included 18 studies where their prevalence of sexual dysfunction was 53% (95% CI 50–55%, $P < 0.001$) and even higher in individuals undergoing operation [odds ratio (OR), 1.33, 95% CI 1.22–1.45, $P < 0.001$)], suffering from depression (OR 6.14, 95% CI 3.51–10.76, $P < 0.001$), experiencing increased disease activity (OR 2.73, 95% CI 1.32–5.64, $P = 0.007$), afflicted with comorbidities (OR 3.21, 95% CI 2.06–5.00, $P < 0.001$), or requiring corticosteroid therapy (OR 2.62, 95% CI 1.48–4.66, $P = 0.001$) [16]. Of women undergoing a proctectomy for inflammatory bowel disease, their total Female Sexual Function Index score and category-based assessments (i.e., desire, arousal, lubrication, orgasm, satisfaction, pain) do not significantly change after surgery. However, subgroup analysis suggests women undergoing an IPAA tend to experience some improvement but not to a degree that is statistically significant [17].

Unhealed Perineal Wound

A significant proportion of patients (37%–79%) experience delayed perineal wound healing following proctectomy for IBD, and it occurs more commonly in patients with Crohn's disease undergoing proctectomy than in those with ulcerative colitis (Fig. 25.8). While past studies [18] have reported that several factors were associated with delayed healing (e.g., age, the presence of a high-lying anorectal fistula, sex, perioperative corticosteroid usage, degree of contamination at operation, wound management), more recent studies [19, 20] have suggested that the presence of preoperative perineal sepsis and ileal pouch complications are the principal culprits. Accordingly, fecal diversion

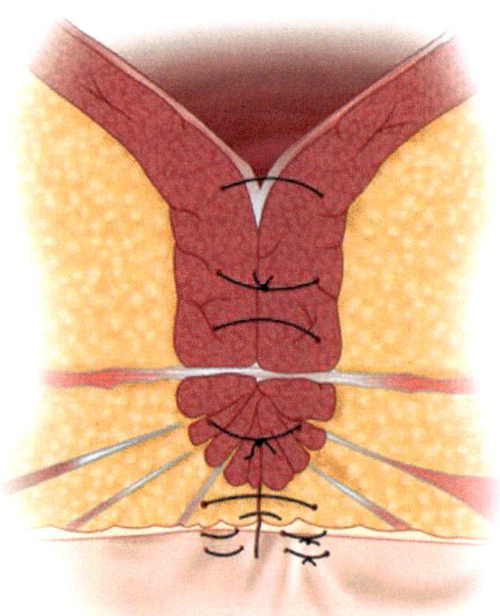

a

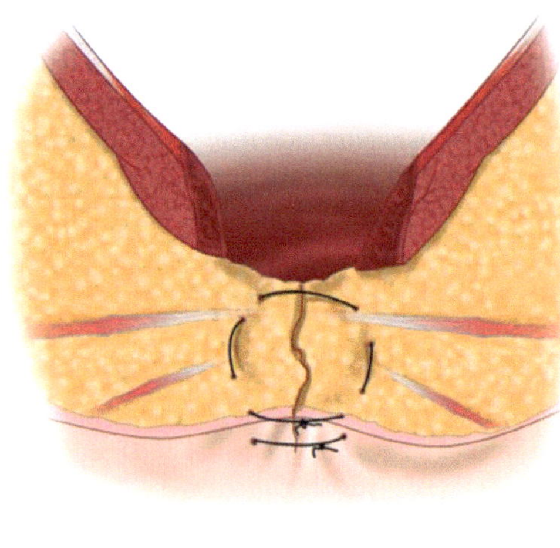

b

Fig. 25.8 Methods for managing excision of the sphincters for patients with inflammatory bowel disease (left: intersphincteric; right: extrasphincteric)

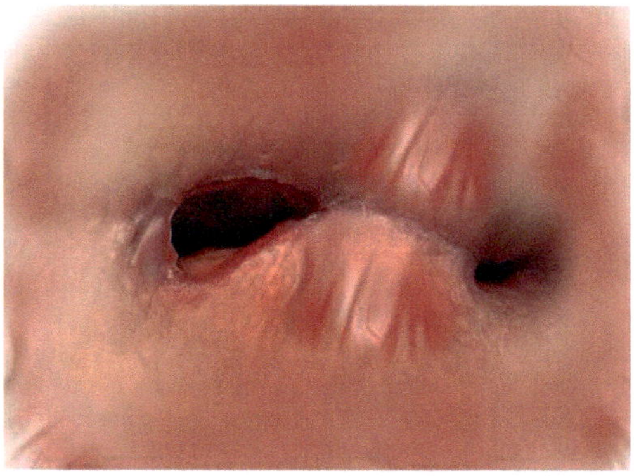

Fig. 25.9 An unhealed perineal wound following proctectomy for Crohn's disease (patient lying in the left lateral decubitus position)

alone is initially recommended followed by subsequent proctectomy or ileal pouch excision with excision or unroofing of all fistula tracts once the local sepsis is adequately controlled. The close rectal dissection discussed earlier actually increases the risk of perineal complications, and, thus, total mesorectal excision is recommended [21].

The management of an unhealed perineal wound—a wound that has failed to heal after 6 months—depends upon the features of the wound and whether a presacral sinus tract is present (Fig. 25.9). A simple wound must be opened to sufficiently expose its depths and then allowed to close by secondary intention, skin grafting, or local flap closure. Presacral sinuses are more difficult to manage because they are associated with a long tract lined by a biofilm that will not heal by secondary intention. In this instance, a transabdominal or transperineal procedure is usually required with the harvesting of an omental or muscular flap to fill the pelvis after all aspects of the perineal wound and sinus tract are thoroughly debrided.

Entrapped Ovary (Inclusion Cyst)

Pelvic cysts can develop several years after proctectomy for IBD, and the cause is likely due to descent of the ovary from an intraperitoneal location to an extraperitoneal position [22]. This condition may be avoided by performing a simple oophoropexy procedure that fixes the ovaries to the lateral wall of the peritoneum with nonabsorbable mattress sutures placed at the time of proctectomy. Affected women typically present with symptoms due to compression of contiguous structures by the enlarging cyst(s), and cross-sectional imaging generally shows cystic masses in the retroperitoneum. Simple cyst aspiration is associated with a high rate of recurrence that occurs soon after the procedure. Instead, the cyst should be excised, and the ovary dissected free and fixed within the peritoneal cavity. If the cyst walls cannot be removed without injury to vital structures, partial resection or marsupialization is recommended along with fixation or removal of the ovary.

Summary

Pelvic surgery for Crohn's disease and ulcerative colitis can be associated with intraoperative complications such as injury to the surrounding structures and bleeding from the vessels located along the pelvic sidewalls or presacral veins. The most bothersome early postoperative complications are infection-related while late complications can result from these infections in the form of a fistula or chronic sinus. Infertility, sexual dysfunction, nonhealing perineal wound, and pelvic cysts are other problems that can manifest themselves months or years after proctectomy for inflammatory bowel disease.

References

1. Practice Committee of the American Society for Reproductive Medicine. Role of tubal surgery in the era of assisted reproductive technology: a committee opinion. Fertil Steril. 2021;115:1143–50.
2. Dolmans MM, von Wolff M, Poirot C, Diaz-Garcia C, Cacciottola L, Boissel N, Liebenthron J, Pellicer A, Donnez J, Andersen CY. Transplantation of cryopreserved ovarian tissue in a series of 285 women: a review of five leading European centers. Fertil Steril. 2021;115:1102–15.

3. Lou Z, Zhang W, Meng RG, Fu CG. Massive presacral bleeding during rectal surgery: from anatomy to clinical practice. World J Gastroenterol. 2013;19:4039–44.
4. Quaresma AB, Yamamoto T, Kotze PG. Biologics and surgical outcomes in Crohn's disease: is there a direct relationship? Ther Adv Gastroenterol. 2020;13:1–15.
5. Quaresma AB, Baraúna FSB, Teixeira FV, Saad-Hossne R, Kotze PG. Exploring the relationship between biologics and postoperative surgical morbidity in ulcerative colitis: a review. J Clin Med. 2021;10:710–24.
6. Bartels SAL, Gardenbroek TJ, Aarts M, Ponsioen CY, Tanis PJ, Buskens CJ, Bemelman WA. Short-term morbidity and quality of life from a randomized clinical trial of close rectal dissection and total mesorectal excision in ileal pouch-anal anastomosis. Br J Surg. 2015;102:281–7.
7. Hicks CW, Hodin RA, Savitt L, Bordeianou L. Does intramesorectal excision for ulcerative colitis impact bowel and sexual function when compared with total mesorectal excision? Am J Surg. 2014;208:499–504.
8. Reijntjes MA, de Jong DC, Bartels S, Wessels EM, Bocharewicz EK, Hompes R, Buskens CJ, d'Haens GR, Duijvestein M, Bemelman WA. Long-term outcomes after close rectal dissection and total mesorectal excision in ileal pouch-anal anastomosis for ulcerative colitis. Coloproctology. 2023;27:297–307.
9. Wasmann KA, Reijntjes MA, Stellingwerf ME, Ponsioen CY, Buskens CJ, Hompes R, Tanis PJ, Bemelman WA. Endosponge assisted early surgical closure of ileal pouch-anal anastomotic leakage preserves long-term function: a cohort study. J Crohns Colitis. 2019;13:1537–45.
10. Kirat HT, Remzi FH, Shen B, Kiran RP. Pelvic abscess associated with anastomotic leak in patients with ileal pouch-anal anastomosis (IPAA): trans-anastomotic or CT-guided drainage? Int J Color Dis. 2011;26:1469–74.
11. Holubar SD, Rajamanickam RK, Gorgun E, Lightner AL, Valente MA, Church J, Hull T, Steele SR. Leaks from the tip of the J-pouch: diagnosis, management, and long-term pouch survival. Dis Colon Rectum. 2023;66:97–105.
12. Pellino G, Celentano V, Vinci D, Romano FM, Pedone A, Vigorita V, Signoriello G, Selvaggi F, do Sciaudone G. Ileoanal pouch-related fistulae: a systematic review with meta-analysis on incidence, treatment options and outcomes. Dig Liver Dis. 2023;55:342–9.
13. Remzi FH, Aytac E, Ashburn J, Gu J, Hull TL, Dietz DW, Stocchi L, Church JM, Shen B. Transabdominal redo ileal pouch surgery for failed restorative proctocolectomy: lessons learned over 500 patients. Ann Surg. 2015;262:675–82.
14. Lee S, Crowe M, Seow CH, Kotze PG, Kaplan GG, Metcalfe A, Ricciuto A, Benchimol EI, Kuenzig ME. The impact of surgical therapies for inflammatory bowel disease on female fertility. Cochrane Database Syst Rev. 2019;7:CD012711.
15. Laube R, Tran Y, Paramsothy S, Leong RW. Assisted reproductive technology in Crohn's disease and ulcerative colitis: a systematic review and meta-analysis. Am J Gastroenterol. 2021;116:2334–44.
16. Zhang J, Wei S, Zeng Q, Wu X, Gan H. Prevalence and risk factors of sexual dysfunction in patients with inflammatory bowel disease: systematic review and meta-analysis. Int J Color Dis. 2021;36:2027–38.
17. Gklavas A, Kyprianou C, Exarchos G, Metaxa L, Dellis A, Ioannis Papaconstantinou I. Sexual function after proctectomy in patients with inflammatory bowel disease: a prospective study. Turk J Gastroenterol. 2019;30:943–50.
18. Grant RK, Elosua-González A, Bouri S, Sahnan K, Brindle WM, Dilke SM, Vincent MLM, Adegbola SOA, Warusavitarne JH, Tozer PJ, Arnott IDR, Hart AL. Prognostic factors associated with unhealed perineal wounds post-proctectomy for perianal Crohn's disease: a two-centre study. Color Dis. 2021;23:2091–9.
19. Li W, Stocchi L, Elagili F, Kiran RP, Strong SA. Healing of the perineal wound after proctectomy in Crohn's disease patients: only preoperative perineal sepsis predicts poor outcome. Coloproctology. 2017;21:715–20.
20. Pooni A, de Buck van Overstraeten A, Cohen Z, HM MR, Kennedy ED, Brar MS. Short-term and long-term outcomes following pelvic pouch excision: the Mount Sinai Hospital experience. Dis Colon Rectum. 2020;63:1621–7.
21. de Groof EJ, van der Meer JHM, Tanis PJ, de Bruyn JR, van Ruler O, D'Haens GRAM, van den Brink GR, Bemelman WA, Wildenberg ME, Buskens CJ. Persistent mesorectal inflammatory activity is associated with complications after proctectomy in Crohn's disease. J Crohns Colitis. 2019;13:285–93.
22. Matthews TM, Kodner IJ, Fry RD, Fazio VW. Entrapped ovary syndrome. Dis Colon Rectum. 1986;29:341–3.

26 Complications of Resection of Retroperitoneal Tumors in the Female Pelvis

Emmanuel Zervos and Nasreen A. Vohra

Introduction

Tumors of the Female Pelvis

Outside of genitourinary pathology, rectal cancer is by far the most common tumor of the female pelvis occurring in about 19,000 women per year in the United States [1]. Rectal adenocarcinoma arises from the mucosa or polyps of the rectum and is, thereby, less conspicuous on axial imaging than most other pelvic pathology. Occasionally, nodal metastases in the mesorectum may manifest as a "pelvic tumor" but these are quickly characterized once the mucosal-based primary reveals itself through symptoms (obstruction or hematochezia) or endoscopy. Less frequently, gastrointestinal stromal tumors (GIST) and carcinoid tumors can also arise from their associated components of the rectum with about 6% of approximately 1500 GISTS in the US each year occurring in the colorectum [2]. GISTs arise from specialized cells within the GI tract known as the interstitial cells of Cajal and, although common in the more proximal GI tract, are relatively rare in the rectum [3]. Rectal carcinoid tumors arise from enterochromaffin (Kulchitsky) cells found in the crypts of Lieberkuhn and are the second most common rectal pathology behind adenocarcinoma [4]. The rectum is the most common site of GI carcinoid tumors and their incidence is rising representing about 3500 cases per year in the United States [5].

Sarcoma is the most common pelvic tumor that does not arise from the rectum. Sarcomas can originate in any of the soft tissue components of the pelvis including: fat (liposarcoma); muscle (leiomyosarcoma); bone (rhabdomyosarcoma); blood vessels (angiosarcoma) and nerve tissue (neurofibroma, neurofibrosarcoma). Most pelvic sarcomas extend into, or out of the pelvis with few confined to the true pelvis. Modern high-resolution imaging (either thin slice CT or MRI) can often distinguish the origin of these tumors based on imaging characteristics and anatomic relationships.

Beyond rectal tumors and sarcomas, all other non-GU pelvic tumors are comparatively rare. Chordomas arise from remnant cells of the embryologic notochord most commonly anterior to the spinal cord at the sacrum. About 33 women are diagnosed each year with sacral (pelvic) chordoma in the United States [6]. Neurofibromas although rare are the most common pelvic tumor in individuals carrying the NF gene mutation and, with the exception of aneurysmal disease, tumors of vascular origin arising from the pelvic vessels are exceedingly rare. Figure 26.1 outlines and characterizes non-urogynecological pelvic masses based on location and malignant potential.

E. Zervos (✉) · N. A. Vohra
Surgery, Division of Surgical Oncology, ECU Health Medical Center, East Carolina University, Greenville, NC, USA
e-mail: ZERVOSE@ecu.edu; VOHRAN@ecu.edu

M. Hoffman et al. (eds.), *Major Complications of Female Pelvic Surgery*,
https://doi.org/10.1007/978-3-031-66772-5_26

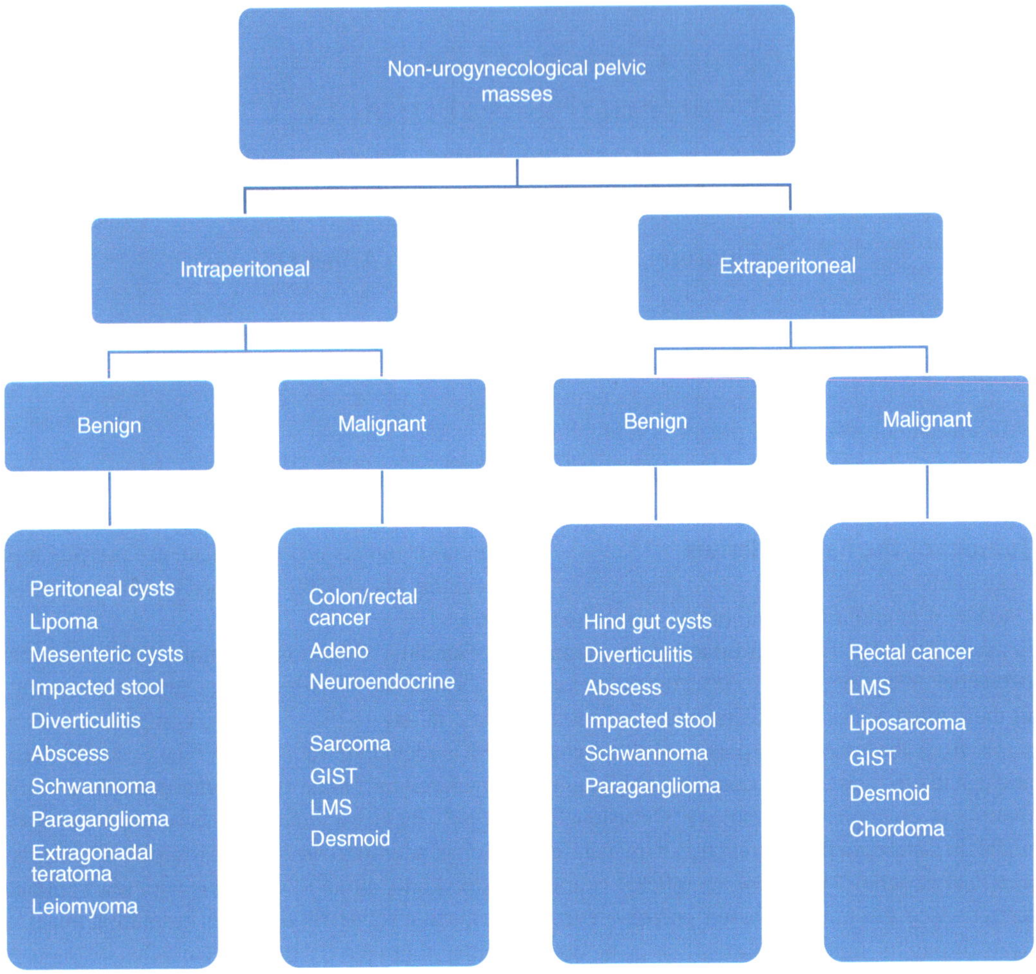

Fig. 26.1 Differential diagnosis of non-urogynecological pelvic masse

The primary treatment for the majority of tumors originating in the pelvis is surgical resection even when they represent locally advanced unresectable or metastatic manifestations of late-stage disease. The narrow confines of the pelvis and symptoms imparted on the daily activities of micturition, defecation and occasionally sexual intercourse by bulky tumor masses often mandate some type of surgical intervention to facilitate these functions and mitigate symptoms. Tumors arising from or invading the pelvic sidewall or sacrum (generally above S3) are usually managed with fecal and or urinary diversion for symptom relief as these are generally unresectable with curative intent due to neurogenic consequences and instability of the pelvis resulting from sacrectomy above that level. In that regard, the complications associated with the surgical management of these tumors are similar for all tumor types. Most are described in detail in other chapters of this book and will be described very superficially in this chapter with references to those other chapters. As such, we will focus on those complications that are most common and not covered elsewhere in this textbook.

Complications of Resection of Non-gynecologic Tumors in the Female Pelvis

The complications of the removal of these tumors can be broadly separated into three categories: (1) Vascular; (2) solid organ and (3) Neurologic. We will describe some injuries and complications in each category and the mechanisms by which they may occur. Understanding these mechanisms will inherently provide insight into some strategies to avoid such complications. Complications and reconstruction of vascular and some genitourinary tract injury (ureter and bladder) are covered extensively in other Chaps. 12, 13, 14, 15, 16, and 17 and will be just briefly mentioned herein with reference to those chapters.

Genitourinary Complications

Background

The genitourinary organs of the female pelvis include the vagina, cervix, uterus, fallopian tubes, ovaries, bladder, urethra, and ureters. Injury to the cervix, uterus, fallopian tubes, and ovaries is most easily dispatched with the removal of the injured organ.

Laceration of the vaginal wall can occur either through sharp or inadvertent intrusion of bipolar thermal energy while separating the tumor from it. Injury to the anterior vagina most commonly occurs during the separation of tumors arising in the space of Retzius and injury to the posterior vagina from anterior rectal tumors that invade it.

Prevention

By the time most tumors (other than rectal cancer) within the true pelvis are diagnosed, total abdominal hysterectomy and salpingo-oophorectomy have either already happened or are unavoidable for oncologic or preventative indications. In such cases, the best strategy to mitigate injury to these organs is either en bloc or isolated resection. Individual and up-front resection offers the advantage of creating space and clarity for primary tumor mobilization. Rarely, preservation of the uterus may be useful when tissue to occupy space created by the resected tumor is required to prevent pelvic herniation. A note of caution is that a uterus utilized for such a purpose will be difficult to remove subsequently should this become necessary. In cases where fertility preservation is a goal and a negative margin is possible with partial removal of the uterus and preservation of at least one tube and ovary, myomectomy/myoplasty can be pursued with the aid of the gynecologic surgeon.

Prevention of injury to the female GU organs is rooted in two principles: an awareness of anatomic relationships between the tumor and the surrounding organs and a low threshold to remove the organs en-bloc with the tumor mass or preemptively to avoid injury. The younger patient wishing to preserve fertility creates a higher level of complexity with regard to the prevention of injury. Absence of invasion must be established with high-resolution imaging prior to resection of any pelvic pathology and, when no invasion is noted, mobilization of the reproductive organs and retraction outside of the direct operative field is the most effective means of preventing injury.

Recognition

Injury to reproductive organs is usually quite obvious, and most of these organs are resilient and quite hardy. Injury to the vagina is easily diagnosed but difficult to manage. Simple digital or speculum exam following tumor extirpation will confirm the integrity of the vagina. In doing so, establishing the length of the vagina and the precise location of the injury is critical in guiding management.

Management

The repair of these defects can range from simple closure to complex vaginoplasty. In cases that involve either obligate (for margin) or inadvertent resection of the vaginal wall, early engagement of the gynecologic oncologist and/or plastic and reconstructive surgery team provides the greatest chance for a good functional outcome. Upper vaginal injuries can often be resolved with hysterectomy and incorporation of the injury in the resection specimen. Injuries occurring in the lower third of the vagina are most problematic owing to their implications for vaginal stenosis at or near the introitus and its impact on sexual intercourse. Figure 26.2 depicts a breakdown of a primary vagi-

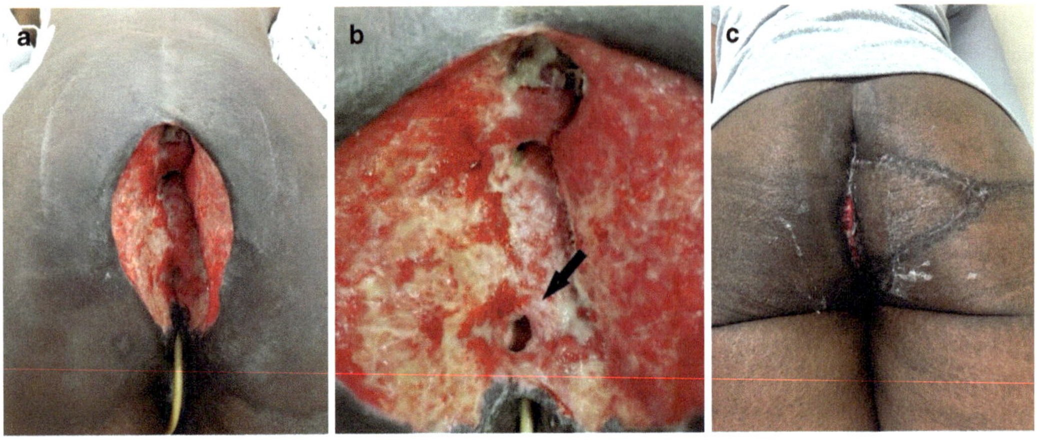

Fig. 26.2 Perineal dehiscence following abdominal perineal resection for anal cancer invading the vagina. (**a**) Dehiscent wound—note foley and attenuated labia and introitus; (**b**) Close up of dehiscence of prior vaginoplasty (arrow); (**c**) Gluteal advancement flap created 38 days after wound dehiscense filled the defect with excellent cosmetic result

nal repair following abdominal perineal resection for rectal cancer that resulted from negative pressure wound therapy in a dehiscent perineal incision. Ultimate reconstruction with skin graft and gluteal advancement flap is shown in the panels. Mid-vaginal injuries are a gray area and must be assessed on an individual basis taking into consideration the precise location and extent of the injury, the length of the vaginal remnant and the patient's desire to engage in sexual intercourse. More complicated vaginal reconstruction using a skin graft or vascularized transposition flaps can be fashioned from the epidermal components of planned transposition flaps mobilized to fill the pelvic void created by radical extirpation. This subject is covered in greater detail in Chap. 41. Figure 26.3 demonstrates vaginal reconstruction using the preserved skin from a vertical rectus myocutaneous flap employed to fill the pelvis in a thin patient with a bulky lower rectal tumor that invaded the vagina.

Perineal Hernia

A perineal hernia is a rare and particularly difficult complication to address. It usually occurs in thin, malnourished patients who undergo partial or total exenteration as part of the resection of their underlying tumor. The presentation in the acute postoperative period is dramatic as it manifests as intestinal herniation through a dehiscent perineal wound. This is a surgical emergency and must be addressed in the operating room immediately due to the high risk of bowel ischemia, incarceration and strangulation. Successful management in the acute setting always involves filling the pelvis with viable, space-occupying tissue. Rectus, gluteal, tensor fascia lata (TFL), or gracilis transposition flaps are the most common with the latissimus dorsi pedicle flap anastomosed to the common iliac vessels as a salvage strategy in patients in whom transposition flaps are otherwise not possible. Perineal hernia in the late postoperative period most commonly manifests as a "bulge" or fullness in the perineum. It may present as a small bowel obstruction-forcing operative intervention sooner rather than later. Again, repair must include obliteration of the pelvic space with vascularized tissue. In the circumstance of delayed presentation, preservation of the healed perineal wound by using a transabdominal approach adds strength to the repair and decreases the potential for evisceration due to skin dehiscence.

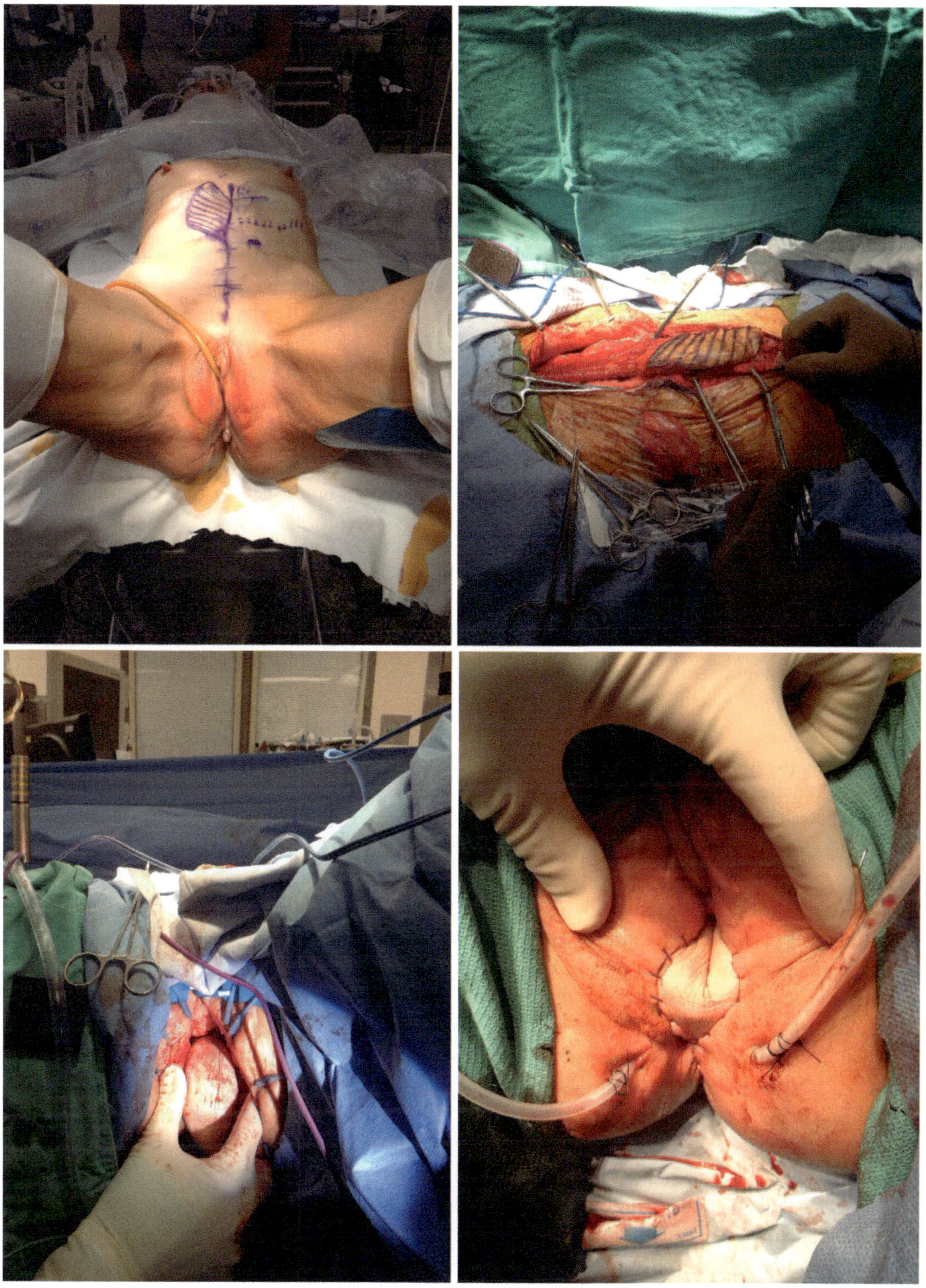

Fig. 26.3 Complete vaginal reconstruction using composite vertical rectus myocutaneous flap

Urinary Tract

Background

Injury to the female urethra is exceedingly rare given its short length and sheltered anatomic location. Cases in which the urethra/base of the bladder is at risk for injury are usually consented for resection with possible anterior or total pelvic exenteration. By far, the most common urinary injury during any pelvic surgery for non-gynecologic pathology is to the ureters given their vertical presence along almost the entire length and both sides of the pelvis. There are a number of mechanisms by which this can occur including laceration or transection with sharp instruments (most common), traction, and thermal injury resulting from the use of cautery or other energy device.

Prevention

For benign or low-grade tumors like schwannoma or paraganglioma, leaving some tumor intact along the cystic or ureteral margin is a preferred strategy over pursuing margin-negative resection that may require complex bladder or ureteral reconstruction especially, when such expertise is not readily available. In cases of sarcoma, margin negative resection is the primary objective of extirpation and should be pursued up to and including total pelvic exenteration when necessary. Unless arising from those organs, most pelvic sarcomas can be separated from surrounding viscera due to the "pushing" (not infiltrating) nature of these tumors. If the tumor extends to the pelvic sidewall or periosteum of the sacrum these structures should be excised with the primary tumor and intraoperative radiotherapy or fiducials placed to facilitate adjunctive radiotherapy.

The adage that an ounce of prevention equates to a pound of cure is particularly relevant in cases of ureteral injury. Due to the narrow confines of the pelvis, ureteral injury should be at the forefront of the pelvic surgeon's consciousness before, during and after he or she endeavors to operate in that space. Identification of both ureters prior to any "blind" or blunt dissection below the sacral promontory is absolutely essential to avoid injury. The ureters are most easily identified as they course over the common iliac vessels (water over the bridge). When one ureter is identified, its unique anatomic relationships to fixed anatomic landmarks such as the common iliac artery and bony pelvis are usually mirrored on the other side informing identification of the contralateral ureter. As such, if the ureter on one side cannot be identified, then attention should be directed to the contralateral ureter for this purpose. Occasionally, the underlying pelvic pathology, prior surgical history or anatomy precludes identification of the ureter at this level and it must then be identified more proximally; evenup to the level of the renal hilum if necessary. Once the ureters are identified, they can be dissected along their length up to their insertion into the bladder and kept out of harm's way. Again, the inseparability of the ureter from the tumor mandates resection and reconstruction in cases of sarcoma and other malignant pathology when margin-negative resection is the goal.

Recognition

Complete transection of the ureter is usually apparent by exposure of preoperatively placed stents, leakage of urine from the proximal cut end of the ureter or unexplained hematuria. Ureteral injury may be subtle, especially in the absence of complete transection. Subtle injury usually results from diathermy and delayed scarring which later presents as ureter obstruction/hydronephrosis. Cystoscopy with retrograde ureterography is the first step in diagnosis in these cases. If the stricture cannot be traversed with a wire, then attempts to pass the stricture through antegrade ureterography should be made before pursuing surgical exploration. Figure 26.4a, b and c shows ureteral blockage at the uretero-cystic junction in a patient who underwent LAR for rectal cancer. If one is concerned about ureteral injury but cannot identify any—a vial of methylene blue or "brilliant blue" can be given by the anesthesia team through the i.v. and the pelvis can be surveyed for extravasation of the dye. Once recognized, then appropriate steps can be taken to repair or mitigate the injury.

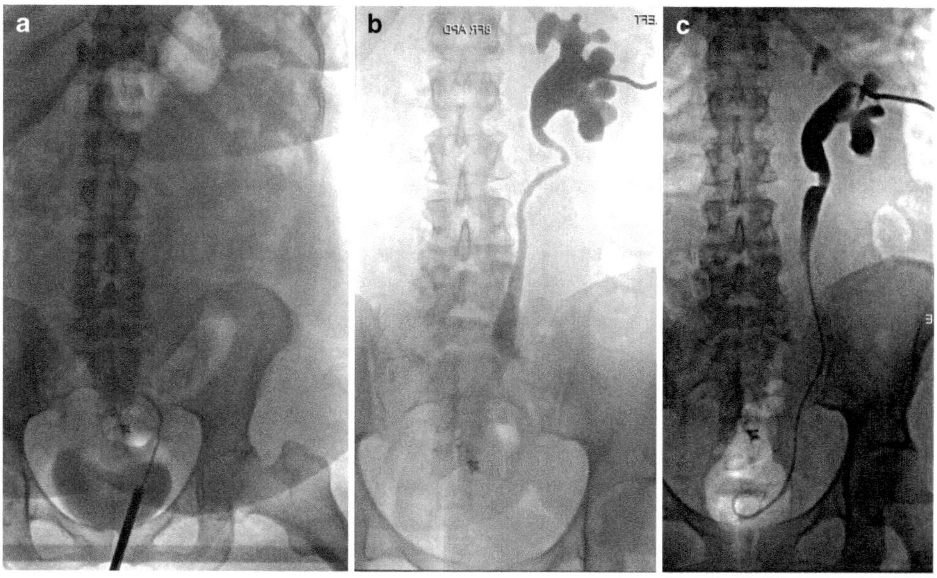

Fig. 26.4 **Delayed ureteral stenosis due to thermal injury**. Retrograde attempt to pass a wire in a patient who sustained thermal injury to the left ureter showing abrubt blockage in the distal ureter (**a**). Antegrade ureterogram establishes a complete obstruction near that level (**b**) and, following operative repair with Broari flap, a stent in place (**c**)

Management

Primary repair by ureteroneocystostomy or end-to-end over a stent is usually possible with transection or short-segment resection. With the mobilization of the bladder and ipsilateral kidney, gaps up to 7 or 8 cm can be bridged. Maintenance of one intact ureter allows such reconstructive options as well as others like uretero-ureterostomy or wet colostomy, which are discussed in greater detail in other chapters in this textbook, particularly Chap. 17.

Bladder Injury

Background

As in real estate, injury to the bladder and its management is heavily dependent on three factors: location, location and location. The higher up and closer to the dome, the better for both the patient and the surgeon. Bladder injury most commonly results from loss of "normal" orientation of the bladder due to primary pelvic pathology. Owing to the relatively thin wall of the bladder, full-thickness injury frequently occurs before one recognizes they are in the wrong anatomic plane. Such inadvertent injury can be a "double edged sword" in the sense that once the lumen is violated, digital palpation from inside the bladder can prevent further injury as the tumor is separated from it and this strategy may even be employed intentionally to minimize bladder injury.

Prevention

Preventing bladder injury is similar to other complications described in this chapter. A keen appreciation and recognition of where the bladder is at all times is the key to avoiding injury. The bladder can even be instilled with saline through the foley and then clamped to define its borders more clearly. This is rarely necessary but is a useful tool in the reoperative or otherwise hostile pelvis.

Recognition

Bladder injury during pelvic dissection is easy to recognize. The first indication is recognition of the shiny, moist and "normal" appearing mucosal lining in the background of significant inflammation and tumor reactive tissue. All one needs to do is insert a finger into the space and palpate the foley balloon to confirm that it is the bladder and not the vagina or rectum that has been violated. In cases where injury is suspected, but can't be proven, filling the bladder with 150 ml of saline (can be doubled if necessary to effect maximal distension) via the foley catheter will expose occult injury through leakage into the pelvis.

Management

This subject is covered more in depth in Chap. 12. Injury at the level of the trigone may require separating the ureter from the bladder at that level and reimplantation over a stent. Resection of the dome of the bladder to mitigate injury or achieve margin is possible as long as there is no significant reduction in bladder volume. As injury extends more distal in the bladder or more length needs to be bridged with a bladder flap, the risk of microbladder increases.. The bladder is forgiving and will tolerate tension and ischemia more readily than the gut. Simple cystotomy can be oversewn in two layers with an absorbable suture to approximate the mucosa and interrupted seromuscular sutures to reinforce the repair. A drain should be left in place in the rare event that a leak does occur in the postoperative period and should be assayed for creatinine prior to removal. A foley catheter should remain in place for at least 7 days following repair and, as a precaution, the drain should be removed only after the patient demonstrates the ability to void normally.

Finally, when utilizing a lower mid-line incision, one must always be cognizant of the risk of bladder injury as the incision extends towards the pubic symphysis. Extra care must be taken in the obese and reoperative patient as the planes of the anterior abdominal wall and bladder may be fused and difficult to separate. Bladder injury of this nature at the very outset of an anticipated complex and difficult planned procedure is particularly dissatisfying and, needless to say, should be avoided. Consideration of the possibility of such injury and close supervision of trainees as the pelvis is exposed is usually sufficient to prevent it.

Vascular Injury

Background

Vascular injury is covered extensively in other chapters in this textbook but warrants some comment here with respect to bulky or locally invasive pelvic tumors.

Prevention

Vascular injury during resection of pelvic tumors usually occurs at the sharp end of a metal instrument such as a fine scissor or scalpel, which are frequently utilized to dissect a solid tumor away from surrounding named blood vessels. Blunt and/or blind dissection deep in the female pelvis can also lead to significant venous hemorrhage as side branches arising from the hypogastric vein are easily avulsed. We use the small- jawed Maryland Ligasure dissector (MedTronic, Inc. St. Paul, MN) deep in the pelvis, following the pelvic sidewall closely to minimize risk of avulsion. This bipolar surgical instrument is better suited to insinuate between tumors and the pelvic sidewall than its larger counterpart and is capable of sealing named and unnamed venous tributaries as large as 7 mm. A word of caution is in order at this time: use of the larger "Impact" Ligasure device reduces precise visualization of the entire length of the active jaws, especially in tight spaces. As such, there is risk of unintended and or unrecognized "side biting" of the named deep pelvic vessels (Fig. 26.5). This area of sealing may be initially hemostatic but can result in catastrophic blowout at any point, especially when venous return increases with resuscitation, normal positioning and normalization of the blood pressure in the postoperative period. Inflammation and abscess formation in the early postoperative period can also weaken an already compromised lengthy vascular seal and lead to dehiscence. Extreme caution should be exercised bearing this specific complication in mind when using this partially blind technique in mobilizing deep attachments of pelvic tumors. Figure 26.6 shows a bulky pel-

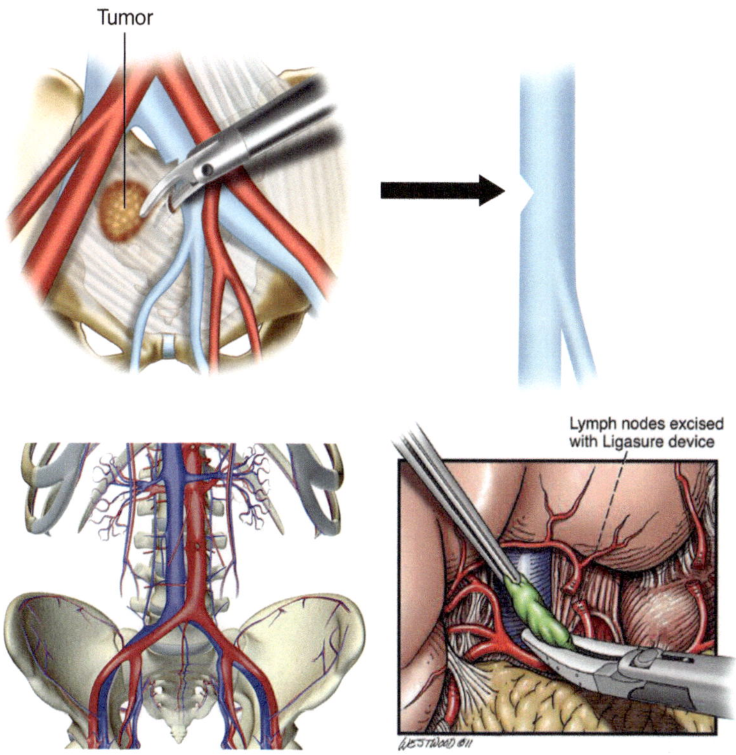

Fig. 26.5 Mechanism of venous injury that can occur with "blind" application of bipolar thermal energy deep in the pelvis

vic liposarcoma where this technique is utilized using the larger instrument.

In cases where the EEA stapler is used to anastamose the rectum to the colon, it is also possible to cause vascular injury as the "spike" from the handle of the stapler is advanced through the stapled distal rectum into an engorged sacral plexus. This usually occurs at the very end of a long and difficult resection and fatigue or inattention can lead to what would seem to be an exquisitely avoidable complication. Awareness that this can and does occur should be sufficient to avoid it in almost every circumstance given the vast space and enhanced visualization that manifests after resection of bulky pelvic pathology. Figure 26.7 illustrates how this injury can occur.

Recognition

Vascular injury is the easiest of any injury for the surgeon to recognize. It declares itself and reminds the surgeon of its presence with each beat of the patient's heart and the relief felt in the heart of both the patient and surgeon is unmistakable. Compromise of arterial inflow to the lower extremity in the setting of arterial injury and repair should be ruled out using Doppler ultrasound anywhere distal to the repair in the arterial tree. Venous injury as described above that is recognized in the recovery room or beyond is likely catastrophic and must be approached as a traumatic injury for there to be any hope of salvage.

Management

First and foremost, hypogastric (internal iliac) arteries and veins can be unilaterally sacrificed with impunity. This is the ultimate exit strategy when other, less radical interventions fail. Bilateral ligation of the hypogastric arteries carries some risk of ischemic proctitis and pelvic

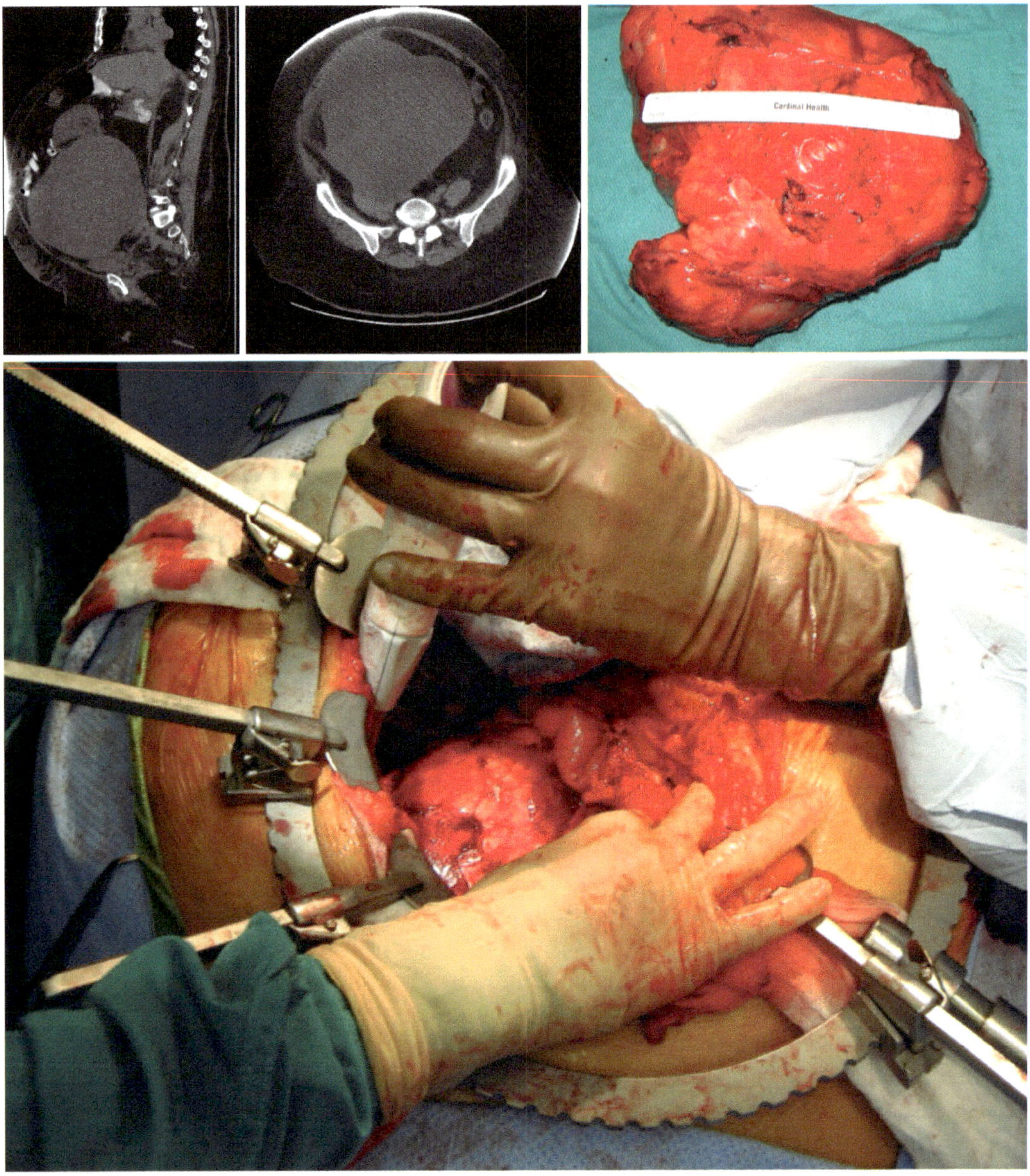

Fig. 26.6 Resection of giant liposarcoma from pelvis using bipolar thermal energy

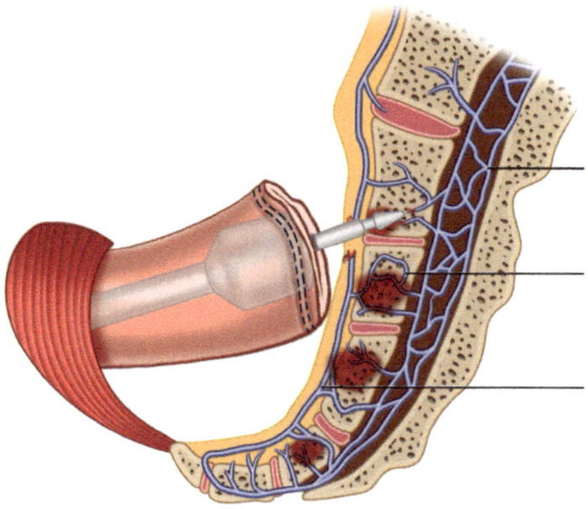

Fig. 26.7 Mechanism of venous laceration with sharp end of EEA anvil

pain syndromes but is a viable strategy in the setting of otherwise unreconcileable life threatening hemorrhage. Bleeding from the sacral plexus is unavoidable to some degree when dealing with any large tumor arising from the rectum or behind it. In most cases, such bleeding is easily managed with simple maneuvers like pressure, excellent visualization and cautery. Inability to safely and expeditiously manage troublesome bleeding from the sacral plexus can usually be attributed to one of these factors. Just as the ability to bag mask ventilate a patient provides time to formulate a plan to manage a difficult airway, control of pelvic hemorrhage from the sacral plexus with pressure alone allows time to: reverse hemodynamic instability; correct coagulopath; gather necessary supplies and equipment; and **call for help**. In cases of problematic bleeding from the sacral plexus, the best help is that which isn't needed—asking for it early rather than later can avoid those factors that turn otherwise manageable hemorrhage into a life-threatening emergency as characterized by the "triad of death": hypothermia, coagulopathy and acidosis. Waiting for help to arrive while pressure is being held gives all members of the surgical team the opportunity to take a breath, avoid premature assessment of the area of hemorrhage by removing pressure too soon and instills a sense of control or calmness in the tense operating environment.

An exit strategy for uncontrollable hemorrhage from the sacral venous plexus is packing, temporary closure and re-exploration. In cases where a perineal wound has been created, a large size (8½) surgical glove can be inserted into the perineal defect and packed with lubricated laparotomy packs or Kerlix gauze to exert pressure on the sacrum and pelvic sidewalls. The abdomen can then be closed definitively and the packs can be removed at the bedside or in the OR once the coagulopathy is corrected. The perineal defect can then be closed without having to re-enter the peritoneal cavity.

Neurologic Injury

Background

Finally, and least commonly, neurologic injury can occur with resection of pelvic tumors. Risk factors for injury include bulky tumors compromising visualization in a confined space, distorted anatomy from direct extension or invasion of tumor, loss of normal tissue planes from prior radiation therapy or pelvic surgery, body habitus, aberrant anatomy, improper placement of retractors and suboptimal patient positioning. Nerve injury can result from traction, compression, entrapment or transection; most commonly traction and compression injuries result from malpositioning the patient or the retractors while entrapment and transection occur from failure to recognize the nerve during the conduct of the operation.

Prevention

The sympathetic, parasympathetic, and somatic (sensory/ motor) nerves in the pelvis control critical functions of micturition, defecation, sexual activity and ambulation. Unless one understands the anatomy of these nerves including their relationship to surrounding structures, during a complex operation their preservation is left to chance or luck. A thorough knowledge of the resulting deficits from division of the nerve allows one to make an informed and balanced intraoperative decision regarding radical extirpation versus preservation while achieving the best oncologic outcome.

Prevention of these injuries starts with a careful evaluation of the patient to assess for any neurological deficits (pain, paresthesia, weakness, incontinence, sexual dysfunction) prior to surgery. A careful review of a pelvic MRI paying particular attention to the nerves as they descend into the pelvis and their relationship to the tumor can alert one to difficulties they may encounter in the operating room. Such preparation helps improve situational awareness during the conduct of the case, thus decreasing the potential for inadvertent partial or complete transection.

Traction or compression injury is the most common nerve injury that occurs with open pelvic surgery and results from lateral retraction of the femoral nerve as it courses along the pelvic sidewall towards the femoral canal. This usually happens with use of a self-retaining retractor such as a Bookwalter retractor, particularly in patients who are thin and when a transverse abdominal incision is used. Owing to the increasing use of minimally invasive approaches to pelvic pathology, the rate of femoral nerve injury is decreasing. Having said that, minimally invasive pelvic surgery can cause ilioinguinal and iliohypogastric nerve injury with placement of trocars below the anterior superior iliac spine. Clinical manifestation of femoral injury can range from pain, paresthesia, sensory loss to weakness and can be transient or permanent. Femoral nerve injury is a frequent source of litigation, especially when symptoms persist. Avoidance of such injury includes avoidance of such retractors altogether and, when not possible, padding blades with laparotomy pads and avoidance of excessive lateral traction when possible. Whenever possible, I avoid using the longer body wall retractors and use the shorter ones to open the surgical incision through retraction of the skin, muscle and subcutaneous fat only and then utilizing hand held retractors when needed only temporarily.

Most sympathetic and parasympathetic nerve injuries occur during dissection along the pelvic fascia which envelops the autonomic nerves that regulate sexual, bladder and bowel function. The retrorectal space described as the "holy plane" by Heald corresponds to the nerve sparing dissection plane that he described in 1996. Adherence to this plane and preservation of the parietal pelvic fascia effectively preserves the superior hypogastric plexus, the hypogastric nerves and the inferior hypogastric plexus.

Recognition

Somatic nerve injury is by far the most conspicuous as it manifests in the recovery room. Injury to sympathetic and parasympathetic nerves is more insidious and may take months or even years to recognize, diagnose and treat when possible. Table 26.1 describes the named somatic nerves of the female pelvis, their component parts and anatomic function.

Management

Complete or partial transection of the nerves of the lumbosacral plexus as they emerge from the spine and course through the pelvis can occur when dissecting large tumors in the pelvis and can result in substantial morbidity postoperatively. Intraoperative recognition of such injury should prompt consideration for reapproximation of the epineurium with fine suture and placement of a neurogenic wrap.

Deficits resulting from traction and compression of the nerves during surgery can result in various degrees of pain, paresthesia, and/or weakness, depending on the severity of injury. In most cases their recognition is delayed and usually managed with physical therapy, with resolution of symptoms over time. Entrapment v can be a major source of pain and may require decompression of the involved nerve.

Table 26.1 Major nerves of the female pelvis and consequence of injury

Nerve	Roots	Sensory function	Motor function	Deficit
Ilioinguinal	L1, L2	Skin of the upper anteromedial thigh and anterior 1/3 of the labium majus and the root of the clitoris	Transversus abdominis and internal oblique muscles	Loss of sensation, pain, weakness of abdominal wall
Iliohypogastric	T12, L1	Sensory fibers to the external abdominal oblique, internal abdominal oblique, and transversus abdominis muscles. Skin of the suprapubic region and the posterolateral aspect of the gluteal region	Transversus abdominis, internal abdominal oblique muscles, conjoint tendon,	Burning pain in the suprapubic and inguinal regions, If injury above ASIS then weakening of posterior wall of the inguinal canal
Genitofemoral	L1, L2	Skin of Mons pubis and labia majora Superior medial aspect of the thigh		Pain along lower abdomen and along its course
Lateral femoral cutaneous	L2, L3	Skin of anterolateral aspects of thigh		
Femoral	L2, L3, L4	Skin of anteromedial thigh, skin of medial leg and foot	Flexors of the hip (pectineus, iliacus, sartorius) Extensors of the knee (quadriceps femoris)	Pain, numbness, tingling, leg weakness, inability to walk, loss of coordination
Obturator	L2, L3, L4	Skin of the proximal part of the medial thigh, hip joint and knee joint	Hip adductors (adductor longus, adductor brevis, gracilis, obturator externus, and ischiocondylar part of adductor magnus muscle)	Numbness of mid and lower third of medial thigh, weak hip adduction, wasting of the medial thigh, wide based gait due to abnormal hip abduction during ambulation
Pudendal	S2, S3, S4	External genitalia and the skin around the anus, anal canal, and perineum	Pelvic muscles, the external urethral sphincter, and the external anal sphincter	Pain, numbness, sexual dysfunction, sphincter dysfunction (micturition, defecation)
Superior gluteal	L4, L5, S1		Gluteus medius, minimus, tensor fasciae latae	Gluteal medius limp or gluteal gait (shifting of the center of gravity to the non-affected limb)
Inferior gluteal	L5, S1, S2		Gluteus maximus muscle	Pain and weakness in the gluteal region, impaired leg extension, lurching gait
Sciatic	L4, L5, S1, S2, S3	Posterior thigh, lateral and posterior leg, dorsum, and sole of the foot	Muscles of the posterior thigh, ischial portion of adductor magnus, muscles of the posterior, anterior and lateral compartments of the leg, foot muscles	Pain in the ipsilateral gluteal area radiating down the lower extremity, Foot drop, impaired knee flexion, difficulty walking, standing, sitting
Posterior femoral cutaneous	S1, S2, S3	Skin of gluteal fold, superomedial thigh, part of external genitalia, posterior thigh, and popliteal fossa		Numbness, tingling posterior thigh, and popliteal fossa

References

1. American Cancer Society Cancer Facts and Figures. 2023. American Cancer Society, Inc.
2. Søreide K, Sandvik OM, Søreide JA, Giljaca V, Jureckova A, Bulusu VR. Global epidemiology of gastrointestinal stromal tumours (GIST): A systematic review of population-based cohort studies. Cancer Epidemiol. 2016:40:39–46. https://doi.org/10.1016/j.canep.2015.10.031. Epub 2015 Nov 24.
3. Kwaan MR, Goldberg JE, Bleday R. Rectal carcinoid tumors: review of results after endoscopic and surgical therapy. Arch Surg. 2008;143(5):471–5. https://doi.org/10.1001/archsurg.143.5.471.
4. Pinchot SN, Holen K, Sippel RS, Chen H. Carcinoid tumors. Oncologist. 2008;13(12):1255–69. https://doi.org/10.1634/theoncologist.2008-0207. Epub 2008 Dec 17.
5. Ahmed M. Gastrointestinal neuroendocrine tumors in. World J Gastrointest Ocol. 2020;12(8):791–807.
6. Das P, Soni P, Jones J, Habboub G, Barnholtz-Sloan JS, Recinos PF, Kshettry VR. Descriptive epidemiology of chordomas in the United States. J Neurooncol. 2020;148(1):173–78. https://doi.org/10.1007/s11060-020-03511-x. Epub 2020 Apr 28.

Part VII

Pregnancy

Cesarean Section

27

Anthony Kendle and Haywood Brown

Introduction

While the exact origin of the cesarean delivery or cesarean section is not known, descriptions of the procedure appear in ancient mythology and early religious practices from both western and non-western cultures [1]. Today, it is the most performed surgical procedure in the United States with over 1.1 million cesarean deliveries performed in 2023 [2]. Although the historic doctrine of "Once a cesarean always a cesarean" was deflated in the 1990s with specific criteria for the trial of labor (TOLAC) and vaginal birth after cesarean (VBAC) peaking at approximately 30 percent, repeat cesarean began to rise again in the 2000's with VBAC rates dropping to below 10 percent by 2010 [3]. As such, currently, the most common indications for cesarean include prior cesarean followed by labor arrest, abnormal fetal heart tracing, and malpresentation [4]. Approximately one-third of all babies are born via cesarean delivery in the United States [5], however, cesarean rates differ greatly across geographic regions and patient demographics. Hospital-level cesarean delivery rates range from 7.1% to 69.9% owing to lack of standardization [6]. Furthermore, racial disparities exist in cesarean delivery rates such that Black birth people are 20–30% more likely to be delivered by cesarean compared to White counterparts [7].

Compared to vaginal delivery, cesarean delivery is consistently associated with higher rates of maternal morbidity and mortality [8–11]. The cesarean epidemic has ushered a generation of reproductive-aged patients undergoing an increasing number of repeat cesarean deliveries resulting in a higher rate of perinatal complications. Injury to maternal bladder and bowel occur in 0.13% and 0.11% of primary cesarean deliveries, respectively, and increases significantly for patients with three or more prior cesarean deliveries [12]. The increased incidence of placenta accreta spectrum disorder with higher-order cesarean deliveries is a substantial source of morbidity and mortality. The approach and management of this condition are described elsewhere. This chapter reviews major complications related to cesarean delivery including postpartum hemorrhage, unintended hysterotomy extension, uterine inversion, bladder injury, and post-cesarean infection.

A. Kendle
Obstetrics and Gynecology, Division of Maternal Fetal Medicine, University of South Florida, Tampa, FL, USA
e-mail: Akendle@usf.edu

H. Brown (✉)
Obstetrics and Gynecology, University of South Florida, Tampa, FL, USA
e-mail: haywoodb@usf.edu

M. Hoffman et al. (eds.), *Major Complications of Female Pelvic Surgery*,
https://doi.org/10.1007/978-3-031-66772-5_27

Postpartum Hemorrhage

Background

The contemporary definition of postpartum hemorrhage is blood loss exceeding 1000 mL after vaginal or cesarean delivery or any blood loss that results in hemodynamic instability [13]. At term, blood flow to the uterus approaches 600 mL per minute [14]. This normal physiologic adaptation also explains why hemorrhage is a leading cause of maternal mortality worldwide. In the United States, postpartum hemorrhage accounts for 11% of maternal deaths [15].

Prevention

The cesarean surgical technique is highly variable. Adherence to a standardized cesarean delivery approach may also reduce blood loss. Specifically, the Joel-Cohen Method, which involves blunt subcutaneous dissection, fascial extension, and peritoneal entry, has demonstrated a reduction in operative blood loss [16]. Low-transverse hysterotomy is preferred to a classical (vertical) incision whenever possible to reduce blood loss. Active management of the third stage of labor (administering a uterine-contracting drug within one minute from the time of delivery until the time of placental delivery) is widely recommended and associated with significantly less blood loss after delivery [17, 18]. Umbilical cord traction and uterine massage are often employed, however, there is less data to support their efficacy. At the time of cesarean, the uterine cavity should be inspected and cleared of any retained placental tissue or membranes.

Recognition

Many cases of postpartum hemorrhage cannot be prevented, however, there are several risk factors that surgeons should be aware of to anticipate the need for additional management and possible transfusion. Prolonged labor induction, administration of magnesium sulfate or general anesthesia, uterine fibroids, and chorioamnionitis impair proper myometrial contraction after delivery. Similarly, uterine overdistension from macrosomia, multifetal gestation, and polyhydramnios increased the risk of uterine atony and resultant hemorrhage. Other maternal comorbidities such as preeclampsia, coagulopathy, and placenta accreta spectrum disorder should be approached with increased caution [19].

Patients with risk factors for postpartum hemorrhage should have vascular access with two large bore IVs as well as type and cross-matched blood readily available. Risk assessment tools have been developed, but low specificity limits their clinical utility [20]. Furthermore, many severe hemorrhages occur in patients without risk factors, thus surgeons must be facile with the management strategies outlined in this section. Management of postpartum hemorrhage begins with anticipation and prevention and the use of effective uterotonics in the third stage of labor. Delayed recognition of hemorrhage is the most common reason for adverse outcomes. Assessing the etiology of excessive bleeding is paramount to successful management. Although 70–80% of postpartum hemorrhage results from uterine atony, blood loss from surgical dissection, vessel injury (uterine artery, inferior epigastric artery, etc.), or adherent placenta must be evaluated since management is distinct [13].

Management

Uterotonics are the first-line treatment for hemorrhage secondary to uterine atony. When recognized, infusion of oxytocin 10–40 units per 500–1000 mL or intramuscular injection of 10 units is the first step of management. Methylergonovine is an ergot alkaloid that acts directly on uterine smooth muscle. It is administered as an intramuscular injection of 0.2 mg every 2–4 hours. Methylergonovine should not be used in patients with hypertension, cardiovascular disease, or in combination with protease inhibitors. Prostaglandin F2α binds to uterine prostaglandin receptors causing smooth muscle contraction and vasoconstriction. It is administered as an intramuscular injection of 0.25 mg every 15 minutes up to eight doses. It should be avoided in people with asthma due to bronchospasm. Misoprostol (Cytotec) 1000 microgram tablets given orally or rectally have a similar, albeit delayed, mechanism of action [21]. Intravenous tranexamic acid inhibits fibrinolysis and is an adjunctive treatment for postpartum hemorrhage. It has been shown to reduce hemorrhage-related mortality by 20% when given within 3 hours of birth [22].

Mechanical tamponade is the next step in management for refractory hemorrhage secondary to atony. Commercially available balloon tamponade kits can be inserted either through the cervix or cesarean incision, inflated with sterile saline, and left in situ and deflated over time to provide tamponade in addition to blood drainage [13]. Approximately one-quarter of patients who receive intrauterine balloon tamponade will require additional intervention or surgery [23]. Balloon tamponade is a temporizing intervention in controlling PPH which allows uterotonic medication and hemodynamic stabilization to occur before coagulopathy further contributes to morbidity and mortality. While tamponade balloons can be placed at the time of cesarean, other intraoperative techniques are effective at reducing blood loss. Uterine compression sutures are commonly employed to address uterine atony and are effective in controlling hemorrhage in 60–75% of cases [23, 24]. The B-Lynch technique [25] is often described. Here, a large, rapidly absorbable (e.g., 1-0 chromic) suture is passed from the cervix/lower uterine segment (to one side of the midline) and over the ipsilateral cornu. The suture is then passed through the posterior lower uterine segment to the contralateral side, draped over the contralateral cornu, and anchored in the anterior lower uterine segment. The suture is then tied in such a fashion that the "suspenders" formed by the suture compress the uterus externally. It is important to use a rapidly absorbable suture to avoid uterine necrosis and bowel herniation as the gravid uterus involutes after delivery.

Vascular ligation techniques can be used to reduce blood flow to the atonic uterus or to directly address injured vasculature from unintended hysterotomy extension. Bilateral uterine artery ligation—known as O'Leary sutures—is a second-line approach to manage hemorrhage and can be rapidly accomplished at the time of cesarean [26] (Fig. 27.1). The uterine artery is first identified based on visualization or palpation of pulsation. An absorbable suture is then passed from the anterior lower uterine segment at a site approximately 2–3 cm medial to the uterine artery through the posterior lower uterine segment. The suture is then passed anteriorly through an avascular space identified in the broad ligament lateral to the uterine artery. The suture is then tied to effectively compress the ascending uterine artery against the lateral uterus. This technique is repeated on the contralateral uterine artery. Ligation of the internal iliac/hypogastric artery ligation has been described historically. In contemporary practice, this technique is rarely employed owing to a 40% failure rate ultimately requiring hysterectomy [27]. Furthermore, many obstetricians avoid the extensive retroperitoneal dissection required to perform this technique, especially in the setting of new, alternative interventional radiological methods to control hemorrhage.

Uterine artery embolization (UAE) is an increasingly utilized intervention that avoids the infertility and morbidity associated with cesarean hysterectomy [28]. While hysterectomy is the preferred option for refractory bleeding during cesarean or when hemodynamic instability is compromised, UAE is particularly useful in stable patients with concern for persistent intraperitoneal bleeding after surgery or in patients who experienced delayed postpartum hemorrhage. Fluoroscopic embolization of uterine and extrauterine vessels with Gelfoam or microparticles has demonstrated a median success rate of 89% from meta-analysis [29], although some large single-center studies report rates of bleeding control that approach 100% [30]. Complications are rare but include rebleeding (5–10%), uterine infarction, and infection [28]. Overall, data regarding future fertility is favorable [31].

Cesarean hysterectomy is reserved for postpartum hemorrhage refractory to techniques described above. Further discussion of this procedure is described in Chap. 30.

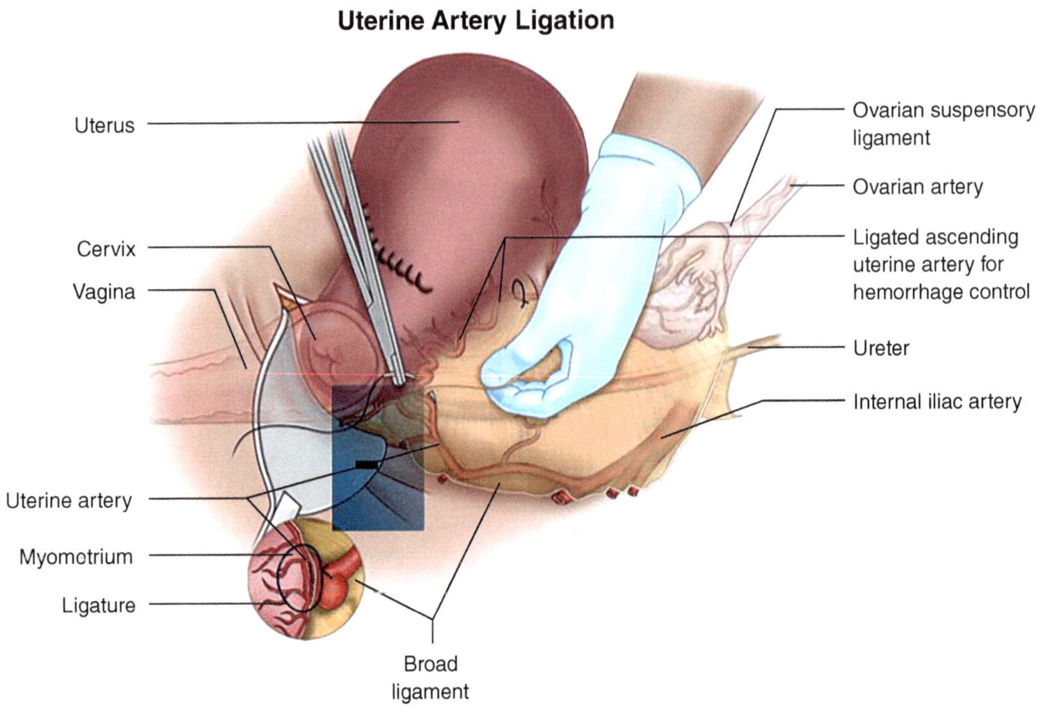

Fig. 27.1 Bilateral uterine artery ligation at time of cesarean delivery. This figure depicts a technique for ligation of the uterine artery to control bleeding at times. An absorbable suture is passed through the myometrium at a site 2–3 cm medial to the uterine artery. The needle is passed from anterior to posterior. The operator's other hand is used to retract the broad ligament and identify an avascular space lateral to the uterine artery. The needle is then passed through this avascular space from posterior to anterior. The suture is then tied down to compress the ascending uterine artery against the lateral uterus. This process can be repeated on the contralateral uterine artery

Unintended Hysterotomy Extension

Background

Contemporary cesarean delivery of a term infant employs a low-transverse hysterotomy whenever possible due to the association with lower blood loss and reduced risk of uterine rupture in subsequent pregnancy compared to classical (or vertical) hysterotomy. Unintended extension of the surgically created hysterotomy occurs in 4–15% of cesarean deliveries [32], and is particularly common following cesarean delivery after a prolonged (>4 hour) second stage [33]. Extension into surrounding tissue such as the contractile myometrium, broad ligament, cervix, and vagina can result in damage to vascular and urinary tract structures, pose unique challenges for surgical repair, and have lasting implications for subsequent pregnancy (Fig. 27.2).

Prevention

Hysterotomy extension may be unavoidable in cases of emergent cesarean delivery when fetal wellbeing supersedes regard for maternal tissue or with complicated extraction of a deeply impacted fetal vertex. Appropriate selection of the location for the low-transverse hysterotomy is paramount. In the labored uterus, the lower uterine segment anatomy is altered and the hysterotomy should be made 1–2 cm superiorly to avoid inadvertent incision into the cervix or vagina. Additionally, it is recommended that expansion of the initial hysterotomy to size to facilitate the fetus should be performed bluntly by pulling in the cephalon-caudad rather

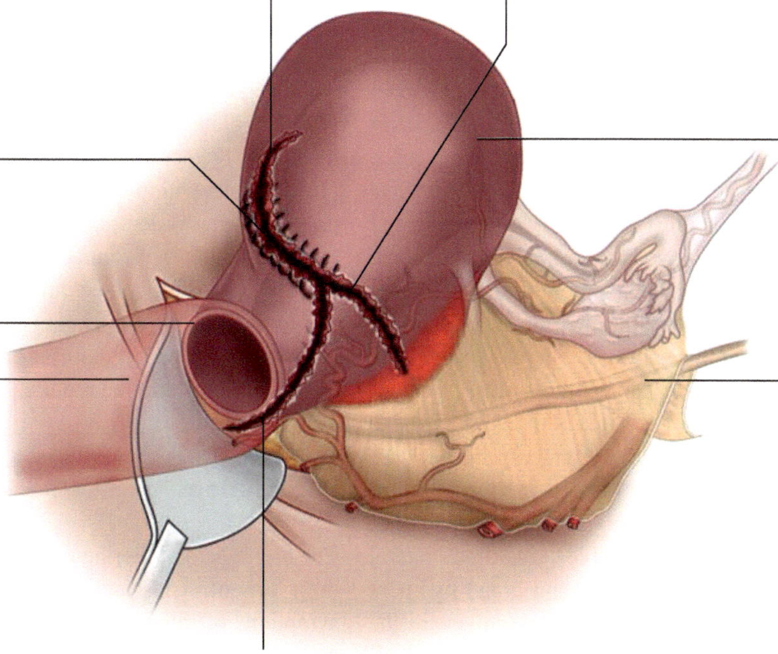

Fig. 27.2 Potential paths of unintended hysterotomy extension at the time of cesarean delivery. This figure depicts the uterus with unrepaired hysterotomy immediately after delivery of the infant and placenta. Unintended extensions of the hysterotomy relative to surrounding anatomy are shown including superior extension into the contractile myometrium, extension into the broad ligament with subsequent injury to the ascending uterine artery, and extension into the deep pelvis that may involve the cervix and/or vaginal fornixes. In the latter extension, attention to the relationship of the potential extension to the uterine artery and ureter is necessary

than laterally [16]. During delivery, the operator should minimize movement at the wrist when rotating the occiput to anterior and lifting the fetal occiput into and through the hysterotomy and instead leverage from the shoulder along the axis of the maternal midline parallel to the operating table. A second operator may assist with elevation of a deeply impacted fetal head from a vaginal approach so that the operator can rotate the occiput and deliver the fetal vertex without lateral motion of the hand and risk of extensions and vascular injury. Vacuum can assist in the delivery of the fetal occiput at cesarean and has been shown to reduce uterine extensions and associated complications [34].

Recognition

The inability to visualize the apices of the hysterotomy suggests an unintended extension. Extensions are often accompanied by persistent bleeding, which further complicates visualization. The appearance of a hematoma at the hysterotomy apex or within the broad ligament may indicate extension. Development of hemoperitoneum, maternal hemodynamic instability, and/or persistent vaginal bleeding in the absence of uterine atony postpartum may indicate an incompletely repaired or unrecognized extension.

Management

The surgical site should be carefully examined to locate the apices of hysterotomy. Palpation can be helpful in identifying an apex that is poorly visualized due to pelvic anatomy or surgical bleeding to understand the extent of repair required. Allis or Pennington clamps can be used to grasp the apex and move it into the surgical field. The apex must be clearly identified and secured with delayed absorbable suture and inspected for hemostasis which, if not identified, can lead to intrabdominal hemorrhage, morbidity, and potential mortality in the immediate hours after delivery. The operator must be mindful when placing these stitches to avoid injury to the uterine artery and ureter, especially with extensions into the deep pelvis. In these circumstances, sutures should be thrown along a craniocaudal axis when possible, avoiding lateral deviation. The uterine artery and broad ligament can be gently retracted posterolaterally with the operator's other hand to facilitate good purchase of uterine tissue when repairing extensions.

A transvaginal inspection of the cervix and fornixes may be necessary to assess for and close extensions that could not be addressed abdominally.

Uterine Scar Dehiscence

Background

Separation of a prior hysterotomy scar during labor is a significant source of maternal and neonatal morbidity. Uterine scar dehiscence occurs during the trial of labor in approximately 0.5–0.9% of people after one prior cesarean and up to 3.7% after more than one cesarean [35].

Prevention

A major risk factor for uterine scar dehiscence and uterine rupture is the closure of the initial low-transverse or classical hysterotomy incision. In the initial closure care should be taken to reapproximate the transverse muscle layer to muscle. Data also suggest that a second imbricating layer adds strength to the healing incision. In a study by Bujold et al of 1768 women with one prior low-transverse cesarean incision findings associated with overt uterine rupture were single layer closure (OR 7.5, 95% CI—3.2–17.6) and inter-delivery interval < 18 months (OR 2.8, 95% CI—1.2–6.6) [36]. Patients with more than two prior cesareans, prior classical hysterotomy (or other hysterotomy extending into the contractile myometrium), or those with prior myomectomy or uterine surgery that resulted in a full-thickness myometrial disruption should not undergo a trial of labor due to the increased risk of uterine rupture.

Recognition

The harbingers of uterine rupture can be subtle or even absent. Classically described signs and symptoms of intrapartum rupture include abnormal fetal heart rate (variable decelerations or bradycardia), sudden loss of fetal station, vaginal bleeding, and acute, severe uterine pain [35].

Management

Repair of silent dehiscence or overt uterine rupture depends on the damage to tissue in the old scar. Attempts should be made to trim the scar until a layer of muscle can be identified to be reapproximated. This may prove to be difficult for the thin inferior transverse scar with an adherent bladder. Hysterectomy should be considered in cases where tissue damage from the rupture is extensive or bleeding is unable to be controlled.

Uterine Inversion

Background

Inversion of the uterine corpus is a rare obstetrical emergency that complicates 1 in 3448 deliveries [37]. Although most cases of uterine inversion are idiopathic, there is an association with certain conditions including fundal placenta, short umbilical cord, placenta accreta, uterine tumors, and uterine atony. Because inversion can provoke massive hemorrhage, it is associated with substantial maternal morbidity. Classical uterine inversion occurs at the time of vaginal delivery during the third stage of labor (after delivery of the infant until the time of placental delivery) by which the uterine fundus herniates through the cervical os. This complication can also arise at the time of cesarean section during or after delivery of the placenta by which the uterine fundus may invert through the open hysterotomy.

Prevention

There is no precipitating factor identified in many cases of uterine inversion. Prevention is dependent upon proper management of the third stage of labor. Avoiding excess traction on the umbilical cord during placental delivery is the primary way to reduce the incidence of inversion.

Recognition

Overt uterine inversion is recognized by a visible or palpable mass at the introitus before or after placental separation. The sudden onset of massive bleeding with rapid progression to shock are ominous signs of a uterine inversion.

Management

The placenta should be left attached to the inverted uterine wall if possible. Gradual pressure is applied to the inverted fundus either with the operator's fist or palm and fingertips to restore usual anatomy through the cervix or hysterotomy. Uterine relaxants such as nitroglycerine, halogenated anesthetic agents, or terbutaline can be administered to facilitate manual replacement [19].

Proceeding to surgical management after unsuccessful attempts to correct inversion must occur quickly via laparotomy, especially if the patient is hemodynamically unstable. For the Huntington procedure [38], the operator places an Allis or Babcock clamp on each round ligament as it enters the defect created by the inversion. Gentle upward traction is placed on the clamps. Additional clamps are placed as the fundus everts until the inversion is corrected. A second operator may assist with manual reduction from a vaginal approach. Alternatively, during the Haultain procedure [39], a 3–4 cm incision is made in the myometrium on the posterior aspect of the constriction ring above the inverted fundus. The fundus can then be reduced either through the newly created posterior uterine defect or vaginally.

After successful reduction of uterine inversion, uterotonic medication should be administered and the patient should be observed until the operator confirms adequate uterine tone. Resuscitation with IV fluids and blood products is continued as needed, and the patient is observed for signs of re-inversion. Strict urinary output is measured to assist with volume resuscitation and assess for ureteral obstruction that may occur with re-inversion.

Bladder and Bowel Injury

Background

Bladder injury can occur at the time of primary or repeat cesarean section. In a prospective cohort study of 30,000 cesarean sections, cystotomy occurred at 0.09% at the first repeat compared to 0.13% with initial cesarean section. Bowel injury occurred at 0.06% for first repeat compared to 0.11% with initial cesarean section [12]. Intraoperative recognition and repair of injury will generally prevent major morbidity.

Prevention

Blunt entry into the peritoneal cavity can reduce the risk of injury to adherent bowel from prior cesarean deliveries, but the operator should enter through a clear peritoneal window when possible [40]. Identification of the bladder is imperative prior to performing hysterotomy, especially in repeat cesarean section where the bladder dome is often pulled up and adherent to the old hysterotomy scar. Fetal distress may preclude careful tissue dissection, and damage to these structures may occur in the course of preventing fetal morbidity.

Recognition

Urine or bowel contents (other than meconium) may be present in the surgical field. Although postoperative oliguria, urinary retention, and ileus may be common after routine cesarean section, a bladder or bowel injury should remain on the differential, especially when the cesarean section was performed emergently or complicated by anterior scarring or bowel adhesions.

Management

Techniques for repairing bowel and bladder injury are outlined elsewhere in this book.

In general, a cystotomy is repaired in two layers by delayed absorbable suture, followed by 1–2 weeks of bladder drainage with a Foley catheter. A small enterotomy requires meticulous one or two-layer closure with care to avoid constriction of the lumen of the bowel.

Post-Cesarean Infection

Background

Surgical site infection (SSI) occurs in 1.4–3.8% of cesarean deliveries [41]. The nature of pregnancy and cesarean delivery impose inherent risk for infection, including immunosuppression of pregnancy, pharmacodynamic changes, the need for inadvertent entry into the genital tract (especially in the patient with ruptured membranes), and the urgent/emergent nature of unscheduled delivery that may preclude proper sterile technique. Most infections after cesarean delivery are polymicrobial, arising from skin or genital tract flora. Endometritis—inflammation and infection of the decidua—can develop after vaginal or cesarean delivery and is distinguished by exquisite uterine tenderness.

Prevention

Risk factors for post-cesarean wound infection include obesity, chorioamnionitis, blood transfusion, and cigarette use [42]. The risk for infection is highest in those who undergo an unscheduled cesarean delivery in the second stage of labor. Evidence-based bundles are effective at reducing surgical site infection by 66% based on a meta-analysis [43]. Components of best practice prevention include antibiotic prophylaxis, use of hair clippers (instead of razors), chlorhexidine abdominal preparation, spontaneous placental removal, and staff education. Appropriate antibiotic prophylaxis is paramount. For patients undergoing scheduled cesarean delivery, cefazolin 1–2 g IV prior to incision provides appropriate coverage. Some evidence suggests that a 3 g dose is appropriate for patients whose weight exceeds 120 kg [42]. For patients with a known diagnosis of chorioamnionitis prior to cesarean delivery, a regimen of ampicillin, clindamycin, and an aminoglycoside provides broader coverage, and should be continued for 24 hours after delivery. The addition of azithromycin 500 mg IV in patients with unscheduled cesareans who are in labor or have ruptured membranes has been shown to reduce the risk of surgical site infection by 50% [44]. Additional evidence-based surgical techniques to reduce infection include non-closure of the peritoneum and re-approximation of the subcutaneous fat when the subcutaneous thickness is ≥2 cm [40]. Careful attention to closure of the abdominal incision, judicious cauterization of subcutaneous bleeding, and closure of the subcutaneous tissue in women with an obese BMI can avert serious wound morbidities including hematomas and infections. Care of the wound in the immediate postpartum period and following within the first weeks facilitates early detection of a wound complication and may avert morbidities.

Recognition

A fever in the postpartum period, especially when associated with increasing abdominal pain and wound erythema or discharge, suggests a surgical site infection. Alternative etiologies such as mastitis, urinary tract infection, endometritis, and atelectasis are also considered. Infections presenting soon (24–48 hours) after delivery characterized by high fevers, necrotic incisions, or sepsis should raise suspicion for causative agents such as Group A beta-hemolytic streptococcus. Without aggressive treatment, these infections progress to necrotizing fasciitis and are associated with substantial maternal mortality.

Management

Treatment of post-cesarean infection relies on antibiotic therapy and source control. The combination of clindamycin and gentamicin is highly effective empiric antibiotic treatment for endometritis after vaginal or cesarean delivery [45]. Ampicillin is added to this regimen if there is no clinical improvement in 48–72 hours, and therapy should continue until fevers and uterine tenderness abate. For incisional infections extended antimicrobial treatment, in addition to surgical drainage, is necessary. It is important to assess fascial integrity and debride devitalized subcutaneous tissue. The wound is left to heal by secondary intention. In addition to broad-spectrum IV antibiotics, necrotizing infections and wound infections resulting in uterine necrosis require extensive surgical debridement and hysterectomy, respectively.

The cost of management of SSI and follow up wound care (especially wound vacuums and secondary closure) is significant. Olsen and colleagues found that the direct cost of each case of cesarean section SSI was approximately $3500. Based on our previous estimate of 27,500 cesarean SSI × $3500 per SSI gives us a conservative estimate of approximately $100 million per year, not factoring in indirect costs including costs of outpatient management and lost productivity [41, 46].

References

1. Sewell J. Cesarean section: a brief history. Bethesda, MD: National Library of Medicine; 1993. Available from: https://www.nlm.nih.gov/exhibition/cesarean/index.html.
2. Osterman MJK, Hamilton BE, Martin JA, Driscoll AK, Valenzuela CP. Births: final data for 2021. Natl Vital Stat Rep. 2023;72(1):1–53.
3. Caughey AB, Cahill AG, Guise JM, Rouse DJ. Safe prevention of the primary cesarean delivery. Am J Obstet Gynecol. 2014;210(3):179–93.
4. Barber EL, Lundsberg LS, Belanger K, Pettker CM, Funai EF, Illuzzi JL. Indications contributing to the increasing cesarean delivery rate. Obstet Gynecol. 2011;118(1):29–38.
5. Hamilton BE, Hoyert DL, Martin JA, Strobino DM, Guyer B. Annual summary of vital statistics: 2010-2011. Pediatrics. 2013;131(3):548–58.
6. Kozhimannil KB, Law MR, Virnig BA. Cesarean delivery rates vary tenfold among US hospitals; reducing variation may address quality and cost issues. Health Aff (Millwood). 2013;32(3):527–35.
7. Teal EN, Anudokem K, Baer RJ, Jelliffe-Pawlowski L, Mengesha B. Racial disparities in the rates of and indications for cesarean delivery in California: are they changing over time? Am J Perinatol. 2024;41(1):31–8.
8. Clark SL, Belfort MA, Dildy GA, Herbst MA, Meyers JA, Hankins GD. Maternal death in the 21st century: causes, prevention, and relationship to cesarean delivery. Am J Obstet Gynecol. 2008;199(1):36.e1-5; discussion 91-2. e7-11.
9. Deneux-Tharaux C, Carmona E, Bouvier-Colle MH, Bréart G. Postpartum maternal mortality and cesarean delivery. Obstet Gynecol. 2006;108(3 Pt 1):541–8.
10. Gregory KD, Jackson S, Korst L, Fridman M. Cesarean versus vaginal delivery: whose risks? Whose benefits? Am J Perinatol. 2012;29(1):7–18.
11. Liu S, Liston RM, Joseph KS, Heaman M, Sauve R, Kramer MS. Maternal mortality and severe morbidity associated with low-risk planned cesarean delivery versus planned vaginal delivery at term. CMAJ. 2007;176(4):455–60.
12. Silver RM, Landon MB, Rouse DJ, Leveno KJ, Spong CY, Thom EA, et al. Maternal morbidity associated with multiple repeat cesarean deliveries. Obstet Gynecol. 2006;107(6):1226–32.
13. Practice bulletin no. 183: postpartum hemorrhage. Obstet Gynecol. 2017;130(4):e168–e86.
14. Wang Y, Zhao S. Integrated systems physiology: from molecules to function to disease. Vascular biology of the placenta. San Rafael: Morgan & Claypool Life Sciences; 2010. Copyright © 2010 by Morgan & Claypool Life Sciences.
15. Pregnancy Mortality Surveillance System: Center for Disease Control and Prevention. Available from: https://www.cdc.gov/reproductivehealth/maternal-mortality/pregnancy-mortality-surveillance-system.

htm#:~:text=Since%20the%20Pregnancy%20Mortality%20Surveillance,100%2C000%20live%20births%20in%202019.
16. Dahlke JD, Mendez-Figueroa H, Rouse DJ, Berghella V, Baxter JK, Chauhan SP. Evidence-based surgery for cesarean delivery: an updated systematic review. Am J Obstet Gynecol. 2013;209(4):294–306.
17. Prendiville WJ, Elbourne D, McDonald S. Active versus expectant management in the third stage of labour. Cochrane Database Syst Rev. 2000;(3):Cd000007.
18. Vogel JP, Williams M, Gallos I, Althabe F, Oladapo OT. WHO recommendations on uterotonics for postpartum haemorrhage prevention: what works, and which one? BMJ Glob Health. 2019;4(2):e001466.
19. Bienstock JL, Eke AC, Hueppchen NA. Postpartum Hemorrhage. N Engl J Med. 2021;384(17):1635–45.
20. Bingham D, Lyndon A, Lagrew D, Main EK. A state-wide obstetric hemorrhage quality improvement initiative. MCN Am J Matern Child Nurs. 2011;36(5):297–304.
21. Parry Smith WR, Papadopoulou A, Thomas E, Tobias A, Price MJ, Meher S, et al. Uterotonic agents for first-line treatment of postpartum haemorrhage: a network meta-analysis. Cochrane Database Syst Rev. 2020;11(11):Cd012754.
22. Effect of early tranexamic acid administration on mortality, hysterectomy, and other morbidities in women with post-partum haemorrhage (WOMAN): an international, randomised, double-blind, placebo-controlled trial. Lancet. 2017;389(10084):2105–16.
23. Likis FE, Sathe NA, Morgans AK, Hartmann KE, Young JL, Carlson-Bremer D, et al. AHRQ comparative effectiveness reviews. Management of postpartum hemorrhage. Rockville (MD): Agency for Healthcare Research and Quality (US); 2015.
24. Kayem G, Kurinczuk JJ, Alfirevic Z, Spark P, Brocklehurst P, Knight M. Uterine compression sutures for the management of severe postpartum hemorrhage. Obstet Gynecol. 2011;117(1):14–20.
25. El-Hamamy E, Wright A, C BL. The B-Lynch suture technique for postpartum haemorrhage: a decade of experience and outcome. J Obstet Gynaecol. 2009;29(4):278–83.
26. O'Leary JA. Uterine artery ligation in the control of postcesarean hemorrhage. J Reprod Med. 1995;40(3):189–93.
27. Joshi VM, Otiv SR, Majumder R, Nikam YA, Shrivastava M. Internal iliac artery ligation for arresting postpartum haemorrhage. BJOG. 2007;114(3):356–61.
28. Brown M, Hong M Jr, Lindquist J. Uterine artery embolization for primary postpartum hemorrhage. Tech Vasc Interv Radiol. 2021;24(1):100727.
29. Sathe NA, Likis FE, Young JL, Morgans A, Carlson-Bremer D, Andrews J. Procedures and uterine-sparing surgeries for managing postpartum hemorrhage: a systematic review. Obstet Gynecol Surv. 2016;71(2):99–113.
30. Lee HY, Shin JH, Kim J, Yoon HK, Ko GY, Won HS, et al. Primary postpartum hemorrhage: outcome of pelvic arterial embolization in 251 patients at a single institution. Radiology. 2012;264(3):903–9.
31. Mohan PP, Hamblin MH, Vogelzang RL. Uterine artery embolization and its effect on fertility. J Vasc Interv Radiol. 2013;24(7):925–30.
32. Giugale LE, Sakamoto S, Yabes J, Dunn SL, Krans EE. Unintended hysterotomy extension during caesarean delivery: risk factors and maternal morbidity. J Obstet Gynaecol. 2018;38(8):1048–53.
33. Sung JF, Daniels KI, Brodzinsky L, El-Sayed YY, Caughey AB, Lyell DJ. Cesarean delivery outcomes after a prolonged second stage of labor. Am J Obstet Gynecol. 2007;197(3):306.e1–5.
34. McQuivey RW, Block JE. Vacuum-assisted cesarean section. Int J Women's Health. 2017;9:151–5.
35. ACOG practice bulletin no. 205: vaginal birth after cesarean delivery. Obstet Gynecol. 2019;133(2):e110–e27.
36. Bujold E, Gauthier RJ. Risk of uterine rupture associated with an interdelivery interval between 18 and 24 months. Obstet Gynecol. 2010;115(5):1003–6.
37. Coad SL, Dahlgren LS, Hutcheon JA. Risks and consequences of puerperal uterine inversion in the United States, 2004 through 2013. Am J Obstet Gynecol. 2017;217(3):377.e1-.e6.
38. Huntington JLIF, Kellogg FS. Abdominal reposition in acute inversion of the puerperal uterus. Am J Obstet Gynecol. 1928;(15):34.
39. Haultain FW. Abdominal hysterotomy for chronic uterine inversion. Proc R Soc Med. 1908;1(Obstet Gynaecol Sect):279–90.
40. Berghella V, Baxter JK, Chauhan SP. Evidence-based surgery for cesarean delivery. Am J Obstet Gynecol. 2005;193(5):1607–17.
41. Edwards JR, Peterson KD, Mu Y, Banerjee S, Allen-Bridson K, Morrell G, et al. National Healthcare Safety Network (NHSN) report: data summary for 2006 through 2008, issued December 2009. Am J Infect Control. 2009;37(10):783–805.
42. ACOG practice bulletin no. 199: use of prophylactic antibiotics in labor and delivery. Obstet Gynecol. 2018;132(3):e103–e19.
43. Carter EB, Temming LA, Fowler S, Eppes C, Gross G, Srinivas SK, et al. Evidence-based bundles and cesarean delivery surgical site infections: a systematic review and meta-analysis. Obstet Gynecol. 2017;130(4):735–46.
44. Tita AT, Szychowski JM, Boggess K, Saade G, Longo S, Clark E, et al. Adjunctive azithromycin prophylaxis for cesarean delivery. N Engl J Med. 2016;375(13):1231–41.
45. Mackeen AD, Packard RE, Ota E, Speer L. Antibiotic regimens for postpartum endometritis. Cochrane Database Syst Rev. 2015;2015(2):Cd001067.
46. Olsen MA, Butler AM, Willers DM, Gross GA, Fraser VJ. Comparison of costs of surgical site infection and endometritis after cesarean delivery using claims and medical record data. Infect Control Hosp Epidemiol. 2010;31(8):872–5.

Management of Ectopic Pregnancy and Surgical Considerations

28

Theresa Fisher and Kristin Powell

Background

The term ectopic pregnancy encompasses all pregnancies located outside of the endometrial cavity. While the vast majority of ectopic pregnancies are located within the fallopian tube (93%), they can also be located within the interstitial portion of the fallopian tube or in the ovary, cervix, cesarean section scar, and abdomen (Fig. 28.1) [1]. An ectopic pregnancy is diagnosed by the visualization of an embryo outside of the endometrial cavity either on ultrasound or at the time of surgery; however, it should be considered in the differential diagnosis in any situation where there is a positive human chorionic gonadotropin (hGC) and no evidence of an intrauterine pregnancy (IUP).

T. Fisher
Obstetrics and Gynecology, Platte Valley Medical Center, Brighton, CO, USA

K. Powell (✉)
Obstetrics and Gynecology, Denver Health, Denver, CO, USA
e-mail: kristin.powell@dhha.org

The evaluation of a pregnancy of unknown location and diagnosis of ectopic pregnancy is out of the scope of this chapter. Once a diagnosis of ectopic pregnancy is made; however, it can be managed in one of several ways, including expectant, medical, and surgical management. The following will focus on surgical management and associated complications. Surgical management is indicated for ectopic pregnancy when there is concern for hemodynamic instability or other findings suggestive of tubal rupture. Surgery should also be considered when there is a high risk of medical treatment failure or the presence of contraindications to the administration of methotrexate or expectant management.

For a tubal ectopic pregnancy, a laparoscopic unilateral salpingectomy is the most common surgical treatment. Since the mid-1990s, laparoscopy has been favored over laparotomy for the treatment of ectopic pregnancy due to its reduced recovery time, decreased blood loss, less pain, and shorter length of hospital stay [2]. Linear salpingostomy, where the fallopian tube is incised and the ectopic pregnancy extracted, is another treatment option. This is more commonly utilized when fertility preservation is a priority such as if there has been prior damage to or removal of the contralateral fallopian tube.

M. Hoffman et al. (eds.), *Major Complications of Female Pelvic Surgery*,
https://doi.org/10.1007/978-3-031-66772-5_28

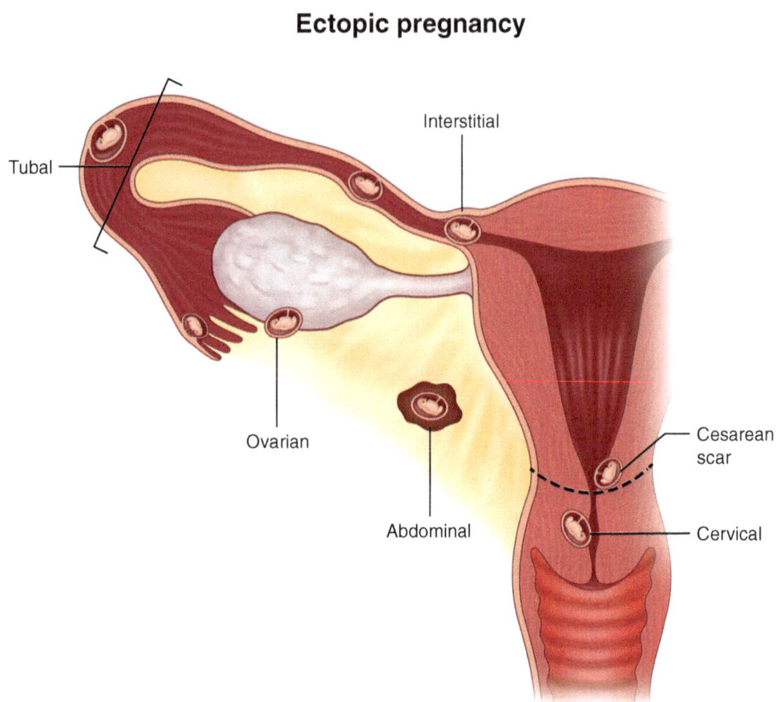

Fig. 28.1 Possible locations of ectopic pregnancy

Tubal Ectopic Pregnancy

Prevention

Avoidance of Surgery with Medical Management

The complications of surgical management for ectopic pregnancy can be drastically reduced by preventing the need for surgery in the first place with medical management. Intramuscular methotrexate is the mainstay of medical treatment for ectopic pregnancy. Methotrexate interferes with the conversion of folate to its active form required for DNA synthesis. Methotrexate is highly effective at resolving ectopic pregnancy with an overall success rate of 89% [3]. However, there are several absolute contraindications to methotrexate therapy including hemodynamic instability, presumed ectopic rupture, intrauterine pregnancy (including heterotopic pregnancy), renal or hepatic impairment, breastfeeding, and certain medical comorbidities such as active pulmonary disease, peptic ulcer disease, and cytopenia [4].

Selection of Appropriate Surgical Candidates

In a hemodynamically stable patient without evidence of tubal rupture, surgery should only be performed when there is clear ultrasonographic evidence of tubal pregnancy or a concerning adnexal mass. Without these findings, there is a risk the ectopic pregnancy will not be identifiable at the time of laparoscopy, resulting in an unnecessary procedure, or worse, inappropriate removal of a normal fallopian tube. In a patient with an hCG trend concerning for ectopic pregnancy *without* ultrasonographic findings, medical management or expectant management should be considered first-line treatment. Expectant management is a reasonable option for patients who are asymptomatic and have a low starting hCG, although there is no consensus on an hCG threshold [5]. If surgical management is highly desired, a repeat transvaginal ultrasound can be performed in a few days, at which time the ectopic may be visualized. Diagnostic dilation and curettage (D&C) can also be utilized when the location of the pregnancy is uncertain.

Bleeding, Infection, and Damage to Surrounding Structures

The risks of surgery for ectopic pregnancy are similar to all surgical procedures and include bleeding, infection, and injury to surrounding structures. Ectopic pregnancy involves the inherent risk of tubal rupture and associated hemorrhage, which will be discussed extensively. Bleeding from procedure-related events is however infrequent. All patients should have an active type and screen, with a low threshold to convert to a type and cross. In the setting of hemodynamic instability, aggressive resuscitation should include blood transfusion rather than crystalloid alone given the risk of significant tubal bleeding. Infection complications are also rare and prophylactic antibiotics are not recommended [6].

Given the location of the fallopian tubes, damage to surrounding structures is also infrequent at the time of surgery for ectopic pregnancy. Nevertheless, the ectopic pregnancy and especially tubal rupture are inflammatory in nature and can cause distortion of normal anatomy. If adhesions are present, adhesiolysis should first be performed to restore normal anatomy and allow full visualization of the fallopian tube and surrounding structures. If a salpingectomy is being performed, care should be taken to identify and avoid the ipsilateral ovary and infundibulopelvic ligament.

Laparoscopy Versus Laparotomy

Laparoscopy is currently the standard of care for the vast majority of gynecologic procedures, including surgery for ectopic pregnancy. The benefits of minimally invasive surgery are numerous when compared to laparotomy, including decreased blood loss, pain, operative time, and length of stay. Historically, concerns were raised regarding the safety of laparoscopy with massive hemorrhage and hemodynamic instability. These concerns included delay in control of bleeding, the hemodynamic effects of laparoscopy, and increased morbidity with the need for conversion to laparotomy.

The establishment of pneumoperitoneum and patient positioning for pelvic surgery can induce physiologic and hemodynamic changes. Pneumoperitoneum increases intrabdominal pressure, decreasing venous return and cardiac output; however, this increased pressure may also provide tamponade to ongoing bleeding from the ectopic. Trendelenburg positioning also increases venous return, possibly balancing the effects of increased intraabdominal pressure [7].

In a study of patients with ruptured ectopic pregnancy and massive (>800 mL) hemoperitoneum, both operating time (50 vs. 60 minutes) and total blood loss (1000 vs 1500 mL) were less in the laparoscopic group [8]. Only two out of 48 patients (4%) required conversion to laparotomy. As experience and comfort with laparoscopy have increased, conversion rates to laparotomy have continued to decrease, including in cases of massive hemoperitoneum and hemodynamic instability [9, 10].

Recognition

Massive Hemorrhage, Hemodynamic Instability

Blood loss from a ruptured ectopic pregnancy encompasses a wide spectrum, from a few milliliters to a catastrophic and life-threatening hemorrhage. Recognition of intrabdominal bleeding prior to the onset of hemodynamic instability can allow for expeditious operative management and resuscitation.

In any patient with a positive pregnancy test and signs or symptoms of hypovolemia, such as tachycardia or hypotension, a ruptured ectopic pregnancy should be considered high on the differential. Nevertheless, normal vital signs can still be observed in cases of ruptured ectopic pregnancy, and in fact normal vital signs are present in the vast majority of cases [11]. The presence of vital sign abnormalities also does not correlate with the volume of the hemoperitoneum at the time of surgery.

Ultrasound can also be used to help recognize hemoperitoneum resulting from ectopic pregnancy. This may be done as a part of a routine pelvic ultrasound or as part of a Focused Assessment with Sonography in Trauma also known as a FAST scan. In one study of patients with a confirmed ectopic pregnancy at the time of surgery, a large amount of pelvic free fluid made rupture likely, however, rupture was still present in 21% of patients with no or trace intraperitoneal fluid on ultrasound [12]. Specific ultrasound findings that may be more associated with higher volume hemoperitoneum (>300 mL) include free fluid extending above the uterine fundus or free fluid in Morison's pouch [13, 14].

A ruptured ectopic pregnancy can also lead to other symptoms, including pain on abdominal and pelvic examination, pain with cervical manipulation, or shoulder pain with inspiration due to referred pain from diaphragmatic irritation.

Laparoscopic Entry and Complications

The general complications of laparoscopic surgery, including laparoscopic entry techniques are discussed in Chap. 23. These risks exist at the time of laparoscopic surgery for ectopic pregnancy and may be further complicated by the presence of large volume hemoperitoneum which can impair visualization. While the choice of abdominal entry technique should be determined by individual experience and preference, it should be noted that hemoperitoneum may be immediately encountered upon entry, making visualization and confirmation of entry more difficult, especially when using a direct vision entry technique.

Nondiagnostic Laparoscopy

If at the time of surgery, bilateral normal-appearing fallopian tubes are visualized, salpingectomy or salpingostomy should not be performed. This situation can be minimized by selecting appropriate candidates for surgery as discussed previously but can still occur. Free fluid visualized on ultrasound may at the time of surgery turn out to be simple physiologic fluid or blood from a ruptured hemorrhagic cyst. An adnexal mass seen on ultrasound may actually be found to be a paratubal cyst or a corpus luteum. In the case of a documented abnormal beta-hCG trend, the patient can be offered a diagnostic D&C or this can be performed simultaneously if it was previously discussed and consent was obtained. The aspirated tissue can be sent to pathology for evaluation or placed into normal saline and examined for floating chorionic villi. The floating villi technique is highly variable and depends on the performer's level of experience. Frozen section is highly sensitive and specific and can still provide the benefit of timely results if the surgeon is examining the specimen themselves [15]. An hCG level should be followed postoperatively and if levels decrease by 15% or more in the 24 hours following the D&C, a completed abortion can be suspected. If the subsequent hCG level rises or plateaus, the diagnosis of an ectopic pregnancy is made, and the patient should be offered methotrexate. In a patient without a preexisting hCG trend, hCG levels should be followed in standard fashion for a pregnancy of an unknown location.

Management

Hemoperitoneum

The key to safe and prompt surgical management of ectopic pregnancy is proper visualization, which can be difficult in the setting of tubal rupture and hemoperitoneum. Immediately upon laparoscopic entry blood may be encountered, completely obscuring the pelvic organs. It is important to slowly place the laparoscope into the abdomen to avoid contact with blood, as this will quickly dirty the lenses and repeated pauses to clean the camera may cause significant delay in treatment. Once the laparoscope is successfully within the abdomen, a few techniques can be used to quickly improve visualization. Extensive suctioning of blood can be time-consuming, especially with large clots, and further slow identification of the bleeding source. A sponge stick can be placed into the vagina or a uterine manipulator can be inserted (if an intrauterine pregnancy has been ruled out) to elevate the uterus and fallopian tubes above the blood and allow rapid identification of the source of bleeding. The patient can also be placed into steep Trendelenburg to quickly facilitate movement of bowel and blood out of the pelvis. In cases of extremely brisk bleeding, the area can be immediately grasped with a nontraumatic instrument to stop further bleeding while additional port access, a coagulation device, etc. is obtained. Once appropriate visualization is secured, hemostasis can be easily achieved with an advanced bipolar device. Afterward, time can be given to evacuating the hemoperitoneum and irrigating the pelvis. Upsizing to a 10 mm port and a 10 mm suction cannula will also facilitate the removal of a large volume of clot and blood.

Choice of Salpingectomy Versus Salpingotomy

There are two options for surgical management of ectopic pregnancy, salpingectomy and salpingostomy. Salpingostomy is contraindicated with tubal rupture, significant tubal damage, or uncontrolled bleeding. Some ectopic pregnancies may also be too large to feasibly remove through a salpingostomy. Salpingostomy should not be used for ectopic pregnancies in the tubal isthmus, due to the risk of trophoblastic infiltration into the muscular layer, leading to significant bleeding and irreparable tubal damage [16] Salpingostomy should also not be performed in cases of recurrent ectopic pregnancy, as the likelihood of subsequent normal tubal function is low.

Given that the entire fallopian tube is usually removed with salpingectomy at the time of surgery, the risk of a persistent ectopic pregnancy (PEP) is extraordinarily low. There are however case reports of PEP in the remaining proximal portion of the ipsilateral tube [17]. This would suggest that minimizing the remaining tubal stump at the time of initial salpingectomy can reduce this risk.

The risk of PEP following salpingostomy is higher, between 5% and 29%, and currently, there are no algorithms that predict who will go on to have a PEP [18]. For this reason, all patients who undergo salpingostomy should have follow-up hCG levels trended. Methotrexate can also be used as an adjuvant therapy in one of three ways. It can be given routinely to all patients undergoing salpingostomy, it can be given on an individualized base postoperatively if there is concern for trophoblastic spill or incomplete tubal evacuation, or it can be given only to those with an abnormal postoperative hCG trend.

Future pregnancy outcomes following salpingostomy and salpingectomy were compared in a 2021 metanalysis. Using data from two randomized controlled trials (RCT), there were no differences in the risk of recurrent ectopic pregnancy (REP) or subsequent intrauterine pregnancy (IUP) between the two methods [18]. However, these RCTs included only low-risk patients with a normal contralateral tube. When a similar analysis of sixteen cohort studies was performed, which contained a more inclusive population, including patients with risk factors for infertility, there was an approximately 50% reduction in subsequent IUP with salpingectomy. In contrast, the risk of REP was greater for salpingostomy when compared with salpingectomy in this population, with an overall odds ratio of 0.732.

In summary, in low-risk patients with a normal-appearing contralateral fallopian tube, salpingectomy minimizes the risk of persistent ectopic pregnancy and the need for additional follow-up. In patients at high risk for infertility or a damaged or absent contralateral tube, salpingostomy can be considered, and the risk of persistent ectopic pregnancy can be minimized by trending hCG levels and adjuvant methotrexate.

Nontubal Ectopic Pregnancy

Prevention

It is important to review the pelvic ultrasound to confirm the ectopic location prior to proceeding with surgery. While implantation in the ampullary portion of the fallopian tube is the most common location for an ectopic pregnancy, implantation in other locations could change the surgical approach and therefore should inform patient consent. Additionally, the surgeon should be prepared to change surgical approaches due to interoperative findings.

Recognition

An ovarian ectopic can be mistaken for tubal pregnancy or aborted tubal pregnancy on ultrasound. Histological diagnosis is based on Spiegelberg criteria. These criteria include that (1) The fallopian tube is undamaged and separate from the ovary on the affected side (2) The gestational sac is in the normal position of the ovary (3) The gestational sac with the ovary is connected to the uterus via the ovarian ligament and (4) Ovarian tissue is located in the wall of the gestational sac [19].

Other presentations that can be more difficult to discern include an interstitial versus an angular pregnancy (Fig. 28.2). Angular pregnancies are less likely to rupture compared to interstitial pregnancies and can go on to be normal-term pregnancies, while interstitial pregnancies require surgical removal. Interstitial pregnancy can be difficult to diagnose on ultrasound and therefore diagnosis of an interstitial pregnancy can be delayed, resulting in a high rate of rupture. On ultrasound, an interstitial pregnancy will look like an eccentric gestational sac, which is not completely surrounded by myometrium and does not communicate or only partially communicates with the endometrium. Angular pregnancies are located in the uterine cavity medial to the outer tubular junction with the gestational sac completely surrounded by endometrium [20]. At the time of surgery, angular pregnancies will be seen medial to the round ligament, while interstitial pregnancies will be lateral.

Cervical and cesarean scar pregnancies are also worth noting as failure to recognize could delay treatment. Cervical pregnancy can be mistaken for incomplete abortion, with cervical ectopic pregnancy being a gestational sac implanted in the cervix with regular contours and without evidence of intrauterine pregnancy. Cesarean scar pregnancy can also be mistaken for either incomplete abortion or cervical ectopic pregnancy. Ultrasound findings for a cesarean scar ectopic pregnancy include a gestational sac and/or placenta at the site of prior hysterotomy [21].

Management

Interstitial

Surgical management of an interstitial pregnancy entails cornuostomy vs cornual resection. Success rates and rates of persistent ectopic pregnancy were similar. The operative time for a cornuostomy tends to be shorter than that of resection [22]. Surgical blood loss at the time of cornuostomy can be reduced with the injection of dilute vasopressin at the site, similar to a myomectomy. Also, similarly, closure of the surgical site with cornuostomy or wedge resection requires multilayer closure. Therefore, the surgical approach in terms of laparotomy vs laparoscopy should be driven by surgeon experience, including comfort with laparoscopic suturing.

Due to disruption of the myometrium, pregnancies after cornuostomy and cornual wedge resection have been known to have an increased

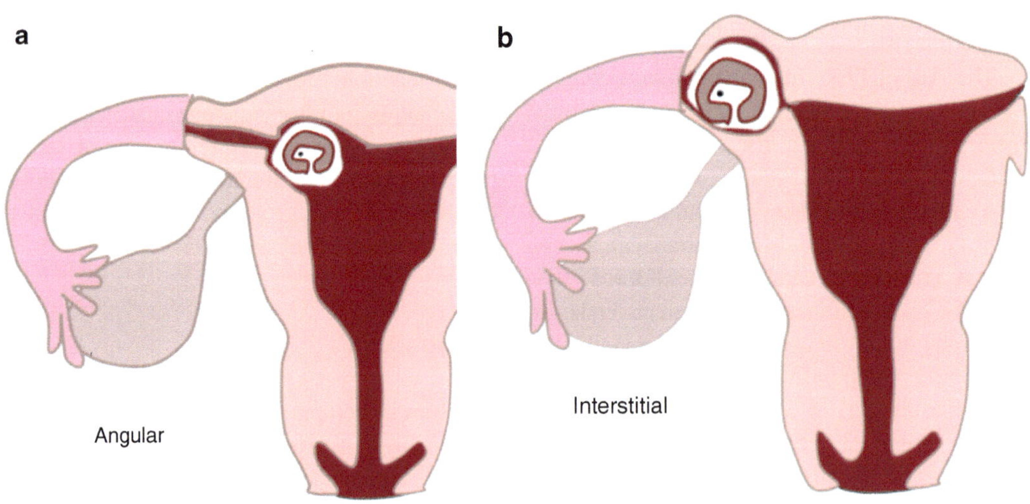

Fig. 28.2 Illustrations of angular vs interstitial ectopic pregnancy

risk of uterine dehiscence and rupture, as high as 30% [23]. These subsequent pregnancies should be managed similarly to pregnancy after full-thickness myomectomy or prior uterine rupture with a recommendation to not labor. Therefore, patients should have a planned cesarean delivery at the gestational age suggested by the most current obstetric guidelines.

Ovarian

Generally, it is recommended to proceed with ovarian sparing surgery for ovarian ectopic pregnancies. This can be achieved in a similar fashion to an ovarian cystectomy. Again, a dilute vasoconstrictor can be injected at the site to aid in the reduction of blood loss. Oophorectomy should only be considered in the case of uncontrolled hemorrhage and hemodynamic instability [24].

Cervical and Cesarean Scar

Cervical and cesarean scar ectopic pregnancy can be managed either medically or surgically. The risk of hemorrhage is high with the evacuation of these pregnancies, especially with using sharp curettage. Uterine artery embolization (UAE) prior to procedure can help to reduce the risk of hemorrhage if performed prior to dilation and curettage with a cervical ectopic pregnancy. UAE has also been shown to be helpful prior to vacuum aspiration or alone for treatment of cesarean scar pregnancies. Hysterectomy can be performed if conservative management fails, or in the case of life-threatening bleeding. Expectant management of cesarean scar pregnancy can result in an increased risk of placenta accreta spectrum disorder and cesarean hysterectomy at the time of delivery [21].

References

1. Hoffman BL, Schorge JO, Halvorson LM, Hamid CA, Corton MM, Schaffer JI. Ectopic pregnancy. In: Williams gynecology. 4e ed. McGraw-Hill Education; 2020. Accessed 27 Sept 2021. accessmedicine.mhmedical.com/content.aspx?aid=1171528516.
2. Takacs P, Chakhtoura N. Laparotomy to laparoscopy: changing trends in the surgical management of ectopic pregnancy in a tertiary care teaching hospital. J Minim Invasive Gynecol. 2006;13(3):175–7. https://doi.org/10.1016/j.jmig.2006.01.007.
3. Barnhart K. The medical management of ectopic pregnancy: a meta-analysis comparing "single dose" and "multidose" regimens. Obstet Gynecol. 2003;101(4):778–84. https://doi.org/10.1016/S0029-7844(02)03158-7.
4. Medical treatment of ectopic pregnancy: a committee opinion. Fertil Steril. 2013;100(3):638–44. https://doi.org/10.1016/j.fertnstert.2013.06.013.
5. Trio D, Strobelt N, Picciolo C, Lapinski RH, Ghidini A. Prognostic factors for successful expectant management of ectopic pregnancy. Fertil Steril. 1995;63(3):469–72. https://doi.org/10.1016/S0015-0282(16)57410-X.
6. Prevention of infection after gynecologic procedures: ACOG practice bulletin, number 195. Accessed 11 Apr 2023. https://oce-ovid-com.proxy.hsl.ucdenver.edu/article/00006250-201806000-00055/PDF.
7. Atkinson TM, Giraud GD, Togioka BM, Jones DB, Cigarroa JE. Cardiovascular and ventilatory consequences of laparoscopic surgery. Circulation. 2017;135(7):700–10. https://doi.org/10.1161/CIRCULATIONAHA.116.023262.
8. Cohen A, Almog B, Satel A, Lessing JB, Tsafrir Z, Levin I. Laparoscopy versus laparotomy in the management of ectopic pregnancy with massive hemoperitoneum. Int J Gynecol Obstet. 2013;123(2):139–41. https://doi.org/10.1016/j.ijgo.2013.05.014.
9. Rizzuto MI, Oliver R, Odejinmi F. Laparoscopic management of ectopic pregnancy in the presence of a significant haemoperitoneum. Arch Gynecol Obstet. 2008;277(5):433–6. https://doi.org/10.1007/s00404-007-0473-7.
10. Odejinmi F, Sangrithi M, Olowu O. Operative laparoscopy as the mainstay method in management of hemodynamically unstable patients with ectopic pregnancy. J Minim Invasive Gynecol. 2011;18(2):179–83. https://doi.org/10.1016/j.jmig.2010.11.005.
11. Birkhahn RH, Gaeta TJ, Van Deusen SK, Tloczkowski J. The ability of traditional vital signs and shock index to identify ruptured ectopic pregnancy. Am J Obstet Gynecol. 2003;189(5):1293–6. https://doi.org/10.1067/S0002-9378(03)00663-X.
12. Frates MC, Doubilet PM, Peters HE, Benson CB. Adnexal sonographic findings in ectopic pregnancy and their correlation with tubal rupture and human chorionic gonadotropin levels. J Ultrasound Med. 2014;33(4):697–703. https://doi.org/10.7863/ultra.33.4.697.
13. Popowski T, Huchon C, Toret-Labeeuw F, Chantry AA, Aegerter P, Fauconnier A. Hemoperitoneum assessment in ectopic pregnancy. Int J Gynecol Obstet. 2012;116(2):97–100. https://doi.org/10.1016/j.ijgo.2011.09.019.
14. Fauconnier A, Mabrouk A, Salomon LJ, Bernard JP, Ville Y. Ultrasound assessment of haemoperitoneum in ectopic pregnancy: derivation of a prediction

model. World J Emerg Surg. 2007;2(1):23. https://doi.org/10.1186/1749-7922-2-23.
15. Spandorfer SD, Menzin AW, Barnhart KT, LiVolsi VA, Pfeifer SM. Efficacy of frozen-section evaluation of uterine curettings in the diagnosis of ectopic pregnancy. Am J Obstet Gynecol. 1996;175(3):603–5. https://doi.org/10.1053/ob.1996.v175.a73599.
16. Donnez J, Nisolle M. 2 endoscopic management of ectopic pregnancy. Baillières Clin Obstet Gynaecol. 1994;8(4):707–22. https://doi.org/10.1016/S0950-3552(05)80051-3.
17. Rizzuto MI, Macrae R, Odejinmi F. Persistent ectopic pregnancy following ipsilateral "salpingectomy". Gynecol Surg. 2007;4(4):305–7. https://doi.org/10.1007/s10397-007-0298-1.
18. Ozcan MCH, Wilson JR, Frishman GN. A systematic review and meta-analysis of surgical treatment of ectopic pregnancy with salpingectomy versus salpingostomy. J Minim Invasive Gynecol. 2021;28(3):656–67. https://doi.org/10.1016/j.jmig.2020.10.014.
19. Spiegelberg O. Zur casuistik der ovarialschwangerschaft. Arch Gynaekol. 1878;13:73.
20. Bollig KJ, Schust DJ. Refining angular pregnancy diagnosis in the first trimester: a case series of expectant management. Obstet Gynecol. 2020;135(1):175–84. https://doi.org/10.1097/AOG.0000000000003595.
21. Grandelis A, Shaffer R, Tonick S. Uncommon presentations of ectopic pregnancy. J Gynecol Surg. 2022;38(3):185–92. https://doi.org/10.1089/gyn.2022.0016.
22. Lee MH, Im SY, Kim MK, Shin SY, Park WI. Comparison of laparoscopic cornual resection and cornuotomy for interstitial pregnancy. J Minim Invasive Gynecol. 2017;24(3):397–401. https://doi.org/10.1016/j.jmig.2016.11.016.
23. Liao CY, Tse J, Sung SY, Chen SH, Tsui WH. Cornual wedge resection for interstitial pregnancy and postoperative outcome. Aust N Z J Obstet Gynaecol. 2017;57(3):342–5. https://doi.org/10.1111/ajo.12497.
24. Kaur N, Reid F, Ma K. Ovarian ectopic pregnancy: laparoscopic excision and ovarian conservation. J Minim Invasive Gynecol. 2019;26(6):1006. https://doi.org/10.1016/j.jmig.2018.12.017.

Surgical Abortion

29

Christy M. Boraas and Jessika A. Ralph

Introduction

Induced abortion and early pregnancy loss in the United States are common. One in four pregnant people will have an induced abortion in their lifetime and roughly one tenth of clinically recognized pregnancies end in miscarriage [1, 2]. Though not all cases are managed surgically, induced abortion remains the second most common procedure for people of reproductive age after cesarean section [1, 3]. Surgical uterine evacuation for induced abortion or pregnancy loss in the United States is safe, and complications are infrequent. Abortion by any method is safer than childbirth; major complication (transfusion, unplanned hospitalization, further surgical procedures) rates for surgical uterine evacuation are less than 1% in the first trimester and less than 5% in the second trimester [4]. Other potential complications include hemorrhage, uterine and cervical injury, infection, and incomplete abortion. Because of the rarity of such events, many clinicians do not have direct experience managing complications of surgical abortion. This chapter details their management so all surgeons, regardless of training, can understand evidence-based procedural abortion care.

C. M. Boraas (✉) · J. A. Ralph
Department of Obstetrics, Gynecology and Women's Health, University of Minnesota Medical School, Minneapolis, MN, USA
e-mail: bora0021@umn.edu; ralph044@umn.edu

Hemorrhage

Hemorrhage after dilation and curettage (D&C) or dilation and evacuation (D&E) is rare, occurring less than 1% of the time and generally considered to be clinically relevant when requiring intervention (such as transfusion or hospital admission) and/or greater than 500 mL total blood loss [5]. Despite its low incidence, post-abortion hemorrhage is one of the most common causes of abortion-related morbidity and mortality, particularly in the second trimester [5]. Etiologies of hemorrhage are similar to those at the time of childbirth, including uterine atony, cervical laceration, retained products of conception, abnormal placentation, uterine perforation, and coagulopathy.

Uterine Atony

Background

Research suggests that atony, or hypercontractility of the uterus, is the most frequent cause of hemorrhage after abortion, identified in approximately 50% of cases [5]. Older patient age and increasing gestational duration were independent risk factors for hemorrhage due to atony, specifically in the second trimester [5]. Other risk factors include prior cesarean section, history of obstetric hemorrhage, underlying bleeding disorders, uterine leiomyomata, and obesity [5].

M. Hoffman et al. (eds.), *Major Complications of Female Pelvic Surgery*,
https://doi.org/10.1007/978-3-031-66772-5_29

Prevention

Hemorrhage prevention measures include the use of vasopressin or epinephrine in the paracervical block, which has been shown to decrease blood loss with dilation and evacuation procedures, especially in the second trimester [6]. Prophylactic use of methylergonovine does not reduce blood loss at the time of surgical abortion, but the use of prophylactic oxytocin has been shown to reduce hemorrhage frequency for second-trimester procedures [4, 7]. The use of halogenated anesthetic gas is also associated with atony and thus is not recommended in the setting of surgical abortion [8].

Recognition

If hemorrhage after surgical abortion does occur, a general approach should start with a physical exam, including inspection of the cervix and vagina to look for lacerations, a bimanual exam to assess uterine tone, and bedside ultrasonography to help identify hematometra, free fluid in the pelvis, or retained tissue.

Management

In the absence of other identifiable causes, poor uterine tone should be considered the primary etiology and bimanual massage should be initiated. Concurrent administration of uterotonic medications should occur if the tone does not rapidly improve and can successfully treat bleeding much of the time. Most used medications for uterine atony are listed in Table 29.1 [9]. There is little evidence to recommend one agent over another. However, due to its rapid onset, administration of methylergonovine maleate is frequently used first unless contraindicated. If heavy bleeding persists, multiple medications and/or doses should be administered, while also reassessing for other potential causes (Figs. 29.1, 29.2, and 29.3).

When bleeding is refractory, additional immediate interventions include placement of additional intravenous access, fluid resuscitation, laboratory evaluation, and consideration of potential transfusion. Intrauterine tamponade with a Foley catheter or intrauterine balloon is often a logical next step; balloons are left in place for up to 24 hours while ensuring hemodynamic stability. Intrauterine tamponade may be similarly achieved with the packing of plain or medication-soaked (vasopressin or thrombin) gauze. If all the above-listed interventions are insufficient, more intensive and invasive procedures may be required, such as uterine artery embolization (UAE), laparoscopy, laparotomy, and rarely, hysterectomy.

Table 29.1 Commonly used medications for surgical abortion hemorrhage[a]

Medication	Dose and route of administration	Dosing frequency	Contraindications[b]
Methylergonovine maleate	0.2 mg PO, IM, IV	Every 2–4 hours	Hypertension
Misoprostol (PGE1 analog)	800 mcg buccal or sublingual	Every 4 hours	Rare
Carboprost (15-methyl PGF2alpha)	0.25 mg IM	Every 15–90 minutes, not to execeed eight doses	Asthma
Oxytocin[c]	10 units IM 10–40 units per 500–1000 mL IV bolus then as continuous infusion	Once	Rare
Tranexamic acid	1 g in 10 mL IV given over 10 minutes	Second dose after 30 minutes if ongoing bleeding	Caution with concurrent antifibrinolytic therapy
Vasopressin[d]	2–8 units per 10–30 mL of saline or local anesthetic	Once	Rare

PO per os, *IM* Intramuscular, *IV* Intravenous, *PGF* prostaglandin F, *PGE* prostaglandin E

[a] Adapted from [9, 15]

[b] In addition to known hypersensitivity to any of the medications

[c] For prevention and treatment

[d] Primarily for prevention, no clear role in acute treatment of hemorrhage

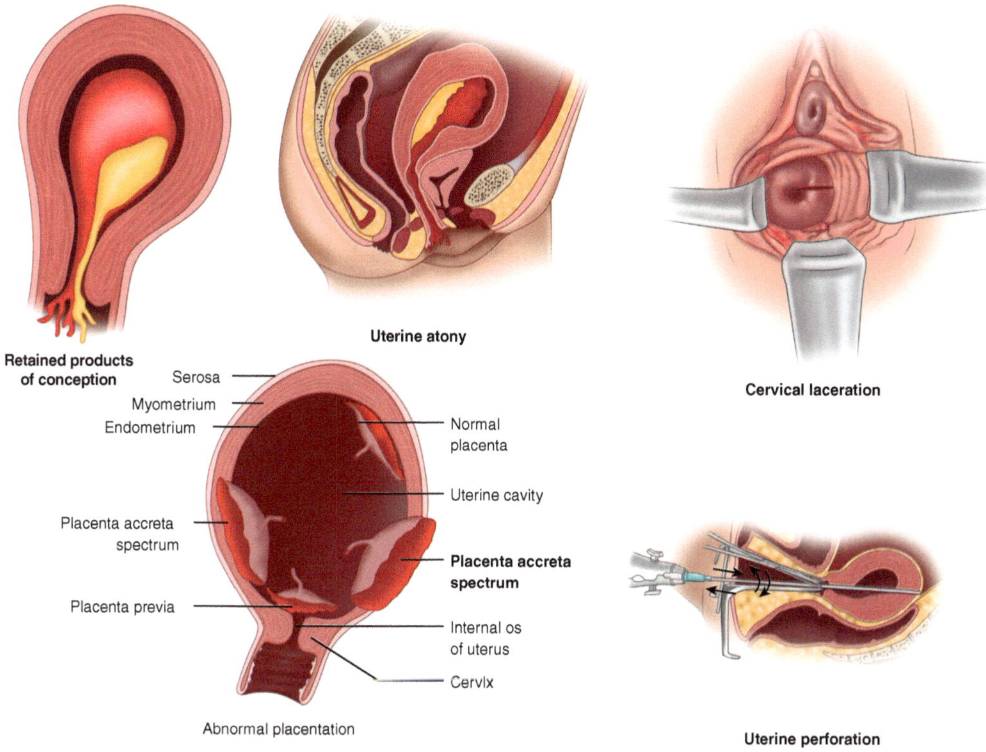

Fig. 29.1 Etiologies of surgical abortion hemorrhage

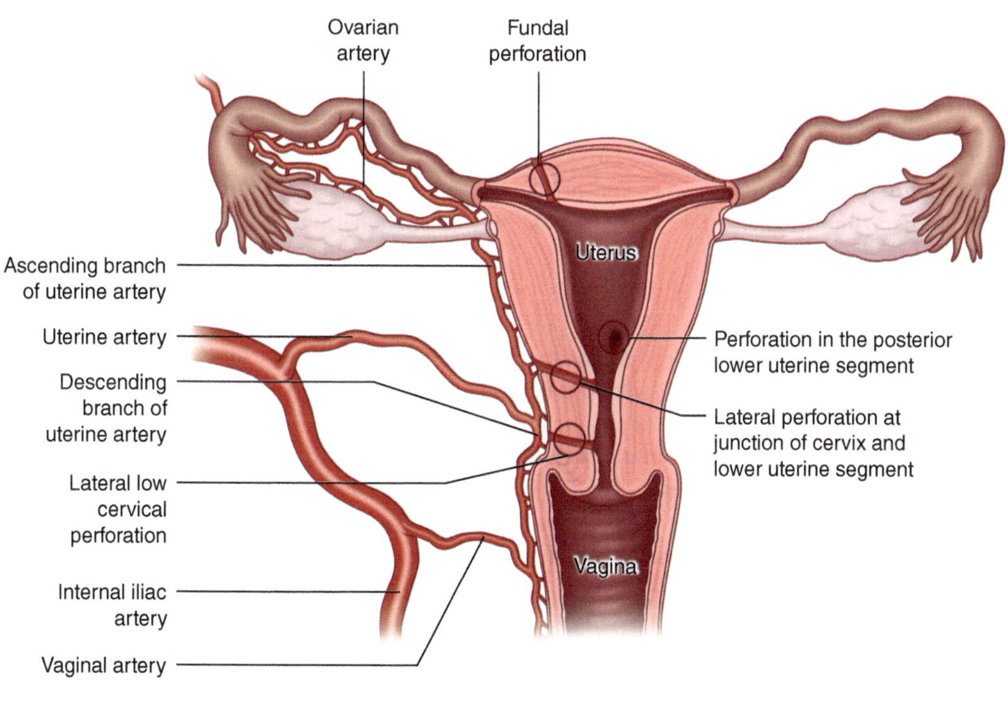

Fig. 29.2 Sites of uterine perforation during surgical abortion

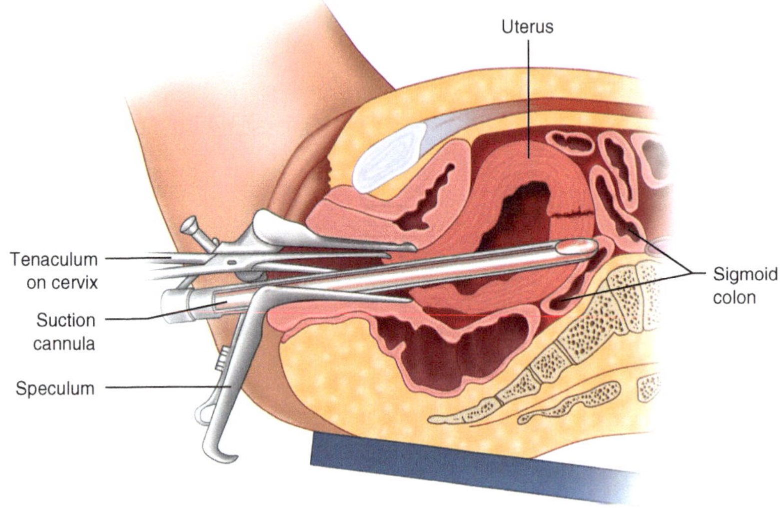

Fig. 29.3 Mechanism of uterine perforation during surgical abortion

Abnormal Placentation

Background

Abnormal placentation, formerly called placenta accreta, increta, and percreta, is now known as placenta accreta spectrum (PAS) disorder and is associated with potentially massive and life-threatening hemorrhage. With a rising incidence, surgeons should maintain a high index of suspicion for PAS, particularly for patients with prior cesarean section or other uterine surgery that involves the full thickness of the myometrium [10].

Prevention

Preoperative identification of PAS is associated with significantly less blood loss and should be evaluated with ultrasonography and/or magnetic resonance imaging in patients presenting with a complete placenta previa and a history of prior uterine surgery or any other concerning findings on ultrasonography. Second-trimester placenta previa is diagnosed in about 2–6% of pregnancies, however, previa alone (without PAS) does not complicate surgical uterine evacuation, including D&E [8].

Patients with suspected PAS have an increased risk of hemorrhage at the time of surgical uterine evacuation and may be best served in a hospital setting with experienced surgeons and the capacity for large-volume blood product transfusion. Access to hospital-based care for induced abortion varies greatly across the United States given the political landscape and restrictive abortion care policy. For those patients desiring future fertility, D&E may be considered depending upon patient and team level factors, operative setting, preoperative imaging, etc. Given the ability of the placenta to invade the uterine myometrium, serosa, parametrium, bladder, and rarely other organs such as the ureters, rectum, and vagina, multidisciplinary care planning, including anesthesia, maternal-fetal medicine, gynecologic oncology, urology, and interventional radiology may help preoperatively in these cases.

Recognition and Management

Hemorrhage during surgical abortion in the setting of PAS should prompt a quick escalation of intervention. Occasionally, UAE alone may be successful in controlling bleeding, but laparoscopy or laparotomy with hysterectomy may be required. Alternatively, for patients that do not desire future fertility, hemorrhage may be reduced or avoided by offering gravid hysterectomy, with or without preoperative UAE, rather than D&E.

Acute Coagulopathy

Background
Disseminated intravascular coagulation (DIC), the extreme activation of the coagulation cascade that leads to depletion of clotting factors and platelets is a rare but serious complication of D&E and is rarely seen after D&C. DIC at the time of surgical abortion tends to be consumptive, in response to massive hemorrhage. DIC associated with late first or second-trimester uterine evacuation is more likely to occur in the setting of an intrauterine fetal demise, especially if the demise occurred at a more advanced gestational duration and when there has been a longer interval between demise and uterine evacuation [11–13]. Amniotic fluid embolism is an even more rare etiology of post-abortion DIC that is not preventable, is characterized by hemodynamic and respiratory collapse, and requires emergent resuscitation [14]. The overall incidence of DIC is roughly 2% for D&E cases performed for fetal demise and 0.2% for other indications, and onset typically occurs within 2 hours of the procedure [12, 13].

Prevention
No known preoperative measures alter the risk of DIC at the time of D&E but surgeons should consider preoperative laboratory evaluation including blood typing, complete blood count, coagulation studies including prothrombin time, fibrinogen level, and consideration of blood crossmatching.

Recognition
No universally recognized diagnostic criteria or single laboratory test can diagnose DIC and clinical recognition remains the mainstay. Laboratory evaluation of platelets, fibrinogen, and D-dimer are useful for diagnosis and evaluation of resuscitation efforts. DIC should be suspected with persistent bleeding from uterine atony or cervical laceration or other etiology, especially when it is failing to clot, and with any signs of cardiovascular compromise.

Management
Given most DIC occurs secondary to another etiology of bleeding, identifying and addressing the primary cause of bleeding is paramount. Concurrently, preparing for blood product replacement therapy is critical. Many D&E procedures take place in outpatient settings without access to blood banking and thus, the next steps are stabilizing the patient with intravenous fluid resuscitation and initiating emergent transfer to a higher acuity setting. In the hospital setting, surgeons should maintain ongoing communication with anesthesia and support teams in the operating room and consider activating the massive transfusion protocol. Recommendations for optimal timing of transfusion for pregnant patients are limited but generally recommended to be a 1:1:1 ratio of red blood cells:fresh frozen plasma:platelets and in the setting of DIC, consideration of early use of cryoprecipitate [15]. Surgeons should be aware of specific protocols at their institutions. Continued clinical and lab assessments are recommended to assess response to blood components.

Cervical Injury

Background

Cervical injury occurs in fewer than 1% of D&Cs and roughly 2% of D&Es [16, 17]. The risk of cervical laceration is increased in individuals without a prior vaginal birth, as well as in cases of more advanced gestation [16].

Prevention

During D&C, the diameter of the required instruments is small and pregnancy tissue is pliable; thus, the cervix may be opened safely with mechanical dilation alone. However, during D&E, the dilation needed to accommodate forceps and fetal tissue is greater, and mechanical dilation alone frequently results in laceration. Preparation of the cervix, either with osmotic dilators, medications, or both reduces the likelihood of cervical laceration [18]. Protocols for cervical preparation vary widely and may occur over hours or days; no one method has been demonstrated to be superior. While a review of potential methods of preparation is beyond the scope of this chapter, they may include mifepristone and/or misoprostol to produce cervical softening and effacement; dilation may be achieved mechanically with a foley balloon or via osmotic dilators such as Dilapan-S or laminaria tents [19, 20].

Recognition

Distal cervical lacerations near the external os are directly visible on an exam. Lacerations of the proximal cervix, near the internal os, can be more difficult to diagnose, both because the internal os is likely not directly visible, and because its injury can create continuity with the abdominal cavity or the retroperitoneal space. Lacerations of the proximal cervix should be suspected if bleeding continues from the endocervical canal in the presence of a firm uterus [8].

Management

Small distal cervical lacerations can often be treated with direct pressure, sometimes combined with the application of silver nitrate or ferric subsulfate solution. Larger lacerations may require re-approximation with absorbable suture [8]. Proximal cervical lacerations can be managed with cervical stay sutures at 3 and 9 o'clock combined with tamponade, which can be achieved with packing or a Foley catheter. If these measures are not sufficient, uterine artery embolization should be considered [8].

Uterine Injury

Background

Uterine perforation is an uncommon complication during surgical abortion. The rate of occurrence ranges from 0.09 to 15 per 1000 cases [16]. Risk factors for perforation are advanced parity, increasing gestational duration, and the use of a uterine sound [8, 16, 17].

Prevention

Like cervical lacerations, appropriate preparation of the cervix helps prevent uterine perforation from occurring. Ultrasound guidance for D&E procedures is reasonable but has not been definitively shown to reduce rates of perforation given the rarity of this complication [8, 19, 20].

Recognition

A surgeon may have increased suspicion for perforation when an instrument passes further than expected without resistance or the gritty sensation is no longer appreciated with the aspiration curette. Patients may develop hypotension, bowel/omentum may be visualized in the instrument, and patients who are awake may express sudden onset pain. The small bowel is the most common viscera injury and can occur through anterior or fundal uterine perforations, while the large bowel is primarily injured through posterior perforations [8].

Management

Low-risk perforation patients (blunt instruments without suction, typically in the first or early second trimesters) can be discharged home after extended observation to ensure no hemodynamic instability; the perforations will resolve without further treatment or sequelae. Higher-risk perforations tend to be: lateral; 1 to 2 cm in diameter; occurring after the first trimester; and associated with acute abdominal pain, symptomatic blood loss, or bowel injury. Ultrasound can be used to observe if there is free fluid in the pelvis, however, laparoscopy or laparotomy may be required if injury to the adnexa or bowel is suspected or if blood loss leads to hemodynamic instability [8, 16, 17].

Infection

Background

Postabortal infection is rare in safe abortion settings, occurring after less than 1% of induced abortions at any gestation in the United States. Most commonly, patients present with endometritis due to translocation of skin, vaginal, and/or gastrointestinal flora into the endometrial cavity; rarely, patients present with sepsis. Risk factors for postabortal infection include an active, untreated sexually transmitted infection or bacterial vaginosis at the time of the procedure [21].

Prevention

Routine antibiotic prophylaxis is the mainstay of prevention and reduces the rate of postoperative infection significantly [8]. The Society of Family Planning recommends a single dose of doxycycline 200 mg pre-operatively; other potential choices are listed in Table 29.2 [22]. Vaginal preparation with either povodine-iodine or chlorhexidine solution does not reduce infection rates. Preoperative screening for *N. gonorrhea* and *C. trachomatis* should be recommended for those with risk factors such as younger age [21].

Recognition

Typically, patients present within a few days of the procedure with some combination of pelvic pain, uterine tenderness, fever, and leukocytosis. These criteria are subjective and likely cause overdiagnosis, but as potential sequelae include infertility and sepsis, a low threshold for treatment is acceptable. Rarely do patients present with toxic shock; these patients may not have specific pelvic complaints but instead manifest general malaise and refractory hypotension [8, 21].

Table 29.2 Commonly used antibiotics for surgical abortion infection prophylaxis[a]

Medication	Dose and route of administration
Doxycycline	200 mg PO or IV
Metronidazole	500 mg PO or IV
Tinidazole	2 g PO or IV
Azithromycin	1 g PO or IV

PO per os, *IM* Intramuscular, *IV* Intravenous
[a]Adapted from [8, 21]

Management

Treatment of postoperative uterine infection typically follows treatment for pelvic inflammatory disease (PID) as it is usually polymicrobial in nature; coverage for *C. trachomatis* should be included. A frequently prescribed combination is ceftriaxone and doxycycline (see the Centers for Disease Control and Prevention PID guidelines for others). Imaging should be considered to rule out retained products of conception as well as pelvic abscess. If identified, retained tissue in the endometrial cavity should be promptly evacuated; an abscess may require percutaneous drainage. Patients who present with sepsis or toxic shock should be given supportive care with aggressive fluid resuscitation, and/or vasopressors, as needed [8, 21].

Retained Products of Conception

Background

Residual pregnancy tissue (incomplete abortion) and/or blood products (hematometra) retained within the uterus following surgical abortion, while uncommon, may cause patients discomfort and predispose them to further complications of ongoing bleeding and infection. The incidence of re-aspiration is low, 0.29–1.96% of patients in the first trimester and 0.40–2.70% in the second trimester, most commonly for hematometra [8].

Prevention

Immediate postoperative inspection of tissue removed from the uterus is standard practice and confirms abortion procedure completion in most cases[7]. Formal pathology evaluation of evacuated tissue is not routinely indicated. It is also crucial for surgeons to note a "gritty" texture with the suction cannula on all intrauterine surfaces and the resolution of any brisk bleeding from the cervical os prior to terminating the procedure. Ultrasound guidance, while not routinely necessary, may be helpful to confirm procedure completion, particularly in anatomically variant or logistically challenging cases, as well as those performed at more advanced gestational durations.

Recognition and Management

Diagnosis and treatment are typically guided by clinical presentation, as it can be normal to observe heterogeneous endometrial tissue and/or small collections of clotted blood on ultrasound examination following clinically complete surgical abortion. Patients presenting with persistent pelvic pain, fever, or ongoing heavy bleeding should undergo prompt imaging and consideration of re-aspiration or treatment with misoprostol to empty uterine contents and avoid further complications.

Conclusions

Overall, surgical evacuation of pregnancy in the first and second trimesters either with dilation and curettage or dilation and evacuation is safe, and complications are rare. Risk generally increases with advancing gestational duration of pregnancy. Understanding risk factors, steps to minimize risk, and overall management of more common potential complications can help decrease surgical morbidity.

References

1. Jones RK, Jerman J. Population group abortion rates and lifetime incidence of abortion: United States, 2008–2014. Am J Public Health. 2017;107(12):1904–9.
2. ACOG practice bulletin no. 200: early pregnancy loss. Obstet Gynecol. 2018;132(5):e197–207.
3. Kortsmit K, Mandel MG, Reeves JA, et al. Abortion surveillance—United States, 2019. MMWR Surveill Summ. 2021;70(SS-9):1–29.
4. National Academies of Sciences, Engineering, and Medicine. The safety and quality of abortion care in the United States. Washington, DC: The National Academies Press. Online document at; 2018. https://doi.org/10.17226/24950. Accessed 7 Mar 2022.
5. Kerns J, Steinauer J. Management of postabortion hemorrhage: release date November 2012 SFP Guideline #20131. Contraception. 2013;87(3):331–42.
6. Frick AC, Drey EA, Diedrich JT, Steinauer JE. Effect of prior cesarean delivery on risk of second-trimester surgical abortion complications. Obstet Gynecol. 2010;115:760–4.
7. Whitehouse K, Tschann M, Soon R, Davis J, Micks E, Salcedo J, Savala M, Kaneshiro B. Effects of prophylactic oxytocin on bleeding outcomes in women undergoing dilation and evacuation: a randomized controlled trial. Obstet Gynecol. 2019;133(3):484–91.
8. Lichtenberg ES, Grimes DA. Surgical complications: prevention and management. In: Paul M, Lichtenberg ES, Borgatta L, Grimes DA, Stubblefield PG, Creinin MD, editors. Management of unintended and abnormal pregnancy: comprehensive abortion care. John Wiley & Sons, Ltd.: Chichester; 2009. http://ebookcentral.proquest.com/lib/umn/detail.action?docID=437417.
9. Harris LH, Grossman D. Complications of unsafe and self-managed abortion. N Engl J Med. 2020;382(11):1029–40.
10. Jauniaux E, Bunce C, Grønbeck L, Langhoff-Roos J. Prevalence and main outcomes of placenta accreta spectrum: a systematic review and meta-analysis. Am J Obstet Gynecol. 2019;221:208–18.
11. Kerns JL, Ti A, Aksel S, Lederle L, Sokoloff A, Steinauer J. Disseminated intravascular coagulation and hemorrhage after dilation and evacuation abortion for fetal death. Obstet Gynecol. 2019;134(4):708–13.
12. Fontenot Ferriss AN, Weisenthal L, Sheeder J, Teal SB, Tocce K. Risk of hemorrhage during surgical evacuation for second-trimester intrauterine fetal demise. Contraception. 2016;94(5):496–8.
13. York S, Lichtenberg ES. Characteristics of presumptive idiopathic disseminated intravascular coagulation during second-trimester induced abortion. Contraception. 2012;85(5):489–95.
14. Clark SL, Romero R, Dildy GA, Callaghan WM, Smiley RM, Bracey AW, et al. Proposed diagnostic criteria for the case definition of amniotic fluid embolism in research studies. Am J Obstet Gynecol. 2016;215:408–12.
15. ACOG practice bulletin no. 183: postpartum hemorrhage. Obstet Gynecol. 2017;130(4):e168–86.
16. Diedrich J, Steinauer J. Complications of surgical abortion. Clin Obstet Gynecol. 2009;52(2):205–12. https://doi.org/10.1097/GRF.0b013e3181a2b756.
17. White K, Carroll E, Grossman D. Complications from first-trimester aspiration abortion: a systematic review of the literature. Contraception. 2015;92(5):422–38.

https://doi.org/10.1016/j.contraception.2015.07.013. Epub 2015 Aug 1.
18. Peterson WF, Berry FN, Grace MR, Gulbranson CL. Second-trimester abortion by dilation and evacuation: an analysis of 11,747 cases. Obstet Gynecol. 1983;62(2):185–90.
19. Diedrich JT, Drey EA, Newmann SJ. Society of Family Planning clinical recommendations: cervical preparation for dilation at 20–24 weeks' gestation. Contraception. 2020;101(5):286–92.
20. Fox MC, Krajewski CM. Cervical preparation for second-trimester surgical abortion prior to 20 weeks' gestation. Contraception. 2014;89(2):75–84.
21. Achilles SL, Reeves MF. Prevention of infection after induced abortion. Contraception. 2010;83(4):295–309.
22. Achilles SL, Reeves MF, Society of Family Planning (SFP). Prevention of infection after induced abortion: released date October 2010: SFP guideline 20102. Contraception. 2011(83):295.

Cesarean Hysterectomy

30

Brett D. Einerson and Andrew P. Soisson

Introduction

The incidence of cesarean hysterectomy, defined as hysterectomy associated with cesarean delivery, is reported to occur in approximately 71–82 cases per 100,00 deliveries worldwide. The prevalence of cesarean hysterectomy is directly related to the increasing incidence of cesarean delivery which is now performed in at least 30% of all births [1]. The most common indication for cesarean hysterectomy is maternal hemorrhage associated with uterine atony (35.3% of cases), placental accreta spectrum (34.8% of cases), and uterine rupture/trauma [2, 3]. Uterine atony is the most common cause of hemorrhage although abnormal placentation is increasingly recognized as a key contributor.

Placenta accreta spectrum (PAS) is defined as abnormal adherence of the placenta to the uterine myometrium. Abnormal attachment of the placenta directly to the myometrium prevents its complete removal leading to almost immediate hemorrhage [4]. This condition develops due to disruption of decidualized endometrium in areas of the uterus that have undergone surgical trauma such as prior dilation and curettage, prior myomectomy, endometrial ablation, and especially cesarean section. The incidence of placenta accreta has now risen to almost 1 in 500 births [5].

Uterine scar rupture is another cause of cesarean hysterectomy and occurs in approximately 0.7–1.6% of those with prior cesarean deliveries undergoing labor. In patients undergoing a trial of labor after cesarean (TOLAC), hysterectomy for uterine rupture is required in 0.19–0.56% [6].

This is a review of the common complications of cesarean hysterectomy, both in those with and those without placenta accreta spectrum.

Complications of Simple Cesarean Hysterectomy

The most common complications associated with simple cesarean hysterectomy, which we will define as hysterectomy due to uterine atony or rupture and not PAS, are hemorrhage and surgical site infection (SSI). Injury to the urologic tract is also common and will be discussed in the section on the placenta accreta spectrum.

B. D. Einerson
Department of Obstetrics & Gynecology, University of Utah, Salt Lake City, UT, USA
e-mail: brett.einerson@hsc.utah.edu

A. P. Soisson (✉)
Division of Gynecologic Oncology, Department of Obstetrics & Gynecology, University of Utah, Salt Lake City, UT, USA
e-mail: andrew.soisson@hci.utah.edu

M. Hoffman et al. (eds.), *Major Complications of Female Pelvic Surgery*,
https://doi.org/10.1007/978-3-031-66772-5_30

Obstetric Hemorrhage

Background

Hemorrhage is by far and away the most common complication of cesarean hysterectomy. Uncomplicated cesarean delivery is associated with approximately a 1000 cc blood loss whereas blood loss associated with hysterectomy is significantly higher [7].

Prevention

Uncontrolled obstetric hemorrhage is often *the indication for* cesarean hysterectomy, and so prevention may not be possible. Even so, severe obstetric hemorrhage can be prevented by prompt recognition of bleeding during cesarean section and by thorough evaluation of the cause and possible treatments. In our experience, a delay in recognizing the need for definitive treatment of obstetric hemorrhage with hysterectomy is often the source of preventable morbidity.

Recognition

Estimation of blood loss during surgery by the surgeon has been shown in multiple studies to be largely inaccurate. Quantitative methods to measure blood loss are better but do not appear to alter clinical outcomes and probably are unnecessary [7]. We recommend close monitoring and communication of blood loss during the case, and if the procedure is taking longer than 90 minutes we would advise serial hematocrit measurements every 15 minutes until completion of the hysterectomy.

Management

Surgeons should anticipate at least a 1500 cc blood loss associated with a simple cesarean hysterectomy and therefore we would recommend that two units of packed red blood cells be available for the procedure. We would not anticipate the need for fibrinogen or platelets. Furthermore, we would not anticipate the need for intra-arterial catheters to temporarily occlude the aorta or the iliac vessels.

Should significant hemorrhage occur during the operative procedure we would recommend consideration of internal iliac or uterine artery ligation. Should the surgeon elect to perform internal iliac (hypogastric) ligation, we recommend ligation of the round ligament followed by retro-peritoneal exploration to identify and locate the ureter. The internal iliac artery can be either clipped with a medium-sized Hema-clip or ligated with a #1 or 0-sized permanent suture such as silk [8]. The vessel should be ligated more than 2 cm beyond the bifurcation of the common and internal iliac artery to avoid disruption of the posterior branch.

Prevention and management of massive hemorrhage related to PAS are discussed further in the section below.

Surgical Site Infection

Background

The incidence of surgical site infections (SSI), defined as wound infection or pelvic abscess, is less than 1% in women undergoing cesarean delivery [9] but much higher in obese and diabetic women [10]. In women undergoing cesarean hysterectomy, SSI occurs in 6–10%, similar to the rate in women undergoing abdominal hysterectomy (4–10%) [3, 11].

Prevention

The most significant clinical factor associated with a reduction in the risk of SSI after is the appropriate use of prophylactic antibiotics. Extrapolating from ACOG committee opinions and studies, we recommend a single dose of a second-generation cephalosporin plus metronidazole or clindamycin prior to initiating surgery [12, 13].

Finally, it is the opinion of the authors that the use of a prophylactic negative pressure wound device should be considered in obese women who undergo cesarean hysterectomy. Studies of cesarean hysterectomy are lacking, but a Cochrane literature review of patients undergoing laparotomy [14] and a prospective randomized trial in cesarean section [15] both suggest that these devices will reduce the incidence of SSI in high-risk individuals.

Recognition

Recognition of an SSI is primarily through physical examination of the wound for the appearance of erythema, fluctuance of the tissues, crepitus, and the presence of dead and devitalized tissue. Other signs such as fever and leukocytosis are often helpful for diagnosis. Pelvic abscess following hysterectomy often presents with fever and lower abdominal pain, and examination may reveal a fluctuant mass or severe tenderness in the pelvis or at the vaginal cuff. Imaging with CT is recommended to evaluate for the presence of a rim-enhancing, thick-walled fluid structure in the pelvis.

Management

As with all surgical wounds that are infected, treatment consists of antibiotics, incision and drainage of the wound if an abscess exits, and surgical debridement to remove devitalized tissues. Pelvic abscesses should be treated with broad-spectrum intravenous antibiotics. Larger abscesses (e.g., those measuring >7 cm) or smaller abscesses that fail to respond to a 48-hour course of broad-spectrum intravenous antibiotics may need drainage which can be accomplished vaginally or by an interventional radiologist percutaneously, although the indications and criteria for pelvic abscess drainage are controversial.

Cesarean Hysterectomy with Placenta Accreta Spectrum (PAS)

In addition to the complications listed above, PAS presents specific challenges to the surgical team performing cesarean hysterectomy. As a result of distorted anatomy and pelvic hypervascularity, strategies to prevent and manage complications in patients with PAS differ substantially from those undergoing cesarean hysterectomy without PAS.

Massive Obstetric Hemorrhage

Background

The most important and life-threatening complication of cesarean hysterectomy for placenta accreta spectrum (PAS) is rapid and massive obstetric hemorrhage. Massive hemorrhage, which can be described as the need for >8 units of red blood cell transfusion within a 24-hour period, occurs in 7%-25% depending on disease severity, the surgical approach, and the surgical team experience [16].

Patients with PAS are at particularly high risk for massive bleeding during cesarean hysterectomy for several reasons including [1] significantly increased blood flow to the pregnant uterus, [2] distortion of the lower uterine segment and pelvic anatomy by an abnormally attached and highly vascular placenta, and [3] recruitment of sometimes enormous and typically numerous collateral pelvic blood vessels. Dissection and ligation of main and collateral arteries during hysterectomy is therefore potentially hazardous with even small surgical missteps resulting in rapid placental bleeding or vascular bleeding.

Prevention

To prevent massive obstetric bleeding in PAS, there is no substitute for surgical experience and team-based care. Interdisciplinary team-based surgical care in high-volume centers is associated with a marked reduction in the risk of massive bleeding and other immediate surgical morbidities [17, 18]. Data are lacking to inform the minimum number of cases to ensure adequate volume, but ideally, the PAS surgical team should perform several cases per year. Many of the busiest centers in the United States now perform PAS surgery for 20–70 cases per year. When possible, patients with PAS should be cared for in high-volume centers with PAS experience.

Preventing massive bleeding from PAS is considerably easier than managing it. Experience enables the surgical team to avoid the surgical missteps that occur in cesarean hysterectomy for the placenta accreta spectrum. Common surgical missteps [19, 20] are:

- **Disrupting or bisecting the placenta during delivery** of the newborn, resulting in bleeding from the placenta. If PAS is identified at the time of laparotomy for cesarean delivery, do not cut through it or near it. Fundal or even posterior hysterotomy may be needed to avoid the placenta. (Fig. 30.1). During delivery of the newborn, take care to avoid placental disruption that can occur manually with difficult delivery or with excessive fundal pressure.
- **Attempting to forcibly deliver the placenta** when PAS is suspected. Attempted delivery of the placenta in known cases of PAS most commonly results in massive and difficult-to-control bleeding. Make no attempt to deliver the placenta when PAS is identified.
- **Excessive bleeding from a fundal or classical hysterotomy** during delivery. One approach to reducing bleeding from the hysterotomy itself is sequential clamping of engorged sinuses along the length of the incision. Another approach we have adopted is the use of a linear stapling-cutting device [21] to create an avascular uterine incision large enough to deliver the fetus(es). (Fig. 30.2a–f).
- **Attempting difficult bladder dissection before securing sources of arterial blood flow**. After securing the utero-ovarian circulation, the team should attempt to ligate the uterine arteries *prior to proceeding with bladder dissection*. The intent here is to reduce blood flow to the placenta as much as possible before it could potentially be disrupted (and fill the pelvis with blood).
- **Operating too slowly after bleeding has started**. Once brisk placental bleeding has started, it is incredibly difficult to contain and may, over the course of a long operation, result in additional liters of blood loss. The most experienced surgeons available should move quickly to complete the hysterectomy to avoid this misstep. If the cervix is not involved with PAS, a supracervical hysterectomy can be performed to expedite specimen removal.

***Prophylactic* use of endovascular interventions** to prevent massive bleeding during cesarean hysterectomy is controversial. Balloon occlusion can be applied at multiple levels from the distal aorta to common and internal iliac and uterine arteries (Fig. 30.3). Any time after delivery of the newborn, balloons can be inflated to reduce flow to the uterus and pelvis. Most prospective studies show no benefit in reducing blood loss [22], although a meta-analysis of uncontrolled studies

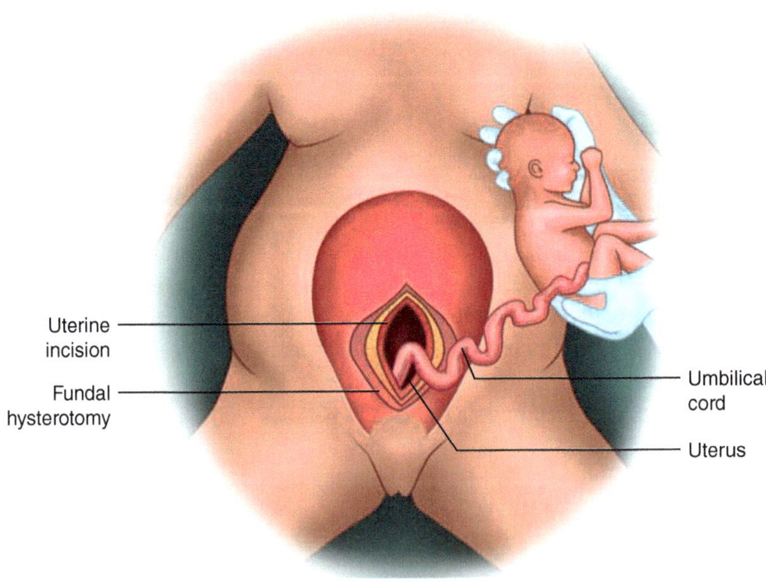

Fig. 30.1 Fundal hysterotomy may be needed to avoid the placenta

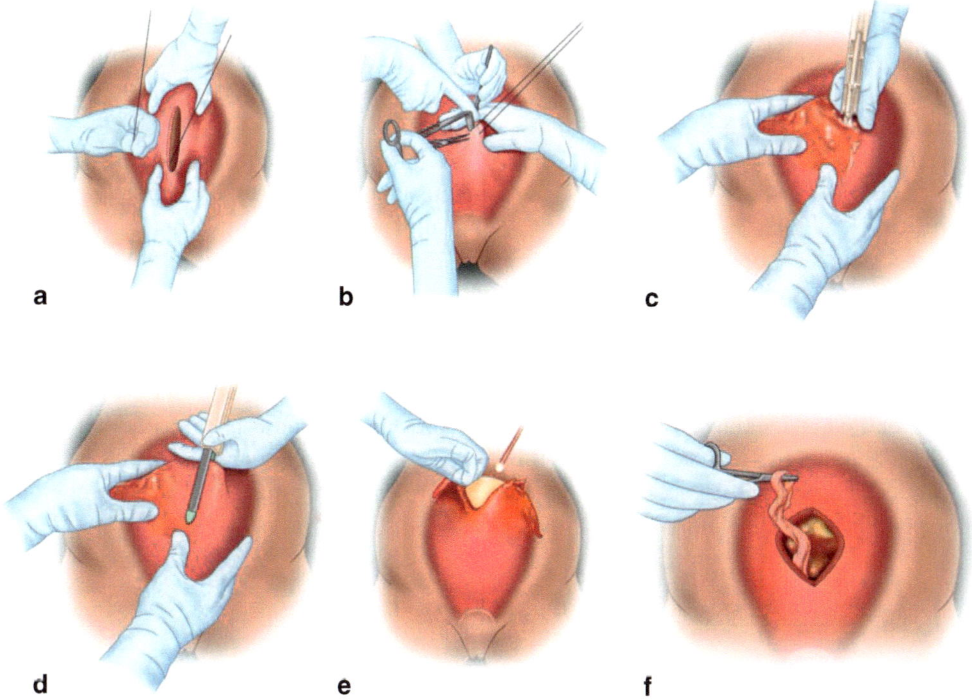

Fig. 30.2 (**a**–**f**) Use of a linear stapling-cutting device to create an avascular uterine incision large enough to deliver the fetus

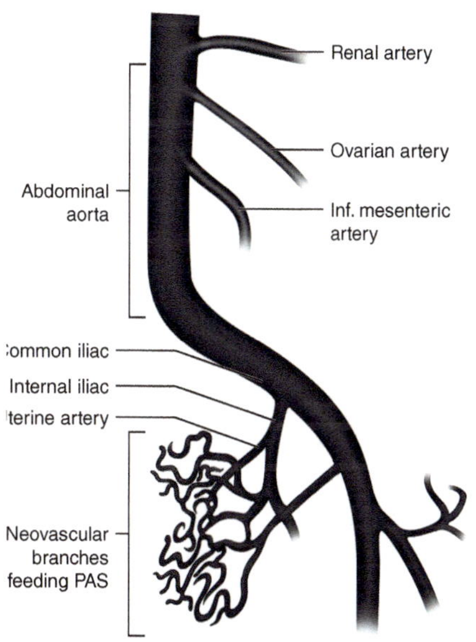

Fig. 30.3 Vascular anatomy related to prophylactic use of endovascular interventions

with highly variable approaches suggests possible benefit [23]. More research is needed before widespread adoption, particularly since serious complications have been reported, including arterial thrombosis with limb ischemia, balloon rupture or migration, and vessel injury [24].

Alternative approaches to immediate cesarean hysterectomy for PAS are still considered investigational. *Delaying hysterectomy* until weeks later may allow for partial involution of the pregnant uterus and reduction in hypervascularity. Outcomes of delayed hysterectomy suggest that total blood loss is lower with this approach (750 mL vs 2500 mL), although total operating time and hospital length of stay are longer [25, 26]. Another alternative is *conservative* in situ *management* wherein the placenta is left undisturbed in the uterus, hysterectomy is intentionally avoided, and the patient is monitored closely over time as the placenta slowly is absorbed or passed out of the body [27]. Conservative in situ management may reduce the immediate risk of major bleeding and transfusion by up to 70% [28]. However, patients face prolonged follow-up over the course of months, a higher rate of hospital readmission and endometritis, and, in the end, 15–20% will require hysterectomy.

Recognition

Massive placental or vascular bleeding during cesarean hysterectomy is unmistakable if it occurs in the surgical field. But beware: large volumes of blood can be lost vaginally and not recognized if the surgical team is unaware of this possibility or is not looking. We position the patient in lithotomy (not supine) and perform timed surgical check-ins to assess for vaginal bleeding periodically (Fig. 30.4).

Management

If brisk placental bleeding is encountered and the hysterectomy is far from complete, the surgical team has several options that may help to reduce blood loss.

A bleeding **placenta extruding from the uterus can be compressed** manually by one of the surgeons or assistants. This is an imperfect but suitable method in helping the team move along to the next steps of the hysterectomy without delay. Spending time suturing, oversewing the placenta, or applying compression sutures is less effective in our opinion, since the surrounding uterus is typically thin and distorted and the placenta hemorrhages briskly once released regardless of these techniques. (Fig. 30.5).

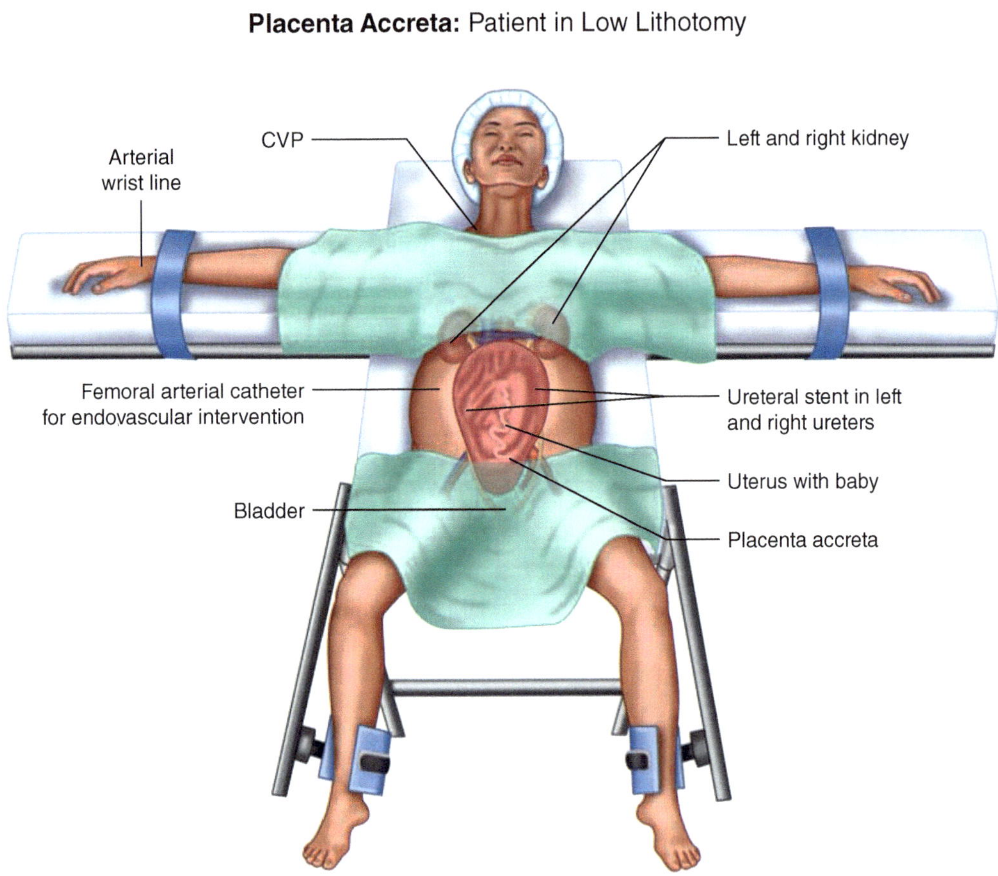

Fig. 30.4 Placenta accreta: Patient in low lithotomy

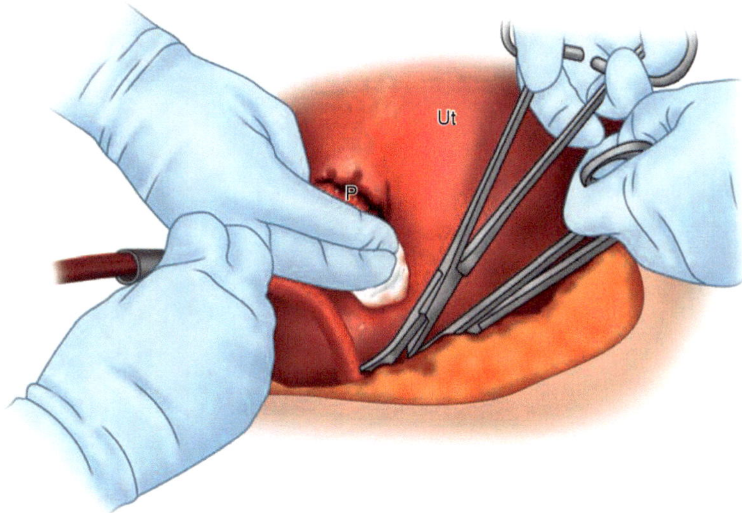

Fig. 30.5 A bleeding placenta extruding from the uterus can be compressed

Another option is **endovascular balloon occlusion or embolization**. Arterial access (typically femoral) can be achieved prior to surgery to allow for more rapid application of arterial catheters (aorta, common iliac, or internal iliac) or embolization during a hemorrhage. This approach, applying endovascular interventions *in response to hemorrhage*, contrasts with the *prophylactic* use of these devices as mentioned above.

When the rate or volume of blood loss is truly critical and life-threatening, as when there are several liters lost in a matter of minutes or when there is cardiovascular collapse due to hypovolemic shock, the surgical team can consider **manual aortic compression** (pressing down directly on the aorta) or aortic cross-clamping to reduce blood flow to the pelvis temporarily while quickly completing the hysterectomy (Fig. 30.6).

Disseminated Intravascular Coagulopathy (DIC)

Background

PAS surgeons often encounter DIC, which is characterized by systemic activation of the coagulation cascade and hyperfibrinolysis [29]. The true rate of DIC in PAS surgery is unknown but some degree of coagulopathy or DIC occurs in up to one-third of patients undergoing hysterectomy for PAS [17].

Prevention

Rapid or high-volume hemorrhage is usually the cause—and typically the result—of DIC in PAS surgery. Consequently, efforts to reduce the volume and rate of blood loss in PAS surgery are the primary means of prevention of DIC (see section on Massive Obstetric Hemorrhage). Additionally, *early*, *aggressive*, and *balanced* transfusion of blood products is critically important to prevent DIC in patients with ongoing hemorrhage due to PAS [30]. Waiting to transfuse until laboratory testing confirms worsening anemia or coagulopathy is not prudent, owing to the rapid changes in coagulation and blood loss that can occur during cesarean hysterectomy for PAS.

Recognition

Diagnosis is a combination of clinical and laboratory findings. The surgeon may observe diffuse bleeding from all cut surfaces despite arterial control. Coagulopathy may manifest as blood within the surgical field that appears thin (like Kool-Aid) or does not clot as expected. Bleeding

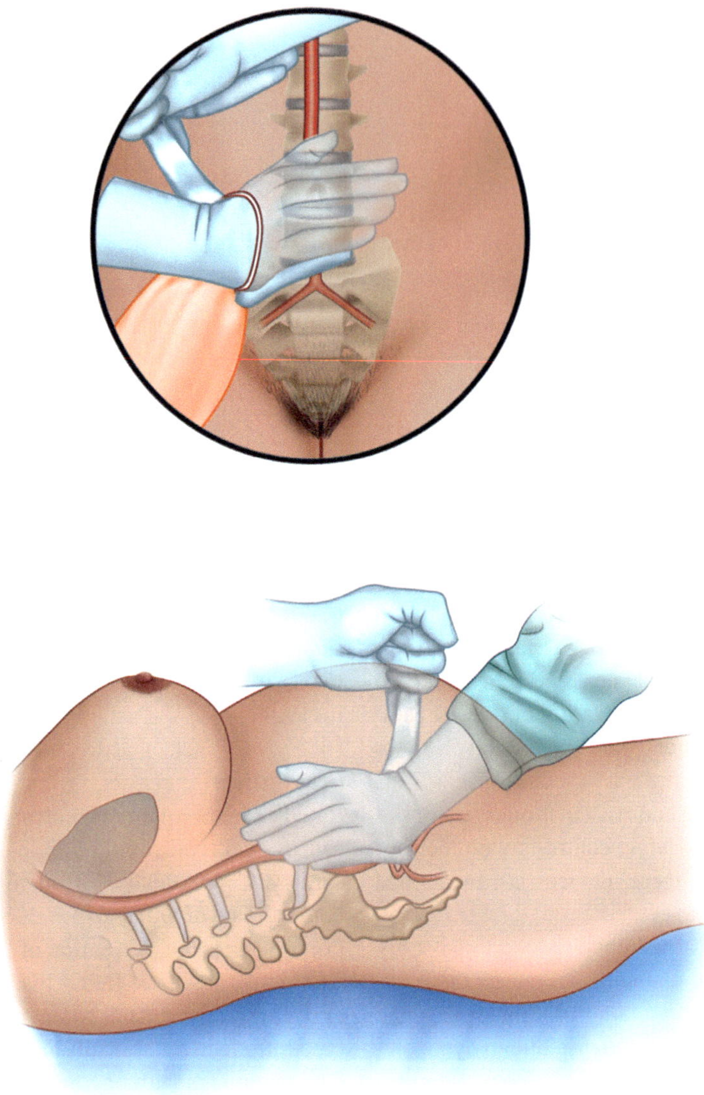

Fig. 30.6 Manual aortic compression

from IV and catheter sites or petechiae may be present. Organ damage occurs as a result of vascular thrombosis and hypoperfusion and may manifest as kidney failure, liver dysfunction, acute lung injury, neurologic injury, or adrenal failure.

When clinical signs of coagulopathy are present in the setting of major bleeding, DIC should

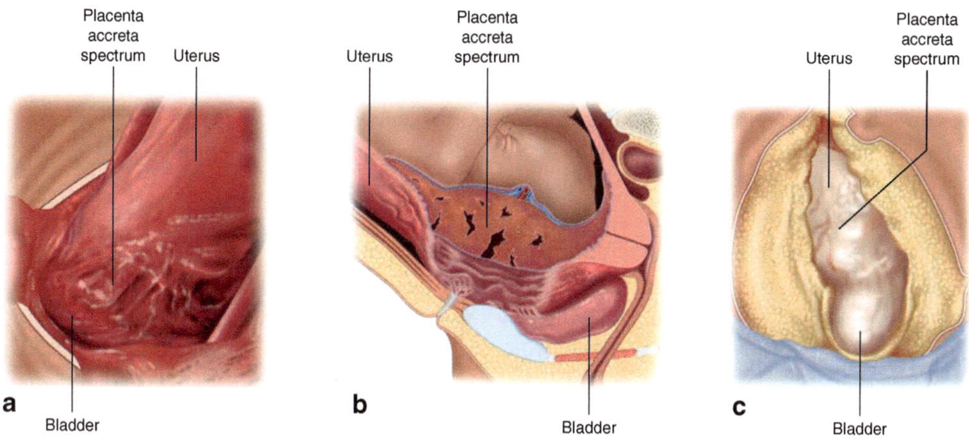

Fig. 30.7 (**a**–**c**) Identifying bladder in relation to PAS

be presumed. Stat laboratory or point-of-care fibroelastic assays should be obtained. New-onset thrombocytopenia, prolonged PT or PTT, and hypofibrinogenemia help to support the presumed clinical diagnosis.

Management

When coagulopathy or DIC is encountered, the highest priorities should be ongoing aggressive blood transfusion and immediate control of hemorrhage.

Whole blood transfusion or the combination of packed red blood cells (RBC) with fresh frozen plasma (FFP) or cryoprecipitate and platelets in a balanced ratio is superior to RBC alone. Use of a specialized **rapid blood warmer-infuser** (e.g. The Belmont) should be considered. To avoid worsening coagulopathy, prevent hypothermia with warming devices and correct hypocalcemia which occurs frequently with multi-unit transfusion [31].

Clinical coagulopathy or DIC that persists after completion of the hysterectomy can be managed with **abdomino-pelvic packing** with or without a vacuum-assisted device [32]. This allows the patient to be transferred out of the operating theater to the intensive care unit for the many hours it takes to monitor and replace coagulation factors.

Urologic Injury

Background

Bladder injury occurs in 7–9% of cesarean hysterectomies, whereas ureteral injury is much less common in simple cesarean hysterectomies (<0.5%) [3, 33]. Patients with PAS are at even higher risk owing to distortion of the anatomy when PAS is located in the lower uterine segment. Significant remodeling of the lower uterine segment and dense vesicouterine adhesive disease often result in the bladder being surgically inseparable from the placenta and scar tissue (Fig. 30.7a–c). Bladder dissection away from the lower uterine segment is often the most difficult and time-consuming part of cesarean hysterectomy for PAS (Fig. 30.7a–c). As a result, PAS patients are at high risk of cystotomy and ureteral injury (9–37%) [34, 35].

Prevention

Identifying the bladder during PAS surgery helps to avoid injury. This can be done visually and with the aid of cystoscopy or bladder backfilling (Fig. 30.7a–c). Bladder filling has been shown to decrease bladder injury in prospective [36] and retrospective [37] studies and should be considered especially in women who have undergone multiple prior cesarean sections. Finally, sharp meticulous dissection should be performed during hysterectomy to separate the bladder from the uterus rather than any type of blunt dissection. In some cases (e.g., percreta with bladder involvement) avoiding bladder injury is not possible since it can be inseparable from the placenta or densely encased in pelvic adhesion. In these cases, intentional cystotomy to define the area of placental involvement may aid in the safe removal of the specimen *with* a small area of attached bladder to avoid causing massive bleeding from placental disruption. When possible, the surgeon should preserve as much bladder as possible and avoid excising the bladder near the trigone and ureteral orifices.

Steps to prevent ureteral injury during cesarean hysterectomy include exploration of the retroperitoneum to identify and locate the ureter as well as the prophylactic use of ureteral stents. Knowledge of the anatomy of the retroperitoneum and the relationship of the ureter to the uterine vessels is essential.

Whether routine cystoscopy and ureteral stenting prevent urinary tract injury is unclear from the literature [38], but at least one study suggests that routine use results in a lower chance of bladder injury as well as ureteral injury [39]. Finally, for PAS, some uncontrolled studies suggest the use of conservative in situ management may reduce the risk of bladder and other urinary tract injury [28], although this finding requires a prospective study to be validated.

Recognition

Bladder defects may be easily identified visually as the bladder opens to the field during abdominal entry or more commonly during bladder dissection. Identification of the bladder catheter bulb or ureteral stents within the bladder confirms the diagnosis. Bladder defects may also be subtle and only recognized when surgeons perform backfilling of the bladder with sterile saline or dye. Saline or dye leaking into the field confirms that an occult injury has occurred. Routine post-hysterectomy evaluation of bladder integrity with some combination of visual inspection and bladder backfilling or cystoscopy is prudent since bladder anatomy is often distorted by PAS and pelvic tissues of pregnant individuals are edematous and hypervascular compared to the non-pregnant state.

Recognition of ureteral injuries is further covered in Chaps. 6 and 17.

Management

Closure of the cystotomy should be performed in two layers incorporating a running non-locking absorbable suture for both layers. Care should be taken to place the sutures well beyond the lateral limit of the injury and at least a.5 cm in the superior and posterior direction to provide adequate tissue closure. Primary repair of a simple dome cystotomy can be performed in two layers incorporating a running non-locking absorbable suture followed by a second absorbable suture. When a bladder injury is large (perhaps >8 cm), involves significant resection or denuding of the bladder, is associated with ureteral injury, or is in close proximity to the ureteral orifices, it is important to involve a surgeon experienced in urologic repair.

Management of complex bladder and ureteral injury is covered in Chaps. 12 and 17.

References

1. Tsolakidis D, Zouzoulas D, Pados G. Pregnancy-related hysterectomy for peripartum hemorrhage: a literature narrative review of the diagnosis, management, and techniques. Biomed Res Int. 2021;2021:9958073.
2. Rattanakanokchai S, Kietpeerakool C, Srisomboon J, Jampathong N, Pattanittum P, Lumbiganon P. Perioperative complications of hysterectomy after a previous cesarean section: a systematic review and meta-analysis. Clin Epidemiol. 2019;11:1089–98.
3. Wright JD, Herzog TJ, Shah M, et al. Regionalization of care for obstetric hemorrhage and its effect on maternal mortality. Obstet Gynecol. 2010;115(6):1194–200.
4. Silver RM, Branch DW. Placenta accreta spectrum. N Engl J Med. 2018;378(16):1529–36.
5. Jauniaux E, Chantraine F, Silver RM, Langhoff-Roos J. FIGO consensus guidelines on placenta accreta spectrum disorders: Epidemiology. Int J Gynaecol Obstet. 2018;140(3):265–73.
6. Tanos V, Toney ZA. Uterine scar rupture – prediction, prevention, diagnosis, and management. Best Pract Res Clin Obstet Gynaecol. 2019;59:115–31.

7. Quantitative blood loss in obstetric hemorrhage: ACOG COMMITTEE OPINION, number 794. Obstet Gynecol. 2019;134(6):e150–6.
8. Sanders AP, Hobson SR, Kobylianskii A, et al. Internal iliac artery ligation-a contemporary simplified approach. Am J Obstet Gynecol. 2021;225(3):339–40.
9. Saeed KB, Corcoran P, Greene RA. Incisional surgical site infection following cesarean section: a national retrospective cohort study. Eur J Obstet Gynecol Reprod Biol. 2019;240:256–60.
10. Dias M, Dick A, Reynolds RM, Lahti-Pulkkinen M, Denison FC. Predictors of surgical site skin infection and clinical outcome at caesarean section in the very severely obese: a retrospective cohort study. PLoS One. 2019;14(6):e0216157.
11. Uppal S, Harris J, Al-Niaimi A, et al. Prophylactic antibiotic choice and risk of surgical site infection after hysterectomy. Obstet Gynecol. 2016;127(2):321–9.
12. Practice bulletin no. 199: use of prophylactic antibiotics in labor and delivery: correction. Obstet Gynecol. 2019;134(4):883–4.
13. Seaman SJ, Han E, Arora C, Kim JH. Surgical site infections in gynecology: the latest evidence for prevention and management. Curr Opin Obstet Gynecol. 2021;33(4):296–304.
14. Meyer J, Roos E, Davies RJ, Buchs NC, Ris F, Toso C. Does prophylactic negative-pressure wound therapy prevent surgical site infection after laparotomy? A systematic review and meta-analysis of randomized controlled trials. World J Surg. 2023;47(6):1464–74.
15. Gillespie BM, Webster J, Ellwood D, et al. Closed incision negative pressure wound therapy versus standard dressings in obese women undergoing caesarean section: multicentre parallel group randomised controlled trial. BMJ. 2021;373:n893.
16. Jauniaux E, Bunce C, Grønbeck L, Langhoff-Roos J. Prevalence and main outcomes of placenta accreta spectrum: a systematic review and meta-analysis. Am J Obstet Gynecol. 2019;221(3):208–18.
17. Eller AG, Bennett MA, Sharshiner M, et al. Maternal morbidity in cases of placenta accreta managed by a multidisciplinary care team compared with standard obstetric care. Obstet Gynecol. 2011;117(2 Pt 1):331–7.
18. Warshak CR, Ramos GA, Eskander R, et al. Effect of predelivery diagnosis in 99 consecutive cases of placenta accreta. Obstet Gynecol. 2010;115(1):65–9.
19. Einerson BD, Branch DW. Surgical management of placenta accreta spectrum. Clin Obstet Gynecol. 2018;61(4):774–82.
20. Kingdom JC, Hobson SR, Murji A, et al. Minimizing surgical blood loss at cesarean hysterectomy for placenta previa with evidence of placenta increta or placenta percreta: the state of play in 2020. Am J Obstet Gynecol. 2020;223(3):322–9.
21. Belfort MA, Shamshiraz AA, Fox K. Minimizing blood loss at cesarean-hysterectomy for placenta previa percreta. Am J Obstet Gynecol. 2017;216(1):78.e71–2.
22. Salim R, Chulski A, Romano S, Garmi G, Rudin M, Shalev E. Precesarean prophylactic balloon catheters for suspected placenta accreta: a randomized controlled trial. Obstet Gynecol. 2015;126(5):1022–8.
23. Dai M, Zhang F, Li K, Jin G, Chen Y, Zhang X. The effect of prophylactic balloon occlusion in patients with placenta accreta spectrum: a Bayesian network meta-analysis. Eur Radiol. 2022;32(5):3297–308.
24. Hawthorn BR, Ratnam LA. Role of interventional radiology in placenta accreta spectrum (PAS) disorders. Best Pract Res Clin Obstet Gynaecol. 2021;72:25–37.
25. Gatta LA, Weber JM, Gilner JB, et al. Transfusion requirements with hybrid management of placenta accreta spectrum incorporating targeted embolization and a selective use of delayed hysterectomy. Am J Perinatol. 2022;29(14):1503–13.
26. Zuckerwise LC, Craig AM, Newton JM, Zhao S, Bennett KA, Crispens MA. Outcomes following a clinical algorithm allowing for delayed hysterectomy in the management of severe placenta accreta spectrum. Am J Obstet Gynecol. 2020;222(2):179.e171–9.
27. Pineles BL, Sibai BM, Sentilhes L. Is conservative management of placenta accreta spectrum disorders practical in the United States? Am J Obstet Gynecol MFM. 2022:100749.
28. Sentilhes L, Seco A, Azria E, et al. Conservative management or cesarean hysterectomy for placenta accreta spectrum: the PACCRETA prospective study. Am J Obstet Gynecol. 2022;226(6):839.e831–24.
29. Levi M, Ten Cate H. Disseminated intravascular coagulation. N Engl J Med. 1999;341(8):586–92.
30. Butwick A, Lyell D, Goodnough L. How do I manage severe postpartum hemorrhage? Transfusion. 2020;60(5):897–907.
31. Einerson BD, Weiniger CF. Placenta accreta spectrum disorder: updates on anesthetic and surgical management strategies. Int J Obstet Anesth. 2021;46:102975.
32. Pacheco LD, Lozada MJ, Saade GR, Hankins GDV. Damage-control surgery for obstetric hemorrhage. Obstet Gynecol. 2018;132(2):423–7.
33. Wei G, Harley F, O'Callaghan M, Adshead J, Hennessey D, Kinnear N. Systematic review of urological injury during caesarean section and hysterectomy. Int Urogynecol J. 2023;34(2):371–89.
34. Erfani H, Salmanian B, Fox KA, et al. Urologic morbidity associated with placenta accreta spectrum surgeries: single-center experience with a multidisciplinary team. Am J Obstet Gynecol. 2022;226(2):245.e241–5.
35. Tam Tam KB, Dozier J, Martin JN Jr. Approaches to reduce urinary tract injury during management of placenta accreta, increta, and percreta: a systematic review. J Matern Fetal Neonatal Med. 2012;25(4):329–34.
36. Özcan H, Balat Ö, Uğur MG, Sucu S, Tepe NB, Kazaz TG. Use of bladder filling to prevent urinary system complications in the management of placenta percreta: a randomized prospective study. Geburtshilfe Frauenheilkd. 2018;78(2):173–8.

37. Kuznetsova N, Bushtyreva I, Barinova V, Shmakova K. Bladder filling technique to prevent complications of the urinary system during placenta accrete surgery. J Matern Fetal Neonatal Med. 2022;35(3):607–9.
38. Collins SL, Alemdar B, van Beekhuizen HJ, et al. Evidence-based guidelines for the management of abnormally invasive placenta: recommendations from the International Society for Abnormally Invasive Placenta. Am J Obstet Gynecol. 2019;220(6):511–26.
39. Scaglione MA, Allshouse AA, Canfield DR, et al. Prophylactic ureteral stent placement and urinary injury during hysterectomy for placenta accreta spectrum. Obstet Gynecol. 2022;140(5):806–11.

Part VIII

Cancer

Inguinal Lymphadenectomy, Radical Vulvectomy

31

Clarissa Lam and Mario M. Leitao

Background of Lymphedema After Inguinofemoral Lymphadenectomy

Lower extremity lymphedema (LEL) is a relatively common complication of inguinofemoral lymphadenectomy (IFL). Rates of LEL after IFL in patients with melanoma have been reported between 13% and 55% [1]. Lymphedema can either be a temporary or a chronic and debilitating condition. In one series of 204 patients with melanoma, 58 patients underwent IFL and 26% of patients had measurable LEL six months postoperatively, with 8% of patients having significant functional deficits [104]. In the GROINSS-V-1 prospective trial, the rate of LEL was 25.2% after sentinel lymph node (SLN) dissection with lymphadenectomy versus 1.9% after SLN dissection alone [105].

Vulvectomy and IFL are typically performed using separate incisions. In one study, approximately three-quarters of patients who underwent modified radical vulvectomy and inguinal lymphadenectomy with separate incisions had one or more documented complications, with 28% of patients experiencing lymphedema [33]. The next sections will cover methods identified in the literature to recognize, prevent, and manage lymphedema.

C. Lam
Gynecology Service, Department of Surgery, Memorial Sloan Kettering Cancer Center, New York, NY, USA
e-mail: LamC2@mskcc.org

M. M. Leitao (✉)
Gynecology Service, Department of Surgery, Memorial Sloan Kettering Cancer Center, New York, NY, USA

Department of Obstetrics and Gynecology, Weill Cornell Medical College, New York, NY, USA
e-mail: leitaom@mskcc.org

Recognition of Lymphedema Following Inguinofemoral Lymphadenectomy

Radionuclide lymphoscintigraphy is the gold standard imaging modality for the diagnosis of lymphedema; it is also useful in surgical planning. Other imaging modalities include magnetic resonance lymphangiography and indocyanine green lymphangiography. Medical history and physical examination by qualified health care practitioners, however, have been used to accurately diagnose patients in approximately 90% of cases [39]. Secondary lymphedema after lymphadenectomy typically presents 12 to 18 months after the inciting injury. Lymphedema almost universally involves the distal extremity and leads to pitting edema on examination. Grading and/or staging can be performed for lymphedema (Table 31.1, Fig. 31.1). Lymphedema after IFL, however, can manifest in the upper thigh, vulva, and/or

M. Hoffman et al. (eds.), *Major Complications of Female Pelvic Surgery*,
https://doi.org/10.1007/978-3-031-66772-5_31

Table 31.1 Grading systems for lymphedema (Dessources et al. 2020)

ISL stage	ISL grading	CTCAE grade
0: Subclinical impaired lymphatic transport without lymphedema	Mild, <20% increase in volume	Grade 1: Trace thickening or faint skin discoloration
1: Relatively high protein edema that reverses with elevation +/– pitting +/– increase in proliferating cells	Moderate, 20%–40% increase in volume	Grade 2: Limits activities of daily living. Characterized by marked skin discoloration, leathery texture, and papillary formation
2: High protein edema with dermal fibrosis that does not easily reverse with elevation. Usually no pitting		
3: Trophic skin changes: warty overgrowths, acanthosis, fat deposits, usually without pitting. Also known as lymphatic elephantiasis	Severe, >40% increase in size	Grade 3: Severe symptoms limiting self-care and activities of daily living

ISL International Society of Lymphology, *CTCAE* Common Terminology Criteria for Adverse Events

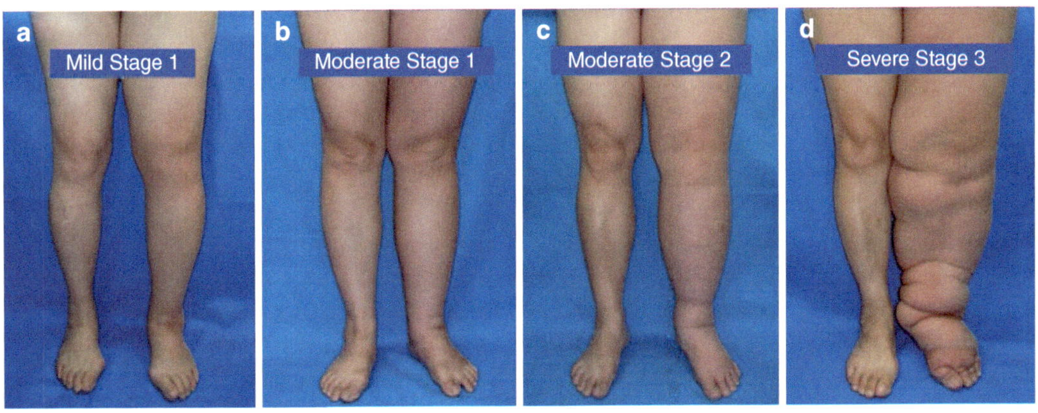

Fig. 31.1 International Society of Lymphology stages/grade of lymphedema. (**a**) Stage 1 mild lymphedema with 40% limb difference, and abnormal fat deposits; (**b**) Stage 1 moderate lymphedema with a 20%–40% difference in limb size; (**c**) Stage 2 moderate lymphedema with a 20%–40% difference in limb size with associated fibrosis and irreversible edema; (**d**) Stage 3 severe lymphedema with >40% limb difference, and abnormal fat deposits (Dessources et al. 2020)

mons pubis. The Stemmer sign, or the inability to pinch up the skin on the dorsum of the foot, is also a sensitive and specific sign of lymphedema. The presence of these factors in the history and on physical examination can help rule out other diagnoses such as a venous thromboembolic event, heart failure, renal failure, or venous insufficiency. Of note, adult-onset primary lymphedema is rare. Lymphedema is a chronic condition that progresses through four stages and can be assessed on physical examination [53].

Prevention of Lymphedema Following Inguinofemoral Lymphadenectomy

Some data suggest there is no benefit to the routine prescription of graduated compression stockings in the prevention of lymphedema after IFL [100]. Findings from other studies, however, suggest that the use of compression stockings combined with patient education delays the onset or even reduces the risk of lymphedema [47, 95].

A historical study of interest that randomized patients with vulvar cancer with positive nodes after radical vulvectomy and IFL to either adjuvant radiation therapy or pelvic lymph node dissection found that adjuvant radiation therapy was associated with a decreased risk of lymphedema and improved two-year survival rates [51]. On the topic of radiotherapy, adjuvant radiation after IFL increases the risk of lymphedema by way of decreased lymphatic proliferation potential, interstitial fibrosis compressing lymphatic vessels, and precipitating mechanical insufficiency of the lymphatic system [4]. Thus, avoiding adjuvant radiation unless clearly clinically indicated can help prevent LEL. To decrease the use of unnecessary pelvic radiation, one study demonstrated that performing minimally invasive pelvic lymphadenectomy was an effective method to screen for patients who do not need adjuvant whole pelvic radiation after IFL [58].

Whenever feasible and indicated, SLN dissection without full IFL is the best method to prevent lower extremity edema. In general, the indication for lymph node sampling includes any tumor greater than stage IA. Omitting full IFL is reasonable in vulvar tumors <4 cm. Full lymphadenectomy after SLN dissection depends on the size of the SLN metastases. In the GROINSS-V-I study, 135 patients with positive SLNs were identified; 115 underwent IFL with a 6% groin recurrence rate, 14 underwent radiation therapy with a 14% groin recurrence rate, and 4 had no treatment with a 25% groin recurrence rate. Omitting IFL in patients with negative SLNs was found to be safe and was associated with a decreased rate of LEL (1.9% with SLN sampling alone versus 25.2% with SLN sampling and IFL, $P < 0.0001$) [105]. GROINSS-V-II, a subsequent prospective phase II trial examining radiation therapy in patients with positive SLNs without IFL, found the risk of groin recurrence was significantly lower in patients with an SLN metastasis ≤ 2 mm ($P = 0.008$). This study also found significantly lower rates of lymphedma in the radiotherapy-only group compared to patients who had IFL with or without adjuvant radiation therapy [72]. Patients who underwent IFL had lymphedema rates of 32% and 22.9% at 6 months and 12 months, respectively.

Saphenous vein preservation has been shown to be associated with less morbidity. A meta-analysis of four studies demonstrated that preservation of the saphenous vein was associated with a decreased risk of LEL (OR: 0.24, 95% CI: 0.11–0.53), wound necrosis (OR: 0.34, 95% CI: 0.19–0.59), and acute cellulitis (OR: 0.4, 95% CI: 0.16–0.96) [1]. In a retrospective evaluation of patients with vulvar squamous cell carcinoma who underwent IFL, saphenous vein preservation was associated with reduced risk of wound cellulitis, wound breakdown, and chronic lymphedema [23]. A systematic literature review of 36 studies on IFL morbidity found that sparing the saphenous vein decreased wound infections, wound breakdown, cellulitis/erysipelas, and lymphedema (Table 31.2) [23, 81, 87, 110, 25].

Preservation of the fascia lata of the major anterior thigh muscles of the femoral triangle during IFL has also been associated with a decreased risk of postoperative LEL. The proposed mechanism for this association is the maintenance of the unidirectional valves of the veins and lymphatics [40, 109]. In one study investigating this fascia-preserving technique, the researchers made a curvilinear incision at the base of the femoral triangle, creating a flap between the superficial and deep layers of the Camper's fascia. At the completion of nodal dissection, the flap was sutured to the fascia lata to eliminate dead space [109]. With this technique, the authors noted a 12% rate of lymphedema. Skin necrosis and local infection made up 5.5% and 2.5% of the postoperative complications in this study, respectively, and oncological outcomes were not compromised.

Pedicled omentoplasty is another technique to decrease the risk of LEL after IFL. This technique, which has been reported after pelvic lymph node dissections, is thought to decrease LEL by altering the absorption or transport of lymph fluids. The benefit of pedicled omentoplasty in IFL was tested in a pilot study of four women and three men with inguinal metastatic lymph nodes [11]. After IFL, four of the seven patients had mild asymptomatic lymphedema,

Table 31.2 Summary of rates of short-term and long-term complications separated by saphenous vein sparing and saphenous vein ligating techniques [81]

		Short term									Long term						
		Wound infection			Wound breakdown			Lymphocele			Lymphedema			Cellulitis/erysipelas			
Study	*N*	Sparing	Ligation	P-value	Sparing	Ligation	P-value	Sparing	Ligation	P-value	Sparing	Ligation	P-value	Sparing	Ligation	P-value	Overall ≥1 complication
Per groin																	
Dardarian 2006	49	0	45	<0.001	0	25	<0.02	0	0	–	11	39	<0.05	0	6	NS	–
Rouzier 2003	355	18	30	0.01	16	36	<0.001	–	–		23	45	<0.001	–	–		–
Zhang 2000	139	–	–		13	38	0.001	10	4	NS	32	70	–	18	39	0.006	–
Zhang 2007	128	68	73	NS	–	–		26	32	NS	25	48	<0.01	21	41	<0.05	–

and the remaining three, who were noted to have lymphedema preoperatively, had improvement in their symptoms postoperatively. To achieve this flap, surgeons in this study made both an abdominal and an inguinal incision, mobilized an omental flap, passed the flap deep to the inguinal ligament through the femoral canal, and sutured it into place. In this study, the saphenous vein was ligated at its proximal and distal ends. One difficulty that surgeons encountered with this technique was the inadequate length of the omental flap. This technique has yet to be validated in larger trials. Omental nodal harvest can also be achieved via a free-flap method, which does not require passage through the femoral canal and eliminates concern about adequate length; however, it would require an adequately vascularized flap with microsurgical anastomosis to vessels in the groin [11].

Lymphovenous anastomosis (LVA) is another technique to help prevent the development of LEL. This approach involves simultaneously preparing an accessory branch of the femoral vein at the time of lymphadenectomy of the groin (or axillary vein in the case of axillary lymph node dissection) followed by an anastomosis with one or more afferent lymphatic vessels (Fig. 31.2). Jørgensen et al. conducted a systematic meta-analysis of studies treating patients with prophylactic LVA following lymphadenectomy to prevent lymphedema. In a quantitative analysis of studies including a control group, the authors found patients treated with prophylactic LVA had a relative risk of 0.33 (95% CI: 0.19–0.56) for developing lymphedema compared to controls [56]. Of note, five of these studies involved patients with gynecologic cancer, two of which involved patients with vulvar cancer specifically. Morotti et al. performed one of the two studies and assessed microsurgical LVA in the prevention of lymphedema in patients with vulvar cancer. This study demonstrated the feasibility of LVA at the time of IFL. LVA appears to be a promising technique for decreasing lymphedema in high-risk patients, although more studies are needed.

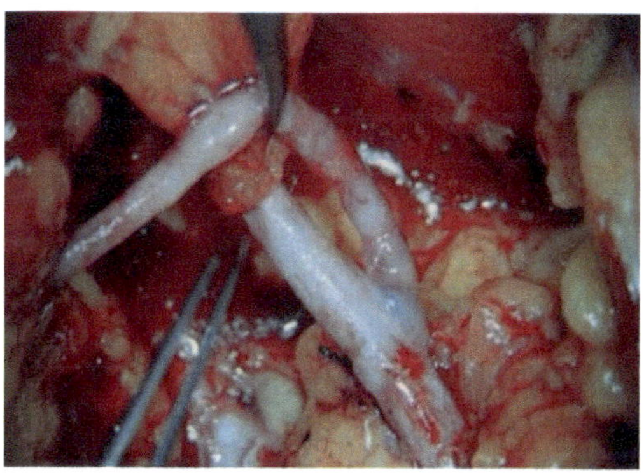

Fig. 31.2 Lymphovenous anastomosis. (Courtesy of Dr. Mario M. Leitao, Jr.)

Laparoendoscopic single-site surgery (LESS) is a minimally invasive technique that has recently been used for IFL in gynecologic oncology diseases, including vulvar and vaginal cancers. A small single-site study, which evaluated six patients with vulvar or vaginal cancer who underwent LESS for inguinal lymphadenectomy from July 2018 to March 2019, demonstrated LESS is a feasible and safe technique for the management of these gynecologic malignancies, with no reported postoperative complications [108]. However, this is an extremely small series to make definitive recommendations.

Robotic-assisted video endoscopic inguinal lymphadenectomy (RAVEIL) is another minimally invasive technique used for IFL. The feasibility of this modality was demonstrated in a study by Josephson et al. [57]. In a retrospective study, reduced complication rates were noted with RAVEIL for the management of penile carcinoma compared with an open approach, while maintaining adequate surgical outcomes [89]. In this study, saphenous vein preservation was more likely with RAVEIL compared to standard-approach inguinal lymphadenectomy. Video endoscopic inguinal lymphadenectomy (VEIL) without robotic assistance was studied in 46 patients with vulvar cancer, and VEIL was associated with reduced postoperative complications compared to traditional open technique for inguinal lymphadenectomy [64]. Therefore, the use of VEIL by trained surgeons, with or without robotic assistance, may be considered in patients with vulvar cancer to decrease the risk of postoperative complications. This approach, however, requires more investigation before routine adoption.

Management of Lymphedema Following Inguinofemoral Lymphadenectomy

Conservative options for the management of lymphedema include lower extremity elevation when at rest, compression techniques, manual lymphatic drainage, exercise, intermittent pneumatic compression devices, and low-level laser therapy. There are no clear data to suggest which, if any, of these measures is most effective in the treatment of lymphedema; although, there does not seem to be any harm documented as a result of these treatments [73].

Surgical management of lymphedema includes two approaches: physiologic and ablative. Physiologic surgical options attempt to improve lymph flow by supporting lymphatic pathways, whereas ablative surgical options aim to debulk lymphedematous areas and reduce morbidity [60]. Lymphaticovenular anastomosis, also known as lymphovenous bypass, is a physiologic surgical technique to reroute lymphatic fluid into the venous system; however, there are mixed data regarding the efficacy of this technique (Fig. 31.3) [18, 22, 32, 52, 59]. Vascularized lymph node transfer is the preferred modality to restore lymphatic drainage in dysfunctional lymph node basins after lymphadenectomy or radiation therapy. This technique entails the transfer of vascularized lymph nodes to the desired area either via free flaps or in a pedicled fashion. Although there is a rare risk of iatrogenic lymphedema due to lymphatic disruption at the transfer site [78, 101, 106, 107], most studies have demonstrated improvement in lymphedema symptoms and quality of life [19, 66, 74, 83]. For advanced-stage chronic lymphedema, ablative procedures such as the Charles procedure, which involves the removal of skin and subcutaneous tissue followed by skin grafts, may restore functional deficits and provide relief in debilitating lymphedema. Suction-assisted lipectomy can be useful in patients who do not have significant pitting edema and who are not candidates for other surgical techniques. Although this method is limited, good patient satisfaction has been reported with suction-assisted lipectomy [13, 14].

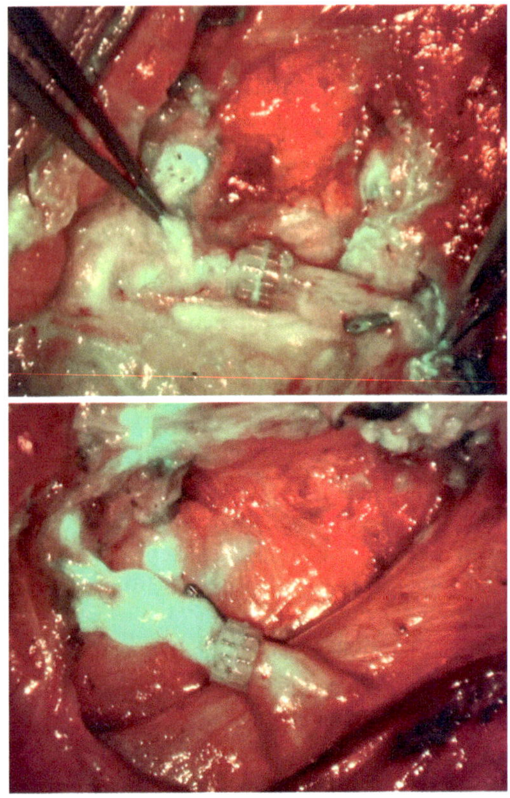

Fig. 31.3 Lymphovenous bypass. (Courtesy of Dr. Mario M. Leitao, Jr.)

Background of Infectious Morbidity Following Radical Vulvectomy and Inguinofemoral Lymphadenectomy

Vulvectomy has long been known to have high rates of postoperative complications due to several host factors, including the specific microbial flora of the genital tract and its surrounding structures, decreased host immunity due to malignancy and other potential comorbidities, prior chemotherapy or radiation in the area, and difficulty of wound care at the surgery site. One study noted a wound infection rate of 7%, and the most common pathogens isolated from wound sites were *Pseudomonas aeruginosa*, *Enterococcus*, and *Escherichia coli* [29].

Although SLN mapping is now an accepted standard for vulvar cancer staging, there are still instances when full IFL is warranted, particularly in patients with vulvar tumors ≥4 cm or multifocal disease. IFL performed for the purpose of sampling enlarged groin lymph nodes is associated with a complication rate as high as 60% [40, 98], with the most common complications being lymphorrea, seroma, infection, and wound breakdown. Some suggested predictors of postoperative complications include number of lymph nodes removed, pathologically positive nodes, patient age, and disease stage [36]. Groin dissection is associated with a high risk of infection due to the inherent moisture in the area and the risk of contamination. Rates of wound infection after groin surgery range from 6% to 29% [10]. Wound infection invariably increases the risk of wound breakdown. Gaarenstroom et al. [33] examined modified radical vulvectomy with IFL through separate incisions and found the incidence of wound breakdown was up to 39%, with or without infection [33]. The next sections will cover methods identified in the literature to recognize, prevent, and manage the complications of wound infection.

Recognition of Infectious Morbidity Following Radical Vulvectomy and Inguinofemoral Lymphadenectomy

Clinical signs of infection, including leukocytosis and fever, should be used in conjunction with physical examination findings including erythema, edema/induration, and/or purulent discharge. Wound breakdown can also be present. Necrotizing infection, which will usually present with pain out of proportion to physical examination findings, crepitus on palpation, skin discoloration, and imaging findings suggestive of gas in the area of interest, is important to rule out.

Prevention of Infectious Morbidity Following Radical Vulvectomy and Inguinofemoral Lymphadenectomy

As mentioned previously, the GROINSS-V-I study demonstrated a significantly decreased risk of postoperative morbidity with SLN sampling alone versus SLN sampling with IFL, with rates of wound breakdown of 11.7% versus 34.0%, respectively ($P < 0.0001$), and rates of cellulitis of 4.5% versus 21.3%, respectively ($P < 0.0001$) [105].

Preoperative preparation of the skin and vagina with povidine-iodine or chlorhexidine gluconate is universally recommended to prevent infection [5], and should be performed for patients who undergo radical vulvectomy and/or IFL. A randomized controlled trial comparing the use of chlorhexidine gluconate and iodine for vaginal preparation prior to hysterectomy in 85 patients demonstrated decreased vaginal bacteria count in patients who underwent chlorhexidine preparation; although, no surgical site infections were identified in either group [46]. In a propensity score-matched analysis, however, povidine-iodine was shown to be preferable to chlorhexidine in vaginal preparation before hysterectomy due to lower rates of infection and fewer emergency department visits [97]. Thus, the choice of preparation solution can be left to the surgeon's preference due to the limited data supporting one over the other.

Aside from open versus endoscopic modalities, there is clear variation in actual surgical technique for groin surgery. One randomized controlled trial compared postoperative complication rate with the use of LigaSure technology versus conventional (sharp/diathermia) technique and found the estimated incidence of ≥1 postoperative complications was 29% after LigaSure versus 70% after conventional inguinal lymphadenectomy ($P < 0.001$) [80]. Creating separate incisions for radical vulvectomy and lymphadenectomy has been shown to decrease risk of infectious morbidity in several studies [29, 41].

The use of groin drains has been investigated in several studies. One retrospective cohort study by Pontre et al. showed the use of groin drains significantly reduced the incidence of postoperative groin cellulitis (8.7% versus 25.4%, $P = 0.039$) [79]. Duration of drain use does not seem to have an effect on the development of postoperative complications [37]. In a Dutch nationwide prospective study by Pouwer et al., using volume-based standards for drain removal was found to be superior to time-based removal

(removal of drain on postoperative day five) in decreasing complication rates (46% versus 75%, respectively, $P = 0.006$) [82]. Of note, no randomized controlled trials have compared surgical outcomes of inguinal lymphadenectomy with and without use of drains.

In a prospective clinical study examining postoperative outcomes after radical lymphadenectomy or SLN procedure, Asciutto et al. employed negative pressure wound therapy (NPWT) in conjunction with groin drains [6]. Surgical site complications were identified in 11 of the 20 patients (55%) who underwent NPWT; one patient suffered a wound rupture, six patients developed lymphoceles, and four patients had a surgical site infection. Although no statistical tests were performed, the use of NPWT in this small cohort was thought to reduce the severity of surgical site complications after inguinal lymphadenectomy. The efficacy of NPWT was evaluated in a meta-analysis of studies looking at its use in various other surgery types (orthopedic, abdominal, colorectal, and obstetric) and was associated with a significant reduction in surgical site infection, wound dehiscence, and length of stay [99].

Modest weight loss preoperatively can potentially decrease the risk of development of at least one complication. In a study of 204 patients with melanoma, the risk of developing at least one complication for all patients who underwent regional lymph node dissection of the neck, axilla, and groin was increased in obese patients ($P = 0.05$) [104].

It is common to recommend frequent sitz baths or loose-fitting underwear postoperatively, but there are limited data to support these practices for the prevention of infection and wound breakdown after vulvectomy in patients with gynecologic cancer. One randomized controlled trial examining sitz baths after episiotomy did not find a statistically significant decrease in the rate of wound breakdown [70]. Prospective data are still needed to optimize postoperative vulvar hygiene and wound care regimens in patients with gynecologic cancers. In addition to the above measures, some clinicians prescribe sitting restrictions to prevent direct pressure on the incisional area for four to six weeks postoperatively. Inflatable donut-like devices or soft pillows provide support and maintain quality of life for patients while following sitting restrictions during recovery. However, no data are available that specifically address the efficacy of sitting restrictions in preventing wound complications after vulvectomy.

Management of Infectious Morbidity Following Radical Vulvectomy and Inguinofemoral Lymphadenectomy

Infection should be managed with antibiotics, either parenteral or oral, and the antibiotic regimen should be tailored based on the clinician's judgement of infection severity. Wound culture should be obtained if applicable to the clinical scenario. Antibiotics should be started empirically and tailored to wound culture results if obtained. In the setting of infection, there may be clinical utility to reopen the incision if the wound has not already opened on its own. The incision should then be allowed to close by secondary intention, whether with wet-to-dry dressing or NPWT, whichever is feasible. NPWT has the benefit of evacuating wound fluid, stimulating granulation tissue formation, and decreasing bacterial colonization of the wound; although, in one retrospective study of the use of vacuum-assisted closure in complex wound failures, patients with gynecologic cancer complained of pain with wound dressing changes [94]. In this study, 96% of patients had complete wound healing. Extensive surgical debridement is the mainstay of treatment for necrotizing soft-tissue infections of the vulva [21]. If this is suspected, early and aggressive surgical resection is critical to minimizing morbidity and mortality.

Background of Functional Impairments After Radical Vulvectomy

Vulvectomy has the potential to result in significant anatomic distortion, leading to a number of functional impairments, including difficulties with micturition, defecation, and sexual activity [48].

In one questionnaire study, fecal incontinence was reported in 43% of survivors of gynecologic cancer [90]; however, rates of fecal incontinence in patients who underwent vulvectomy specifically were not reported.

Various forms of sexual dysfunction have been reported after a vulvectomy, including sexual aversion disorder, hypoactive sexual disorder, and arousal disorder. Factors associated with posttreatment sexual dysfunction in patients who underwent surgical treatment for vulvar cancer include increased age, poor overall well-being, history of depression or anxiety, and excision size of vulvar malignancy [2]. Compared to healthy controls, patients with vulvar cancer are at increased risk for sexual dysfunction, both before and after surgical excision [3]. Extent of surgery or type of vulvectomy has not been found to be correlated with the degree of sexual dysfunction present postoperatively [38].

Recognition of Functional Impairments After Radical Vulvectomy

Functional impairments can be diagnosed based on patient-reported symptoms postoperatively. These symptoms can present immediately or even one year after primary surgery. According to a questionnaire-based study, only 40% of survivors of gynecologic cancer reported having been asked about urinary/fecal incontinence or sexual function by their oncologist [90], which highlights the importance of obtaining a thorough history and physical examination to recognize and treat these functional impairments.

Urinary incontinence is very common in postmenopausal patients, with or without radical vulvectomy. Urinary incontinence should be separated by type, namely, urge, stress, or mixed incontinence. Because treatment will depend on the type of incontinence present, it is important to take a thorough history and perform a detailed physical examination, including specific tests such as the Q-tip test for urethral mobility and the Pelvic Organ Prolapse Quantification system (POP-Q) to assess for pelvic organ prolapse contributing to urinary symptoms. Urinary tract infection should be ruled out in patients presenting with new-onset urinary incontinence postoperatively. Anatomic distortions, particularly in patients who underwent urethrectomy as part of radical vulvar surgery, can be identified on physical examination as contributing factors to urinary incontinence; these patients can present with total incontinence (Fig. 31.4).

When a patient presents with sexual dysfunction, it is important to screen for psychosocial factors that may be contributing factors, including depression and relational discord. Physical examination can elucidate whether there is an anatomical aberration related to vulvar surgery, including introital stenosis or clitoral distortion (Fig. 31.4).

Once again, performing a thorough history and physical examination are crucial to diagnosing fecal incontinence. Fistula can be an etiology

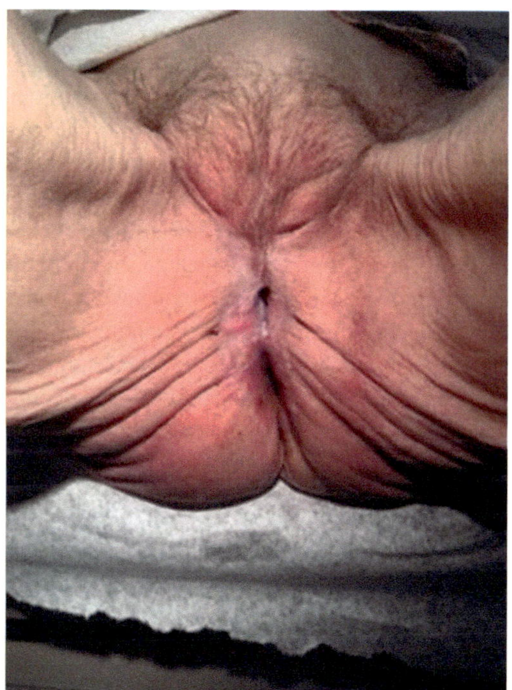

Fig. 31.4 Introital stenosis with urethral hooding and fecal incontinence after radical vulvectomy. (Courtesy of Dr. Mitchel Hoffman)

of fecal incontinence, particularly in patients with previous irradiation. The digital rectal examination is a rudimentary way to assess quality of anal tone. Fecal incontinence has been evaluated using anorectal manometry, pudendal nerve latency studies, and electromyography [55]. The Wexner fecal incontinence scale is likely the most widely used tool to assess for presence of fecal incontinence and to measure the severity of symptoms.

Prevention of Functional Impairments After Radical Vulvectomy

Radical vulvectomy by itself does not cause incontinence, but according to a prospective study of 21 patients who underwent a radical vulvectomy, removal of a portion of the urethra is a risk factor for urinary incontinence, with estimated rates of severe/total urinary incontinence ranging from 22% to 100% [85]. Appropriate patient selection based on imaging and examination findings, as well as adequate preoperative and postoperative patient counseling, are recommended for all patients. Resection of the external anal sphincter is a risk factor for postoperative fecal incontinence. According to one retrospective study, two patients with resection of most of the anus developed severe fecal incontinence postoperatively, four of eight patients with partial resection of the external anal sphincter developed persistent postoperative fecal incontinence, and no patients with preserved external anal sphincter developed new-onset postoperative fecal incontinence [50]. Extensive perianal resection followed by primary anal reconstruction using local skin flaps, such as unilateral or bilateral rhomboid flaps or local advancement flaps, should be considered for preservation of fecal continence [9, 49]. Primary repair of the external anal sphincter by anal sphincteroplasty, most commonly used in the setting of obstetrical lacerations, can also be considered at the time of radical vulvectomy to preserve function of the external anal sphincter and to prevent postoperative fecal incontinence. Among the obstetric population, postoperative results are felt to be better with delayed repair rather than primary repair, which is likely due to edematous tissues [35]; however, this may not apply to oncologic procedures involving resection of the anal sphincter.

Although the primary aim of surgery is to achieve local control of cancer or precancerous lesions, as alluded to above, vulvar reconstruction has also become an area of interest for improved outcomes for our patients. Reconstructive surgery can provide aesthetic and functional benefits while maintaining the integrity of the oncologic resection with safe surgical margins. In large defects, wound closure with reconstructive flaps is suggested to be superior to direct wound closure for cosmetic and functional purposes.

Various flaps have been evaluated for reconstruction after extensive vulvovaginal carcinoma surgery. Of 12 patients with gynecologic cancer who underwent vulvovaginal surgery with simultaneous reconstruction, seven maintained satisfactory sexual function postoperatively. All of these patients had been treated with the innervated pudendal-thigh flap [61]. In this study, the gracilis myocutaneous flap was thought to be better suited for patients with a large defect after excision procedure. In a systematic review of various fascio-cutaneous flaps for vulvovaginal reconstruction, the lotus petal flap, which includes the pudendal nerves in the pedicle, the gluteal-fold fascio-cutaneous flap (Fig. 31.5), which includes the cutaneous branches of the internal pudendal nerve, the V-Y advancement gluteal-fold flap (Fig. 31.6), which includes branches of the cutaneous nerve from the femoral and obturator nerves, and the medial thigh fascio-cutaneous flap all support restoration of sensitivity in the area, and, therefore have the potential to promote satisfactory sexual function after surgery [26]. One cross-sectional study assessing quality of life and sexual function after vulvovaginal surgery with concurrent lotus petal flap procedure demonstrated overall satisfaction in sexual function in this patient population [44]; this finding has been confirmed in other studies [93]. Additionally, compared to the V-Y advancement flap, the lotus petal flap was deemed to be

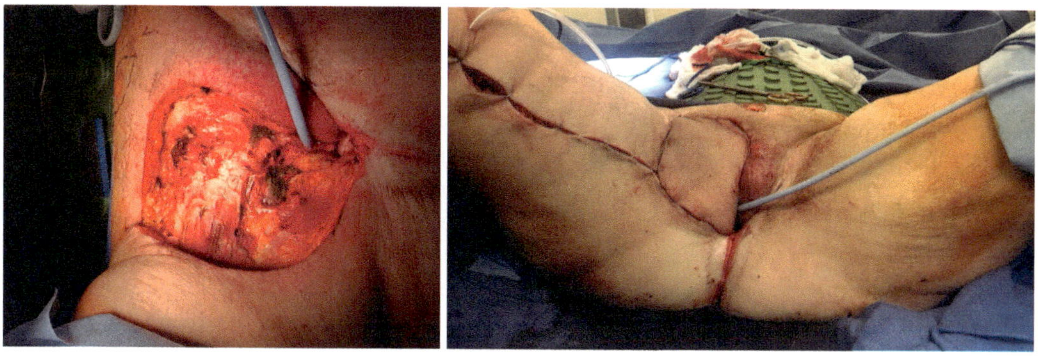

Fig. 31.5 Gluteus fasciocutaneous rotational flap. (Courtesy of Dr. Mario M. Leitao, Jr.)

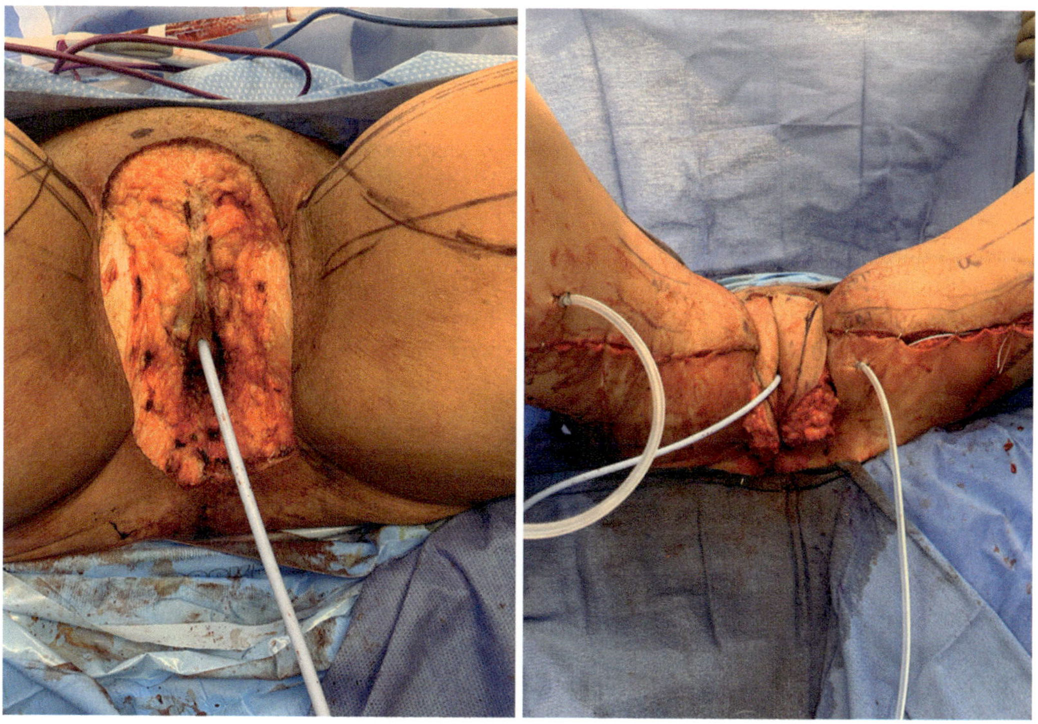

Fig. 31.6 V-Y advancement flap (Courtesy of Dr. Mario M. Leitao, Jr.)

superior in terms of functional and cosmetic results in patients who underwent vulvovaginal oncologic surgery [20].

Several algorithms have been proposed to help surgeons determine the best reconstructive plan [92, 54, 31, 91, 34]. Further data of postoperative outcomes, specifically sexual function, are necessary to inform physicians and patients alike.

Postoperative sexual function after extensive perineal excision may be particularly compromised due to posterior introital scarring. Many flaps have been evaluated in the closure of perineal defects specifically, including the inferior gluteal flap, V-Y flap, lotus petal flap, and rhomboid transposition flap [16, 45, 67, 93]. Repair of perineal defects after radical vulvar surgery is best performed with skin flaps versus direct closure to reduce postoperative morbidity and provide better anatomical and functional results [62].

Management of Functional Impairments After Radical Vulvectomy

Urinary incontinence related to anatomical distortions from radical vulvectomy warrants a different treatment approach. Urethral resection is sometimes necessary in the surgical treatment of locally advanced vulvar cancer, which leads to a pathology similar to type III stress urinary incontinence related to intrinsic sphincter deficiency. Management options for urinary incontinence due to radical vulvectomy with urethrectomy are similar to those used to treat intrinsic sphincter deficiency. This includes artificial sphincter implantation, pubovaginal sling, midurethral tension-free vaginal tape, or bulking agent injection. One unique treatment modality is transurethral Macroplastique implantation, which was shown to be safe and effective in oncologic patients with total urinary incontinence after radical vulvar surgery [76].

Urethral eversion can be seen specifically after a radical vulvectomy. It is important to perform a thorough physical examination to rule this out, as urethral eversion is a cause of urinary incontinence and general difficulty with micturition can be managed surgically. In one case report, a patient who underwent radical vulvectomy with direct wound closure presented with severe pain due to urethral orifice eversion one year after primary surgery; the patient subsequently underwent a secondary vulvar reconstruction using bilateral gluteal-fold flaps three years after primary surgery [86]. Although primary reconstruction is ideal, this case report supports the feasibility of secondary reconstruction should it be necessary.

Fecal incontinence after radical vulvectomy is most commonly observed in patients with anal sphincter resection or damage. Conservative measures should be attempted first; these include dietary adjustments, fiber supplementation or other bulking agents, constipating agents, anal plugs, and biofeedback therapy [28]. Avoiding food and drink that cause loose stool or increasing the intake of constipating agents are key dietary adjustments that have been shown to be effective in some cases of fecal incontinence. Fiber and bulking agents, such as psyllium, methyl cellulose, and synthetic polycarbophil, can change stool consistency to decrease symptoms of fecal incontinence [12, 102]. Loperamide increases anal resting pressure, impairs the recto-anal inhibitory reflex, and increases transit time in the small and large intestines, and has been well-documented to have efficacy in cases of fecal incontinence associated with loose stool [43, 63, 69, 71, 84, 88]. Pelvic floor rehabilitation plays a crucial role in the management of anal incontinence, often in conjunction with surgical procedures such as sphincteroplasty [75].

Pudendal nerve terminal motor latencies can be used to assess pudendal neuropathy. Once standard evaluation has been completed, if the determined etiology of fecal incontinence is not pudendal neuropathy, sphincteroplasty may be an option to restore anal continence, depending on the availability of the anal sphincter muscle. If there is inadequate sphincter muscle due to resection, encirclement procedures using synthetic materials or muscle transfer techniques can be employed. Implantation of a stimulating electrode can be helpful in certain clinical scenarios, particularly when using a gracilis neosphincter or artificial sphincter [55]. Sacral nerve stimulation and posterior tibial nerve modulation are neuromodulatory techniques that can decrease incontinence episodes, and there does not seem to be a difference in efficacy between the two methods [103]. Antegrade colonic irrigation through an appendicostomy was first described in children but has been shown to have some long-term efficacy in adults [65, 77]. Fecal diversion can be pursued if all other options are exhausted, or if the patient desires this option or is not a candidate for other therapeutic options.

General emotional support in the preoperative and postoperative phases has been shown to be necessary for patients who undergo surgical treatment for vulvar cancer [7]. With depression and anxiety affecting up to one-third of all patients with vulvar cancer, the complex correlation between psychosocial status and sexual dysfunction cannot be ignored [68]. Preoperative relational dissatisfaction is more common in patients with vulvar malignancy and can continue or even worsen postoperatively, regardless of the extent of surgical excision [8, 68]. Depending on the type of sexual dysfunction the patient presents with, psychotherapy can be tailored to fit their needs.

In addition to psychosocial risk factors, anatomic distortions can also contribute to sexual dysfunction in patients with vulvar cancer. Introital stenosis is one such example that can occur after vulvectomy. As in the case of urethral eversion, introital stenosis can also be managed surgically if conservative treatment with dilators is not sufficient to provide adequate relief of symptoms. A case report demonstrated the lotus petal flap was a safe and effective technique for reconstruction in the case of severe introital stenosis after primary vulvovaginal surgery with direct wound closure [15]. Given the crucial role of the clitoris in sexual function, clitoral-sparing surgical procedures have been evaluated for safety and efficacy in the management of vulvar carcinomas. One retrospective study examining clitoral-sparing modified vulvectomies found no loco-regional recurrences [17]. In fact, when compared to complete radical vulvectomy, modified radical vulvectomy is generally associated with the same rate of recurrence and decreased risk of sexual dysfunction [27, 30, 96]. One retrospective study, however, demonstrated an increased risk of loco-regional recurrence after wide local excision compared to radical vulvectomy, suggesting that less radical surgery was associated with a higher risk of recurrence. Although, in this study, there was no difference in survival between the two groups, which suggests that such loco-regional recurrences can be successfully salvaged [24]. Thus, clitoral-sparing surgery can preserve sexual function while maintaining oncologic integrity of the excisional procedure.

Physiological changes, present both preoperatively and potentially enhanced postoperatively, including anorgasmia, difficulty in lubrication, and pain, can contribute to sexual dysfunction and should be addressed as indicated [68].

References

1. Abbas S, Seitz M. Systematic review and meta-analysis of the used surgical techniques to reduce leg lymphedema following radical inguinal nodes dissection. Surg Oncol. 2011;20:88–96. https://doi.org/10.1016/j.suronc.2009.11.003.
2. Aerts L, Enzlin P, Vergote I, et al. Sexual, psychological, and relational functioning in women after surgical treatment for vulvar malignancy: a literature review. J Sex Med. 2012;9:361–71. https://doi.org/10.1111/j.1743-6109.2011.02520.x.
3. Aerts L, Enzlin P, Verhaeghe J, et al. Psychologic, relational, and sexual functioning in women after surgical treatment of vulvar malignancy: a prospective controlled study. Int J Gynecol Cancer. 2014;24:372–80. https://doi.org/10.1097/IGC.0000000000000035.
4. Allam O, Park KE, Chandler L, et al. The impact of radiation on lymphedema: a review of the literature. Gland Surg. 2020;9:596–602. https://doi.org/10.21037/gs.2020.03.20.
5. American College of Obstetricians and Gynecologists Women's Health Care Physicians, Committee on Gynecologic Practice. Committee opinion no. 571: solutions for surgical preparation of the vagina. Obstet Gynecol. 2013;122:718–20. https://doi.org/10.1097/01.AOG.0000433982.36184.95.
6. Asciutto KC, Acosta S, Borgfeldt C. Negative Pressure Wound Therapy (NPWT) in groin wounds after lymphadenectomy in vulvar cancer patients. Vivo Athens Greece. 2020;34:3511–7. https://doi.org/10.21873/invivo.12192.
7. Avery W, Gardner C, Palmer S. Vulvectomy. Am J Nurs. 1974;74:453–5.
8. Barlow EL, Hacker NF, Hussain R, Parmenter G. Sexuality and body image following treatment for early-stage vulvar cancer: a qualitative study. J Adv Nurs. 2014;70:1856–66. https://doi.org/10.1111/jan.12346.
9. Barton DPJ, Hoffman MS, Roberts WS, et al. Use of local flaps in the preservation of fecal continence following resection of perianal neoplasias. Int J Gynecol Cancer. 1993;3:318–23. https://doi.org/10.1046/j.1525-1438.1993.03050318.x.
10. Beitsch P, Balch C. Operative morbidity and risk factor assessment in melanoma patients undergoing inguinal lymph node dissection. Am J Surg. 1992;164:462–6. https://doi.org/10.1016/S0002-9610(05)81181-X.
11. Benoit L, Boichot C, Cheynel N, et al. Preventing lymphedema and morbidity with an omentum flap after ilioinguinal lymph node dissection. Ann Surg Oncol. 2005;12:793–9. https://doi.org/10.1245/ASO.2005.09.022.
12. Bliss DZ, Jung HJ, Savik K, et al. Supplementation with dietary fiber improves fecal incontinence. Nurs Res. 2001;50:203–13. https://doi.org/10.1097/00006199-200107000-00004.

13. Boyages J, Kastanias K, Koelmeyer LA, et al. Liposuction for advanced lymphedema: a multidisciplinary approach for complete reduction of arm and leg swelling. Ann Surg Oncol. 2015;22(Suppl 3):S1263–70. https://doi.org/10.1245/s10434-015-4700-3.
14. Brorson H. Liposuction in lymphedema treatment. J Reconstr Microsurg. 2016;32:56–65. https://doi.org/10.1055/s-0035-1549158.
15. Buda A, Confalonieri PL, Rovati LCV, et al. Tunneled modified lotus petal flap for surgical reconstruction of severe introital stenosis after radical vulvectomy. Int J Surg Case Rep. 2012;3:299–301. https://doi.org/10.1016/j.ijscr.2012.03.024.
16. Carramaschi F, Ramos ML, Nisida AC, et al. V-Y flap for perineal reconstruction following modified approach to vulvectomy in vulvar cancer. Int J Gynaecol Obstet. 1999;65:157–63. https://doi.org/10.1016/s0020-7292(99)00016-8.
17. Chan JK, Sugiyama V, Tajalli TR, et al. Conservative clitoral preservation surgery in the treatment of vulvar squamous cell carcinoma. Gynecol Oncol. 2004;95:152–6. https://doi.org/10.1016/j.ygyno.2004.07.004.
18. Chang DW. Lymphaticovenular bypass for lymphedema management in breast cancer patients: a prospective study. Plast Reconstr Surg. 2010;126:752–8. https://doi.org/10.1097/PRS.0b013e3181e5f6a9.
19. Cheng M-H, Chen S-C, Henry SL, et al. Vascularized groin lymph node flap transfer for postmastectomy upper limb lymphedema: flap anatomy, recipient sites, and outcomes. Plast Reconstr Surg. 2013;131:1286–98. https://doi.org/10.1097/PRS.0b013e31828bd3b3.
20. Confalonieri PL, Gilardi R, Rovati LC, et al. Comparison of V-Y advancement flap versus lotus petal flap for plastic reconstruction after surgery in case of vulvar malignancies: a retrospective single center experience. Ann Plast Surg. 2017;79:186–91. https://doi.org/10.1097/SAP.0000000000001094.
21. Courtney-Brooks M, Scalici J, Henretta MS, et al. Vulvar necrotizing soft tissue infection: a review of a multi-disciplinary surgical emergency and management in the modern era. Gynecol Oncol Case Rep. 2013;5:6–9. https://doi.org/10.1016/j.gynor.2013.02.002.
22. Damstra RJ, Voesten HGJ, van Schelven WD, van der Lei B. Lymphatic venous anastomosis (LVA) for treatment of secondary arm lymphedema. A prospective study of 11 LVA procedures in 10 patients with breast cancer related lymphedema and a critical review of the literature. Breast Cancer Res Treat. 2009;113:199–206. https://doi.org/10.1007/s10549-008-9932-5.
23. Dardarian TS, Gray HJ, Morgan MA, et al. Saphenous vein sparing during inguinal lymphadenectomy to reduce morbidity in patients with vulvar carcinoma. Gynecol Oncol. 2006;101:140–2. https://doi.org/10.1016/j.ygyno.2005.10.002.
24. De Hullu JA, Hollema H, Lolkema S, et al. Vulvar carcinoma: the price of less radical surgery. Cancer. 2002;95:2331–8. https://doi.org/10.1002/cncr.10969.
25. Dessources K, Aviki E, Leitao MM Jr. Lower extremity lymphedema in patients with gynecologic malignancies. Int J Gynecol Cancer. 2020;30(2):252–260. https://doi.org/10.1136/ijgc-2019-001032.
26. Di Donato V, Bracchi C, Cigna E, et al. Vulvo-vaginal reconstruction after radical excision for treatment of vulvar cancer: evaluation of feasibility and morbidity of different surgical techniques. Surg Oncol. 2017;26:511–21. https://doi.org/10.1016/j.suronc.2017.10.002.
27. DiSaia PJ, Creasman WT, Rich WM. An alternate approach to early cancer of the vulva. Am J Obstet Gynecol. 1979;133:825–32. https://doi.org/10.1016/0002-9378(79)90119-4.
28. Duelund-Jakobsen J, Worsoe J, Lundby L, et al. Management of patients with faecal incontinence. Ther Adv Gastroenterol. 2016;9:86–97. https://doi.org/10.1177/1756283X15614516.
29. Elg SA, Carson LF, Brooker DC, et al. Infectious morbidity after radical vulvectomy. Infect Dis Obstet Gynecol. 1994;2:130–5. https://doi.org/10.1155/S1064744994000529.
30. Farias-Eisner R, Cirisano FD, Grouse D, et al. Conservative and individualized surgery for early squamous carcinoma of the vulva: the treatment of choice for stage I and II (T1-2 N0-1 M0) disease. Gynecol Oncol. 1994;53:55–8. https://doi.org/10.1006/gyno.1994.1087.
31. Friedman J, Dinh T, Potochny J. Reconstruction of the perineum. Semin Surg Oncol. 2000;19:282–93. https://doi.org/10.1002/1098-2388(200010/11)19:3<282::aid-ssu10>3.0.co;2-b.
32. Furukawa H, Osawa M, Saito A, et al. Microsurgical lymphaticovenous implantation targeting dermal lymphatic backflow using indocyanine green fluorescence lymphography in the treatment of postmastectomy lymphedema. Plast Reconstr Surg. 2011;127:1804–11. https://doi.org/10.1097/PRS.0b013e31820cf2e2.
33. Gaarenstroom KN, Kenter GG, Trimbos JB, et al. Postoperative complications after vulvectomy and inguinofemoral lymphadenectomy using separate groin incisions. Int J Gynecol Cancer. 2003;13:522–7. https://doi.org/10.1046/j.1525-1438.2003.13304.x.
34. Gentileschi S, Servillo M, Garganese G, et al. Surgical therapy of vulvar cancer: how to choose the correct reconstruction? J Gynecol Oncol. 2016;27:e60. https://doi.org/10.3802/jgo.2016.27.e60.
35. Goetz LH, Lowry AC. Overlapping sphincteroplasty: is it the standard of care? Clin Colon Rectal Surg. 2005;18:22. https://doi.org/10.1055/s-2005-864072.
36. Gopman JM, Djajadiningrat RS, Baumgarten AS, et al. Predicting postoperative complications of inguinal lymph node dissection for penile cancer in an international multicentre cohort. BJU

Int. 2015;116:196–201. https://doi.org/10.1111/bju.13009.
37. Gould N, Kamelle S, Tillmanns T, et al. Predictors of complications after inguinal lymphadenectomy. Gynecol Oncol. 2001;82:329–32. https://doi.org/10.1006/gyno.2001.6266.
38. Green MS, Naumann RW, Elliot M, et al. Sexual dysfunction following vulvectomy. Gynecol Oncol. 2000;77:73–7. https://doi.org/10.1006/gyno.2000.5745.
39. Greene AK, Goss JA. Diagnosis and staging of lymphedema. Semin Plast Surg. 2018;32:12–6. https://doi.org/10.1055/s-0038-1635117.
40. Gupta MK, Patel AP, Master VA. Technical considerations to minimize complications of inguinal lymph node dissection. Transl Androl Urol. 2017;6:820–5. https://doi.org/10.21037/tau.2017.06.06.
41. Hacker NF, Leuchter RS, Berek JS, et al. Radical vulvectomy and bilateral inguinal lymphadenectomy through separate groin incisions. Obstet Gynecol. 1981;58:574–9.
42. Hanauer SB. The role of loperamide in gastrointestinal disorders. Rev Gastroenterol Disord. 2008;8:15–20.
43. Hellinga J, te Grootenhuis NC, Werker PMN, et al. Quality of life and sexual functioning after vulvar reconstruction with the lotus petal flap. Int J Gynecol Cancer. 2018;28(9):1728. https://doi.org/10.1097/IGC.0000000000001340.
44. Helm CW, Hatch KD, Partridge EE, Shingleton HM. The rhomboid transposition flap for repair of the perineal defect after radical vulvar surgery. Gynecol Oncol. 1993;50:164–7. https://doi.org/10.1006/gyno.1993.1186.
45. Hill AM, Pauls RN, Basil J, et al. Chlorhexidine versus iodine for vaginal preparation before hysterectomy: a randomized clinical trial. Urogynecology. 2022;28:77. https://doi.org/10.1097/SPV.0000000000001066.
46. Hnin YK, Ong LX, Tsai CC-C, et al. Does initial routine use of a compression garment reduce the risk of lower limb lymphedema after gynecological cancer treatment? A randomized pilot study in an Asian institution and review of the literature. Lymphology. 2018;51:174–83.
47. Höckel M, Dornhöfer N. Vulvovaginal reconstruction for neoplastic disease. Lancet Oncol. 2008;9:559–68. https://doi.org/10.1016/S1470-2045(08)70147-5.
48. Hoffman MS, LaPolla JP, Roberts WS, et al. Use of local flaps for primary anal reconstruction following perianal resection for neoplasia. Gynecol Oncol. 1990;36:348–52. https://doi.org/10.1016/0090-8258(90)90140-g.
49. Hoffman MS, Roberts WS, LaPolla JP, et al. Carcinoma of the vulva involving the perianal or anal skin. Gynecol Oncol. 1989;35:215–8. https://doi.org/10.1016/0090-8258(89)90046-2.
50. Homesley HD, Bundy BN, Sedlis A, Adcock L. Radiation therapy versus pelvic node resection for carcinoma of the vulva with positive groin nodes. Obstet Gynecol. 1986;68:733–40.
51. Ince C, Temple-Oberle C, Leitao MM, et al. Immediate lymphatic reconstruction: the time is right to prevent lymphedema following lymphadenectomy for vulvar cancer. Int J Gynecol Cancer. 2021;31:943. https://doi.org/10.1136/ijgc-2021-002666.
52. International Society of Lymphology. The diagnosis and treatment of peripheral lymphedema: 2013 Consensus Document of the International Society of Lymphology. Lymphology. 2013;46:1–11.
53. John HE, Jessop ZM, Di Candia M, et al. An algorithmic approach to perineal reconstruction after cancer resection—experience from two international centers. Ann Plast Surg. 2013;71:96–102. https://doi.org/10.1097/SAP.0b013e3182414485.
54. Jorge JM, Wexner SD. Etiology and management of fecal incontinence. Dis Colon Rectum. 1993;36:77–97. https://doi.org/10.1007/BF02050307.
55. Jørgensen MG, Toyserkani NM, Sørensen JA. The effect of prophylactic lymphovenous anastomosis and shunts for preventing cancer-related lymphedema: a systematic review and meta-analysis. Microsurgery. 2018;38:576–85. https://doi.org/10.1002/micr.30180.
56. Josephson DY, Jacobsohn KM, Link BA, Wilson TG. Robotic-assisted endoscopic inguinal lymphadenectomy. Urology. 2009;73:167–70; discussion 170–171. https://doi.org/10.1016/j.urology.2008.05.060.
57. Klemm P, Marnitz S, Köhler C, et al. Clinical implication of laparoscopic pelvic lymphadenectomy in patients with vulvar cancer and positive groin nodes. Gynecol Oncol. 2005;99:101–5. https://doi.org/10.1016/j.ygyno.2005.05.027.
58. Koshima I, Inagawa K, Urushibara K, Moriguchi T. Supermicrosurgical lymphaticovenular anastomosis for the treatment of lymphedema in the upper extremities. J Reconstr Microsurg. 2000;16:437–42. https://doi.org/10.1055/s-2006-947150.
59. Kung TA, Champaneria MC, Maki JH, Neligan PC. Current concepts in the surgical Management of Lymphedema. Plast Reconstr Surg. 2017;139:1003e. https://doi.org/10.1097/PRS.0000000000003218.
60. Lai YL, Chang CJ. Vulvovaginal reconstruction following radical tumor resection: report of 12 cases. Chang Yi Xue Za Zhi. 1999;22:253–8.
61. Landoni F, Proserpio M, Maneo A, et al. Repair of the perineal defect after radical vulvar surgery: direct closure versus skin flaps reconstruction. A retrospective comparative study. Aust N Z J Obstet Gynaecol. 1995;35:300–4. https://doi.org/10.1111/j.1479-828x.1995.tb01987.x.
62. Lauti M, Scott D, Thompson-Fawcett MW. Fibre supplementation in addition to loperamide for faecal incontinence in adults: a randomized

trial. Color Dis. 2008;10:553–62. https://doi.org/10.1111/j.1463-1318.2007.01439.x.
63. Le A, Xiong J, Wang Z, et al. Endoscopy-assisted inguinal lymphadenectomy in vulvar cancer. Arch Gynecol Obstet. 2018;297:1277–83. https://doi.org/10.1007/s00404-018-4732-6.
64. Lefèvre JH, Parc Y, Giraudo G, et al. Outcome of antegrade continence enema procedures for faecal incontinence in adults. Br J Surg. 2006;93:1265–9. https://doi.org/10.1002/bjs.5383.
65. Leung N, Furniss D, Giele H. Modern surgical management of breast cancer therapy related upper limb and breast lymphoedema. Maturitas. 2015;80:384–90. https://doi.org/10.1016/j.maturitas.2015.01.012.
66. Loree TR, Hempling RE, Eltabbakh GH, et al. The inferior gluteal flap in the difficult vulvar and perineal reconstruction. Gynecol Oncol. 1997;66:429–34. https://doi.org/10.1006/gyno.1997.4790.
67. Malandrone F, Bevilacqua F, Merola M, et al. The impact of vulvar cancer on psychosocial and sexual functioning: a literature review. Cancers. 2022;14:63. https://doi.org/10.3390/cancers14010063.
68. Musial F, Enck P, Kalveram KT, Erckenbrecht JF. The effect of loperamide on anorectal function in normal healthy men. J Clin Gastroenterol. 1992;15:321–4. https://doi.org/10.1097/00004836-199212000-00011.
69. Oladokun A, Babarinsa IA, Adewole IF, et al. A Sitz bath does not improve wound healing after elective episiotomy. J Obstet Gynaecol. 2000;20:277–9. https://doi.org/10.1080/01443610050009601.
70. Ooms LA, Degryse AD, Janssen PA. Mechanisms of action of loperamide. Scand J Gastroenterol Suppl. 1984;96:145–55.
71. Oonk MHM, Slomovitz B, Baldwin PJW, et al. Radiotherapy versus inguinofemoral lymphadenectomy as treatment for vulvar cancer patients with micrometastases in the sentinel node: results of GROINSS-V II. J Clin Oncol Off J Am Soc Clin Oncol. 2021;39:3623–32. https://doi.org/10.1200/JCO.21.00006.
72. Oremus M, Dayes I, Walker K, Raina P. Systematic review: conservative treatments for secondary lymphedema. BMC Cancer. 2012;12:6. https://doi.org/10.1186/1471-2407-12-6.
73. Patel KM, Lin C-Y, Cheng M-H. A prospective evaluation of lymphedema-specific quality-of-life outcomes following vascularized lymph node transfer. Ann Surg Oncol. 2015;22:2424–30. https://doi.org/10.1245/s10434-014-4276-3.
74. Pescatori LC, Pescatori M. Sphincteroplasty for anal incontinence. Gastroenterol Rep. 2014;2:92–7. https://doi.org/10.1093/gastro/gou003.
75. Plotti F, Zullo MA, Palaia I, et al. Urinary incontinence after radical vulvectomy treated with macroplastique implantation. J Minim Invasive Gynecol. 2008;15:113–5. https://doi.org/10.1016/j.jmig.2007.08.607.
76. Poirier M, Abcarian H, Nelson R. Malone antegrade continent enema: an alternative to resection in severe defecation disorders. Dis Colon Rectum. 2007;50:22–8. https://doi.org/10.1007/s10350-006-0732-x.
77. Pons G, Masia J, Loschi P, et al. A case of donor-site lymphoedema after lymph node-superficial circumflex iliac artery perforator flap transfer. J Plast Reconstr Aesthet Surg. 2014;67:119–23. https://doi.org/10.1016/j.bjps.2013.06.005.
78. Pontre J, Harding J, Chivers P, et al. Do groin drains reduce postoperative morbidity in women undergoing Inguinofemoral lymphadenectomy for vulvar cancer? Int J Gynecol Cancer. 2018;28:183–7. https://doi.org/10.1097/IGC.0000000000001146.
79. Pouwer A-FW, Arts HJ, Koopmans CM, et al. Reduced morbidity by using LigaSure compared to conventional inguinofemoral lymphadenectomy in vulvar cancer patients: a randomized controlled trial. Surg Oncol. 2020;35:149–55. https://doi.org/10.1016/j.suronc.2020.08.011.
80. Pouwer A-FW, Arts HJ, van der Velden J, de Hullu JA. Limiting the morbidity of inguinofemoral lymphadenectomy in vulvar cancer patients; a review. Expert Rev Anticancer Ther. 2017a;17:615–24. https://doi.org/10.1080/14737140.2017.1337513.
81. Pouwer AW, Hinten F, van der Velden J, et al. Volume-controlled versus short drainage after inguinofemoral lymphadenectomy in vulvar cancer patients: a Dutch nationwide prospective study. Gynecol Oncol. 2017b;146:580–7. https://doi.org/10.1016/j.ygyno.2017.06.031.
82. Raju A, Chang DW. Vascularized lymph node transfer for treatment of lymphedema: a comprehensive literature review. Ann Surg. 2015;261:1013–23. https://doi.org/10.1097/SLA.0000000000000763.
83. Read M, Read NW, Barber DC, Duthie HL. Effects of loperamide on anal sphincter function in patients complaining of chronic diarrhea with fecal incontinence and urgency. Dig Dis Sci. 1982;27:807–14. https://doi.org/10.1007/BF01391374.
84. Reid GC, DeLANCEY JOL, Hopkins MP, et al. Urinary incontinence following radical vulvectomy. Obstet Gynecol. 1990;75:852.
85. Roh S, Miyamoto S, Kitamura Y, et al. Secondary vulvar reconstruction using bilateral gluteal fold flaps after radical vulvectomy with direct closure. Plast Reconstr Surg Glob Open. 2021;9:e3550. https://doi.org/10.1097/GOX.0000000000003550.
86. Rouzier R, Haddad B, Dubernard G, et al. Inguinofemoral dissection for carcinoma of the vulva: effect of modifications of extent and technique on morbidity and survival. J Am Coll Surg. 2003;196:442–50. https://doi.org/10.1016/S1072-7515(02)01895-1.
87. Ruppin H. Review: loperamide—a potent antidiarrhoeal drug with actions along the alimentary tract. Aliment Pharmacol Ther. 1987;1:179–90. https://doi.org/10.1111/j.1365-2036.1987.tb00617.x.

88. Russell CM, Salami SS, Niemann A, et al. Minimally invasive inguinal lymphadenectomy in the management of penile carcinoma. Urology. 2017;106:113–8. https://doi.org/10.1016/j.urology.2017.04.022.
89. Rutledge TL, Heckman SR, Qualls C, et al. Pelvic floor disorders and sexual function in gynecologic cancer survivors: a cohort study. Am J Obstet Gynecol. 2010;203:514.e1–7. https://doi.org/10.1016/j.ajog.2010.08.004.
90. Saleh DB, Liddington MI, Loughenbury P, et al. Reconstruction of the irradiated perineum following extended abdomino-perineal excision for cancer: an algorithmic approach. J Plast Reconstr Aesthet Surg. 2012;65:1537–43. https://doi.org/10.1016/j.bjps.2012.05.011.
91. Salgarello M, Farallo E, Barone-Adesi L, et al. Flap algorithm in vulvar reconstruction after radical, extensive vulvectomy. Ann Plast Surg. 2005;54:184–90. https://doi.org/10.1097/01.sap.0000141381.77762.07.
92. Sawada M, Kimata Y, Kasamatsu T, et al. Versatile lotus petal flap for vulvoperineal reconstruction after gynecological ablative surgery. Gynecol Oncol. 2004;95:330–5. https://doi.org/10.1016/j.ygyno.2004.07.038.
93. Schimp VL, Worley C, Brunello S, et al. Vacuum-assisted closure in the treatment of gynecologic oncology wound failures. Gynecol Oncol. 2004;92:586–91. https://doi.org/10.1016/j.ygyno.2003.10.055.
94. Shallwani SM, Towers A, Newman A, et al. Feasibility of a pilot randomized controlled trial examining a multidimensional intervention in women with gynecological cancer at risk of lymphedema. Curr Oncol. 2021;28:455–70. https://doi.org/10.3390/curroncol28010048.
95. Siller BS, Alvarez RD, Conner WD, et al. T2/3 vulva cancer: a case-control study of triple incision versus en bloc radical vulvectomy and inguinal lymphadenectomy. Gynecol Oncol. 1995;57:335–9. https://doi.org/10.1006/gyno.1995.1152.
96. Skeith AE, Morgan DM, Schmidt PC. Vaginal preparation with povidone-iodine or chlorhexidine before hysterectomy: a propensity score matched analysis. Am J Obstet Gynecol. 2021;225:560.e1–9. https://doi.org/10.1016/j.ajog.2021.08.035.
97. Söderman M, Thomsen JB, Sørensen JA. Complications following inguinal and ilioinguinal lymphadenectomies: a meta-analysis. J Plast Surg Hand Surg. 2016;50:315–20. https://doi.org/10.3109/2000656X.2016.1173560.
98. Strugala V, Martin R. Meta-analysis of comparative trials evaluating a prophylactic single-use negative pressure wound therapy system for the prevention of surgical site complications. Surg Infect. 2017;18:810–9. https://doi.org/10.1089/sur.2017.156.
99. Stuiver MM, de Rooij JD, Lucas C, et al. No evidence of benefit from class-II compression stockings in the prevention of lower-limb lymphedema after inguinal lymph node dissection: results of a randomized controlled trial. Lymphology. 2013;46:120–31.
100. Sulo E, Hartiala P, Viitanen T, et al. Risk of donor-site lymphatic vessel dysfunction after microvascular lymph node transfer. J Plast Reconstr Aesthet Surg. 2015;68:551–8. https://doi.org/10.1016/j.bjps.2014.11.016.
101. Sze EHM, Hobbs G. Efficacy of methylcellulose and loperamide in managing fecal incontinence. Acta Obstet Gynecol Scand. 2009;88:766–71. https://doi.org/10.1080/00016340902993320.
102. Thin NN, Taylor SJC, Bremner SA, et al. Randomized clinical trial of sacral versus percutaneous tibial nerve stimulation in patients with faecal incontinence. Br J Surg. 2015;102:349–58. https://doi.org/10.1002/bjs.9695.
103. Urist MM, Maddox WA, Kennedyy JE, Balch CM. Patient risk factors and surgical morbidity after regional lymphadenectomy in 204 melanoma patients. Cancer. 1983;51:2152–6. https://doi.org/10.1002/1097-0142(19830601)51:11<2152::AID-CNCR2820511134>3.0.CO;2-7.
104. Van der Zee AGJ, Oonk MH, De Hullu JA, et al. Sentinel node dissection is safe in the treatment of early-stage vulvar cancer. J Clin Oncol. 2008;26:884–9. https://doi.org/10.1200/JCO.2007.14.0566.
105. Vignes S, Blanchard M, Yannoutsos A, Arrault M. Complications of autologous lymph-node transplantation for limb lymphoedema. Eur J Vasc Endovasc Surg. 2013;45:516–20. https://doi.org/10.1016/j.ejvs.2012.11.026.
106. Viitanen TP, Mäki MT, Seppänen MP, et al. Donor-site lymphatic function after microvascular lymph node transfer. Plast Reconstr Surg. 2012;130:1246–53. https://doi.org/10.1097/PRS.0b013e31826d1682.
107. Xu J, Duan K, Guan X, et al. Laparoendoscopic single-site inguinal lymphadenectomy in gynecology: preliminary experience at a single institution. Arch Gynecol Obstet. 2020;302:497–503. https://doi.org/10.1007/s00404-020-05649-5.
108. Yao K, Zou Z, Li Z, et al. Fascia lata preservation during inguinal lymphadenectomy for penile cancer: rationale and outcome. Urology. 2013;82:642–7. https://doi.org/10.1016/j.urology.2013.05.021.
109. Zhang SH, Sood AK, Sorosky JI, et al. Preservation of the saphenous vein during inguinal lymphadenectomy decreases morbidity in patients with carcinoma of the vulva. Cancer. 2000;89:1520–5.
110. Zhang X, Sheng X, Niu J, et al. Sparing of saphenous vein during inguinal lymphadenectomy for vulval malignancies. Gynecol Oncol. 2007;105:722–6. https://doi.org/10.1016/j.ygyno.2007.02.011.

Pelvic and Paraaortic Lymphadenectomy

32

Mitchel Hoffman, Murray Shames,
and Bernard H. Bochner

Introduction

Removal of pelvic and/or paraaortic lymph nodes is an integral part of surgery for gynecologic and urologic cancers. For gynecologic malignancies paraaortic lymph nodes are divided into infra- and supramesenteric relative to the bifurcation of the aorta, inferior mesenteric artery (IMA), and left renal vein (Fig. 32.1). For women with high-risk bladder cancer undergoing a radical cystectomy, the pelvic lymphadenectomy is routinely performed and is divided into limited, extended and super-extended with the proximal limit of dissection at the common iliac bifurcation, aortic bifurcation, or the base of the IMA respectively [1]. Lymphadenectomy may be performed by open or laparoscopic surgery.

Major complications related to pelvic and paraaortic lymphadenectomy (PPLND) include vascular injury, lymphedema, nerve injury, ureteral injury, compromise of blood supply to the intestinal tract, injury to the duodenum, arterial embolization, lymphocyst and chylous ascites.

M. Hoffman (✉)
Department of Gynecologic Oncology, Moffitt Cancer Center, USF Morsani College of Medicine, Tampa, FL, USA
e-mail: mitchel.hoffman@moffitt.org

M. Shames
Department of Surgery, Division of Vascular Surgery, USF Morsani College of Medicine, Tampa, FL, USA
e-mail: mshames@usf.edu

B. H. Bochner
Urology Service, Department of Surgery, Memorial Sloan Kettering Cancer Center, New York, NY, USA
e-mail: bochnerb@mskcc.org

M. Hoffman et al. (eds.), *Major Complications of Female Pelvic Surgery*,
https://doi.org/10.1007/978-3-031-66772-5_32

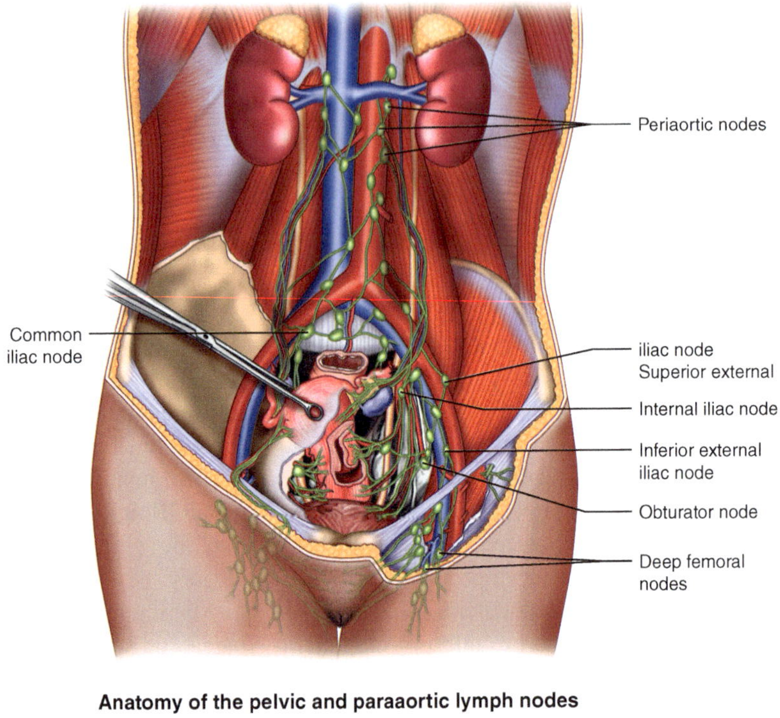

Fig. 32.1 Anatomy of the lymphatic system as it relates to pelvic and paraaortic lymphadenectomy. The relationships of the major vasculature, urinary tract and obturator nerves are shown

Vascular Injury

Background

Risk factors for major vascular injury include obesity, obliteration of the retroperitoneum or pelvic planes (prior surgery, radiation therapy), tumor involvement of the vasculature either via direct extension or involved regional lymph nodes, aberrant anatomy, and utilization of an energy device that may impact tissue beyond what is intended [2]. Although uncommon, major vascular injury is the most serious and life-threatening complication of PPLND [3]. Therefore, much of this chapter will focus on vascular injury during the performance of a PPLND.

Prevention

The internal iliac venous plexus is complex, relatively delicate, and not easily visualized. This plexus progressively coalesces into the short internal iliac vein. Several venous branches to the internal iliac vein travel in an anterior/posterior plane as they arise from the gluteal compartment. Injury to the more cephalad and coalescing portion of this plexus is more likely to result in substantial hemorrhage that may be difficult to control due to the caliber, anatomic complexity, thin walls, and relative surgical inaccessibility. Control of bleeding is best done prophylactically. The plexus is mainly at risk during the dissection of internal iliac and obturator lymph nodes. Prevention of injury to this plexus begins with appropriate development of the relatively avascular paravesical space, exposing the obturator fossa. When reasonable based on clinical findings, the surgeon should limit dissection to remain superficial to the obturator nerve, with caution moving the cephalad toward the venous confluence. If deeper dissection is needed, a layered approach to dissection of the obturator fossa is optimal [4]. A split and roll technique can be used to free the lymphatic tissues anterior to the obturator nerve. The nerve can then be mobilized by freeing from the membranous attachments posterior to the nerve. This will then expose the obturator vessels, that can be traced toward the obturator foramen distally. These vessels can be isolated and secured with hemoclips or a vessel-sealing energy device. This will then expose the hypogastric nodal packet lateral to the internal iliac artery and overlying the internal iliac vein. Careful dissection of these lymph nodes will allow for identification of the origin of the obturator vessels, particularly the vein which must be re-secured at its origin. Careful dissection around the internal iliac veins is required to avoid injury to the posteriorly located hypogastric venous channels. When extensive involvement of this region is encountered, ligation and resection of the internal iliac vein may be required as clinically indicated.

Branches or the main divisions of the internal iliac artery may likewise be injured during the dissection of the obturator fossa. The arteries are less delicate and therefore less prone to injury, which is best prevented by the development of the paravesical and pararectal spaces and prophylactic ligation as clinically indicated.

The external iliac vein is a large bore with a visible and predictable location and course. It may be obscured by retroperitoneal fat or nodal tissue. Prevention of injury to this vein during a pelvic lymphadenectomy requires adequate development of the retroperitoneal spaces, cautious dissection parallel to the wall of the vein, and prudence regarding the risk-benefit of attempted removal of densely adherent positive nodes. Laterally located psoas branches will be encountered during dissection of the external iliac vessels. Multiple branches may be present and are paired arterial and venous channels. Securing these with clips or energy ligation may be needed to completely free the external iliac vessels from the surrounding lymphatic tissues.

Injury of the common or external iliac arteries during lymphadenectomy may occur when resection of densely adherent positive nodes is attempted. Weighing risk versus benefit is particularly important given the potential loss of blood supply to an extremity. Attempting resection in such cases begins with securing proximal and distal access (vessel loops) followed by cautious, precise arteriolysis. An anterior split and roll technique can facilitate the identification of the vessel wall.

Lymph nodes along the right (versus left) common iliac vein are much more likely to be involved with metastatic disease from gynecologic malignancy. Injury of this vein or the inferior vena cava (IVC) during lymphadenectomy is commonly the result of shearing of a venule entering these veins, which may be avoided by dissecting in a cephalad to caudal direction and meticulous prophylactic control of the venules as they are encountered. As with the external iliac vein, resection of densely adherent lymph nodes must be approached with great caution. The left common iliac vein is at risk of injury when the left side is approached from the midline and dissection is misdirected during the development of the left retroperitoneal space. Initial identification of the right common iliac artery and laterally the IVC formation can provide optimal visualization needed to clear the left common iliac vein. Anatomic relationships are key to understanding this region. The left common iliac vein will travel posterior (dorsal) to the right common iliac artery. The initial clearing of the aortic bifurcation and right common iliac artery will allow for the dissection to proceed medially along the right common iliac artery. At this location, the anterior wall of the left common iliac vein can be identified. A careful split and roll of the lymphatics along its anterior wall will facilitate the freeing of the remaining vein. Care should be taken as small venous branches of the left common iliac vein may be present. They can variably arise anteriorly or along the cephalad groove just medial to the left common iliac artery. Initial Identification of the left common iliac artery helps identify the correct plane of dissection.

Considering the risk/benefit ratio based on the biology of the patient's tumor type, resection of tumor densely adherent to the aorta must be carefully considered. During paraaortic lymphadenectomy, the IMA may be avulsed from the aorta. This may occur during mobilization and retraction of the sigmoid colon.

Recognition

"There will be blood" [5].

Management

When hemorrhage from the internal iliac veins is encountered, gentle tissue handling is important in order to prevent further injury to the plexus and exacerbation of the problem. Pressure (judiciously applied), hemostatic agents, sutures and clips may all be useful. The obturator nerve and the lumbosacral nerve plexus are in harm's way.

Injury to internal iliac arterial branches is more easily identified than those of the veins but with the same issue of limited surgical accessibility. However, such injuries are more easily controlled.

A small injury to one of the major veins (less than 1–2 mm) is likely to require pressure only, with or without hemostatic agents. Some advanced hemostatic agents are now available that may at least temporarily control significant bleeding. It is important to know which agents are available in the operating room and have familiarity with their use. Have patience and apply gentle pressure for 10–15 minutes without trying to explore the area for bleeding. Blind dissection or attempts to suture the area without control will lead to excessive hemorrhage and the potential to make the injury worse. With a larger defect, suture repair will be necessary. At times this can be accomplished expeditiously during control by gentle pressure and avoidance of further trauma to the vein. Temporary closure of the hole with Allis clamps or isolation of the hole from the venous stream are useful techniques. Proximal and distal control with vessel loops or even vascular clamps may be necessary. Suture repair should be perpendicular to the lumen if possible, to avoid constriction (Fig. 32.2). Caution should be taken to include an adequate bite of the vein and to avoid excessive tension on the vein when tying the suture to prevent tearing the vein and creating a larger defect. It is important to generously hydrate the monofilament suture (5–0 or 6–0) and the surgeons' hands when tying knots to prevent breaking the suture. Exposure and visualization of the defect is critical when repairing venous injuries and calling for experienced help should be considered before attempting repair. Skillful placement of the suction cannot be underestimated. Our experience suggests that these patients are at high risk for subsequent deep vein thrombosis [6, 7]. Ligation of the vein is a lifesaving measure when conservative efforts fail [8]. Distal and proximal control as well as repair are approached

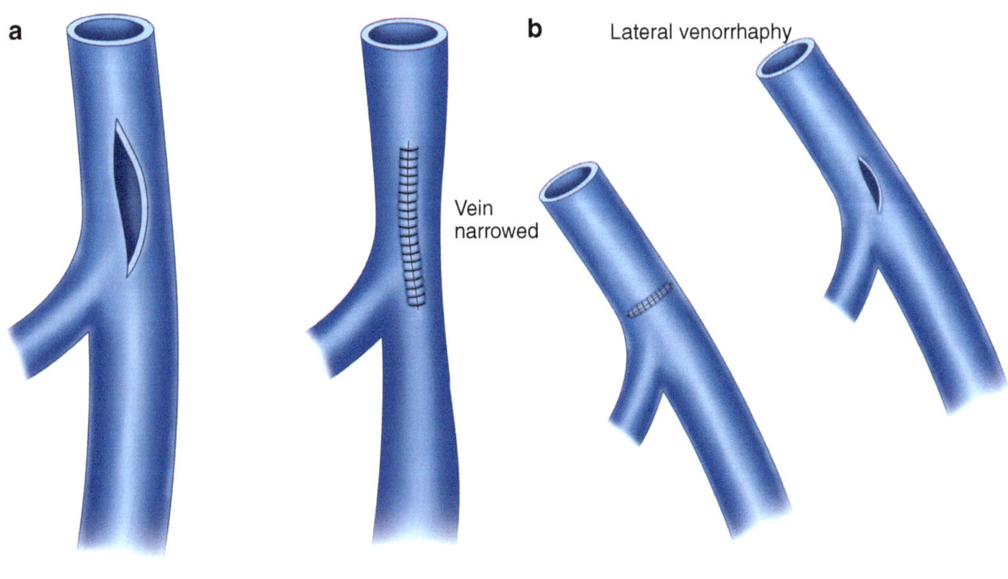

Fig. 32.2 (**a** and **b**) Lateral venorrhaphy. (**a**) Venous laceration repaired parallel to the lumen, resulting in constriction of the caliber. (**b**) Venous laceration repaired perpendicular to the lumen, with preservation of the caliber

with caution to avoid exacerbating a tear of the rather delicate vein wall. f direct repair of the vein is likely to cause stenosis then patch repair can be considered with autogenous saphenous vein or if necessary bovine pericardium. The patch should be sewn in longitudinally. It is typical to extend the venotomy to allow adequate caliber to the vein. Patch repair should be started in the proximal and distal ends with 5–0 or 6–0 polypropylene sutures. Bring each suture to the middle of the patch and tie to the opposite end.

Injury of the external or common iliac artery or aorta during lymphadenectomy requires immediate focal or proximal and distal control, followed by suture repair. Surgical repair of a focal arterial injury can be easily achieved with simple transverse interrupted stitches. Care should be taken to include the intima and adventitia to avoid delayed pseudoaneurysm formation. If possible a double needle 5–0 monofilament suture placed from intima to adventitia under direct vision provides assurance of a durable repair. Placing multiple individual sutures prior to tying the knots rather than a running suture is recommended for larger injuries. For larger defects (>50% of the lumen) patch angioplasty should be considered to avoid vessel stenosis and occlusion. With avulsion of the IMA, it may be possible to secure the stump with clips or suture. With complete avulsion there will be a significant (2 mm) hole in the aorta with rapid and life-threatening hemorrhage.

Immediate control and suture repair are critical. Partial aortic occlusion can be obtained with a Satinsky or similar vascular clamp (Fig. 32.3). Direct pressure should control bleeding until adequate help can be called in. Loss of the IMA at this level is rarely of consequence regarding intestinal blood supply due to extensive collateral circulation from the celiac, SMA and internal iliac arteries. If the colon side of the transected

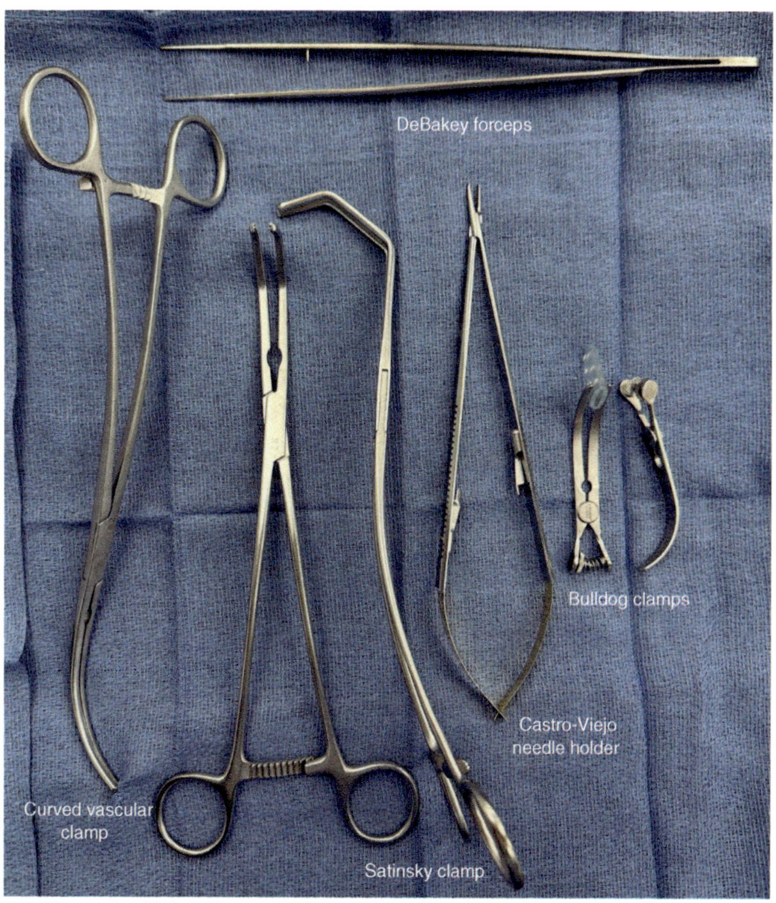

Fig. 32.3 Some useful vascular instruments. Curved vascular clamp, Statinsky clamp, Castro-Viejo needle holder, bulldog clamps, Debakey forceps

artery demonstrates brisk back-bleeding then good collateral circulation is likely. If the colon exhibits evidence of ischemia after IMA ligation, the IMA should be reconstructed either directly or with a vascular bypass. Assessment of the blood supply of the colon with intravenous injection of indocyanine green dye and intraoperative fluorescence angiography may be considered if this is available.

Lymphedema

Background

Factors that increase the likelihood of lymphedema subsequent to PPLND include the extent of lymph node dissection, removal of lymph nodes lateral to the external iliac vessels, removal of lymph nodes distal to the circumflex iliac vein (suprainguinal), and prior or planned postoperative external beam pelvic radiation therapy [9–11].

Prevention

Limiting the extent of pelvic lymphadenectomy, particularly by confining dissection to the sentinel lymph nodes, has the greatest impact on the prevention of subsequent lower extremity lymphedema [12–14]. When a more complete pelvic lymphadenectomy is indicated, dependent upon the clinical findings, the risk of lymphedema is reduced by avoiding disruption of the lymphatics lateral to the external iliac artery and distal to the circumflex iliac vein [14]. In addition, nonclosure of the pelvic peritoneum after pelvic lymphadenectomy has been shown to reduce the incidence of lower extremity lymphedema [15]. Lymphedema is one of the risks when weighing the risk versus benefit of adjuvant external beam pelvic radiation therapy [15]. Prior to and subsequent to surgery, well-fitted support stockings may provide some additional level of prevention. It is also worth mentioning that there have been *reports of early successes of microsurgery and immediate lymphatic reconstruction in lymphedema prevention for breast cancer patients* [16].

Recognition

Unilateral or bilateral lower extremity edema will generally present early in the postoperative course and progress over time. Deep vein thrombosis must be ruled out and other causes of lower extremity edema (bilateral) should be considered, such as chronic venous insufficiency, fluid overload, and congestive heart failure.

Management

Mild lymphedema should be managed proactively with leg elevation while resting and well-fitted support stockings while ambulatory [17]. Avoidance of even minor trauma to the extremity is important due to the susceptibility to lymphangitis. Prompt recognition and management of lymphangitis reduces the likelihood of sepsis and exacerbation of the lymphedema. For more severe cases, referral to a lymphedema specialty clinic should be considered. Additional measures that are of potential benefit include lymphatic massage, wrapping of the extremity, and an intermittent compression device. Microsurgical lymphatic bypass has been shown to result in modest improvement in selected patients although this approach is not widely available [16, 17].

Nerve Injury

Background

Nerves that are most commonly injured during a PPLND are the obturator nerve and the genitofemoral nerve [18–20]. Infrequently the sciatic nerve roots may be injured, most commonly from sutures used for controlling deep bleeding from the hypogastric venous plexus. With an open procedure, injury of the femoral nerve may occur from compression by the lateral blade of a self-retaining retractor.

Prevention

Identification and dissection of the lymphatic bundle away from the obturator nerve should be the initial step during resection of the obturator fossa lymph nodes. A systematic dissection from anterior to posterior will facilitate optimal visualization of the obturator nerve while clearing all lymphatic tissues from the fossa. Initial control of the small lateral perforating vessels from the obturator vessels laterally to the obturator internus muscle will allow for minimizing early bleeding that would otherwise obscure visualization of the nerve. Avoid excessive traction on the nerve during this dissection.

The genitofemoral nerve or a branch of it may be difficult to identify even with normal anatomy, particularly when obscured by retroperitoneal fat or positive lymph nodes. Early identification, avoidance of dissection lateral to the external iliac artery, and dissection with minimal manipulation away from the nerve when necessary are all measures that may prevent injury to this nerve.

When utilizing a self-retaining retractor, the lateral blade should be placed above the psoas muscle—particularly at the caudal location where the femoral nerve becomes superficial as it exits under the inguinal ligament. Overly tightening these retractor blades should also be avoided, and period loosening during a long case is a good practice.

Recognition

Obturator neuropathy is readily recognized by the development postoperatively of unilateral adductor muscle weakness. Numbness or paresthesia of the medial thigh may also be present. Injury of the genitofemoral nerve presents postoperatively as numbness or paresthesia of the skin overlying the upper anterior thigh. Femoral nerve injury may, unfortunately, be recognized after the patient falls with her first attempt at postoperative ambulation. Flexion of the thigh and extension of the knee will be compromised.

Management

Following intraoperative recognition of partial or complete transection of the obturator nerve, reapproximation of the epineurium with fine suture is considered (Fig. 32.4). Wrapping the repair with a local neural regenerative agent may be of some value as well, but the cornerstone of management is physical therapy. There is no specific management for genitofemoral nerve injury except reassurance that the majority of these will resolve over time.

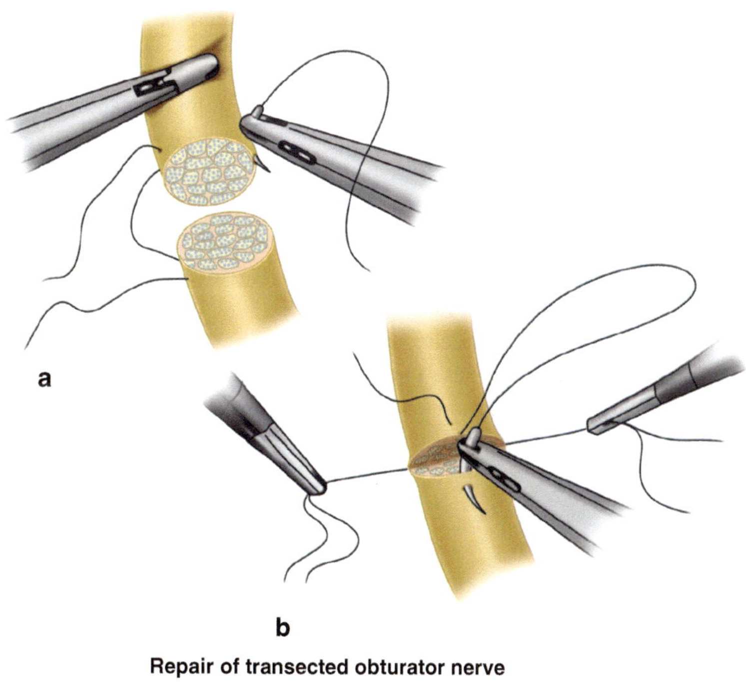

Fig. 32.4 (**a** and **b**) Repair of transected obturator nerve by approximation of the epineurium utilizing fine suture

Femoral nerve injury is managed by physical therapy, and complete recovery occurs in the majority of cases within 3 to 6 months.

Ureteral Injury

Background

The pelvic ureter crosses and lies against the bifurcation of the common iliac artery and remains in close proximity to the major pelvic vasculature up to the ureteric tunnel (Fig. 32.1). During pelvic lymphadenectomy, it is at risk of injury during this entire course [21]. Likewise, the abdominal ureter travels just lateral to the inferior vena cava on the right side and just lateral to the aorta on the left side. During a left paraaortic lymphadenectomy approached from the midline, the left ureter may be difficult to identify and keep out of harm's way due to its somewhat hidden position dorsal to the sigmoid colon mesentery. The ureteral blood supply is segmental, coming from multiple vessels from the aorta, renal, common, and internal iliac arteries. The blood travels cephalad and caudad along the ureter via fine arterioles located in the periureteral adventitial sheath. Careful manipulation of the ureter with a noncrushing technique is important to minimize damage to this collateral circulation within the ureteral wall.

Prevention

Identify and mobilize the ureters prior to beginning the lymphadenectomy, and keep them retracted out of the operative field during the dissection. When unusual difficulty is encountered (left paraaortic nodes in obese patients, grossly positive nodes), consideration can be given to pre-procedural stenting or the use of ureteral ICG dye in concert with a near-infrared camera.

Recognition

Continual focus on the operative field throughout the procedure and careful inspection of the ureters immediately upon completion will usually allow intraoperative recognition. Additional adjuvant methods to facilitate intraoperative recognition of ureteral injury include administration of intravenous dye (such as fluorescein) that is excreted by the urinary tract (allowing for identification of a gross leak into the peritoneal cavity or lack of efflux from a ureteral orifice visualized cystoscopically.

Management

Management of ureteral injury is covered in Chap. 17.

Disruption of the Mesentery

Background

The mesentery of the sigmoid colon may inadvertently be damaged during paraaortic lymphadenectomy, especially from the midline approach as the surgeon attempts to gain exposure to the left paraaortic and common iliac lymph nodes.

Prevention

Proceed cautiously when exposing the left common iliac and paraaortic region from the midline and when retracting in a cephalad direction under the inferior mesenteric artery (IMA). Misdirected dissection into the sigmoid colon mesentery may be avoided by following the right common iliac artery to the bifurcation and then exposing the left common iliac artery.

Recognition

Laceration or avulsion of the IMA will result in hemorrhage, which may be severe. Damage to the sigmoid colon mesentery may only be recognized after re-directing an initial incorrect pane of dissection. Inspection of the tissues that have been disrupted may reveal damage to mesenteric blood vessels supplying the sigmoid colon.

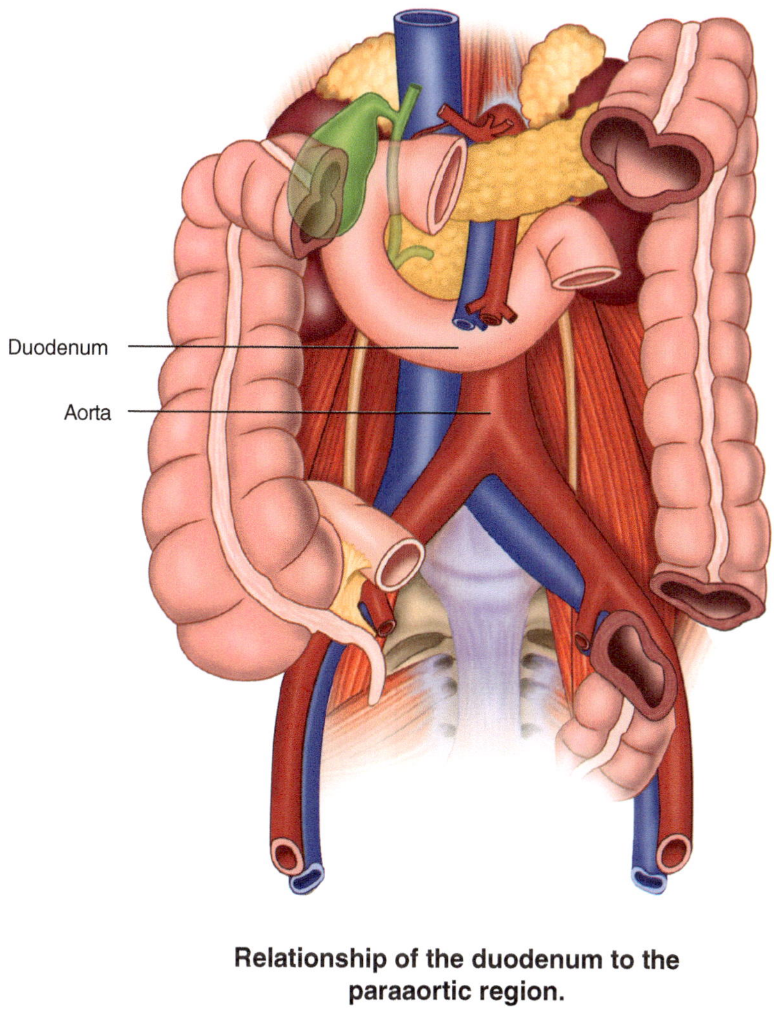

Fig. 32.5 Anatomic relationship of duodenum to paraaortic basin

Management

Management of injury to the IMA has already been addressed. Damage to the sigmoid colon mesentery requires careful clinical assessment of the adequacy of the remaining blood supply. In the unlikely event of loss of viability, surgical resection is required.

Duodenum

Background

The third portion of the duodenum begins to emerge from the retroperitoneum and typically crosses the aorta at about the level of the IMA (Fig. 32.5). The level of crossing is variable and may be as low as the common iliac vessels. During exposure of the retroperitoneum to access the common iliac and paraaortic lymph nodes (especially on the right side), the duodenum may not be recognized or otherwise inadvertently injured [22].

Prevention

As lymphadenectomy proceeds cephalad to the aorta, it is important to recognize the crossing of the duodenum and mobilize it out of harm's way.

Recognition

Spillage of bilious material during dissection of the paraaortic region should prompt an immediate search for the source. Assuming the remainder of the bowel has been kept out of the operative field, injury to the duodenum is likely.

Management

Mobilize the defect in the duodenum so that the full extent of the injury can be assessed and properly repaired. Assuming a small hole on the caudal side of the bowel, repair proceeds as with any enterotomy. The placement of a drain is considered depending on the clinical scenario.

Arterial Embolization

Background

During the course of a pelvic lymphadenectomy, manipulation of an arteriosclerotic external iliac artery may rarely result in the dislodging of a plaque, which embolizes and obstructs the distal arterial supply to a portion of the lower extremity [23].

Prevention

When performing a lymphadenectomy in a patient with known or suspected arteriosclerotic vascular disease, manipulation of the major arteries should be avoided to the extent possible.

Recognition

Very early in the postoperative course, the patient may develop evidence of progressive loss of viability of the lower extremity.

Management

This is a medical emergency requiring immediate evaluation by a vascular surgeon.

Lymphocyst and Chylous Ascites

Background

During PPLND, lymphatic channels are invariably disrupted. Leakage of lymphatic fluid is generally self-limited and of no clinical consequence. Small areas of trapped lymphatic fluid or low-volume chylous ascites are common and require no intervention. A lymphocyst may become large and problematic and require intervention. This is more likely in patients who have also received radiation therapy or have lymph node metastases. Likewise, chylous ascites may persist in large volumes and be clinically problematic.

Prevention

Avoiding closure of the peritoneum following pelvic lymphadenectomy has been shown to reduce the incidence of a subsequent lymphocyst [15]. Meticulous ligation or clipping of afferent and efferent lymphatic channels may reduce the likelihood of these complications. The low likelihood of a problematic lymphocyst or chylous ascites and the prevalence of performing lymphadenectomy with an energy device, particularly with minimally invasive surgery, are among the factors that may dissuade surgeons from these methods. The surgical approaches described earlier to reduce the likelihood of lymphedema, especially limiting the extent of dissection, apply here as well. However, randomized trial data in bladder cancer patients undergoing limited versus extended pelvic lymphadenectomy have found relatively small added morbidity associated with the more extensive dissection [24]. Only a modest increase in lymphoceles requiring drainage was observed.

Management

Small asymptomatic lymphocysts are common following lymphadenectomy and are often seen on imaging done for unrelated reasons. Indications for drainage of a lymphocyst include the development of deep vein thrombosis, attributable ureteral obstruction or lymphedema, pain, or secondary infection. An infected lymphocyst is managed as any abscess. Following drainage of a lymphocyst, a drain should be left in place until reimaging suggests resolution. When persistent or recurrent, a sclerosing agent or marsupialization is considered [25].

Chylous ascites is often self-limited and resolves spontaneously or with conservative management (diet modification +/− Somatostatin, paracentesis) [26]. If these measures fail lymphangiography with embolization is performed, and very occasionally surgery is considered.

References

1. Tarin TV, Power NE, Ehdaie B, Sfakianos JP, Silberstein JL, Savage CJ, et al. Lymph node positive bladder cancer treated with radical cystectomy and lymphadenectomy: effect of the level of node positivity. Eur Urol. 2012;61(5):1025–30.
2. Buras AL, Chern JY, Chon HS, Shahzad MM, Wenham RM, Hoffman MS. Major vascular injury during gynecologic cancer surgery. Gynecol Oncol Rep. 2021;37:100815.
3. Herraiz Roda JL, Llueca A, Maazouzi Y, Piquer Simó D, Guijarro Colomer M, Sentís MJ. Complications of laparoscopic lymphadenectomy for gynecologic malignancies. Experience of 372 patients. Res Rep Gynaecol Obstet. 2017;1:12–6.
4. Bochner BH, Quek M, Skinner DG. Radical cystectomy and pelvic lymph node dissection. In: Scardino PT, Linehan MW, Zelefsky MJ, Vogelzang N, Rini BI, Bochner BH, Sheinfeld J, editors. Comprehensive textbook of genitourinary oncology. 4th ed. Philadelphia: Lippincott Williams and Wilkins; 2011.
5. "There will be blood". Ghoulardi Film Company, 2007.
6. Greene K, Shames M, Grundy S, Hoffman M. Case report: use of endovascular techniques for management of iatrogenic iliac vein injuries. J Gynecol Surg. 2012;28:134–5.
7. Hoffman MS, Humphrey MM. Venous injury during lymphadenectomy: management without laparotomy. J Robot Surg. 2012;6(3):267–8.
8. Magee GA, Cho J, Matsushima K, Strumwasser A, Inaba K, Jazaeri O, et al. Isolated iliac vascular injuries and outcome of repair versus ligation of isolated iliac vein injury. J Vasc Surg. 2018;67(1):254–61.
9. Abu-Rustum NR, Alektiar K, Iasonos A, Lev G, Sonoda Y, Aghajanian C, et al. The incidence of symptomatic lower-extremity lymphedema following treatment of uterine corpus malignancies: a 12-year experience at Memorial Sloan-Kettering Cancer Center. Gynecol Oncol. 2006;103(2):714–8.
10. Volpi L, Sozzi G, Capozzi VA, Ricco M, Merisio C, Di Serio M, et al. Long term complications following pelvic and para-aortic lymphadenectomy for endometrial cancer, incidence and potential risk factors: a single institution experience. Int J Gynecol Cancer. 2019;29(2):312–9.
11. Yost KJ, Cheville AL, Al-Hilli MM, Mariani A, Barrette BA, McGree ME, et al. Lymphedema after surgery for endometrial cancer: prevalence, risk factors, and quality of life. Obstet Gynecol. 2014;124(2 Pt 1):307–15.
12. Rossi EC, Kowalski LD, Scalici J, Cantrell L, Schuler K, Hanna RK, et al. A comparison of sentinel lymph node biopsy to lymphadenectomy for endometrial cancer staging (FIRES trial): a multicentre, prospective, cohort study. Lancet Oncol. 2017;18(3):384–92.
13. Hamilton CA, Pothuri B, Arend RC, Backes FJ, Gehrig PA, Soliman PT, et al. Endometrial cancer: a society of gynecologic oncology evidence-based review and recommendations. Gynecol Oncol. 2021;160(3):817–26.
14. Abu-Rustum NR, Barakat RR. Observations on the role of circumflex iliac node resection and the etiology of lower extremity lymphedema following pelvic lymphadenectomy for gynecologic malignancy. Gynecol Oncol. 2007;106(1):4–5.
15. Tanaka T, Ohki N, Kojima A, Maeno Y, Miyahara Y, Sudo T, et al. Radiotherapy negates the effect of retroperitoneal nonclosure for prevention of lymphedema of the legs following pelvic lymphadenectomy for gynecological malignancies: an analysis from a questionnaire survey. Int J Gynecol Cancer. 2007;17(2):460–4.
16. Weinstein B, Le NK, Robertson E, Zimmerman A, Tavares T, Tran T, et al. Reverse lymphatic mapping and immediate microsurgical lymphatic reconstruction reduces early risk of breast cancer-related lymphedema. Plast Reconstr Surg. 2022;149(5):1061–9.
17. de Sire A, Losco L, Lippi L, Spadoni D, Kaciulyte J, Sert G, et al. Surgical treatment and rehabilitation strategies for upper and lower extremity lymphedema: a comprehensive review. Medicina (Kaunas). 2022;58(7):954.
18. Cardosi RJ, Cox CS, Hoffman MS. Postoperative neuropathies after major pelvic surgery. Obstet Gynecol. 2002;100(2):240–4.
19. Tanaka T, Terai Y, Ono YJ, Fujiwara S, Tanaka Y, Sasaki H, et al. Genitofemoral neuropathy after pelvic lymphadenectomy in patients with uterine corpus cancer. Int J Gynecol Cancer. 2015;25(3):533–6.

20. La Riva A, Sayegh AS, Perez LC, Poncel J, Medina LG, Adamic B, et al. Obturator nerve injury in robotic pelvic surgery: scenarios and management strategies. Eur Urol. 2023;83(4):361–8.
21. Martin A, Wells A, Anderson ML, Chern JY, Rutherford TJ, Shahzad MM, et al. Trends in ureteral surgery on an academic gynecologic oncology service. Gynecol Oncol. 2021;163(3):552–6.
22. Choi JS, Bae J, Lee WM, Jung US, Eom JM, Lee H. 2274 laparoscopic primary repair of duodenal perforation after laparoscopic para-aortic lymphadenectomy. J Minim Invasive Gynecol. 2019;26(7, Supplement):S105–S6.
23. Tounsi S, Zhang Y, Moufarrij S, Costales AB. Postoperative arterial thromboembolism resulting in acute limb ischemia after staging surgery for endometrial carcinoma: a case report. Gynecol Oncol Rep. 2022;41:100983.
24. Gschwend JE, Heck MM, Lehmann J, Rübben H, Albers P, Wolff JM, et al. Extended versus limited lymph node dissection in bladder cancer patients undergoing radical cystectomy: survival results from a prospective, randomized trial. Eur Urol. 2019;75(4):604–11.
25. Logmans A, Trimbos JB, van Lent M. The omentoplasty: a neglected ally in gynecologic surgery. Eur J Obstet Gynecol Reprod Biol. 1995;58(2):167–71.
26. Rose KM, Huelster HL, Roberts EC, Manley BJ, Gilbert SM, Sexton WJ. Contemporary management of chylous ascites after retroperitoneal surgery: development of an evidence-based treatment algorithm. J Urol. 2022;208(1):53–61.

Radical Hysterectomy

33

Mitchel Hoffman, Nadim Bou Zgheib,
Monica Avila, and Jing-Yi Chern

Introduction

Radical hysterectomy is an extended hysterectomy that is intended to remove the uterus as well as a variable amount of soft tissue, for the purpose of achieving appropriate oncologic resection of a pelvic malignancy. While mainly utilized as primary surgical treatment of early stage cervical cancer, this operation may also be incorporated into the surgical management of extended operations for ovarian, colorectal or urologic malignancies.

When utilized to treat cervical cancer, radical hysterectomy includes surgical assessment of the pelvic and sometimes paraaortic lymph nodes. Pelvic and paraaortic lymphadenectomy is covered in Chap. 32. When performed as a primary operation for cervical cancer, the oncologic margins include the endopelvic fascia ventrally, the lymph node-bearing tissue associated with the uterine vessels as well as the paravaginal portion of the cardinal ligament laterally, the uterosacral and rectovaginal ligaments dorsally, and the upper vagina distally. Resection of this addition soft tissue requires extensive mobilization of the distal ureters and bladder from the cervix and upper vagina. The upper rectum must be separated from the upper vagina. Variations of this operation are performed to resect other pelvic malignancies, depending on their extent. Radical hysterectomy may be performed by open or laparoscopic surgery.

Major complications of radical hysterectomy include urinary tract injury, bladder dysfunction, rectal injury, colorectal dysfunction, vaginal dehiscence, surgical site infection and sexual dysfunction.

Ureteral Injury

Background

Freeing the ureter from its course through the parametria (Fig. 33.1) is a major part of the effort in performing a radical hysterectomy. The extent of ureteral dissection varies according to the radicality of the operation, but invariably results in some loss of ureteral vasculature.

The incidence of ureteral injury (immediate and delayed) is reported to be 1–2% [1–17]. The risk is much higher in those who have received prior pelvic radiotherapy [18, 19].

M. Hoffman (✉) · M. Avila · J.-Y. Chern
Department of Gynecologic Oncology, Moffitt Cancer Center, USF Morsani College of Medicine, Tampa, FL, USA
e-mail: mitchel.hoffman@moffitt.org; Monica.Avila@moffitt.org; Jing-Yi.Chern@moffitt.org

N. B. Zgheib
Department of Oncology, Edwards Comprehensive Cancer Center and Joan C. Edwards School of Medicine, Huntington, WV, USA
e-mail: nadim.bouZgheib@chhi.org

M. Hoffman et al. (eds.), *Major Complications of Female Pelvic Surgery*,
https://doi.org/10.1007/978-3-031-66772-5_33

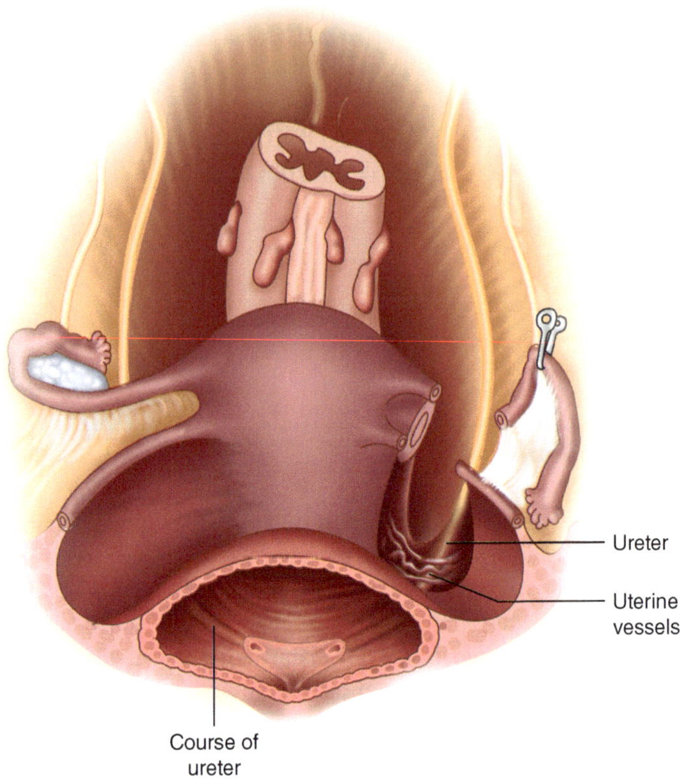

Fig. 33.1 Course of the ureter through the parametrium

Prevention

Thorough knowledge of the surgical anatomy of the pelvic ureter is a critical factor in the safe performance of a radical hysterectomy. There must be gentle, meticulous dissection of the ureter with avoidance of thermal energy in proximity to this structure. It is the opinion of the authors that stents may have a deleterious effect during radical hysterectomy by making the ureters stiff and more susceptible to shearing of feeder vessels and the adventitia.

The degree of ureteral dissection will vary according to the radicality of the hysterectomy, which should be tailored to an oncologically appropriate resection (Fig. 33.2). Regardless, it is of paramount importance that the integrity of the ureteral adventitia be preserved and that dissection lateral to the distal most aspect of the ureter be avoided (Fig. 33.3) [1]. Finally, for women who have received prior full dose radiotherapy, radical hysterectomy that will involve anything beyond minimal ureteral dissection should only be considered in highly selected cases [18, 19].

Recognition

During radical hysterectomy, the surgeon must maintain a high level of vigilance with the ureters, both during dissection and resection. Thermal damage may not be readily appreciable and any concern regarding this possibility must be managed accordingly. Loss of adventitia is equally concerning. Clear fluid appearing in the operative field must be investigated with careful inspection, aided by intravenous injection to dye the urine. Cystoscopy with the passage of a stent and/or retrograde pyelography are also options.

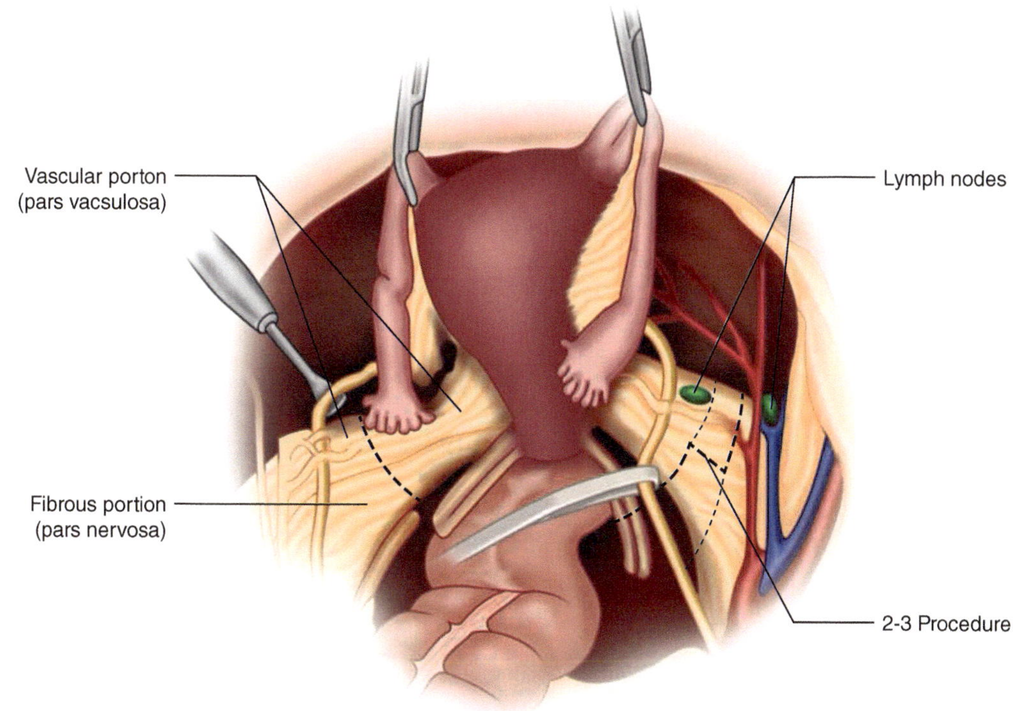

Fig. 33.2 Extent of radical hysterectomy. Right lateral line represents Class III and left line represents Class II radical hysterectomy. "Zigzag" line on right represents a hybrid or Class II/III radial hysterectomy. The latter operation includes resection of the entire vascular cardinal ligament but spares the lateral and deep portions of the fibrous, nerve-containing ligament

Unrecognized complete transection or ligation of a ureter is highly unlikely given that the ureter is dissected out and in direct view of the surgeon. At the completion of surgery, the operative field should always be carefully inspected for injuries and hemostasis.

Following surgery, a ureteral injury may present within days or weeks depending on the mechanism of the insult. Thermal injury tends to be more delayed. With unilateral obstruction there may be a transient rise in the serum creatinine during the first several days after surgery. A large volume of clear fluid from a drain or the vagina is concerning and is initially evaluated by sending a sample for creatinine and dying the urine. A CT urogram is the definitive test to evaluate for and identify the location of a ureteral injury, as well as to look for the presence of a urinoma. Unfortunately, the silent death of a kidney secondary to obstruction is a well-known phenomenon.

Management

This is covered in detail in Chap. 17. Briefly, the vast majority of ureteral injuries that are recognized intraoperatively are managed with a ureteroneocystostomy. For minimal damage (loss of a small area of adventitia) or suspected mild injury (questionable mild thermal insult), ureteral stenting alone may be considered. For management of an injury diagnosed postoperatively, please refer to Chap. 17.

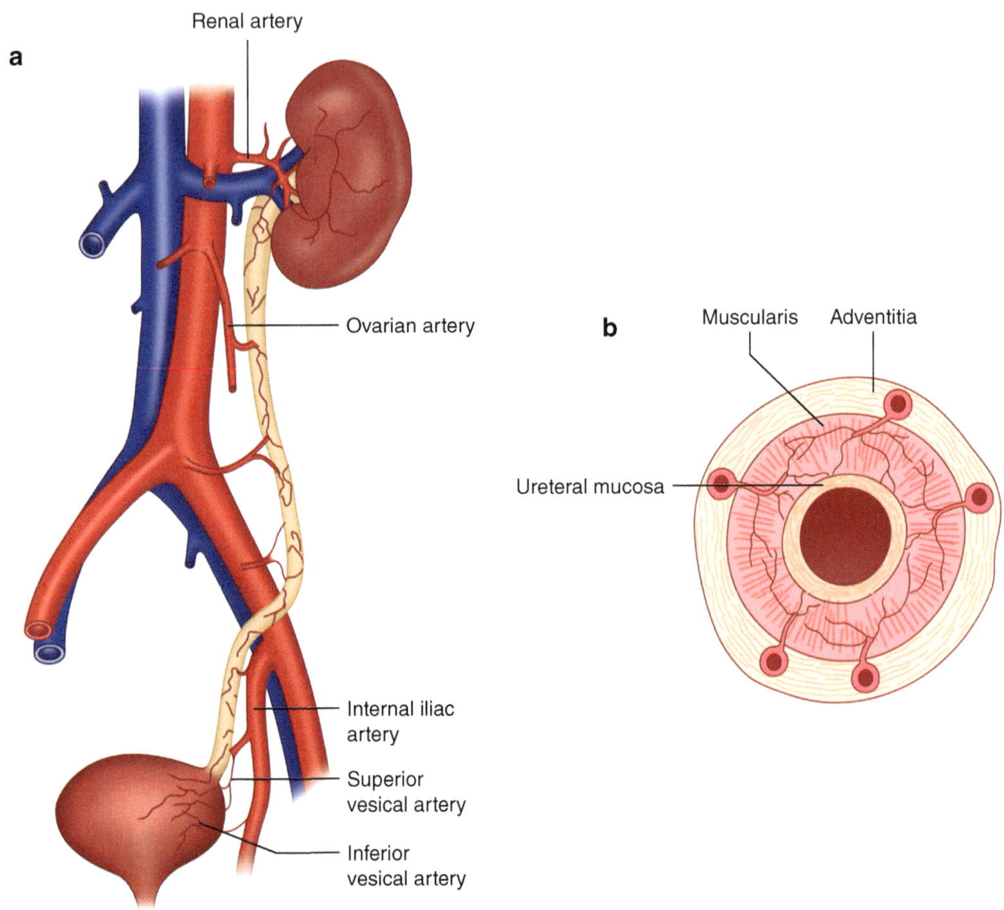

Fig. 33.3 Blood supply of the ureter

Bladder Injury

Background

During radical hysterectomy, the bladder must be mobilized to a much greater extent than required for a simple hysterectomy. This is necessary to achieve adequate vaginal and parametrial margins. The incidence of bladder injury associated with radical hysterectomy is up to 4% [17, 20, 21]. Significantly, some of these injuries are close to the trigone due to the need for more distal dissection.

Prevention

Due to the oncologic importance of maintaining the integrity of the endopelvic fascia with the specimen, it is not appropriate to direct dissection away from the bladder and into the cervix or vagina. Prevention of injury requires cautious dissection, including the lateral aspects of the bladder that might otherwise be damaged during paravaginal resection. Backfilling the bladder is occasionally useful in challenging cases. Minimal and judicious use of thermal injury is important here.

Recognition

As with the ureters, the surgeon must maintain a high level of vigilance with the bladder, both during dissection and resection. Similarly, thermal damage may not be readily appreciable and any concern regarding this possibility must be managed accordingly. Clear fluid appearing in the operative field must be investigated with careful inspection, aided by backfilling the bladder under observation.

Following surgery, a bladder injury may present within days or weeks depending on the mechanism of the insult. As with the ureter, thermal injury tends to be more delayed. Large volume clear drainage from the vagina is concerning and is initially evaluated by backfilling the bladder with a dyed solution while observing the vaginal cuff with a speculum. A CT urogram is the definitive test to evaluate for and define the location of a bladder injury, and to look for a concomitant ureteral injury and/or urinoma.

Management

This subject is covered in detail in Chap. 12. Following a radical hysterectomy, bladder sensation is often impaired. An overdistended bladder may lead to failure of repair of even a minor injury. This requires special consideration when determining the length of time for postoperative bladder rest.

Rectal Injury

Background

During radical hysterectomy, it is necessary to mobilize the rectum from the upper vagina and medial aspect of the rectovaginal ligaments in order to obtain appropriate margins. Injury of the rectum may occur during dissection or resection. Injury of the rectum (immediate or delayed) is uncommon and underreported. However, it is presumed to be comparable to benign hysterectomy where it has been shown to occur in less than 1% of cases [17, 22, 23].

Prevention

Identification and incision of the rectal reflection must be accomplished, followed by maintaining the correct path of dissection in the rectovaginal space and off of the rectovaginal ligaments. This may be challenging in cases of Pouch of Douglas obliteration (endometriosis, diverticulitis). An instrument in the rectum such as an EEA sizer may occasionally be useful in challenging cases. Judicious use of thermal energy is a must when in proximity to the rectum.

Recognition

As with the previously discussed urinary tract injuries, constant vigilance is required during dissection and resection if the surgeon is to recognize this uncommon intraoperative complication. Stool in the field or noting the rectal lumen makes the injury apparent. Sudden loss of resistance during development of the rectovaginal space should lead to prompt investigation for this possibility. When any level of concern exists, the "air bubble" or "flat tire" test is useful in ruling a rectal injury in or out.

With delayed injury, the patient will almost always present with stool per vagina. Examination and a contrast enema will be confirmatory.

Management

A rectal injury identified at the time of surgery is temporarily closed to reduce contamination while the hysterectomy is completed. After controlled irrigation, the defect is closed in two layers as described in several other chapters.

When presenting as a delayed rectal injury, diversion is required followed by later repair.

Bladder Dysfunction

Background

Radical hysterectomy partially denervates the bladder (Fig. 33.4). Following radical hysterec-

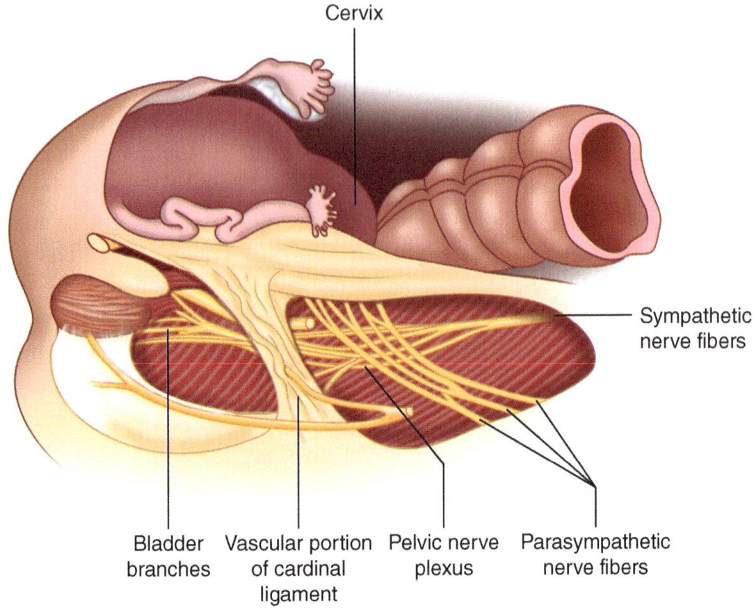

Fig. 33.4 Neuroanatomy clinically relevant to radical hysterectomy

tomy, a majority of patients experience some degree of lower urinary tract dysfunction, although the reported incidence varies greatly in the literature [15, 24–39]. The most common morbidity related to the extent of radicality is lower urinary tract dysfunction [12, 15, 40–44]. This is mainly a short-term difference (first 3 months) although the infrequent occurrence of long-term (greater than 6–12 months) severe voiding dysfunction also appears to be greater with the Class III operation (Fig. 33.2) [13, 14]. The pathophysiology of lower urinary tract dysfunction after radical hysterectomy is not clearly understood. Plausible theories include direct surgical trauma, subsequent perivesical fibrosis, interruption of afferent sensory, parasympathetic and sympathetic autonomic motor nerves (Fig. 33.4), and an impaired detrusor reflex [15, 24–26, 28–35]. Overall, the likelihood of chronic urinary tract dysfunction following a radical hysterectomy may be related to preoperative function, the degree of surgical neurological injury, and subsequent injury by bladder overdistention.

Better case selection, an improved understanding of contributing surgical factors, appropriate oncologic surgical modifications, extended bladder rest in some cases, and highly selective use of adjuvant radiotherapy have all contributed to a reduction in both the incidence and severity of this problem.

A smaller percentage of patients will develop stress or mixed urinary incontinence, especially when adjuvant radiotherapy has been administered [28, 32, 33, 43, 44]. Prevention and management of these types of voiding dysfunction are less clear, but probably follow the same principles outlined for the denervation-related dysfunction described.

Prevention

Prevention of postoperative bladder dysfunction begins with careful case selection. Large tumors require more extensive resection. These and deeply invasive tumors are more likely to have indications for postoperative adjuvant radiotherapy and are better managed primarily with chemoradiotherapy [45].

Modifications of radical hysterectomy markedly reduce the incidence and severity of subsequent bladder dysfunction (Fig. 33.2) [12–15, 26, 28, 40–42, 46–61]. The specific modifications include avoiding very lateral and caudal resection of the paravaginal, vesicovaginal and rectovaginal ligaments as well as limiting the extent of bladder mobilization and vaginal resection [45]. These modifications are consistent with an appropriate oncologic resection [62–65]. A recent study has suggested that radicality involving less extensive vaginal resection (<3 cm) will minimize the need for ongoing postoperative catheterization [66]. Therefore, larger vaginal resections should be limited as they can cause more damage to the pelvic floor. If resection leaves only the urethral vagina, the posterior urethro-vesical angle may be lost, which will predispose to lower urinary tract symptoms or LUTS (especially incontinence) [67]. Another recent study (prospective, randomized) concluded that simple hysterectomy is non-inferior to radical hysterectomy for women with low-risk cervical cancer (lesions of ≤2 cm with limited stromal invasion) [68].

Minimizing the use of postoperative adjuvant pelvic radiotherapy to appropriate indications is also an important factor in reducing the incidence of postoperative bladder dysfunction.

Postoperative bladder overdistention is a major contributing factor to short and especially long-term bladder dysfunction. The length of recommended bladder rest following radical hysterectomy varies among studies and practices. Prior to discontinuation, an active voiding trial should be performed. Additionally, given the potential decrease in bladder sensation, the patient should be instructed to "void by the clock" in order to avoid bladder overdistention. Counseling on using Valsalva to aid in bladder emptying is also reasonable. When difficulty with bladder emptying persists during the first 6 weeks after surgery, having the patient perform intermittent self-catheterization (ISC) is more likely to result in a degree of bladder recovery than further complete bladder rest.

Recognition

After an initial period of bladder rest, failure to pass an active voiding trial alerts the surgeon that more time for bladder recuperation is needed. If the patient is still not able to empty her bladder (<100 cc post-void residual [PVR]) after 6 weeks, then consideration should be given to instituting ISC until the PVR is consistently <100 cc. Additional recovery of bladder function may occur over the next 6 months, but beyond that, the problem is likely to be permanent [69].

An initially successful voiding trial may occasionally be followed, usually within days to weeks, by incomplete voiding. The problem accumulates until the patient presents with overflow incontinence or inability to void, with a markedly overdistended bladder.

Management

For women with persistent inability to adequately void following radical hysterectomy, the mainstay of management is some form of catheterization. It is important to avoid both acute and chronic bladder overdistention, which will lead to infection and further decompensation of bladder function. Pharmacologic agents may be tried but have been met with limited success. Catheter options are an indwelling Foley, ISC, or a suprapubic tube.

Colorectal Dysfunction

Background

As with the bladder, extensive pelvic resection during radical hysterectomy may denervate the rectosigmoid colon. Unlike voiding dysfunction, this problem appears to be very uncommon [12, 56, 57]. Subsequent to surgery, the patient has a segment of the rectosigmoid colon with poor peristaltic function.

Risk factors are unclear but likely include the extent of resection and associated pelvic nerve plexus denervation (as previously described) and preexisting chronic constipation and/or defecatory dysfunction. Whether specific aspects of the radical hysterectomy radicality, such as more extensive rectovaginal ligament resection, contribute to the development of this problem is not known. Survivorship studies suggest that the long-term effects of bowel dysfunction tend to be mild in isolated radical hysterectomy and are not significantly impacted by the need for a radical procedure [70]. However, other studies comparing surgical radicality suggest that a more extensive procedure such as total mesorectal excision tends to have higher rates of dysfunction than radical hysterectomy alone [71].

Prevention

As with the prevention of bladder dysfunction, case selection that precludes the oncologic necessity of an extensive wide and deep resection of the paravaginal tissues would likely prevent most instances of significant colorectal dysfunction following radical hysterectomy. Regardless, extensive resection of the uterosacral and rectovaginal ligaments for cervical cancer does not have an oncologic basis [49, 62–65].

During the weeks following a radical hysterectomy, there is a tendency toward bowel dysfunction and constipation. It is good practice to maintain these patients on a bowel regimen that will help avoid severe constipation, which may be an additional contributing factor to the development of colorectal dysfunction.

Recognition

Women with significant colorectal dysfunction following radical hysterectomy present in a manner similar to those who have undergone colorectal anastomosis, although the problem may involve a longer bowel segment and be more severe and persistent. There is a "functional obstruction", with the ineffective passage of stool past this area resulting in chronic and severe constipation [72]. The problem persists despite conservative measures. The combination of a colon transit study and defecography helps confirm the diagnosis.

Management

When women initially present postoperatively following radical hysterectomy, the mainstay of management is a good bowel regimen that includes a bulking agent combined with adequate hydration and supplemented by a combination of laxatives and stool softeners. If studies confirm a defect in transition across the rectosigmoid colon, consideration is given to intensifying this regimen. A small case series reported good results with segmental resection [73]. This should only be considered in severe, recalcitrant cases and after informed consent regarding both the potential for a major complication (leak) and failure to improve the problem.

Vaginal Dehiscence and Evisceration

This topic is covered in Chap. 6. The incidence of vaginal cuff dehiscence with or without evisceration does not appear to be significantly different with radical versus simple hysterectomy.

Surgical Site Infection

Background

Surgical site infection (SSI) is the most common complication of gynecologic surgery and has been associated with mortality, prolonged hospitalization, increased readmission rate, and long-term disability. SSIs are defined as "an infection related to an operative procedure that occurs at or near the surgical incision within 30 days" [74, 75]. With the implementation of routine preoperative antibiotics along with bundled surgical site infection preventions there have been decreased infection rates in gynecologic cancer surgery [74]. There are several risk factors that contribute to SSIs such as obesity, hyperglycemia, poor nutritional status, tobacco use, steroid use, and untreated infections. These are modifiable risk factors and should be evaluated and addressed prior to surgery, which may impact the outcome [75, 76].

Radical hysterectomy is classified as a clean-contaminated operation due to entry into the vagina. Cervical tumors may become infected, adding to the field contamination. Following radical hysterectomy, surgical site infection may take the form of urinary tract infection (UTI), abdominal wound infection, pelvic cellulitis, or pelvic abscess. The pathogens that are attributed to SSIs are endogenous microbes of the skin, vagina, and gastrointestinal tract. When considering antimicrobial agents for gynecologic procedures, it is important to consider the three sites of infection: superficial incisional- involves the skin and subcutaneous layer, deep incisional- involves the deeper soft tissues of the incision such as muscle or fascia, and organ/space which involves any part of the anatomy other than the incised body layer [75, 77]. During a radical hysterectomy, the surgical site is exposed to gram-positive, gram-negative, and anaerobic organisms. To effectively prevent SSIs, interventions are directed at broadly covering these sites. Current studies and intervention strategies demonstrate a multi-modal approach has provided the greatest benefit in decreasing complications.

Prevention

The most effective method of preventing SSIs is incorporating a bundled approach of administering effective preoperative antibiotics and thorough preoperative surgical sterile measures. The components of this bundling method include patient factors such as optimization of modifiable risk factors as briefly mentioned above. Personal skin preparation prior to surgery includes avoiding hair removal (ie. shaving) and preoperative shower with 4% chlorhexidine gluconate. If hair removal is deemed necessary, this should be done in the operating room prior to surgery using hair clippers.

Generally, the routine use of intravenous cefazolin and metronidazole is recommended at least 1 hour prior to skin incision and redosing of cefazolin at four hours or blood loss >1500 mL, with increased dosing of cephalosporin for obese patients [74, 78, 79]. The addition of metronidazole additionally addresses the common problem of bacterial vaginosis which occurs in a third of patients [74, 78, 80]. Preoperative treatment can decrease the rate of vaginal cuff infections after hysterectomy.

Skin preparation prior to surgical incision should be with chlorhexidine gluconate and isopropyl alcohol 70%. The vaginal tract should be prepped with either a povidone-iodine solution or chlorhexidine gluconate with 4% of isopropyl alcohol.

Wound infections are less common with active maintenance of intraoperative normothermia by pre-warming patients and avoiding a decrease in body temperature.

In a radical hysterectomy, there can be disruption of autonomic innervation of the bladder which can cause voiding dysfunction. Prior to starting the procedure, a urethral catheter is placed into the bladder and historically the catheter is maintained into the postoperative period. Unfortunately, catheter-associated urinary tract infections (CAUTI) are common and carry serious morbidity. CAUTIs are urinary tract infection symptoms with no other source of infection and with bacteriuria diagnosed within 48 hours of a catheter left in situ. Preventative measures such as prophylactic antibiotics have not been shown to decrease CAUTIs [81, 82]. One of the most notable postoperative factors related to urinary tract infections is the duration of catheterization, and early catheter discontinuation should be considered depending on the radicality of the surgery and the judgment of the surgeon.

Surgery should be meticulous, including avoidance of excess thermal damage to tissues and attention to hemostasis, while operating with pace. Abdominal wound closure should include subcutaneous layer approximation for obese women. Placing a vacuum device on the closed wound may be considered in high-risk cases, but the benefit in terms of preventing wound infection remains unclear.

Recognition

CAUTI is the most common hospital-acquired condition following gynecologic surgery, more so after a radical hysterectomy. While an indwelling urinary catheter is in place, symptoms of urinary tract infection (UTI) may not be apparent. Hematuria, although not uncommon secondary to mild trauma, may be a sign of infection cystitis. Following removal of the catheter, the patient may develop clinical UTI days to weeks later, which at times is chronic and difficult to eradicate. Fever, flank pain, costovertebral angle tenderness, and leukocytosis are suggestive of pyelonephritis.

Following radical hysterectomy, clinically apparent pelvic cellulitis may develop days to weeks following surgery. The diagnosis is somewhat subjective and made largely on clinical impression. Lower abdominal or pelvic discomfort, tenderness on lower abdominal and especially pelvic exam, fever, and leukocytosis may all be present. Vaginal discharge and/or a partially disrupted vaginal cuff may be present. Findings on imaging are nonspecific.

Abdominal wound infection (a common occurrence in obese women) typically presents 1–2 weeks after surgery with tender, red, warm surrounding skin. Initially, there may be cellulitis with surrounding induration. This may progress to or initially present with fluctuance or even purulent drainage. Imaging may be helpful in selected cases when the presence of a drainable abscess is unclear. Fever and leukocytosis may be present.

A pelvic abscess may develop in a small percentage of patients, usually within 2–3 weeks postoperatively. The common presentation is lower abdominal or pelvic discomfort, fever, malaise, purulent vaginal drainage, leukocytosis, and an abscess found on imaging.

Management

Fevers in the first 48 hours are conservatively managed as this is most often related to cytokine release from tissue injury or atelectasis. The patient should be encouraged to ambulate, use incentive spirometry, and respiratory toilet. After this time period if a fever persists, a thoughtful work-up should be completed for a postoperative patient.

When it is the clinical impression that an early abdominal wound infection has been identified (cellulitis only), then management with antibiotics and warm compresses is initiated. If there is progression to or presentation with a wound abscess (or drainage with subcutaneous dehiscence), then the wound should be opened. This can usually be done in the clinic or bedside setting but occasionally needs to be done in the operating room, especially when extensive debridement is required. After thorough drainage and washout of the wound, care may consist of moist-to-dry dressings or a wound vacuum system. Some patients are candidates for subsequent secondary closure.

UTI that is clinically confined to cystitis is treated, ideally, with a culture-directed antibiotic in addition to a urinary anesthetic. Pyelonephritis with signs of systemic infection requires initial hospitalization for supportive care and intravenous antibiotics. Ureteral obstruction should be ruled out in such cases.

Clinically diagnosed pelvic cellulitis is treated with broad-spectrum antibiotics. Hospitalization may not be necessary.

Pelvic abscess that develops following radical hysterectomy requires antibiotics and drainage. The route of drainage is individualized and generally can be accomplished percutaneously by interventional radiology or transvaginally.

Sexual Dysfunction

Background

A standard part of a radical hysterectomy is the removal of a portion of the upper vagina. The length of the vagina removed depends on the radicality of the operation, varying from approximately 2–4 cm. The loss of this portion is rarely of clinical significance in terms of sexual function, likely due to the distensibility of the vagina and its ability to stretch. Associated factors that may impair vaginal health and function include concomitant removal of the ovaries in premenopausal women, adjuvant radiation therapy (more so if this includes vaginal brachytherapy), and the radicality of the operation [38, 70, 71].

Prevention

As discussed in previous sections, radical hysterectomy is modified when oncologically appropriate in an attempt to reduce surgical complications. Avoiding excess removal of vagina should reduce the likelihood of a symptomatically shortened vagina. Adequate suspension of the vaginal cuff may be of further benefit. When ovaries are retained, we routinely suspend them to the lateral aspect of the round ligament (or transpose them in selected cases). This is done to preclude subsequent proximity to the vaginal apex as well as to facilitate later oophorectomy should this become necessary. Use of adjuvant radiotherapy should be limited to strict evidence-based criteria, and vaginal brachytherapy is rarely indicated. In premenopausal women who have undergone concomitant oophorectomy, estrogen replacement therapy will generally help maintain vaginal health.

Women who have undergone radical hysterectomy for cervical cancer may have some apprehension regarding resumption of intercourse, and preemptive counseling is good medical practice. This should occur both preoperatively and at the postoperative visit when examination suggests that intercourse may safely and comfortably resume. A recent prospective study suggests that while desire, arousal and orgasm may not be impacted there may be some dysfunction in the act of intercourse itself. However, for those undergoing nerve-sparing radical hysterectomy, one-year outcomes suggests no impact to quality of life which suggests that dysfunction is (1) lessened by perseveration of hypogastric nerve plexua and (2) can improve over time [83].

Recognition

Following radical hysterectomy, women who present with dyspareunia require a thoughtful and directed history and physical exam. Insertional must be differentiated from deep-thrust dyspareunia.

There are many possible related and unrelated causes of insertional dyspareunia. These include an unrecognized and poorly healed introital tear that occurred during surgery, a chronic inflammatory condition involving the vaginal opening, lack of lubrication which may be due to atrophy or suboptimal sexual response, or levator spasm (primary or secondary).

Deep-thrust dyspareunia following radical hysterectomy may be secondary to a tender cuff scar, proximity of ovaries, hypoestrogenism or suboptimal sexual response.

Management

Management begins with preoperative and postoperative counseling as previously discussed, preferably to include the patient and her partner, regarding post-treatment expectations with regard to sexual relations. For premenopausal women who lose ovarian function, strong consideration is given to estrogen replacement.

Introital issues are managed according to the perceived problem based on history and physical exam. Examples included medical management of vulvovaginitis, estrogen, artificial lubricant and/or introital revision.

Reflexive levator tightening is managed with reassurance, pelvic floor therapy and addressing any underlying contributing factors (source of pain, psychosocial issues, etc.).

Apical tenderness that is associated with a prominent and tender scar ("M" or "W" shaped deformity) may eventually require vaginal cuff revision. Apical tenderness that appears (on transvaginal ultrasound) to be related to proximally situated ovaries may ultimately require ovarian suspension or even removal.

In recalcitrant cases, referral to a sexual medicine practice should be considered.

References

1. Kiran A, Hilton P, Cromwell DA. The risk of ureteric injury associated with hysterectomy: a 10-year retrospective cohort study. BJOG. 2016;123(7):1184–91.
2. Green TH Jr, Meigs JV, Ulfelder H, Curtin RR. Urologic complications of radical Wertheim hys-

terectomy: incidence, etiology, management, and prevention. Obstet Gynecol. 1962;20:293–312.
3. Piver MS, Rutledge F, Smith JP. Five classes of extended hysterectomy for women with cervical cancer. Obstet Gynecol. 1974;44(2):265–72.
4. Burghardt E. Radicality in gynecologic cancer surgery: a historical perspective. Gynecol Oncol. 1998;70(2):172–5.
5. Hoskins WJ, Ford JH Jr, Lutz MH, Averette HE. Radical hysterectomy and pelvic lymphadenectomy for the management of early invasive cancer of the cervix. Gynecol Oncol. 1976;4(3):278–90.
6. Webb MJ, Symmonds RE. Wertheim hysterectomy: a reappraisal. Obstet Gynecol. 1979;54(2):140–5.
7. Underwood PB Jr, Wilson WC, Kreutner A, Miller MC 3rd, Murphy E. Radical hysterectomy: a critical review of twenty-two years' experience. Am J Obstet Gynecol. 1979;134(8):889–98.
8. Powell JL, Burrell MO, Franklin EW 3rd. Radical hysterectomy and pelvic lymphadenectomy. Gynecol Oncol. 1981;12(1):23–32.
9. Artman LE, Hoskins WJ, Bibro MC, Heller PB, Weiser EB, Barnhill DR, et al. Radical hysterectomy and pelvic lymphadenectomy for stage IB carcinoma of the cervix: 21 years experience. Gynecol Oncol. 1987;28(1):8–13.
10. Kenter GG, Ansink AC, Heintz AP, Aartsen EJ, Delemarre JF, Hart AA. Carcinoma of the uterine cervix stage I and IIA: results of surgical treatment: complications, recurrence and survival. Eur J Surg Oncol. 1989;15(1):55–60.
11. Averette HE, Nguyen HN, Donato DM, Penalver MA, Sevin BU, Estape R, et al. Radical hysterectomy for invasive cervical cancer. A 25-year prospective experience with the Miami technique. Cancer. 1993;71(4 Suppl):1422–37.
12. Magrina JF, Goodrich MA, Weaver AL, Podratz KC. Modified radical hysterectomy: morbidity and mortality. Gynecol Oncol. 1995;59(2):277–82.
13. Fotiou S, Tserkezoglou A, Hatzieleftheriou G, Apostolikas N. Class III vs class II radical hysterectomy in stage IB cervical carcinoma: a comparison of morbidity and survival. Int J Gynecol Cancer. 1997;7(2):117–21.
14. Landoni F, Maneo A, Cormio G, Perego P, Milani R, Caruso O, et al. Class II versus class III radical hysterectomy in stage IB-IIA cervical cancer: a prospective randomized study. Gynecol Oncol. 2001;80(1):3–12.
15. Buller RE, Tamir IL, DiSaia PJ, Berman ML. Early evaluation of the urinary tract following radical hysterectomy: structure and function relationships. Obstet Gynecol. 1991;78(5 Pt 1):840–4.
16. Liu P, Liang C, Lu A, Chen X, Liang W, Li D, et al. Risk factors and long-term impact of urologic complications during radical hysterectomy for cervical cancer in China, 2004–2016. Gynecol Oncol. 2020;158(2):294–302.
17. Obermair A, Asher R, Pareja R, Frumovitz M, Lopez A, Moretti-Marques R, et al. Incidence of adverse events in minimally invasive vs open radical hysterectomy in early cervical cancer: results of a randomized controlled trial. Am J Obstet Gynecol. 2020;222(3):249.e1–249.e10.
18. Touboul C, Uzan C, Mauguen A, Gouy S, Rey A, Pautier P, et al. Prognostic factors and morbidities after completion surgery in patients undergoing initial chemoradiation therapy for locally advanced cervical cancer. Oncologist. 2010;15(4):405–15.
19. van Kol KGG, Ebisch RMF, Piek JMJ, Zusterzeel PLM, Vergeldt TFM, Bekkers RLM. Salvage surgery for patients with residual disease after chemoradiation therapy for locally advanced cervical cancer: a systematic review on indication, complications, and survival. Acta Obstet Gynecol Scand. 2021;100(7):1176–85.
20. Limón Luque LM, Alva Trujillo HN, Delgado Urdapilleta J. Urologic lesions in gynecologic and uro-gynecologic surgery. Two years of hospital experience. Ginecol Obstet Mex. 1995;63:410–3.
21. Likic IS, Kadija S, Ladjevic NG, Stefanovic A, Jeremic K, Petkovic S, et al. Analysis of urologic complications after radical hysterectomy. Am J Obstet Gynecol. 2008;199(6):644.e1–3.
22. Jo EJ, Lee YY, Kim TJ, Choi CH, Lee JW, Bae DS, et al. Management and outcome of rectal injury during gynecologic laparoscopic surgery. J Minim Invasive Gynecol. 2013;20(2):166–71.
23. Hoffman MS, Lynch C, Lockhart J, Knapp R. Injury of the rectum during vaginal surgery. Am J Obstet Gynecol. 1999;181(2):274–7.
24. Fraser AC. The late effects of Wertheim's hysterectomy on the urinary tract. J Obstet Gynaecol Br Commonw. 1966;73(6):1002–7.
25. Low JA, Mauger GM, Carmichael JA. The effect of Wertheim hysterectomy upon bladder and urethral function. Am J Obstet Gynecol. 1981;139(7):826–34.
26. Carenza L, Nobili F, Giacobini S. Voiding disorders after radical hysterectomy. Gynecol Oncol. 1982;13(2):213–9.
27. Lewington W. Disturbances of micturition following Wertheim hysterectomy. J Obstet Gynaecol Br Emp. 1956;63(6):861–4.
28. Kristensen GB, Frimodt-Møller PC, Poulsen HK, Ulbak S. Persistent bladder dysfunction after surgical and combination therapy of cancer of the cervix uteri stages Ib and IIa. Gynecol Oncol. 1984;18(1):38–42.
29. Kadar N, Saliba N, Nelson JH. The frequency, causes and prevention of severe urinary dysfunction after radical hysterectomy. Br J Obstet Gynaecol. 1983;90(9):858–63.
30. Fishman IJ, Shabsigh R, Kaplan AL. Lower urinary tract dysfunction after radical hysterectomy for carcinoma of cervix. Urology. 1986;28(6):462–8.
31. Scotti RJ, Bergman A, Bhatia NN, Ostergard DR. Urodynamic changes in urethrovesical function after radical hysterectomy. Obstet Gynecol. 1986;68(1):111–20.
32. Bandy LC, Clarke-Pearson DL, Soper JT, Mutch DG, MacMillan J, Creasman WT. Long-term effects on

bladder function following radical hysterectomy with and without postoperative radiation. Gynecol Oncol. 1987;26(2):160–8.
33. Farquharson DI, Shingleton HM, Soong SJ, Sanford SP, Levy DS, Hatch KD. The adverse effects of cervical cancer treatment on bladder function. Gynecol Oncol. 1987;27(1):15–23.
34. Garris PD, Gallup DC, Gallup DG, Johnson MH, Messing MJ, King LA. The cystometric evaluation of bladder function before and after radical hysterectomy. Urogynecology. 1997;3(1):15–8.
35. Vervest HA, Barents JW, Haspels AA, Debruyne FM. Radical hysterectomy and the function of the lower urinary tract. Urodynamic quantification of changes in storage and evacuation function. Acta Obstet Gynecol Scand. 1989;68(4):331–40.
36. Chun N, Noh GO, Song HJ, Kim SH. Frequency, intensity and daily life distress of urinary dysfunction in women with cervical cancer after radical hysterectomy. J Korean Acad Nurs. 2016;46(3):400–8.
37. Aoun F, Roumeguère T. Lower urinary tract dysfunction following radical hysterectomy. Prog Urol. 2015;25(17):1184–90.
38. Wang X, Chen C, Liu P, Li W, Wang L, Liu Y. The morbidity of sexual dysfunction of 125 Chinese women following different types of radical hysterectomy for gynaecological malignancies. Arch Gynecol Obstet. 2018;297(2):459–66.
39. Hoffman MS. Extent of radical hysterectomy: evolving emphasis. Gynecol Oncol. 2004;94(1):1–9.
40. Hoffman MS, Cardosi RJ. Intraoperative measurements to determine the extent of radical hysterectomy. Gynecol Oncol. 2002;87(3):281–6.
41. Ralph G, Winter R, Michelitsch L, Tamussino K. Radicality of parametrial resection and dysfunction of the lower urinary tract after radical hysterectomy. Eur J Gynaecol Oncol. 1991;12(1):27–30.
42. Yang YC, Chang CL. Modified radical hysterectomy for early Ib cervical cancer. Gynecol Oncol. 1999;74(2):241–4.
43. Landoni F, Maneo A, Colombo A, Placa F, Milani R, Perego P, et al. Randomised study of radical surgery versus radiotherapy for stage Ib-IIa cervical cancer. Lancet. 1997;350(9077):535–40.
44. Sartori E, Fallo L, La Face B, Bianchi UA, Pecorelli S. Extended radical hysterectomy in early-stage carcinoma of the uterine cervix: tailoring the radicality. Int J Gynecol Cancer. 1995;5(2):143–7.
45. Bansal N, Herzog TJ, Shaw RE, Burke WM, Deutsch I, Wright JD. Primary therapy for early-stage cervical cancer: radical hysterectomy vs radiation. Am J Obstet Gynecol. 2009;201(5):485.e1–9.
46. Forney JP. The effect of radical hysterectomy on bladder physiology. Am J Obstet Gynecol. 1980;138(4):374–82.
47. Trimbos JB, Maas CP, Deruiter MC, Peters AA, Kenter GG. A nerve-sparing radical hysterectomy: guidelines and feasibility in Western patients. Int J Gynecol Cancer. 2001;11(3):180–6.
48. Michalas S, Rodolakis A, Voulgaris Z, Vlachos G, Giannakoulis N, Diakomanolis E. Management of early-stage cervical carcinoma by modified (type II) radical hysterectomy. Gynecol Oncol. 2002;85(3):415–22.
49. Campbell RM. The anatomy and histology of the sacrouterine ligaments. Am J Obstet Gynecol. 1950;59(1):1–12, illust.
50. Twombly GH, Landers D. The innervation of the bladder with reference to radical hysterectomy. Am J Obstet Gynecol. 1956;71(6):1291–300.
51. Smith PH, Ballantyne B. The neuroanatomical basis for denervation of the urinary bladder following major pelvic surgery. Br J Surg. 1968;55(12):929–33.
52. Asmussen M, Ulmsten U. Effects of radical hysterectomy with lymph nodes dissection on the lower urinary tract. Zentralbl Gynakol. 1982;104(14):868–73.
53. Sakamoto S, Takizawa K. An improved radical hysterectomy with fewer urological complications and with no loss of therapeutic results for invasive cervical cancer. Baillieres Clin Obstet Gynaecol. 1988;2(4):953–62.
54. Tong XK, Huo RJ. The anatomical basis and prevention of neurogenic voiding dysfunction following radical hysterectomy. Surg Radiol Anat. 1991;13(2):145–8.
55. Yabuki Y, Asamoto A, Hoshiba T, Nishimoto H, Kitamura S. Dissection of the cardinal ligament in radical hysterectomy for cervical cancer with emphasis on the lateral ligament. Am J Obstet Gynecol. 1991;164(1 Pt 1):7–14.
56. Yabuki Y, Asamoto A, Hoshiba T, Nishimoto H, Satou N. A new proposal for radical hysterectomy. Gynecol Oncol. 1996;62(3):370–8.
57. Höckel M, Konerding MA, Heussel CP. Liposuction-assisted nerve-sparing extended radical hysterectomy: oncologic rationale, surgical anatomy, and feasibility study. Am J Obstet Gynecol. 1998;178(5):971–6.
58. Ercoli A, Delmas V, Gadonneix P, Fanfani F, Villet R, Paparella P, et al. Classical and nerve-sparing radical hysterectomy: an evaluation of the risk of injury to the autonomous pelvic nerves. Surg Radiol Anat. 2003;25(3–4):200–6.
59. Butler-Manuel SA, Buttery LD, A'Hern RP, Polak JM, Barton DP. Pelvic nerve plexus trauma at radical hysterectomy and simple hysterectomy: the nerve content of the uterine supporting ligaments. Cancer. 2000;89(4):834–41.
60. Possover M, Stöber S, Plaul K, Schneider A. Identification and preservation of the motoric innervation of the bladder in radical hysterectomy type III. Gynecol Oncol. 2000;79(2):154–7.
61. Ito E, Kudo R, Saito T, Koizumi M, Noda M. A new technique for radical hysterectomy with emphasis on preservation of bladder function. J Gynecol Surg. 2000;16(4):133–40.
62. Burghardt E, Haas J, Girardi F. The significance of the parametrium in the operative treatment of

cervical cancer. Baillieres Clin Obstet Gynaecol. 1988;2(4):879–88.
63. Girardi F, Pickel H, Winter R. Pelvic and parametrial lymph nodes in the quality control of the surgical treatment of cervical cancer. Gynecol Oncol. 1993;50(3):330–3.
64. Benedetti-Panici P, Maneschi F, D'Andrea G, Cutillo G, Rabitti C, Congiu M, et al. Early cervical carcinoma: the natural history of lymph node involvement redefined on the basis of thorough parametrectomy and giant section study. Cancer. 2000;88(10):2267–74.
65. Girardi F, Lichtenegger W, Tamussino K, Haas J. The importance of parametrial lymph nodes in the treatment of cervical cancer. Gynecol Oncol. 1989;34(2):206–11.
66. Gallotta V, Conte C, Federico A, Vizzielli G, Gueli Alletti S, Tortorella L, et al. Robotic versus laparoscopic radical hysterectomy in early cervical cancer: a case matched control study. Eur J Surg Oncol. 2018;44(6):754–9.
67. Wang S, Wang R, Wen H, Gao Y, Lv Q, Li H, et al. Association of pelvic floor function with postoperative urinary incontinence in cervical cancer patients after the radical hysterectomy. Neurourol Urodyn. 2021;40(1):483–92.
68. Plante M, Kwon JS, Ferguson S, Samouëlian V, Ferron G, Maulard A, et al. Simple versus Radical Hysterectomy in Women with Low-Risk Cervical Cancer. N Engl J Med. 2024;390(9):819–29.
69. Campbell P, Casement M, Addley S, Dobbs S, Harley I, Nagar H. Early catheter removal following laparoscopic radical hysterectomy for cervical cancer: assessment of a new bladder care protocol. J Obstet Gynaecol. 2017;37(7):970–2.
70. Brooks RA, Wright JD, Powell MA, Rader JS, Gao F, Mutch DG, et al. Long-term assessment of bladder and bowel dysfunction after radical hysterectomy. Gynecol Oncol. 2009;114(1):75–9.
71. Baessler K, Windemut S, Chiantera V, Köhler C, Sehouli J. Sexual, bladder and bowel function following different minimally invasive techniques of radical hysterectomy in patients with early-stage cervical cancer. Clin Transl Oncol. 2021;23(11):2335–43.
72. Barnes W, Waggoner S, Delgado G, Maher K, Potkul R, Barter J, et al. Manometric characterization of rectal dysfunction following radical hysterectomy. Gynecol Oncol. 1991;42(2):116–9.
73. Vierhout ME, Schreuder HW, Veen HF. Severe slow-transit constipation following radical hysterectomy. Gynecol Oncol. 1993;51(3):401–3.
74. Kuznicki M, Mallen A, McClung EC, Robertson SE, Todd S, Boulware D, et al. Dual antibiotic prevention bundle is associated with decreased surgical site infections. Int J Gynecol Cancer. 2020;30(9):1411–7.
75. Steiner HL, Strand EA. Surgical-site infection in gynecologic surgery: pathophysiology and prevention. Am J Obstet Gynecol. 2017;217(2):121–8.
76. Guo XM, Runge M, Miller D, Aaby D, Milad M. A bundled intervention lowers surgical site infection in hysterectomy for benign and malignant indications. Int J Gynaecol Obstet. 2020;150(3):392–7.
77. Cowley ES, Jacques L, Powell AM, Al-Niaimi A, Pop-Vicas A. Characterization of bacterial composition of surgical site infections after gynecologic surgery. Am J Obstet Gynecol. 2022;227(2):345–7.
78. Till SR, Morgan DM, Bazzi AA, Pearlman MD, Abdelsattar Z, Campbell DA, et al. Reducing surgical site infections after hysterectomy: metronidazole plus cefazolin compared with cephalosporin alone. Am J Obstet Gynecol. 2017;217(2):187.e1–187.e11.
79. Nelson G, Altman AD, Nick A, Meyer LA, Ramirez PT, Achtari C, et al. Guidelines for pre- and intra-operative care in gynecologic/oncology surgery: enhanced recovery after surgery (ERAS®) society recommendations—part I. Gynecol Oncol. 2016;140(2):313–22.
80. Soper DE. Bacterial vaginosis and surgical site infections. Am J Obstet Gynecol. 2020;222(3):219–23.
81. Cardosi RJ, Cardosi RP, Grendys EC Jr, Fiorica JV, Hoffman MS. Infectious urinary tract morbidity with prolonged bladder catheterization after radical hysterectomy. Am J Obstet Gynecol. 2003;189(2):380–3; discussion 3–4.
82. Mercadel AJ, Holloway SB, Saripella M, Lea JS. Risk factors for catheter-associated urinary tract infections following radical hysterectomy for cervical cancer. Am J Obstet Gynecol. 2023;228(6):718.e1–7.
83. Novackova M, Pastor Z, Chmel R Jr, Mala I, Chmel R. Sexuality and quality of life after nerve-sparing radical hysterectomy for cervical cancer: a prospective study. Taiwan J Obstet Gynecol. 2022;61(4):641–5.

34 Composite Pelvic Resection for Ovarian Cancer

Beverly Long and William A. Cliby

Vascular Injury

Background

Because ovarian cancer tends to spread along the surface of the peritoneum and pelvic organs, direct extension into large vessels is uncommon. However, injury to the external or internal iliac vessels or presacral venous plexus may occur during the mobilization of an ovarian mass from the sidewall or posterior pelvis.

Prevention

The external iliac vessels should be identified during the initial steps of composite pelvic resection when the pararectal and paravesical spaces are developed after incising the peritoneum overlying the psoas muscle or the lateral portion of the round ligament. At this point, any adnexal masses will be mobilized from lateral to medial, mobilizing them away from the pelvic sidewall and external iliac vessels. When a pelvic mass is morbidly adherent to or invading the vessels, the surgeon should first skeletonize the vessels proximal and distal to the area of invasion to allow for vascular control in the event of vascular injury. It is then safer to explore and/or resect this area of disease without the risk of uncontrolled hemorrhage. Vessel loops and/or vascular clamps should be immediately available.

The uterine artery, a major branch of the internal iliac artery, can be ligated at the site where the uterine artery crosses anteriorly to the ureter to lateralize the ureter and resect the involved pararectal peritoneum en bloc with the adnexa and uterus. Care should also be taken to avoid laceration of the hypogastric venous plexus, as this can result in bleeding that is difficult to control.

When en bloc rectosigmoid resection is required, the presacral venous plexus may be encountered. Careful dissection of the retrorectal space is important to prevent the tearing of these vessels, which can also result in massive blood loss. Gaining wide exposure to this area before dissection is critical to managing possible hemorrhage.

Recognition

Intra-operative hemorrhage from major vessels is immediately evident. The operating room team should be alerted to massive bleeding so that blood products can be prepared, and any neces-

B. Long
Division of Gynecologic Oncology, Sarasota Memorial Healthcare System, Sarasota, FL, USA
e-mail: Beverly-long@smh.com

W. A. Cliby (✉)
Division of Gynecologic Oncology, Mayo Clinic, Rochester, MN, USA
e-mail: Cliby.william@mayo.edu

M. Hoffman et al. (eds.), *Major Complications of Female Pelvic Surgery*,
https://doi.org/10.1007/978-3-031-66772-5_34

sary vascular instruments can be made available. Blood loss should be quantified by both visual inspection and objective methods including using graduated suction canisters or weighing saturated laparotomy pads.

Management

When a small defect in a vein or artery is encountered, primary repair is typically performed. Vascular repair is described in Chap. 39.

Small vessel bleeding and/or low pressure, low volume (i.e., venous) bleeding can usually be controlled with pressure or hemostatic agents (see below, 'Post-operative bleeding/hematoma: prevention'). However, these methods may be insufficient for the control of pelvic hemorrhage from the presacral venous plexus. In these cases, pelvic packing with re-operation for removal in 24–48 hours, metallic tacks with or without hemostatic agents, or an overlay autogenous tissue patch may be necessary [1].

Post-Operative Bleeding/ Hematoma

Background

Post-operative hemorrhage or hematomas are usually the result of bleeding from pedicles or small vessel branches.

Prevention

Hemostasis must be ensured before the closure of the abdomen. A systematic approach to checking all pedicles and pelvic spaces for hemostasis is critical, and having a checklist can avoid omitting this step late in a tiring case. Irrigating the pelvis with sterile water can be helpful in identifying individual bleeding vessels before closure. For minimally invasive surgeries with diffuse dissection, evaluating for hemostasis after lowering the intraperitoneal pressure to 5 mm can unmask small bleeders tamponaded by the elevated intraperitoneal pressures. Topical hemostatic agents (i.e. oxidized regenerated cellulose, microfibrillar collagen, gelatin matrix, or thrombin agents) can be used to obtain hemostasis at the site of diffuse low-volume, low-pressure bleeding when cautery, surgical clips, or suture ligation is not safe or effective; however, these agents have not been shown to lower the rate of post-operative bleeding, transfusion, or return to the operating room and are not recommended for routine prophylaxis of post-operative bleeding, as they are associated with higher cost and possible increased risk of infection and adhesion formation [2].

Recognition

Early recognition of post-operative bleeding allows for appropriate resuscitation and immediate return to the operating room when necessary. Low to no urine output is typically the first sign of intra-abdominal bleeding, and tachycardia and hypotension will follow if bleeding continues, though cardiovascular changes are subtle until 25% of the circulating volume is lost. Anecdotally, symptomatic bleeding within 6 hours of surgery typically requires return to the operating room, while bleeding recognized 12 or more hours post-operatively can often be managed with supportive care and blood transfusion as necessary, since tamponade or coagulation will typically occur within this time frame.

Delayed, low-pressure bleeding typically presents as a pelvic hematoma. Many hematomas are asymptomatic but can present with pelvic or abdominal pain, malaise, nausea/vomiting, low-grade fever, leukocytosis, or vaginal bleeding, as the hematoma liquifies and drains through the vaginal incision. A pelvic hematoma can also become infected and present as an abscess (see below).

Management

When active bleeding with hemorrhagic shock occurs within 6–12 hours post-operatively, re-operation is usually necessary to identify and ligate a bleeding vessel. Coagulation status should be immediately checked and corrected if grossly abnormal. Re-operation on a patient who is in fulminant disseminated intravascular coagulopathy (DIC) is likely to be fruitless, and correction itself may stop bleeding for some patients. When bleeding is noted later in the post-operative period, it can usually be managed with supportive care including blood transfusion and fluid resuscitation. Resulting hematomas can be symptomatic but will resolve over time. Rarely, re-operation is necessary to evacuate a very large or symptomatic hematoma.

Hematomas can become secondarily infected and present as a post-operative abscess. In those cases, computed tomography (CT) or ultrasound-guided drain placement is usually adequate for source control with short-term intravenous or oral antibiotics.

Urinary Tract Injury

Background

The bladder peritoneum is frequently involved in ovarian cancer, and stripping of the bladder peritoneum may be required for complete gross resection. Invasion into the bladder mucosa is rare, but bladder injury can occur when tumor nodules invade into the bladder serosa or muscularis when anatomy is distorted, or due to inadvertent thermal injury. This dissection can be difficult in cases of prior hysterectomy or cesarean delivery.

Ureteral injury is another complication of pelvic surgery that carries significant consequences, due to the need for re-operation in the case of delayed or unrecognized injury or risk of ureteral stricture even when repaired intra-operatively. The pelvic ureters are frequently adherent to fixed ovarian masses or involved peritoneum, and ureterolysis is usually necessary.

Prevention

Prevention of bladder injury during composite pelvic resection begins with knowledge of anatomy, appropriate development of the paravesical spaces and vesicouterine space, and inspection of the bladder prior to closure. Instillation of normal saline (with or without indigo carmine, methylene blue, or sterile milk) can distend the bladder during dissection to better delineate the bladder contour.

Identification and isolation of bilateral ureters is an important step during composite pelvic resection for ovarian cancer, and most injuries can be prevented in this manner. However, this is difficult with bulky pelvic disease, prior radiation, or prior pelvic/retroperitoneal surgery including prior lymphadenectomy. Pre-operative ureteral stent placement (conventional stents with or without intraureteral indocyanine green (ICG) or lighted ureteral stents) has been proposed to reduce ureteral injury during complex pelvic surgery, and they can be particularly useful in cases where previous retroperitoneal surgery and fibrosis has occurred. No randomized data exist to support this practice, but single institutions have reported no ureteral injuries in small series when ureteral stenting is performed prior ovarian cancer debulking and/or colorectal resections [3–5].

Recognition

Urinary tract injuries may be recognized intra-operatively by direct visualization of an injury or during inspection of the bladder or ureters prior to closure. Urine or bladder mucosa noted in the surgical field, air in the catheter bag, or persistent hematuria may also alert the surgeon to a possible injury, though transient blood in the urine is common during ureterolysis or bladder manipulation. Sterile water, diluted methylene blue, or sterile milk can also be instilled via the Foley catheter to fill the bladder to uncover occult injuries and leaks. Partial thickness injuries including serosal or muscularis defects are also more easily recognized with this technique.

Some surgeons perform routine cystoscopy after composite pelvic resection to confirm integrity of the bladder and patency of bilateral ureters. Indigo carmine, methylene blue, or sodium fluorescein can be injected intravenously for improved visualization of ureteral efflux during cystoscopy and to inspect the ureters for leaks in the pelvis. Oral phenazopyridine can also be given pre-operatively if cystoscopy is planned. While the efficacy of cystoscopy to prevent delayed ureteral or bladder injury in composite pelvic resection has not been studied, routine cystoscopy after hysterectomy increases the intra-operative detection of urinary tract injury but does not decrease the rate of delayed urinary tract injuries in most studies. This is likely due to the low rate of urinary tract injuries, the detection of clinically insignificant injuries, and the large sample size that would be required to detect a difference in the post-operative injury rate [6]. Cystoscopy is probably less useful in composite pelvic resection compared to simple hysterectomy since the ureters are dissected nearly to their insertions into the bladder. We reserve cystoscopy for cases where there is concern for occult urinary tract injury that is unable to be visualized abdominally.

In cases of unrecognized urinary tract injury, thermal injury, or failed repairs, patients may present with ileus, malaise, fever, nausea/vomiting, or flank pain. Intraperitoneal urine leakage will also transiently raise the serum creatinine. Symptoms may be vague and will depend on the nature of the injury. Computed tomography (CT) scan is typically performed in the post-operative setting, but renal ultrasound could also identify a urinoma, hydronephrosis, or free fluid in the pelvis. A CT urogram or cystogram can identify the site of a urinary leak or confirm a urinoma vs. seroma. Paracentesis fluid or aspirate from a suspected urinoma can be tested for creatinine level to confirm a urinary source.

Management

When bladder injuries are diagnosed intra-operatively, primary repair should be performed. When cystotomy is performed with cautery, cold scissors should be used to resect the cauterized edges and ensure healthy tissue is reapproximated during the repair. Injuries at the bladder dome are easily repaired and heal quickly. Injuries in the bladder trigone may be close to one or both ureters, so care must be taken to avoid compromising the ureteral orifice(s). The bladder is reapproximated in two layers using an absorbable synthetic suture. A catheter should be maintained for 3–14 days depending on the size and location of the defect. The catheter can be removed relatively quickly for small injuries at the bladder dome and should be maintained longer for trigone injuries. Cystogram can be considered for cases with prior radiation and trigone injuries. If the injury is involving the trigone, a ureteral stent may be useful. The stent can be placed through the cystotomy during abdominal surgery or can be placed cystoscopically if necessary. The stent can typically be removed in 4–6 weeks. However, injuries close to the trigone may require ureteral reimplantation if the transmural portion of the ureter is impacted.

Post-operative bladder injuries including small fistulas may resolve spontaneously with Foley decompression in patients without prior pelvic radiation, but larger injuries require repeat operation for repair. Immediate repair is typically performed for larger lesions or those involving the trigone.

Repair of ureteral injuries is addressed in Chap. 17. Many delayed ureteral injuries can be managed with ureteral stent placement when a small injury or incomplete transection occurs. The ureteral stent is usually placed cystoscopically and can be removed in 6–12 weeks. If stent placement fails to control a ureteral leak, surgical repair is necessary. Immediate surgical repair can usually be performed, but if abscess, adhesions, or urinary tract infections co-exist with the injury, delayed repair may be required. A nephrostomy tube can be placed in the interim.

Urinomas may also occur after small bladder or ureteral injuries. Urinomas can also become infected, so antibiotic therapy may be necessary. Small, asymptomatic urinomas may resolve without intervention, but large or infected urinomas require drainage. CT or ultrasound-guided drainage catheter placement can be performed with or without ureteral stent placement. A nephrostomy tube can also be used in refractory cases.

Anastomotic Leak

Background

Anastomotic leak is the largest contributor to severe morbidity and prolonged hospitalization after pelvic surgery for ovarian cancer [7]. Multiple patient and procedural factors have been associated with increased risk of anastomotic leak including serum albumin <3 g/dL, prior pelvic radiation, and ultra-low anastomoses (≤6 cm from the anal verge) [8, 9].

Prevention

The consequences associated with anastomotic leak can be mitigated with a diverting ostomy, particularly in high-risk patients. In a study by the Mayo Clinic, the use of diverting loop ileostomy in patients with risk factors for leak (i.e., serum albumin <3 g/dL, prior pelvic radiation, anastomosis ≤6 cm from the anal verge, additional large bowel resections, failed leak test, or gross stool contamination) reduced the rate of clinical anastomotic leak from 7.8% to 1.3% [9]. Appropriate use of diverting ileostomy or colostomy is important to decrease the rate of anastomotic leaks while avoiding the morbidity of ostomies (repeat surgery for reversal, high output ileostomy, etc.) when not necessary.

While patient and procedural factors are important predictors of anastomotic leak, the most common preventable causes of this complication are technical, specifically compromised perfusion of and/or undue tension on the anastomosis. Historically, techniques to assess blood supply to distal and proximal limbs of an anastomosis have included transillumination of the mesentery to identify feeding vessels, visual inspection of the anastomosis, and doppler ultrasound assessment. Indocyanine green (ICG)-enhanced fluorescence angiography has emerged as an effective and reproducible method of assessing perfusion of anastomoses. In this method, 25 mg of ICG (Eisai, Tokyo, JP) is diluted in 10 mL of sterile water (2.5 mg/mL), and 1–3 mL is injected intravenously followed by a 10 mL normal saline flush. Near-infrared fluorescence imaging is used to immediately visualize perfusion to the anastomosis (Fig. 34.1). Randomized data have shown this technique can alter the planned points of resection/anastomosis but have not demonstrated reduced anastomotic

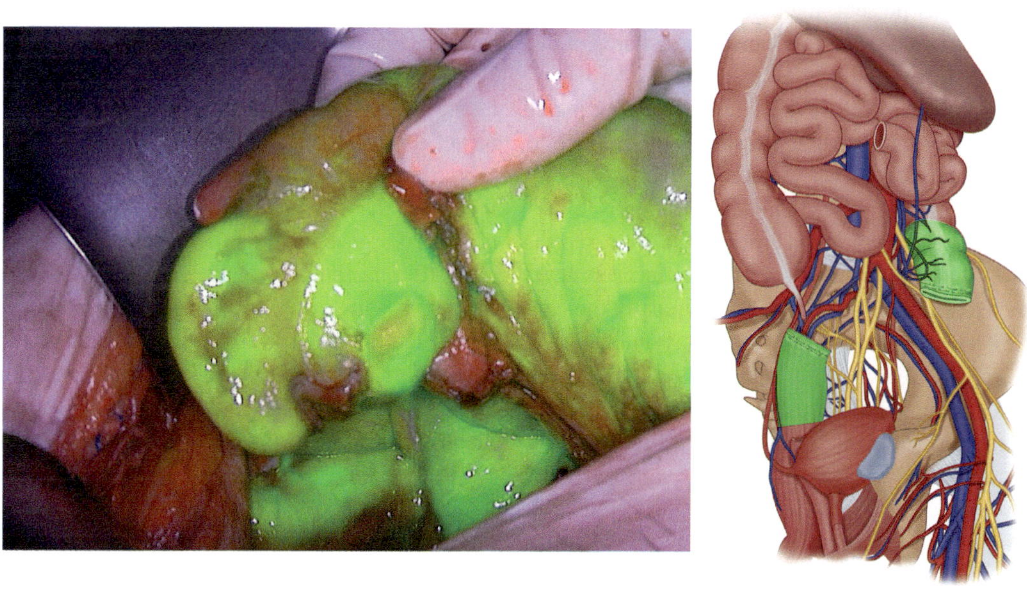

Fig. 34.1 Indocyanine green fluorescence angiography is used to visualize perfusion to the rectosigmoid anastomosis

leaks; however multiple high-volume centers have incorporated this method to assess anastomoses in ovarian cancer surgery and we feel it is a useful adjunct to clinical judgment to assess vascular supply [10–12].

Common ways to reduce tension on the pelvic anastomosis include mobilization of the splenic flexure and division of the inferior mesenteric vein. Further mobilization can be gained by dividing the inferior mesenteric artery while preserving the very proximal origin of the left colic vessel. Surgeons should be cautious in this approach if the middle colic artery has been ligated.

Recognition

Technical failure of a rectosigmoid anastomosis can be recognized intra-operatively with a variety of methods: ensuring two complete rings after completion of a stapled circular anastomosis, proctoscopy, visual inspection, and ICG angiography. A leak test can be performed using a rigid proctoscope to introduce air into the distal rectum while the proximal sigmoid is occluded manually, and the anastomosis is submerged in sterile water or saline to confirm an airtight seal. If a leak is present, the continuous stream of air bubbles can be used to locate the exact area of the defect. Care should be taken to avoid overdistention of the rectum, as this could disrupt an intact anastomosis if the burst pressure of the staple line is exceeded.

In cases of anastomotic leak, early post-operative recognition is crucial to prevent sepsis, end-organ injury, and death. Low urine output, tachycardia, and tachypnea are typically the earliest signs of bowel injury or anastomotic leak. Fever, nausea/vomiting, ileus, hypotension, elevated serum lactate, and acute kidney injury are common late signs. Feculent discharge from the wound is a very late and obvious sign. CT scan should be employed early if anastomotic leak is suspected as plain films of the abdomen are non-specific in the early post-operative period. While (non-barium) oral contrast will usually identify a more proximal bowel injury it may miss more distal leaks. Gentle instillation of rectal contrast may be required to locate a rectosigmoid anastomotic leak or distal bowel injury but should be done with caution. For patients with signs of peritonitis or sepsis, return to the operating room should not be delayed for advanced imaging.

A pelvic abscess can also occur as the result of a small, contained anastomotic leak or microperforation of the colon or small bowel. Pelvic abscesses typically present with nausea, vomiting, pelvic or abdominal pain, malaise, ileus, or fever.

Management

When anastomotic leak is diagnosed post-operatively, management depends on the location of the defect, the nature of the leak (contained vs. free intraperitoneal contents), and the stability of the patient. A subclinical anastomotic leak (small, asymptomatic abscess diagnosed on imaging) can be managed expectantly. A small (<3 cm abscess) contained anastomotic leak in an otherwise stable patient can be managed with bowel rest and systemic antibiotics, while a larger (>3 cm abscess) contained leak can be managed with antibiotics and percutaneous drain placement. An intraperitoneal leak, either an anastomotic leak, that is not contained (i.e., free intraperitoneal air on cross-sectional imaging or plain film), requires re-operation [13]. A laparotomy should be performed to locate the site of the defect. In cases of small bowel injury or anastomotic leak, small bowel resection and reanastomosis can usually be performed if the surrounding tissues are otherwise healthy. Large bowel injuries, including rectosigmoid anastomotic leaks, typically require diversion with either ileostomy or colostomy performed proximal to the defect, though simultaneous repair or revision of the anastomosis can be performed in some cases (Fig. 34.2). When diversion is performed, management of the anastomosis or injury depends on multiple factors, including the stability of the patient and the condition of the surrounding tissues. It may include oversewing or repair of the anastomosis if possible, and an abdominal washout should be performed. Post-operative antibiotics are typically continued for 5–14 days. CT with oral and rectal

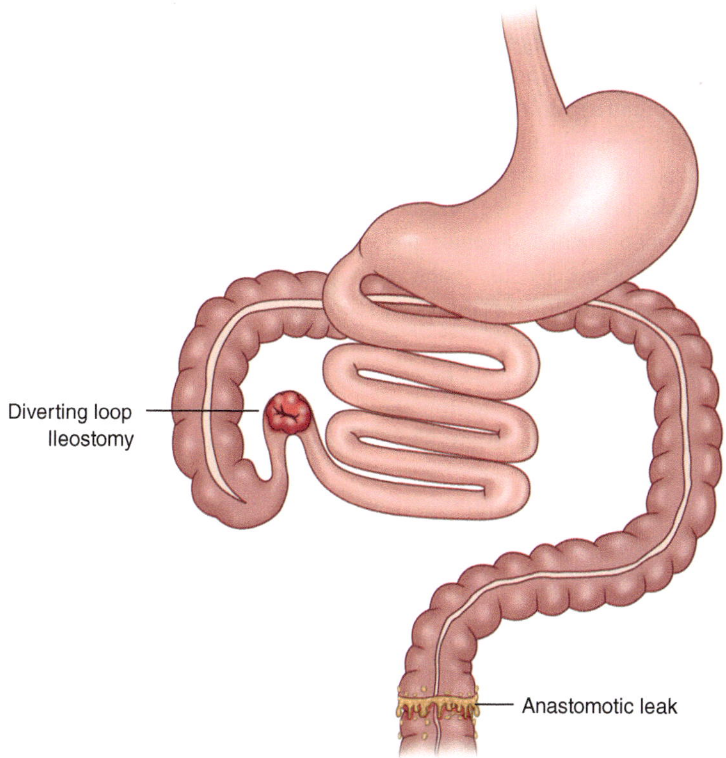

Fig. 34.2 Fecal diversion for post-operative anastomotic leak

contrast should be performed prior to ostomy reversal to ensure no persistent leaks or strictures. Reversal is usually performed about 12 weeks after the initial injury if adequate nutrition and performance status have been re-established.

In some cases, intra-abdominal adhesions or a "frozen abdomen" render the usual diversion and/or repair impossible. Damage control methods including temporary abdominal closure, open abdomen negative pressure therapy, or delayed abdominal closure may be necessary. Collaboration with a colorectal or trauma surgeon is often helpful in these cases.

Bowel Injury

Background

Bowel injury can occur during composite pelvic resection when the colon or small bowel is adherent to or invaded by a bulky pelvic mass or when the serosa or mesentery is involved by miliary disease.

Prevention

Prevention of bowel injury begins with careful tissue handling and sharp rather than cautery or blunt dissection in proximity to the bowel wall. Thermal injuries are especially dangerous since the initial injury may be unrecognized, or its extent minimized, and thus present several days to a week post-operatively. A rectal probe or proctoscopy with insufflation to distend the colon during dissection can better delineate the bowel wall. Inspection of the entire large and small bowel should be performed in order to identify and repair any injuries prior to closure. A systematic approach to examining the bowel can avoid unrecognized injuries.

Recognition

Careful inspection of both the small and large bowel should be performed to rule out inadvertent serosal injuries, colotomies or enterotomies, or thermal injuries. While anastomotic leaks are most feared, it is important to remember that enteric leaks in the absence of bowel resection are a common source of major post-operative morbidity. Proctoscopy to distend the pelvic colon with air can also be useful to recognize occult injuries.

A delayed or unrecognized bowel injury will present similarly to an anastomotic leak, as described above ("Anastomotic leak: recognition").

Management

When bowel injury is noted intra-operatively, primary repair can be performed for small defects. The bowel is typically repaired in two layers, using a running, delayed absorbable suture to reapproximate the mucosa and permanent (silk) Lambert sutures to reapproximate the serosa. The defect should be repaired in a transverse fashion in order to prevent the narrowing of the bowel lumen. Larger defects, thermal injuries or those involving the mesentery of the small or large bowel typically require resection of the damaged segment. Primary anastomosis can be performed in most cases.

Delayed bowel injuries are managed similarly to anastomotic leaks, as described above ('Anastomotic leak: Recognition').

Anastomotic Bleeding

Background

Anastomotic bleeding (often mucosal) after low anterior resection is rare but can result in significant blood loss and/or contribute to failure of the anastomosis.

Prevention

There are no well-established methods for the prevention of anastomotic bleeding. Intra-operative proctoscopy can be used to ensure hemostasis at the anastomosis, but most bleeding is delayed. There is no high-quality evidence to suggest a lower risk of bleeding with hand-sewn or stapled anastomoses.

Recognition

Anastomotic bleeding presents as hematochezia or passage of blood and clots per rectum. This usually occurs within 24–48 hours post-operatively. Given the distal location of the recto-sigmoid anastomosis, the bleeding is typically immediately apparent.

Management

Bleeding from the rectosigmoid anastomosis following composite pelvic resection for ovarian cancer can typically be managed expectantly. Some patients may require transfusion, and anti-coagulation should be held until hemostasis is ensured. If bleeding continues despite conservative measures, colonoscopic clipping or fulguration should be attempted. Re-operation and revision of the anastomosis is rarely required but can be necessary if endoscopic methods are not successful.

Anastomotic Stricture

Background

Anastomotic stricture is typically attributed to tissue ischemia, though the rate of stricture after composite pelvic resection for ovarian cancer is not well-defined. Risk factors for anastomotic stricture include obesity, anastomotic leak, smoking, and low or ultra-low anastomosis.

Prevention

Anastomotic stricture can result from ischemia, tension, or subclinical leaks/tissue remodeling. In addition to the maneuvers described above (see: "Anastomotic leak: prevention"), surgeons should avoid using circular staplers less than 25 mm in diameter: in cases of narrow diameter proximal colon stump an end-to-side anastomosis should be used to avoid this.

Recognition

Anastomotic strictures typically present weeks to months after surgery and should be recognized on imaging when patients present with obstructive symptoms, pain, and/or incontinence.

Management

Anastomotic stricture after rectosigmoid resection typically presents weeks to months after surgery with symptoms of complete or partial obstruction. Low anastomotic strictures can be dilated digitally or with flexible dilators. More proximal strictures can be dilated with endoscopic balloon dilation or stenting. Re-operation for revision of an anastomosis is required in rare cases, and permanent diversion can be performed if symptoms persist and revision is not possible.

References

1. Hammond IG, et al. The control of severe intraoperative bleeding using an overlay autogenous tissue (OAT) patch: case reports. Gynecol Oncol. 2004;94(2):564–6.
2. American College of Obstetricians and Gynecologists' Committee on Gynecologic Practice. Topical hemostatic agents at time of obstetric and gynecologic surgery: ACOG committee opinion, number 812. Obstet Gynecol. 2020;136(4):e81–9.
3. White LA, Joseph JP, Yang DY, Kelley SR, Mathis KL, Behm K, Viers BR. Intraureteral indocyanine green augments ureteral identification and avoidance during complex robotic-assisted colorectal surgery. Color Dis. 2021;23(3):718–23.
4. Boyan WP Jr, Lavy D, Dinallo A, Otero J, Roding A, Hanos D, Dressner R, Arvanitis M. Lighted ureteral stents in laparoscopic colorectal surgery; a five-year experience. Ann Transl Med. 2017;5(3):44.
5. Abu-Zaid A, Abou Al-Shaar H, Azzam A, Alomar O, Al-Otaibi MF, Amin T, Al-Badawi IA. Routine ureteric stenting before cytoreductive surgery plus hyperthermic intraperitoneal chemotherapy in managing peritoneal carcinomatosis from gynecologic malignancies: a single-center experience. Ir J Med Sci. 2017;186(2):269–73.
6. Teeluckdharry B, et al. Urinary tract injury at benign gynecologic surgery and the role of cystoscopy: a systematic review and meta-analysis. Obstet Gynecol. 2015;126(6):1161.
7. Narasimhulu DM, Bews KA, Hanson KT, Chang YH, Dowdy SC, Cliby WA. Using evidence to direct quality improvement efforts: defining the highest impact complications after complex cytoreductive surgery for ovarian cancer. Gynecol Oncol. 2020;156(2):278–83.
8. Richardson DL, Mariani A, Cliby WA. Risk factors for anastomotic leak after recto-sigmoid resection for ovarian cancer. Gynecol Oncol. 2006;103(2):667–72.
9. Kalogera E, Nitschmann CC, Dowdy SC, Cliby WA, Langstraat CL. A prospective algorithm to reduce anastomotic leaks after rectosigmoid resection for gynecologic malignancies. Gynecol Oncol. 2017;144(2):343–7.
10. Liu D, Liang L, Liu L, Zhu Z. Does intraoperative indocyanine green fluorescence angiography decrease the incidence of anastomotic leakage in colorectal surgery? A systematic review and meta-analysis. Int J Color Dis. 2021;36(1):57–66.
11. Pang HY, Chen XL, Song XH, Galiullin D, Zhao LY, Liu K, Zhang WH, Yang K, Chen XZ, Hu JK. Indocyanine green fluorescence angiography prevents anastomotic leakage in rectal cancer surgery: a systematic review and meta-analysis. Langenbeck's Arch Surg. 2021;406(2):261–71.
12. De Nardi P, Elmore U, Maggi G, Maggiore R, Boni L, Cassinotti E, Fumagalli U, Gardani M, De Pascale S, Parise P, Vignali A, Rosati R. Intraoperative angiography with indocyanine green to assess anastomosis perfusion in patients undergoing laparoscopic colorectal resection: results of a multicenter randomized controlled trial. Surg Endosc. 2020;34(1):53–60.
13. Phitayakorn R, Delaney CP, Reynolds HL, et al. Standardized algorithms for management of anastomotic leaks and related abdominal and pelvic abscesses after colorectal surgery. World J Surg. 2008;32:1147–56.

Anal Cancer

35

Anne Macleod and Susan Galandiuk

Introduction

First described in 1974, the Nigro protocol using definitive chemoradiotherapy (CRT) is the primary treatment for most cases of anal squamous cell carcinoma (SCC), which encompasses >90% of anal cancers [1, 2]. Surgery is indicated for the treatment of (i) perianal cancers without sphincter involvement (local excision), (ii) patients with persistent or recurrent disease following initial chemoradiation therapy (salvage surgery), (iii) complications of primary disease, and (iv) complications resulting from chemoradiation therapy (CRT).

This chapter will focus primarily on the management of complications of radical surgery performed for progressive disease including, (i) perineal wound complications; (ii) pelvic fluid collections/abscess/organ space infection; (iii) perineal hernia, and (iv) small bowel obstruction as well as those secondary to primary disease and chemoradiation therapy. Complications of primary disease and nonoperative therapy discussed include large bowel obstruction; fecal incontinence; rectovaginal and anorectal fistulae; sigmoid and ureteral stricture formation and radiation enteritis.

Complications of Local Excision

Local excision for anal squamous cell cancer is indicated in T1N0, well-differentiated peri-anal cancer [3, 4] as well as superficial anal cancer that has been completely excised (T1NX <3 mm deep and < 7 mm horizontal spread) (Fig. 35.1). These are often completely excised at biopsy, and local resection with negative margins may be sufficient [3, 5] (Fig. 35.2). Complications of local excision are uncommon; if healing problems occur, most wounds will heal by secondary intention.

A. Macleod
Price Institute of Surgical Research, University of Louisville, Louisville, KY, USA

S. Galandiuk (✉)
Division of Colon & Rectal Surgery, Hiram C Polk Jr., MD Department of Surgery, University of Louisville, Louisville, KY, USA
e-mail: s0gala01@louisville.edu

M. Hoffman et al. (eds.), *Major Complications of Female Pelvic Surgery*,
https://doi.org/10.1007/978-3-031-66772-5_35

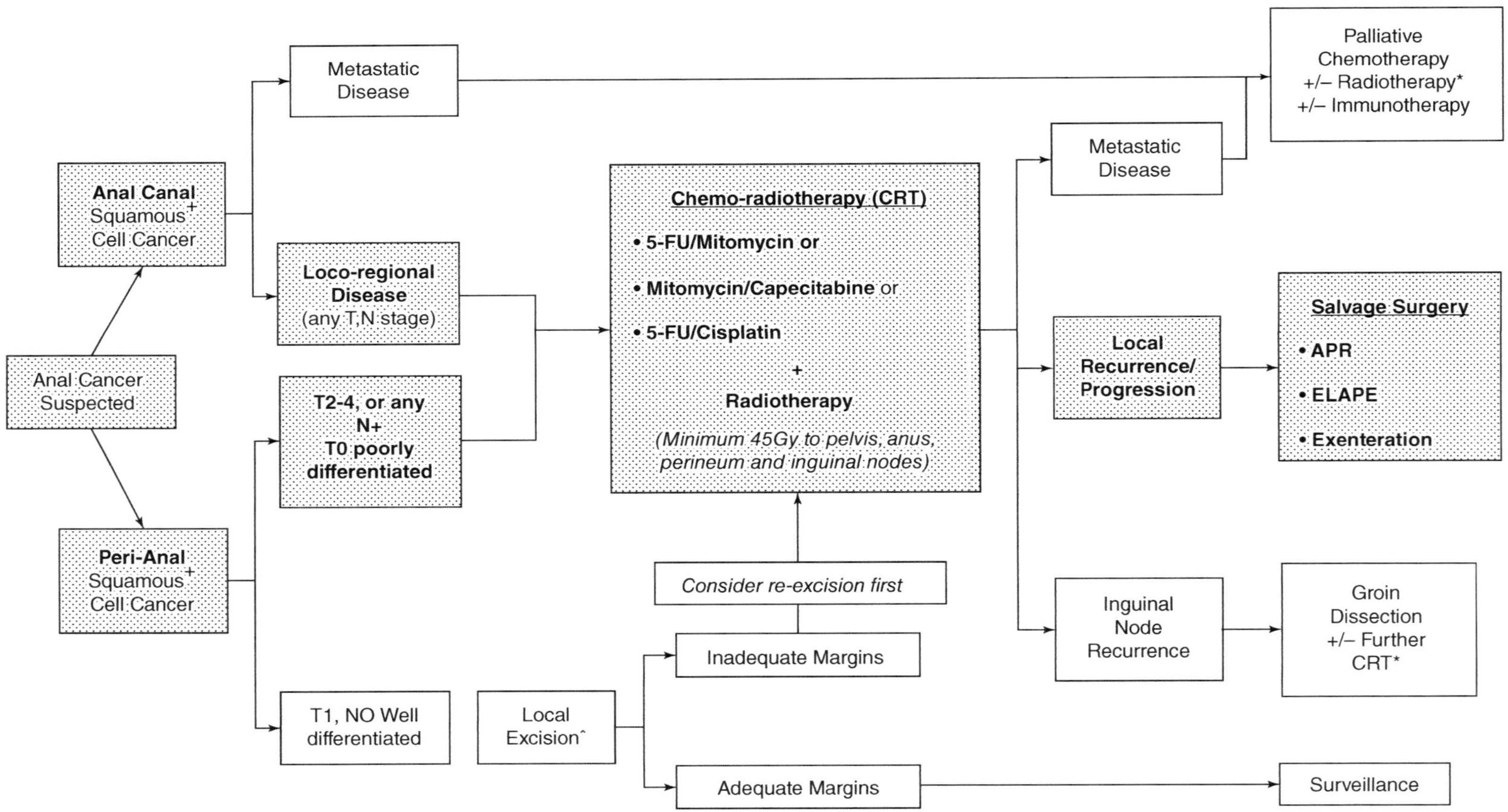

Fig. 35.1 Treatment algorithm following anal SCC diagnosis: Adapted from (3). +Anal adenocarcinoma and melanoma histology- use alternative treatment algorithm. ^Local excision: 1 cm margin recommended. Local excision also recommended in T1Nx superficial cancer completely excised at biopsy; *Additional CRT/radiotherapy depending on prior dose/field included. *APR* Abdominal-erineal resection, *ELAPE* extra-levator abdominal-perineal resection

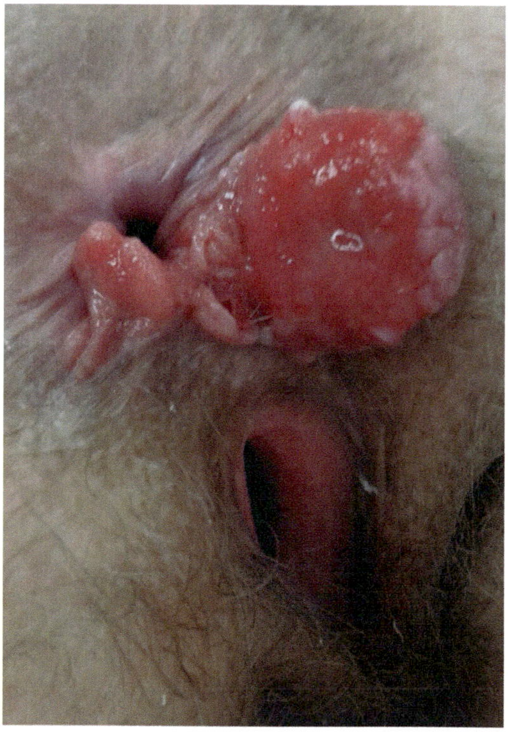

Fig. 35.2 Perianal cancer without sphincter involvement

Complications of Radical Surgery Performed for Persistent or Recurrent Disease

Major pelvic surgery is reserved for locally progressive or recurrent disease, occurring in 10–30% of anal SCC cases [6, 7]. Patients who are HIV positive, those with advanced T or N stage, and incomplete CRT therapy have an increased risk of recurrence and requiring subsequent radical surgery [8, 9]. A conventional APR or ELAPE (if there is an extension beyond the sphincters to the levators) are the most common salvage surgeries performed for anal SCC. The aims of salvage surgery are local disease control and prevention of distant recurrence. Positive resection margins are a reliable predictor of recurrence and poor survival; therefore, en-bloc resection of involved adjacent organs to achieve negative surgical margins may be required [10]. The reader is referred to Chap. 38 "Exenteration" for details specific to pelvic exenteration, which may be required with disease extending to involve the bladder or in cases of severe radiation damage/radiation necrosis.

Due to the high dose of radiation utilized for the primary treatment of anal SCC, healing problems are not uncommon in the postoperative period (see also Chap. 37, Pelvic Radiation Therapy). Added risk factors include malnutrition and the presence of cigarette smoking, which can also lead to impaired wound healing. The latter has been linked to higher HPV16 viral levels [11]. Common complications include perineal wound infection/dehiscence, pelvic fluid collections/abscesses/organ space infections, perineal hernia, and small bowel obstruction. These will be discussed below.

Perineal Wound Infection/Dehiscence

Background

Impaired perineal wound healing is a major source of morbidity following pelvic surgery. APR for anal cancer generally follows the same technique principles as for rectal cancer (see Chap. 36); however, wider perineal margins or an extra-levator (ELAPE) approach may be required. A larger perineal wound in combination with higher doses of perineal radiation may result in an increased risk of wound infection and poor healing [12, 13]. The incidence of wound dehiscence or infection following primary closure varies but has been reported in 15–70% of cases following APR or ELAPE [7, 12, 14].

Prevention

The use of reconstructive muscle or myocutaneous flaps for perineal closure has led to reduced rates and severity of perineal wound complications [15] (see also Chap. 41, Pelvic Reconstructive Procedures). A myocutaneous flap using rectus abdominis (VRAM), gluteal, or gracilis muscle are the most widely reported techniques (Fig. 35.3). Reconstructive flaps aid with wound closure and contribute to reduced wound infections by filling the dead space within the pelvis. A 2016 meta-analysis of primary versus flap closure included 10 studies and 566 patients. Eight studies used rectus abdominis

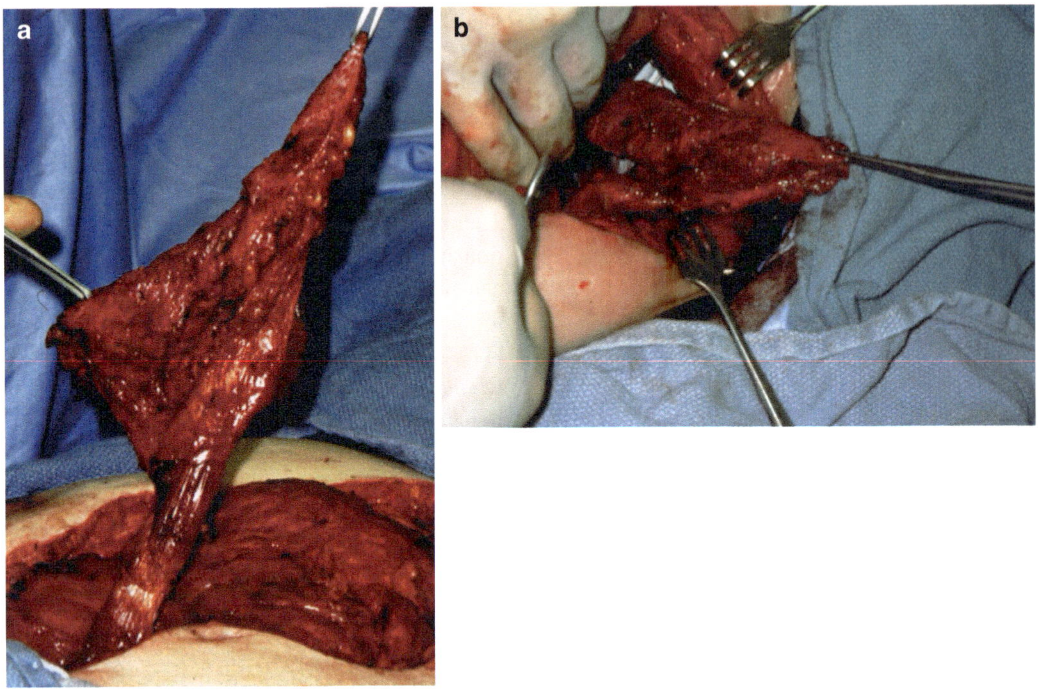

Fig. 35.3 (**a**) Rectus muscle flap harvested to help fill a pelvis and (**b**) following abdominoperineal resection

flaps and two used gracilis flaps. Overall major wound complications were higher in the primary closure groups [16]. In 98 patients undergoing salvage surgery for anal cancer, Baloch et al. reported significantly higher perineal wound healing at 3 months following perineal reconstruction using a vertical rectus abdominis (VRAM) flap, versus primary closure or gluteal flap [17]. A small RCT comparing biologic mesh versus primary closure following ELAPE for rectal cancer found no difference in wound healing at all time intervals measured [18]. Despite many retrospective studies and systematic reviews, the heterogeneity of indication for surgery along with selection bias and confounding patient factors, has resulted in a lack of consensus regarding optimal perineal closure technique [13, 19].

Modifiable risk factors associated with poor wound healing preoperatively should be addressed where possible, including preoperative smoking cessation, optimizing nutrition, and diabetic control [13].

Recognition

Perineal wound dehiscence or poor healing presents similarly to wound complications elsewhere, however, due to the location of the wound, it is at risk of being missed in the early postoperative period. Careful monitoring is crucial to identify early signs of complications such as inflammation, discharge, necrosis, or swelling, which may indicate a nonhealing wound or flap failure. Identification of the depth and extent of dehiscence guides the appropriate management and will be dependent on the perineal reconstruction technique at primary surgery.

Management

Acute

Full-thickness dehiscence with evisceration or flap loss are surgical emergencies and require an immediate return to the operating room for debridement and re-closure. Careful inspection of small bowel and mesentery for evidence of trauma should be performed prior to washout and re-closure [13].

Incomplete dehiscence with evidence of perineal infection should be managed with intravenous antibiotics, local exploration, and debridement of any nonviable tissue. CT scan evaluation for deeper pelvic collections or tracts should be performed and managed as per the section on pelvic fluid collections below.

Chronic

A chronic nonhealing wound of >6 months duration is defined as a persistent perineal sinus. Recurrent or residual cancer should be considered in any persistent wound/sinus and an examination under anesthesia performed with biopsies of suspicious areas along with exploring +/− deroofing tracts. MRI is useful in assessing for recurrence or undrained fluid collections. Definitive management is guided by the size of the wound and the involvement of surrounding structures. This can range from conservative local excision and debridement with the use of negative pressure dressings to extensive surgery involving coccygectomy or sacral body resection with muscle flap transposition. Negative pressure or vacuum-assisted closure (VAC) dressings are known to accelerate open wound healing via reduction of edema, mechanically drawing together wound edges, increasing local perfusion, and promoting the formation of granulation tissue [22, 23]. Although positionally more difficult to maintain a vacuum seal, these can be used for open perineal wounds with favorable outcomes. Alternative nonsurgical adjuncts, such as topical application of growth factors and mesenchymal stem cell treatments, are being explored in other chronic wounds, such as diabetic ulcers, and may in the future offer an alternative treatment option in perineal wound management [20, 21].

Pelvic Fluid Collections/Abscesses/Organ Space Infections

Background

Pelvic fluid collections following anorectal excision often result from the accumulation of exudative fluid or hematoma in the pelvic dead space. More extensive excisions such as in ELAPE and pelvic exenteration have increased dead space and are higher risk for organ space infection [13] (Fig. 35.4).

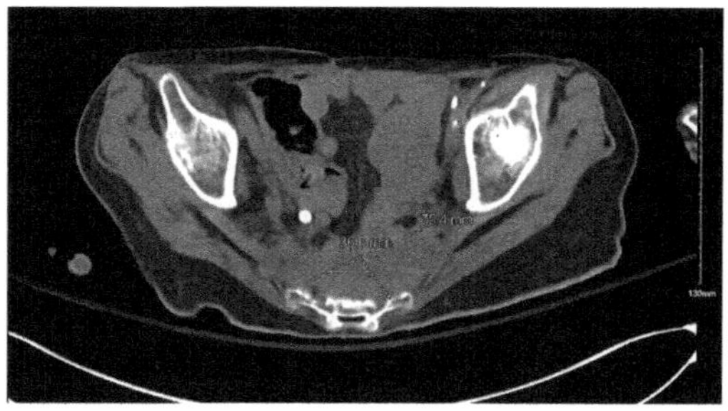

Fig. 35.4 Large infected presacral fluid collection in a woman 10 days following pelvic exenteration for complications due to radiation therapy for anal squamous cell cancer

Prevention

Filling or excluding the empty pelvic space has been shown to improve perineal wound healing and reduce both pelvic fluid collection/abscess formation and perineal hernia rates along with keeping small bowel out of the pelvis. Several techniques for pelvic exclusion have been described, including omentoplasty, mesh or flap reconstruction, prosthesis placement, and the use of terminal ileal mesentery to reconstruct the pelvic peritoneum [24–26].

The use of an omental flap to obliterate the pelvic dead space has been reported in several case series and retrospective studies with contradictory results. The largest recent cohort study examining the benefit of omentoplasty after APR/ELAPE for rectal cancer included a cohort of 477 patients (of which 96% received neoadjuvant CRT) who were found to have no benefit from the omentoplasty + primary closure versus primary closure alone. Thirty-day nonhealing rates, chronic perineal wounds, and presacral abscess formation were similar [26]. These findings were supported by a 2021 systematic review in which omentoplasty was not associated with risk of pelvic abscess formation, wound healing at 30 days, or chronic perineal sinus [27]. A 2022 systematic review of six different techniques for filling the empty pelvis following pelvic exenteration found no consensus on the best method of pelvic exclusion. Mesh reconstruction and breast prosthesis placement were associated with the lowest rates of small bowel obstruction and abscess formation. Flap reconstruction had similar outcomes, although higher rates of perineal wound morbidity and re-operation. Omentoplasty was associated with increased rates of wound infection and morbidity [28]. Some centers have trialed the use of obstetric balloons and silicone expanders, and while outcomes were promising in reported case series, there is insufficient evidence to compare to more traditional techniques.

Recognition

Patients develop pyrexia, leukocytosis often accompanied by abdominal pain, ileus, and a systemic inflammatory response. Perineal wound discharge may increase or become purulent. Imaging with a CT scan can delineate a collection and assess suitability for percutaneous drainage. Imaging <5 days postoperative is likely to show a degree of free pelvic fluid, which must be interpreted cautiously and in clinical context.

The finding of pelvic free fluid in an unwell patient following APR/ELAPE should prompt consideration of inadvertent injury to surrounding structures such as small bowel, bladder, or ureters. Renal function and urinary output should be assessed, a discussion of recognition and management of urinary tract complications can be found in Chap. 17 "Injury/Repair of Pelvic Ureter".

Management

Initial resuscitation and intravenous broad-spectrum antibiotics followed by percutaneous drainage is the primary management in most cases of pelvic abscess. CT-guided percutaneous drainage is the first-line treatment for most abdominal-pelvic collections greater than 3 cm and is successful in >90% of patients, with low complication rates [29, 30]. Following drain placement, regular drain flushing ensures drain patency. Upsizing or re-positing of the drains may be required. Patients should undergo repeat imaging prior to drain removal to evaluate collection resolution along with microbial culture of abscess contents to rationalize antibiotic choice.

Patients without access to interventional radiology or significant hemodynamic instability require a return to theatre for either laparoscopic or open surgical washout. Recurrent, multiloculated, or complex intra-loop abscesses may not respond to conservative management and may require surgical washout. In the case of very low-lying collections, these are sometimes most easily drained transperineally.

In the case of bilious drain output, communication of abscess cavity with small bowel is likely, and the patient should be managed as for an entero-cutaneous fistula. This is a rare complication of APR/ELAPE, although may occur due to a missed, or failed repair of, inadvertent enterotomy, particularly in patients with friable small bowel due to radiation enteritis. Detailed principles of fistula management are beyond the scope of this chapter; however, in brief, these include (i) control of infection, (ii) reduction of fistula output, (iii) optimization of nutrition, and (iv) imaging with oral contrast and/or fistulogram to assess anatomy prior to consideration of surgical repair. Most low output fistula will heal without surgical intervention.

Perineal Hernia

Background

Perineal hernia is a late, and relatively underappreciated, complication following APR/ELAPE. There are little data regarding the incidence and outcomes of treatment, with much evidence reported from expert opinions and small case series with short follow-ups. High-dose radiation along with an extra-levator resection increases the risk of perineal hernia. Many small or minimally symptomatic hernias likely go undiagnosed; however, the overall incidence has been reported in studies between 12–26% [31, 32]. The incidence of this complication appears to be increasing with the increase in minimally invasive surgical approach.

Prevention

Closure of a perineal defect with a reconstructive flap or mesh, and pelvic exclusion as described above for wound complication and pelvic abscess prevention, can also be used to reduce the frequency of perineal hernia. While not the primary aim of the study a prospective randomized controlled trial, comparing primary versus biologic mesh closure following ELAPE for rectal cancer found a significantly lower 1-year perineal hernia rate in the biologic mesh closure patients (13 vs. 27%) [18]. Conversely, a large Dutch observational study found the use of omentoplasty for pelvic space exclusion increased the rate of perineal hernia development [26]. Patients should be aware of modifiable risk factors preoperatively to reduce the risk of perineal hernia, including weight loss, careful postoperative wound care, and avoidance of strenuous daily activities postoperatively.

Recognition

The diagnosis of a perineal hernia is primarily clinical, with patients reporting a bulge or mass, often positional and associated with pain or discomfort. Complications associated with perineal hernia include skin erosion, urinary or sexual dysfunction, and bowel obstruction. CT or MRI imaging may be useful in supporting diagnosis, however, hernias that present on standing or straining may not be detected on imaging.

Management

Given the relative rarity of this complication, there is a lack of consensus on the optimal surgical approach (perineal vs. abdominal) or technique (primary closure, insertion of mesh, reconstructive flap, or combination) for repair. A recent meta-analysis of 29 studies included 325 patients undergoing 347 perineal hernia repairs and found an overall recurrence rate of 22% with no significant difference between the abdominal versus perineal approach. A combined approach was reported in five studies, and results appear to suggest a lower rate of recurrence; however, current evidence is not sufficient to confirm this. Mesh repairs have largely replaced primary repair in recent years; however, at meta-analysis, there was no significant risk difference identified between any repair techniques. Synthetic mesh had the lowest recurrence rate but the highest postoperative morbidity [33].

Small Bowel Obstruction

Background

There is an increased risk of small bowel obstruction (SBO) following surgery due to pre-operative high-dose chemoradiation in anal SCC. The terminal ileum is at particular risk of radiation enteritis (see section "Complications of Therapy (Chemoradiation)" later in this chapter) and is often the site of SBO (Fig. 35.5). Other causes of obstruction include surgical adhesions or small bowel adherent in the pelvis with associated radiation-induced fibrosis.

Prevention

Pelvic exclusion techniques, as described above, aim to keep small bowel out of the pelvis and reduce the risk of SBO, along with the risk of additional injury associated with further radiation. Closure of the pelvic peritoneum using the distal ileal mesentery was first described in

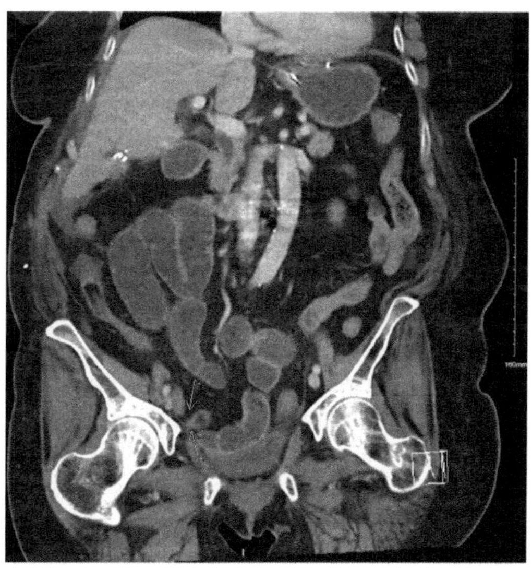

Fig. 35.5 Coronal CT scan showing severely narrowed small bowel (white arrows) due to radiation enteritis resulting in refractory small bowel obstruction

1996, with a recent case series published in 2022 of 10 patients following resection for rectal or gynecological cancer. The distal ileal mesentery is used to close peritoneal defect in a "fan-like" method suturing the mesentery to the peritoneum at the pelvic brim. In the most recent publication of this technique, success was noted by follow-up imaging reporting the absence of a small bowel within the pelvis. At follow-up ranging from 3–28 months, no postoperative perineal hernia or intestinal obstruction had occurred; however, 9/10 patients had no neoadjuvant radiotherapy. Due to the degree of fibrosis and tissue friability following chemoradiation in anal SCC, suturing to residual peritoneum may be difficult, so this technique *may* not be as successful [24, 25].

Recognition

Patients typically present with abdominal pain, distention, emesis, and inability to pass stool or flatus. In the immediate postoperative period, this is commonly secondary to ileus and can usually be managed conservatively. CT imaging can confirm obstruction and may aid in diagnosing the site and etiology of obstruction, while excluding any additional complications.

Management

Initial trial of conservative management with nasogastric tube (NGT) for decompression, fluid and electrolyte replacement, and a gastrograffin small bowel follow-through is first-line treatment provided no concern of bowel viability or perforation. In a stable patient, with suspected adhesional obstruction, a repeat small bowel follow-through following initial failure is reasonable and may resolve obstruction while avoiding surgery. Failure of conservative management warrants surgical intervention, the extent of which varies depending on the site, extent, and etiology of obstruction. Division of adhesions may be sufficient to resolve obstruction, but in the case of significant radiation-induced enteritis, small bowel resection or bypass (if there are prohibitive adhesions) may be required.

Complications of Primary Disease

Complications requiring surgery due to the primary disease itself include large bowel obstruction, fecal incontinence, and the development of rectovaginal or anorectal fistula. Fecal incontinence and development of fistula can also be a result of, or complicated by, chemoradiation therapy, which will be discussed later.

Large Bowel Obstruction

Background

Anal cancer may present as an acute or subacute large bowel obstruction (LBO), with progressive distention, pain, absolute constipation, and feculent vomiting. Large bowel obstruction may also develop in patients with known anal cancer, with poor response and tumor progression whilst undergoing chemoradiation.

Prevention

Patients undergoing chemoradiation therapy should be closely monitored and should be aware of symptoms suggestive of impending obstruction secondary to anal cancer. Patients with near-obstructing cancers either clinically or radiologically may benefit from placement of a diverting ostomy prior to chemoradiation to prevent complete obstruction and its associated complications.

Recognition

Patients with anal cancer with progressive obstructive symptoms should undergo abdominal and digital rectal examination, and CT imaging to evaluate for obstruction.

Management

Obstructing anal cancer should be managed with proximal diverting colostomy, ideally prior to initiation of chemoradiation. Patients presenting with large bowel obstruction as an emergency or during chemoradiation therapy have increased risk of infectious, cardiopulmonary and stoma complications. In the situation of a competent ileocecal valve, there is an added risk of cecal compromise, and the patient may require colectomy. In addition to immediate complications, there is an increased risk of recurrence or primary disease progression due to a treatment break during therapy or being unable to complete chemoradiation.

Fecal Incontinence

Background

Fecal urgency or incontinence is common in patients following radiation treatment for pelvic malignancies. A Danish study of 380 patients found that 95% of patients had fecal urgency; 59% were incontinent to liquid and 33% to solid stool following treatment with pelvic radiation [34]. Fecal incontinence due to anal cancer may develop secondary to tumor invasion into sphincter complex; the residual defect following destruction of tumor with chemoradiation, as well as due to radiation-induced injury and fibrosis. Incontinence can be further exacerbated by radiation-induced proctitis/enteritis causing loose bowel movements and urgency.

Prevention

There are no effective methods to prevent fecal incontinence (FI) in anal cancer treatment, but close monitoring and early recognition allows earlier initiation of treatment.

Recognition

Bowel function and continence should be assessed at all follow-up office visits for patients who have undergone, or are undergoing, treatment for anal cancer. Objective measures of severity, such as the IMPACT score should be used to determine baseline score for patients, and response to therapies [35, 36]. Due to nature of radiation-induced damage, symptoms may continue to evolve and progress several years after completion of treatment.

Management

The primary management of FI includes the use of stool-bulking agents, anti-diarrheals, dietary modification, pelvic floor physical therapy, and biofeedback. Topical treatment for radiation-induced proctitis can be considered, including steroid or anti-inflammatory enemas. For all causes of FI, conservative measures have been found to improve symptoms in 22–54% of patients [36, 37].

Sacral nerve stimulation (SNS) is an effective treatment option and should be considered as a first-line surgical option in those patients in whom conservative measures fail [36, 38]. A systematic review which measured the success rate of SNS, as at least a 50% improvement in incontinence episodes, reported a median of 89% of patients had successful outcomes after a 36-month follow-up [39]. Success of SNS is best predicted by temporary trial stimulation. Clinical parameters such as the presence of a sphincter defect, pudendal neuropathy, or previous repairs shincter were not associated with SNS outcome [36, 40]. Patients in which sacral neuromodulation fails or FI recurs may require colostomy diversion to manage symptoms.

Rectovaginal Fistula

Background

Rectovaginal fistulas (RVFs) can develop as a result of primary disease or secondary to chemoradiation [41]. Due to the location of anal cancer, these are usually low, but can occur in the mid-rectum in the case of higher cancers (Fig. 35.6).

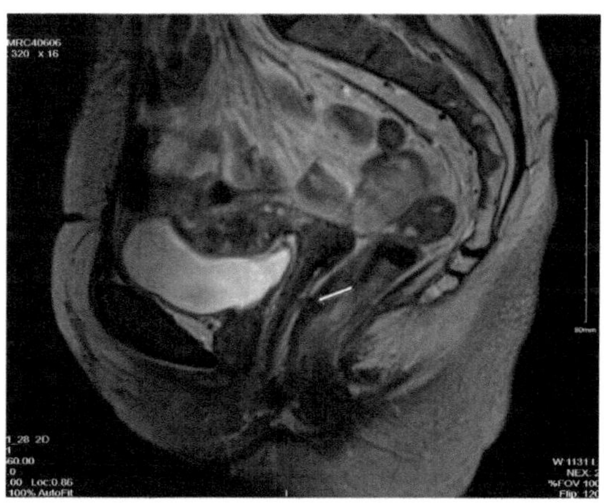

Fig. 35.6 Pelvic MRI, sagittal view showing a rectovaginal fistula (white arrow) resulting from a high anal squamous cell carcinoma within the mid-rectum. This fistula required colostomy diversion prior to beginning chemoradiation

Data on risk of RVF development following definitive CRT for anal cancer specifically is sparse; however, the incidence is reported to be 5–7% in patients following radiation therapy for cervical cancer [41, 42].

Prevention

Avoidance of fistula development is difficult; inflammatory response and fibrosis of irradiated tissue increases the risk of RVF. Fecal diversion with a proximal colostomy, while not preventing RVF development allows for early control of symptoms while treatment is ongoing it permits continuation of chemoradiation therapy and minimizes fistula complications [42].

Recognition

RVF development should be suspected based on patient symptoms of flatus, foul smelling discharge, or stool per vagina. Evaluation by way of examination under anesthesia and radiologic assessment is used to define the anatomy of the tract and the structures involved. Assessment of quality and function of anal sphincter is crucial in decision-making regarding optimal repair technique. This is of particular importance in anal SCC patients who likely have sphincter involvement from their primary disease along with exposure to high dose perineal targeted radiation [41].

Management

Any consideration of repair cannot be undertaken until all cancer treatment has been completed and the patient has no evidence of residual disease. Acute inflammation or infection can be managed with a loose fitting seton, along with appropriate anti-microbial therapy. This may also benefit patients who still require ongoing chemoradiation, prior to consideration of a more definitive repair [41]. Symptomatic relief is achieved with proximal fecal diversion alone. Due to the high dose of radiation given and significant radiation injury typically seen, patients should undergo fecal diversion prior to repair. In addition, they should be counseled regarding preoperative smoking cessation.

Definitive management options include endorectal advancement flap, interposition flap or completion proctectomy; overall success ranges from 41% up to 80% with repeated procedures [41, 43–46]. Pelvic radiation greatly increases the risk of failure of endorectal advancement flap although it is a less invasive, local procedure. Procedures using gracilis or bulbocavernosus flap (Martius flap) are more likely to succeed. More advanced fistulas, particularly in the setting of radiation-induced proctitis and RVF, may require completion proctectomy with or without a coloanal anastomosis (see Chap. 36, Rectal and Rectosigmoid Carcinoma).

Complications of Therapy (Chemoradiation)

High dose pelvic radiation contributes to and worsens many of the surgical and disease-related complications as discussed above. Several complications occur as a direct result of radiation therapy including radiation enteritis and the development of late sigmoid and ureteral strictures. Ureteral strictures and their management are discussed in Chap. 17 "Injury/Repair of Pelvic Ureter".

Radiation Enteritis

Background

Radiation to the small bowel causes proliferating cell apoptosis, denuding of the mucosa, and loss of the intestinal barrier function. The loss of intestinal barrier function leads to disruption in gut microbiota and inflammation causing acute enteritis. Acute enteritis presents with abdominal pain, emesis, diarrhea, and dehydration, and while symptoms may be significant, these usually resolve with supportive treatment. However, around 5–15% of patients with irradiated small bowel will go on to develop severe chronic enteritis [47]. Chronic enteritis results in significant intestinal fibrosis ,which can lead to obstruction or perforation, along with dysregulation of the intestinal microbiome [48, 49].

Prevention

The radiation dose and protocol are the most significant risk factors for developing enteritis. Image-guided or intensity-modulated radiotherapy (IMRT) protocols can better localize tumor with reduced reduce risk to surrounding structures, such as the small bowel, compared to conventional protocols [49–51].

Recognition

Acute radiation-induced enteritis should be suspected in all patients with nausea, emesis, diarrhea, or abdominal pain during, or immediately following, abdominal/pelvic radiation. Chronic enteritis should be considered in patients with chronic diarrhea or malabsorption. This can develop 3 months to 6 years after radiation exposure and should be considered in patients presenting with small bowel obstruction following treatment for anal SCC. Patients may also present with, or develop, short bowel syndrome, or develop anemia secondary to telangiectasia [52].

Management

Acute enteritis is usually managed with supportive therapy. Surgery is indicated for complications of chronic enteritis such as bowel obstruction (discussed previously) and perforation. Fibrosing enteritis causing complete small bowel obstruction requires small bowel resection and primary anastomosis or bypass. In the case of perforation, resection is indicated with the decision to perform an anastomosis dependent on degree of contamination, bowel viability and the patients' general condition and nutritional status. Patients with chronic radiation enteritis often present with malnutrition or anemia. In such cases, or in the case of an a unstable, or immunocompromised patient in which further chemoradiation is planned, a proximal diverting loop, ileostomy may be required.

Novel therapies for radiation-induced enteritis include stem cell therapy, probiotic microbial therapy, and fecal microbiota transplantation. Experimental studies have been reported to show restoration of intestinal microbiota and epithelial repair and regeneration [48, 49].

Sigmoid Stricture Formation

Background

Tissue damage and fibrotic reaction secondary to radiation are progressive, so sigmoid stricture may develop several years following initial chemoradiation treatment [53]. The rectosigmoid junction is particularly susceptible to radiation-induced injury due to its relatively fixed nature [54].

Prevention

Modification of radiotherapy protocols as above may reduce the inadvertent irradiation of surrounding bowel; however, there are no surgical or medical preventative measures to reduce the occurrence of strictures. Early recognition may allow intervention with more favorable treatment options and reduce risk of resection and stoma. To prevent complications of known strictures, ensuring soft stools with a bowel regimen and avoidance of constipation is important.

Recognition

Symptomatic strictures may present as an acute or slowly progressive large bowel obstruction as described above or be found incidentally on follow up imaging or sigmoidoscopy. Radiological severity does not always correlate to clinical or endoscopic severity; therefore, imaging should be interpreted in context of symptoms and endoscopy findings.

Management

All strictures should be biopsied to exclude alternative causes such as malignancy or inflammatory bowel disease. Once benign disease is confirmed treatment is guided based on acuity of symptoms and patients' overall function and goals. Acute complete obstruction management is as per LBO above, which includes gastric decompression, fluid and electrolyte resuscitation and emergent surgery. Surgical options include loop colostomy, resection, and end colostomy or resection and primary anastomosis +/– diverting loop ileostomy.

Patients presenting with partially obstructing strictures may undergo trial of nonoperative interventions such as endoscopic balloon dilatation. In radiation-induced strictures, the degree of fibrosis means strictures commonly recur and repeated interventions, often resulting in colonic resection are required. Fibrotic and inflammatory effects of radiation increase the risks of surgery, with scarring making dissection more difficult, and anatomy of surrounding structures less well-delineated. Following resection, the distal colon or rectum for anastomosis may be free of significant stricture, but it has also been exposed to significant radiation and therefore at increased risk of anastomotic leak. Diverting loop ileostomy is commonly performed in this situation, with reversal once water-soluble enema has confirmed healing and patency of anastomosis [54].

Conclusion

Complications associated with anal squamous cell cancer are varied. They can occur either as a result of the primary disease or following surgery for persistent or recurrent disease or following surgery for complications of treatment. Careful patient assessment is key in achieving good outcomes.

References

1. Nigro ND, Vaitkevicius VK, Buroker T, Bradley GT, Considine B. Combined therapy for cancer of the anal canal. Dis Colon Rectum. 1981;24(2):73–5.
2. Nigro ND, Vaitkevicius VK, Considine BJ. Combined therapy for cancer of the anal canal: a preliminary report. Dis Colon Rectum. 1974;17(3):354–6.
3. Benson AB, Venook AP, Al-Hawary MM, Cederquist L, Chen YJ, Ciombor KK, et al. Anal Carcinoma, Version 2.2018, NCCN Clinical Practice Guidelines in Oncology. J Natl Compr Cancer Netw. 2018;16(7):852–71.
4. Chai CY, Tran Cao HS, Awad S, Massarweh NN. Management of stage I squamous cell carcinoma of the anal canal. JAMA Surg. 2018;153(3):209–15.
5. Arana R, Fléjou JF, Si-Mohamed A, Bauer P, Etienney I. Clinicopathological and virological characteristics of superficially invasive squamous-cell carcinoma of the anus. Color Dis. 2015;17(11):965–72.
6. Northover J, Glynne-Jones R, Sebag-Montefiore D, James R, Meadows H, Wan S, et al. Chemoradiation for the treatment of epidermoid anal cancer: 13-year follow-up of the first randomised UKCCCR Anal Cancer Trial (ACT I). Br J Cancer. 2010;102(7):1123–8.
7. Park IJ, Chang G. Survival and operative outcomes after salvage surgery for recurrent or persistent anal cancer. Ann Coloproctol. 2020;36(6):361–73.
8. Julie DR, Goodman KA. Advances in the Management of Anal Cancer. Curr Oncol Rep. 2016;18(3):20.
9. Osborne MC, Maykel J, Johnson EK, Steele SR. Anal squamous cell carcinoma: an evolution in disease and management. World J Gastroenterol. 2014;20(36):13052–9.
10. Eeson G, Foo M, Harrow S, McGregor G, Hay J. Outcomes of salvage surgery for epidermoid carcinoma of the anus following failed combined modality treatment. Am J Surg. 2011;201(5):628–33.
11. Wei L, Griego AM, Chu M, Ozbun MA. Tobacco exposure results in increased E6 and E7 oncogene expression, DNA damage and mutation rates in cells maintaining episomal human papillomavirus 16 genomes. Carcinogenesis. 2014;35(10):2373–81.
12. Musters GD, Buskens CJ, Bemelman WA, Tanis PJ. Perineal wound healing after abdominoperineal resection for rectal cancer: a systematic review and meta-analysis. Dis Colon Rectum. 2014;57(9):1129–39.
13. Mori GA, Tiernan JP. Management of perineal wounds following pelvic surgery. Clin Colon Rectal Surg. 2022;35(3):212–20.
14. Ghouti L, Houvenaeghel G, Moutardier V, Giovannini M, Magnin V, Lelong B, et al. Salvage abdominoperineal resection after failure of conservative treatment in anal epidermoid cancer. Dis Colon Rectum. 2005;48(1):16–22.
15. Nisar PJ, Scott HJ. Myocutaneous flap reconstruction of the pelvis after abdominoperineal excision. Color Dis. 2009;11(8):806–16.
16. Devulapalli C, Jia Wei AT, DiBiagio JR, Baez ML, Baltodano PA, Seal SM, et al. Primary versus flap closure of perineal defects following oncologic resection: a systematic review and meta-analysis. Plast Reconstr Surg. 2016;137(5):1602–13.
17. Baloch N, Nordenvall C, Johansson H, Nygren J, Nilsson PJ. Perineal healing following salvage surgery for anal cancer. Color Dis. 2021;23(5):1102–8.
18. Musters GD, Klaver CEL, Bosker RJI, Burger JWA, van Duijvendijk P, van Etten B, et al. Biological mesh closure of the pelvic floor after extralevator abdominoperineal resection for rectal cancer: a multicenter randomized controlled trial (the BIOPEX-study). Ann Surg. 2017;265(6):1074–81.
19. Foster JD, Tou S, Curtis NJ, Smart NJ, Acheson A, Maxwell-Armstrong C, et al. Closure of the perineal defect after abdominoperineal excision for rectal adenocarcinoma – ACPGBI position statement. Color Dis. 2018;20(Suppl 5):5–23.
20. Wong AYW, Ong BSY, Lee ARYB, Mai AS, Selvarajan S, Lakshminarasappa SR, et al. Topical biological agents as adjuncts to improve wound healing in chronic diabetic wounds: a systematic review

of clinical evidence and future directions. Cureus. 2022;14(7):e27180.
21. Guillamat-Prats R. The role of MSC in wound healing, scarring and regeneration. Cells. 2021;10(7):1729.
22. Cahill C, Fowler A, Williams LJ. The application of incisional negative pressure wound therapy for perineal wounds: a systematic review. Int Wound J. 2018;15(5):740–8.
23. Enoch S, Grey JE, Harding KG. ABC of wound healing. Non-surgical and drug treatments BMJ. 2006;332(7546):900–3.
24. Luo W, Lu T, Xu Z, Qian C, Li F, Xiao Y, et al. A novel technique with ileal mesentery to reconstruct the pelvic peritoneum after pelvic dissection with end colostomy for rectal cancer. Dis Colon Rectum. 2022;65(9):e910–3.
25. Voros D, Fragoulidis G, Theodosopoulos T, Mavrantonis C, Samanidis L, Papavasiliou C, et al. Pelvic floor reconstruction after major cancer surgery. Dis Colon Rectum. 1996;39(11):1232–4.
26. Blok RD, Musters GD, Borstlap WAA, Buskens CJ, Bemelman WA, Tanis PJ. Snapshot study on the value of omentoplasty in abdominoperineal resection with primary perineal closure for rectal cancer. Ann Surg Oncol. 2018;25(3):729–36.
27. Blok RD, Hagemans JAW, Klaver CEL, Hellinga J, van Etten B, Burger JWA, et al. A systematic review and meta-analysis on omentoplasty for the management of abdominoperineal defects in patients treated for cancer. Ann Surg. 2020;271(4):654–62.
28. Johnson YL, West MA, Gould LE, Drami I, Behrenbruch C, Burns EM, et al. Empty pelvis syndrome: a systematic review of reconstruction techniques and their associated complications. Color Dis. 2022;24(1):16–26.
29. Akıncı D, Ergun O, Topel Ç, Çiftçi T, Akhan O. Pelvic abscess drainage: outcome with factors affecting the clinical success. Diagn Interv Radiol. 2018;24(3):146–52.
30. De Filippo M, Puglisi S, D'Amuri F, Gentili F, Paladini I, Carrafiello G, et al. CT-guided percutaneous drainage of abdominopelvic collections: a pictorial essay. Radiol Med. 2021;126(12):1561–70.
31. Bertrand K, Lefevre JH, Creavin B, Luong M, Debove C, Voron T, et al. The management of perineal hernia following abdomino-perineal excision for cancer. Hernia. 2020;24(2):279–86.
32. Sayers AE, Patel RK, Hunter IA. Perineal hernia formation following extralevator abdominoperineal excision. Color Dis. 2015;17(4):351–5.
33. Maspero M, Heilman J, Otero Piñeiro A, Steele SR, Hull TL. Techniques of perineal hernia repair: a systematic review and meta-analysis. Surgery. 2023;173(2):312–21.
34. Mekhael M, Larsen HM, Lauritzen MB, Thorlacius-Ussing O, Laurberg S, Krogh K, et al. Bowel dysfunction following pelvic organ cancer: a prospective study on the treatment effect in nurse-led late sequelae clinics. Acta Oncol. 2023;62(1):70–9.
35. Bordeianou LG, Anger JT, Boutros M, Birnbaum E, Carmichael JC, Connell KA, et al. Measuring pelvic floor disorder symptoms using patient-reported instruments: proceedings of the consensus meeting of the pelvic floor consortium of the American Society of Colon and Rectal Surgeons, the International Continence Society, the American Urogynecologic Society, and the Society of Urodynamics, Female Pelvic Medicine and Urogenital Reconstruction. Female Pelvic Med Reconstr Surg. 2020;26(1):1–15.
36. Bordeianou LG, Thorsen AJ, Keller DS, Hawkins AT, Messick C, Oliveira L, et al. The American Society of Colon and Rectal Surgeons Clinical Practice Guidelines for the Management of Fecal Incontinence. Dis Colon Rectum. 2023;66(5):647–61.
37. Bliss DZ, Savik K, Jung HJG, Whitebird R, Lowry A, Sheng X. Dietary fiber supplementation for fecal incontinence: a randomized clinical trial. Res Nurs Health. 2014;37(5):367–78.
38. Mellgren A. Expert commentary on management of anal incontinence with implantable sacral neuromodulation. Dis Colon Rectum. 2023;66(6):762–3.
39. Thin NN, Horrocks EJ, Hotouras A, Palit S, Thaha MA, Chan CLH, et al. Systematic review of the clinical effectiveness of neuromodulation in the treatment of faecal incontinence. Br J Surg. 2013;100(11):1430–47.
40. Brouwer R, Duthie G. Sacral nerve neuromodulation is effective treatment for fecal incontinence in the presence of a sphincter defect, pudendal neuropathy, or previous sphincter repair. Dis Colon Rectum. 2010;53(3):273–8.
41. Gaertner WB, Burgess PL, Davids JS, Lightner AL, Shogan BD, Sun MY, et al. The American Society of Colon and Rectal Surgeons Clinical Practice Guidelines for the Management of Anorectal Abscess, Fistula-in-Ano, and Rectovaginal Fistula. Dis Colon Rectum. 2022;65(8):964–85.
42. Zelga P, Tchórzewski M, Zelga M, Sobotkowski J, Dziki A. Radiation-induced rectovaginal fistulas in locally advanced gynaecological malignancies-new patients, old problem? Langenbeck's Arch Surg. 2017;402(7):1079–88.
43. Korsun S, Liebig-Hoerl G, Fuerst A. Gracilis muscle transposition for treatment of recurrent anovaginal, rectovaginal, rectourethral, and pouch-vaginal fistulas in patients with inflammatory bowel disease. Tech Coloproctol. 2019;23(1):43–52.
44. Pinto RA, Peterson TV, Shawki S, Davila GW, Wexner SD. Are there predictors of outcome following rectovaginal fistula repair? Dis Colon Rectum. 2010;53(9):1240–7.
45. Park SO, Hong KY, Park KJ, Chang H, Shin JY, Jeong SY. Treatment of rectovaginal fistula with gracilis muscle flap transposition: long-term follow-up. Int J Color Dis. 2017;32(7):1029–32.
46. Tozer PJ, Balmforth D, Kayani B, Rahbour G, Hart AL, Phillips RKS. Surgical management of rectovaginal fistula in a tertiary referral centre: many techniques are needed. Color Dis. 2013;15(7):871–7.

47. Spyropoulos BG, Misiakos EP, Fotiadis C, Stoidis CN. Antioxidant properties of probiotics and their protective effects in the pathogenesis of radiation-induced enteritis and colitis. Dig Dis Sci. 2011;56(2):285–94.
48. Moraitis I, Guiu J, Rubert J. Gut microbiota controlling radiation-induced enteritis and intestinal regeneration. Trends Endocrinol Metab. 2023;34(8):489–501.
49. Yang Q, Qin B, Hou W, Qin H, Yin F. Pathogenesis and therapy of radiation enteritis with gut microbiota. Front Pharmacol. 2023;14:1116558.
50. Yu C, Zhu W, Ji Y, Guo J, Pan P, Han J, et al. A comparative study of intensity-modulated radiotherapy and standard radiation field with concurrent chemotherapy for local advanced cervical cancer. Eur J Gynaecol Oncol. 2015;36(3):278–82.
51. Tsuchida K, Murakami N, Kato T, Okuma K, Okamoto H, Kashihara T, et al. Postoperative pelvic intensity-modulated radiation therapy reduced the incidence of late gastrointestinal complications for uterine cervical cancer patients. J Radiat Res. 2019;60(5):650–7.
52. Turina M, Mulhall AM, Mahid SS, Yashar C, Galandiuk S. Frequency and surgical management of chronic complications related to pelvic radiation. Arch Surg. 2008;143(1):46–52; discussion 52.
53. Kunkel G, Patel H, Kaldany A, Allu S, Elsamra S, Cancian M. Pelvic radiation-induced urinary strictures: etiology and management of a challenging disease. World J Urol. 2023;41(5):1459–68.
54. Cain BT, Huang LC. Benign colonic strictures. Dis Colon Rectum. 2021;64(9):1041–4.

Rectal and Rectosigmoid Carcinoma

36

Michelle DeLeon and Luca Stocchi

Introduction

Despite advances in surgical technology, there is still significant morbidity associated with rectal cancer surgery. This is in part due to the close proximity of vital structures to the rectum, the effects of radiotherapy and the challenges of operating in the narrow pelvis, particularly in the obese population. This chapter reviews the common postoperative complications of rectal cancer surgery and key strategies for prevention and management.

Anastomotic Leak

Background

The International Study Group of Rectal Cancer has proposed the definition of a colorectal anastomotic leak (AL) as a "defect of the intestinal wall integrity at the colorectal or coloanal anastomotic site (including suture and staple lines of neorectal reservoirs) leading to a communication between the intra- and extraluminal compartments. A pelvic abscess close to the anastomosis is also considered as anastomotic leakage." The definition excludes symptoms that are difficult to uniformly report. A corresponding grading system for the management of colorectal anastomotic leaks based on their severity has also been proposed (Table 36.1) [43].

The sequelae of AL are profound and can lead to permanent colostomy, derangements in bowel function, urinary and sexual dysfunction, reduced fertility and overall worsened quality of life. Recovery from pelvic sepsis and prolonged hospitalizations may cause a delay in chemotherapy, and AL has been arguably associated with increased rates of local recurrence and worse overall survival [22]. Prevention of this devastating complication is paramount.

Prevention

Prevention begins with addressing modifiable patient risk factors preoperatively. This includes

Table 36.1 Classification of anastomotic leakage following anterior resection of the rectum based on severity [43]

Grade	
A	Anastomotic leakage requiring no active therapeutic intervention
B	Anastomotic leakage requiring active therapeutic intervention but manageable without relaparotomy
C	Anastomotic leakage requiring relaparotomy

M. DeLeon · L. Stocchi (✉)
Division of Colon and Rectal Surgery, Mayo Clinic, Jacksonville, FL, USA
e-mail: deleon.michelle@mayo.edu; Stocchi.luca@mayo.edu

M. Hoffman et al. (eds.), *Major Complications of Female Pelvic Surgery*,
https://doi.org/10.1007/978-3-031-66772-5_36

smoking cessation, weight loss, nutritional supplementation/counseling, diabetic control and prehabilitation to improve frailty and functional status. Ideal optimization can be difficult for patients proceeding directly to surgery but is becoming more feasible in the era of total neoadjuvant therapy (TNT) where patients undergo radiation and chemotherapy for several months prior to surgery.

Intraoperatively, prevention focuses on proper assessment of perfusion, lack of tension, surgical technique and endoscopic evaluation.

Blood Supply After high ligation of the inferior mesenteric artery (IMA), the blood supply of the descending colon conduit relies primarily on the middle colic artery and marginal artery of Drummond. A low ligation (a division of the superior rectal artery just distal to the takeoff of the left colic artery) is an acceptable oncologic alternative if tension-free anastomosis can still be achieved. Careful attention to the marginal artery is imperative during mobilization of the descending colon and splenic flexure. In 10–20% of patients, the Arc of Riolan connecting the IMA and SMA is present and contributes to the colonic blood supply [52]. It can cross the IMV near the inferior border of the pancreas (Fig. 36.1). The artery of Moskowitz, found in 11–16% of patients

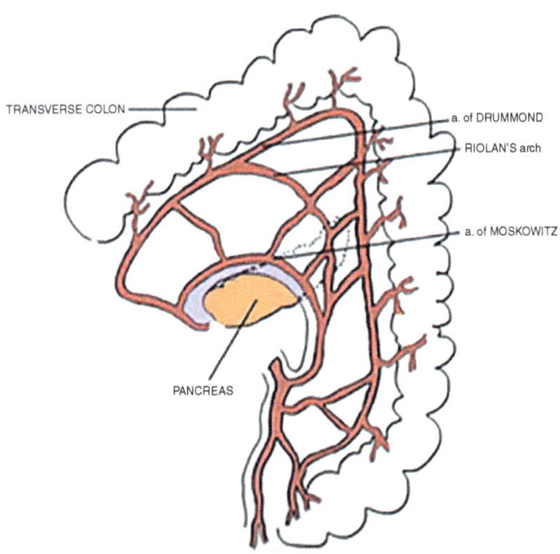

Fig. 36.1 Relation of Arc of Riolan and Moskowitz Artery to the marginal artery of Drummond

may similarly supply the colonic conduit [32] [20]. When mobilizing the splenic flexure, any aberrant vessels encountered near the IMV should be spared if possible.

After mobilization of the splenic flexure, assessment for adequate perfusion can be done by intentional transection and then ligation of the marginal artery seeking visible pulsatile blood flow, with Doppler ultrasound, or the use of indocyanine green (ICG) fluorescence (Fig. 36.2). In a recent randomized controlled trial comparing ICG to marginal artery bleeding, there was no statistically significant difference in AL rates [16] [28]. Therefore, any of the aforementioned adjuncts to visual bowel inspection may be used to ensure adequate perfusion to the descending colon conduit.

Tension Although splenic flexure mobilization is often necessary to attain adequate reach to the pelvis, routine splenic flexure mobilization has not been shown to improve clinical or oncologic outcomes [46], and has been associated with increased operative time and intraoperative complications. We recommend selective splenic flex-

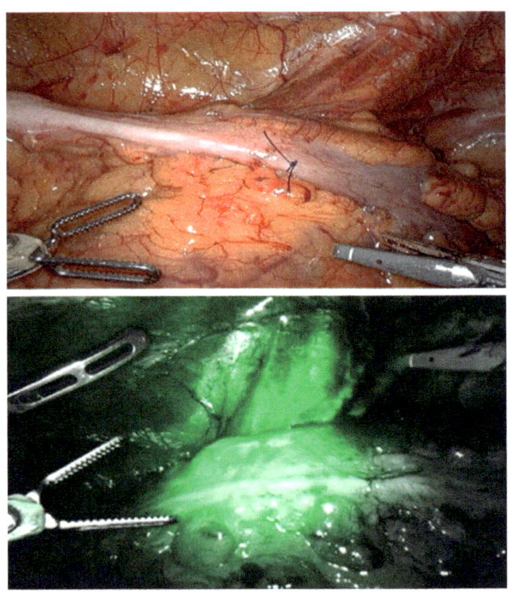

Fig. 36.2 Use of ICG fluorescence to evaluate colonic perfusion. Stitch marks the area of mesenteric transection to the bowel wall. Top panel—visual inspection alone. Bottom panel—visual inspection using ICG fluorescence

ure mobilization and careful evaluation of the anastomosis. If there are any signs suggesting anastomotic tension, full mobilization of the splenic flexure, with the division of the IMV at the inferior border of the pancreas should be performed. In some cases, additional maneuvers may be necessary [54]. If the anastomosis is possible but only after additional lengthening maneuvers, there should be strong consideration for diverting loop ileostomy, if this is not already planned.

Surgical Technique The majority of colorectal anastomoses are completed with a double-stapled technique due to their ease and reproducibility. However, stapling the distal rectum in the narrow pelvis remains a significant challenge, particularly in minimally invasive surgery (MIS). It is important to avoid an angled staple line and limit the number of firings required, as multiple staple lines may increase the risk of AL [8]. For very distal transections, perineal pressure helps to accommodate the stapler in the pelvis and facilitates proper stapling technique. For patients who may require multiple firings of a laparoscopic or robotic stapler, the surgeon should not hesitate to create an incision to insert an open stapler. When using the circular stapler, anastomotic rings should be evaluated for completeness and uniformity. Any disruptions or thinned areas may indicate a dehiscence or weakening of the anastomosis. The anastomosis should be inspected visually—if any obvious defects are seen, the anastomosis should be redone if possible. If anastomotic reconstruction is not possible due to inadequate length, the defect should be repaired and a defunctioning stoma created.

Endoscopic Assessment Assessment of the integrity of the anastomosis should be done in all patients undergoing low anterior resection for rectal cancer. Air leak tests have been shown to help identify intraoperative AL and decrease the risk of clinically significant postoperative AL [61]. The use of routine endoscopic assessment is under debate, but has the advantage of visual inspection of the anastomosis to evaluate for mucosal integrity, viability, and bleeding [31]. We recommend routine flexible endoscopy and especially air leak tests to evaluate all colorectal anastomoses. If an anastomotic air leak test is positive, the anastomosis should be reconstructed or repaired with a defunctioning stoma. Suture repair alone is associated with an increased risk of subsequent clinical AL when compared to either anastomotic reconstruction or additional stoma diversion and is not recommended [45].

Fecal Diversion Risk factors for AL include previous radiotherapy, malnutrition, smoking, obesity, emergency surgery, use of immunosuppressive medications, and a short distance of the anastomosis from the anal verge [38]. Fecal diversion should be considered on a case-by-case basis, taking into account the quality of the anastomosis and the number of risk factors involved. We recommend routine diversion for patients who have undergone neoadjuvant radiation and those with an anastomosis within 7 cm from the anal verge [55].

Recognition

Patients with an AL may present with abdominal pain, distention, fevers and tachycardia. Laboratory evaluation often reveals leukocytosis and increased C-reactive protein (CRP). There is increasing evidence that an elevated CRP is highly predictive of AL and is now being used in many enhanced recovery protocols to facilitate early discharge [12]. A meta-analysis based on 23 studies with 6647 patients identified a cut-off CRP of 148 milligram/liter on postoperative day 3 with sensitivity and specificity of 95% [62]. Computed Tomography (CT) scan may show intraperitoneal free air, extravasation of contrast or abscess. Contrast enema will show extravasation at the level of the anastomosis (Fig. 36.3). Patients with a diverting stoma and radiological AL discovered at the time of preoperative contrast enema are often asymptomatic.

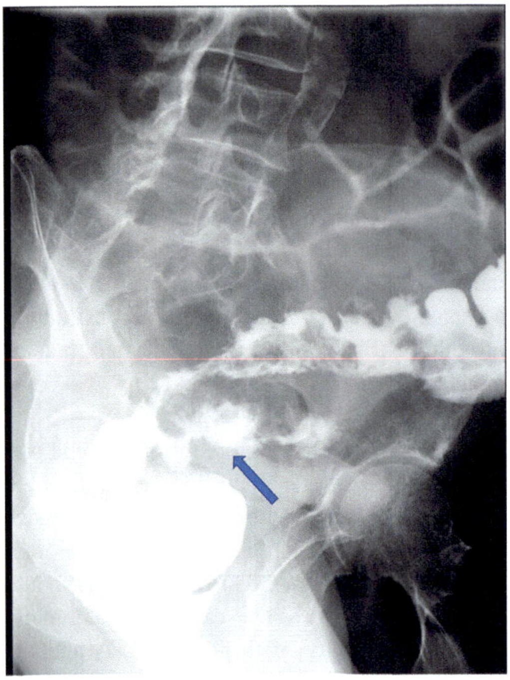

Fig. 36.3 Contrast enema showing contrast extravasation from a colorectal anastomosis. *Arrow indicates contrast extravasation

Management

AL Requiring Operative Intervention

Patients with clinical instability require immediate reoperative intervention. At that time the management depends on intraoperative findings. The anastomosis should be resected if ischemic and/or the anastomotic defect is large and/or there is extensive contamination and an end colostomy created. When a smaller defect is encountered with limited contamination, a primary repair of the defect with placement of drains and proximal stoma diversion is an appropriate approach. However, if the tissues do not hold the stitches, the anastomosis cannot be salvaged and should be treated as in the case of larger defects. The difference between a small and large defect remains subjective. When polling the opinions of several experts using a Delphi technique to standardize both definitions and management of AL, the 2 preferred definitions of minor defect were size less than 1 cm or less than a third of the anastomotic circumference [41]. If an end colostomy is needed, a transanal rectal tube to allow rectal decompression should be considered to help prevent rectal stump dehiscence.

In those cases in which the anastomosis is initially preserved, the AL can ultimately heal with supportive management, including surgical and/or percutaneous drainage and proximal diversion. For those that do not resolve, several techniques have been described to address chronic leaks, sinuses and presacral abscess cavities including endosponge, local repair, and marsupialization of the sinus tract.

Endosponge

The use of an endosponge connected to the suction device was described by Weidenhagen in 2008 [57]. It consists of a sponge placed into the extraperitoneal anastomotic defect connected to a suction device based on the principle of vacuum-assisted closure (VAC) widely used for other wounds. Since then, a number of studies have confirmed its applicability and efficacy [5], with clinical success rates approaching 85% [17]. The Endo-SPONGE® (B. Braun Medical, Melsungen, Germany) is widely available in Europe and elsewhere but is not readily available in the United States despite FDA approval in 2012.

Local Repairs

A number of techniques have been described to treat the anastomotic defect including endorectal advancement flap, dermal flap, or simple debridement [4]. Endoscopic approaches include fibrin glue injection, endosponge insertion or over-the-scope-clip system (OTSC). A recent review suggests that at times a combination of different techniques is necessary to achieve secondary closure of the anastomotic defect leading to stoma closure and return to anorectal function [15]. With a variety of available options, it is difficult to formulate an organized algorithm prescribing clear indications and sequences of the individual techniques. The reported cases remain isolated, therefore clinical decisions should be made on an individual basis.

Marsupialization of the Sinus Tract

A number of short reports have described marsupialization of the sinus tract, also referred to as septotomy or sinusotomy. This consists of division of the colonic wall which constitutes the roof of a posterior anastomotic sinus. This can be carried out under direct vision with electrocautery, endoscopically using the ERCP blade, vessel sealant, or application of a mechanical stapler [1, 9, 60]. The numbers are too small to draw definitive conclusions but anecdotal success justifies this technique as one of the possible options in the treatment of chronic sinus.

Despite these maneuvers and prolonged diversion, the patient remains at risk of permanent stoma. In a study evaluating outcomes after AL, 48% had not healed in 12 months [6]. Ultimately the patient may require either a colostomy after anastomosis takedown and completion proctectomy, or retain an indefinite diverting loop ileostomy created at the time of the index surgery.

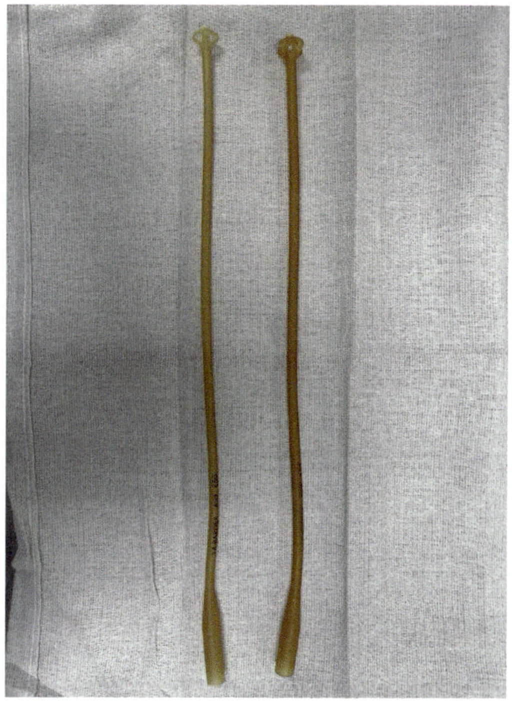

Fig. 36.4 Malecot catheters used for transanal trans-anastomotic drainage of pelvic abscess

Nonoperative Management of AL

If the patient is hemodynamically stable and presents with a contained AL, this may be treated nonoperatively. Abscesses less than 3 cm in diameter can be initially treated with broad-spectrum antibiotics alone, while larger abscesses are generally approached with percutaneous drainage [3]. In cases of inadequate drainage, the catheter can be manipulated or exchanged, which is also associated with a high success rate [21].

Alternatively, transanal trans-anastomotic drainage has been proposed for low colorectal/coloanal anastomoses [49]. The rationale of transanal drainage is to avoid percutaneous drainage, particularly transgluteal drainage which based on data from management of ileal pouch leak [34] can predispose to the iatrogenic creation of an extrasphincteric fistula. Other reported complications include gluteal abscess [53], pain, and bleeding from injury to the gluteal artery [11, 23] A possible approach is to utilize Malecot catheters (Fig. 36.4) tailored to have their head placed through the anastomotic defect and into the extraluminal cavity, often located posteriorly. The straight portion of the catheter is transected so that only a few centimeters are left into the bowel lumen and then secured with transfixing sutures to the bowel wall near the anastomotic defect. The patient is reexamined every 2–3 weeks for a catheter exchange and evaluation of the defect and the associated cavity. As the patient's condition improves, the cavity should reduce in size allowing for replacement with progressively smaller Malecot catheters until ultimate removal.

Subclinical AL For patients with fecal diversion who are found to have an AL on contrast enema, delay of ileostomy closure for 3–6 months often results in spontaneous resolution of small leaks without further intervention. For patients with a persistent leak/sinus beyond 6 months, the aforementioned treatment strategies should be employed. Reoperative intervention with takedown and reconstruction of the anastomosis or permanent colostomy is ultimately the last resort.

Anastomotic Stricture

Background

The incidence of anastomotic strictures varies widely in the literature, ranging from 5–20%. The most commonly described definition is a narrowing unable to allow passage of a standard colonoscope (12 mm in width). Risk factors include AL, pelvic sepsis, radiotherapy, low anastomosis and diverting stomas [42]. The pathophysiology is multifactorial and thought to be due to ischemia that ultimately leads to fibrosis and narrowing of the intestinal lumen.

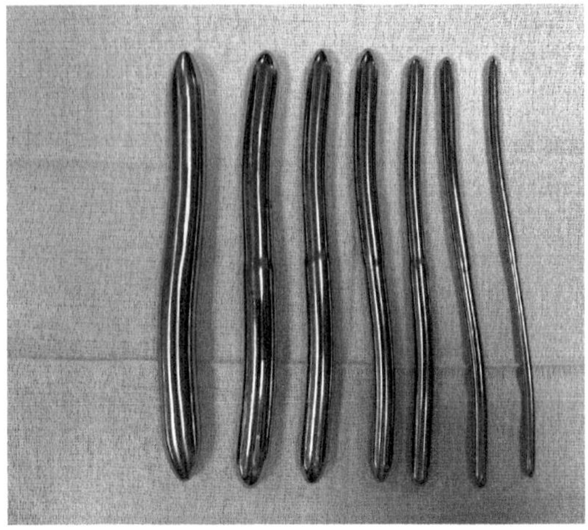

Fig. 36.5 Hegar Dilators

Prevention

Prevention focuses on avoiding ischemia to the colonic conduit and taking measures to prevent AL as discussed previously. It is imperative that appropriate multidisciplinary discussions are held preoperatively to plan radiation in the neoadjuvant setting if indicated and limit the need for adjuvant radiation therapy.

Recognition

Patients may present with constipation, abdominal cramping, distention, difficulty passing stools, and a change in the stool caliber. They may also experience frequency and overflow incontinence due to an inability to pass formed stools. Radiographic imaging may show a dilated colon in cases of severe colonic obstruction. A definitive diagnosis is made with a colonoscopy.

Management

Patients with an anastomotic stricture should have biopsies and radiographic imaging with pelvic MRI to rule out recurrent disease. In the absence of malignancy, the management of anastomotic strictures depends on their location. Low coloanal anastomoses can be dilated digitally or using Hegar dilators (Fig. 36.5). This may require repeated dilations, and many patients can be taught to do this safely at home. The majority of higher anastomotic strictures can be managed successfully with endoscopic balloon dilation (EBD) (Fig. 36.6). Other techniques like endoscopic electrocautery incision [29] and endoscopic stricturotomy can be used as adjuncts to EBD for severe strictures, or strictures refractory to EBD (Figs. 36.7 and 36.8). Metallic stent insertion is described in the literature (Fig. 36.9); however, stent migration limits its long-term efficacy [35]. TAMIS has emerged as a minimally invasive option that may allow for more aggressive stricturotomy compared to an endoscopic approach. Small series in the literature have shown the safety and efficacy of this technique [63].

For those patients who fail endoscopic treatment, reoperative intervention is required. As the majority of strictures are secondary to ischemia and pelvic sepsis in a reoperative and often irradiated field, these operations are technically challenging and associated with significant morbidity. The anastomosis and adjacent rectum will be fibrotic, and surgical planes obscured. There is a high risk for significant pelvic bleeding and iatrogenic injury to surrounding structures. We recommend the routine use of ureteral stents to help with ureteral identification. The anesthesia team should be prepared for the possibility of significant hemorrhage due to presacral venous bleed-

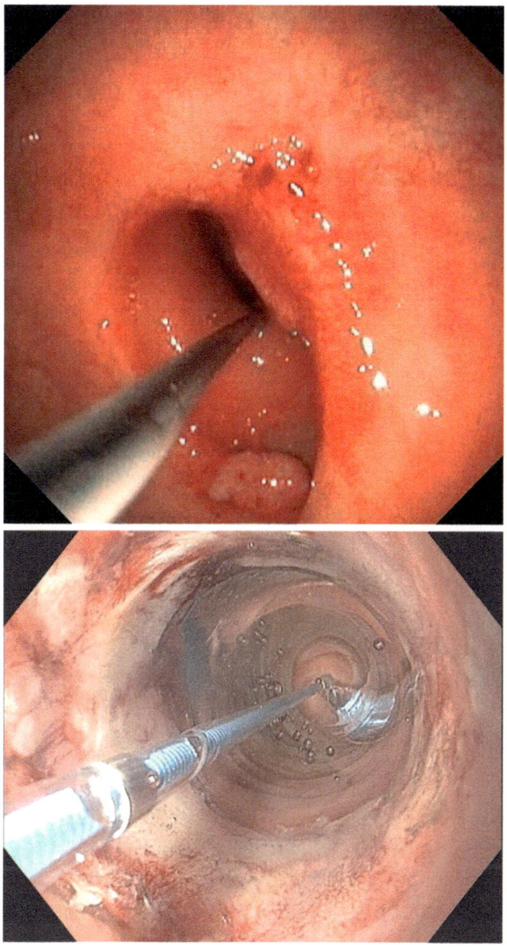

Fig. 36.6 Endoscopic Balloon Dilation. Top panel—A wire is first passed across the anastomotic stricture. Bottom panel—Balloon dilatation at anastomotic stricture. Photo courtesy of: Vivek Kumbhari, MD and Mahmoud Mahfouz, MD

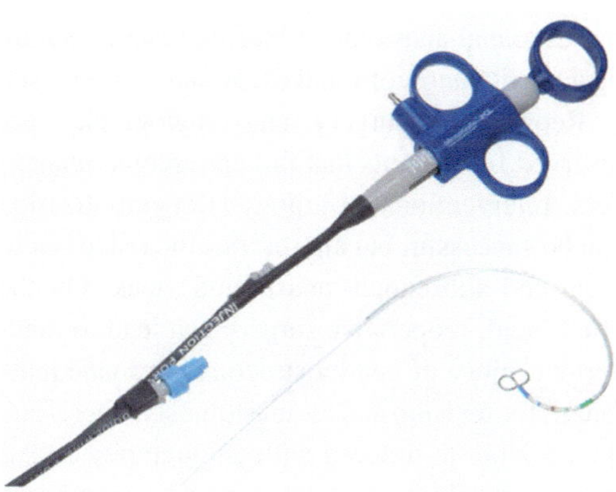

Fig. 36.7 Needle knife used for endoscopic stricturotomy

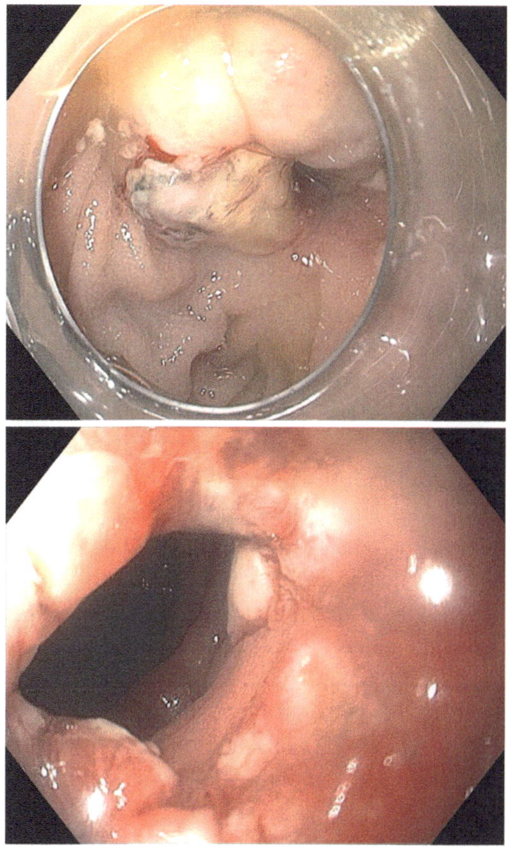

Fig. 36.8 Endoscopic stricturotomy. Top panel before stricturotomy. Bottom panel—after stricturotomy. Photo courtesy of Vivek Kumbhari, MD and Mahmoud Mahfouz, MD

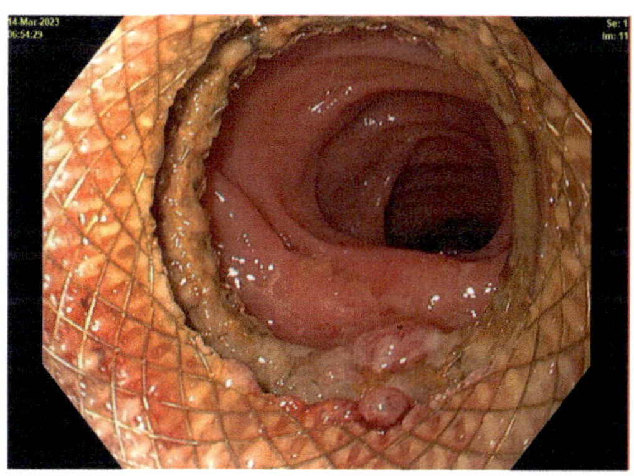

Fig. 36.9 Colonic stent across anastomotic stricture. Photo courtesy of Victoria Gomez, MD

ing. The goal is to resect all areas of fibrosis to normal healthy tissue, which often requires coloanal anastomosis. In cases of severe pelvic sepsis and fibrosis, delayed anastomotic reconstruction with a Turnbull-Cutait technique should be considered [36]. Due to the complexity of these operations, most patients will require temporary diversion. Prior to embarking on surgery, realistic functional expectations should be discussed with the patient, and the option of permanent colostomy should be offered as this may ultimately afford the best quality of life. A significant proportion of patients may suffer from incontinence and low anterior resection syndrome [59]. Elderly individuals with significant comorbidities and suboptimal sphincter function are not good candidates for reconstructive surgery. For patients with significant symptoms who are too frail to undergo a major pelvic operation, proximal diversion alone is recommended. Very obese individuals should lose weight to render this option technically feasible. In the largest series to date including 200 patients, the 1-year success rate was 80%. The authors elaborated a scoring system to estimate success rate based on recognized risk factors including male gender, age greater than 60 years, obesity and history of pelvic radiotherapy. The success rate ranged from 92% if none of these factors were present to 62% if all 4 factors were present [13].

Anastomotic Bleeding

Background

It is very common for patients to experience minor anal bleeding with bowel movements immediately after surgery. The majority of these cases are self-limited and clinically insignificant. The incidence of anastomotic bleeds that require some form of intervention has been reported to be less than 1% [37].

Prevention

Preoperatively, any coagulopathies should be addressed and corrected. Blood thinning medications should be held if possible. Intraoperatively, it is important to ensure that either mesocolon or mesorectum (if applicable) are not incorporated into the staple line. We recommend routine endoscopy to evaluate all anastomoses so that any bleeding encountered can be corrected at the time of surgery either by endoscopic clipping, or extraluminal oversewing of the vessel under endoscopic guidance.

Recognition

Patients with colorectal anastomotic bleeding generally present with bright red blood per rectum and are usually otherwise asymptomatic. Those with clinically significant bleeding may have associated hemodynamic instability, clinical symptoms and a drop in hematocrit.

Management

Minor bleeding episodes can resolve spontaneously without the need for transfusion or intervention. For patients with clinically significant bleeding, management begins with correction of underlying coagulopathies, cessation of medications affecting coagulation and transfusion of packed red blood cells. For persistent bleeding in patients with mid to high anastomoses, endoscopic intervention with clipping is the preferred modality of choice. Electrocautery and epinephrine injection can also be effective but carry a small risk of ischemia and compromise to the anastomosis. Coloanal anastomotic bleeding can be suture ligated with anoscopy and exam under anesthesia.

Reoperative surgery and angiography are reserved for patients that fail endoscopic maneuvers. Interventional radiology (IR) embolization can be successful but also carries the risk of ischemia and subsequent anastomotic leak. On the other hand, reoperative surgery can lead to inadvertent injury of nearby structures or inadequate length for revision and re-anastomosis. Therefore, the decision to proceed with angiography versus surgery should be made on a case-by-case basis, taking into account the predicted hostility of the abdomen, comorbidities and risk factors for reoperation and ability to refashion an anastomosis.

Presacral Venous Bleeding

Background

Presacral venous bleeding is not uncommon, occurring in 0.25–8.6% of rectal cancer operations [14]. It can cause massive hemorrhage, quickly leading to hemodynamic instability and even death if not controlled rapidly. Risk factors for bleeding include history of radiotherapy, previous rectal surgery, distal tumor and locally advanced tumors.

Recognition

Massive hemorrhage during pelvic dissection is indicative of presacral venous plexus bleeding.

Prevention

The presacral venous plexus resides posterior to the presacral fascia (Figs. 36.10 and 36.11). Proper total mesorectal excision (TME) requires the rectal dissection to occur in the avascular plane between the fascia propria and presacral fascia. Dissection outside of the presacral fascia can lead to venous plexus injury and severe hemorrhage. Blunt dissection may also cause inadvertent tearing of the presacral fascia and the underlying venous plexus. Sharp dissection in the proper plane and avoidance of excessive retraction are key to avoiding this devastating complication.

Management

As with any situation with significant hemorrhage, the first step is to control bleeding with direct pressure. The anesthesia team should be

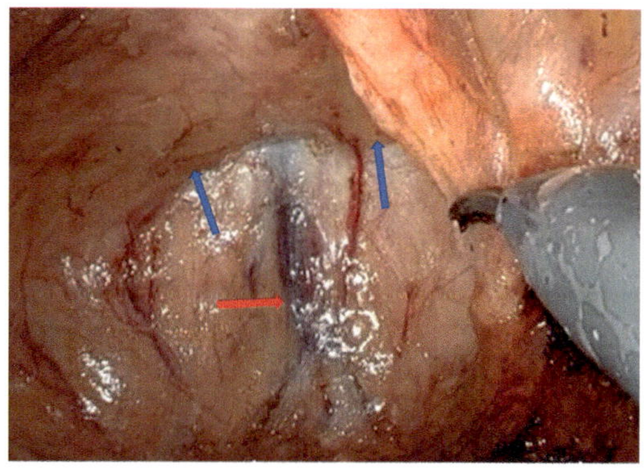

Fig. 36.11 Presacral veins during robotic TME dissection. Blue arrows indicate plane between mesorectum and presacral fascia, red arrow indicates presacral vein

Fig. 36.10 Presacral venous plexus

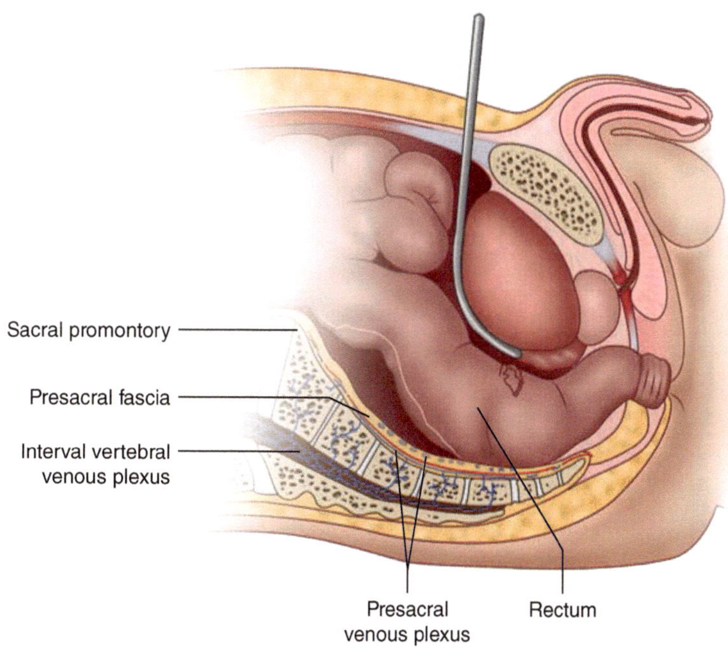

notified immediately to ensure adequate vascular access and availability of blood products. The surgeon should maintain direct pressure until hemodynamic stability can be achieved. At this point, if the area of bleeding can be identified, electrocautery, preferably bipolar energy should be applied. One should avoid the use of monopolar energy directly on the vessel, which can exacerbate bleeding as the vein retracts into the sacral foramina. Instead, indirect monopolar electrocautery should be applied through an epiploica appendix or piece of anterior rectus abdominis muscle. Historically, pins or tacks have been successfully used to address presacral bleeding [56]. However, in practice, these items are not always readily available and can be difficult to place correctly in the narrow deep pelvis. The use of a ProTack™ device on a hemostatic agent like Surgicel® may be more effective and overcome the shortcomings of manual pin/tack placement. The successful use of a free rectus abdominis muscle fragment sutured to the presacral tissue to tamponade the bleeding has been described [44] (Fig. 36.12a, b). A possible alternative or complementary maneuver to suturing of a muscle fragment is muscle fragment welding using electrocautery [24]. Bilateral ligation of the internal iliac artery has been described but is relatively extreme and could lead to ischemia of pelvic muscles or bladder [48]. If bleeding cannot be controlled directly, the surgeon should proceed with pelvic packing. This is traditionally done with laparotomy pads and a planned reoperation to address bleeding after any coagulopathies and hemodynamic instabilities are corrected. Other options for pelvic packing include a filled intravenous saline bag [40] or breast implant sizer [7]. In most cases, pelvic packing with laparotomy pads achieves hemodynamic stability after which the patient can be transferred to the intensive care unit and returned to the operative room in 24–48 hours. If a restorative operation had been originally planned the surgeon should make an effort to remove the specimen at the time of the initial operation and transect the distal anorectum before pelvic packing with the plan of reestablishing intestinal continuity at the time of the planned reoperation.

Low Anterior Resection Syndrome

Background

Low anterior resection syndrome (LARS) refers to the constellation of symptoms and the complexity of anorectal dysfunction that may result in patients undergoing low anterior resection [19]. These symptoms include fecal incontinence, urgency, frequency, clustering, and painful defecation. There is no clear etiology but it is thought to be a combination of radiation-induced mucosal injury, loss of the rectal reservoir, autonomic denervation, decreased recto-anal sensitiv-

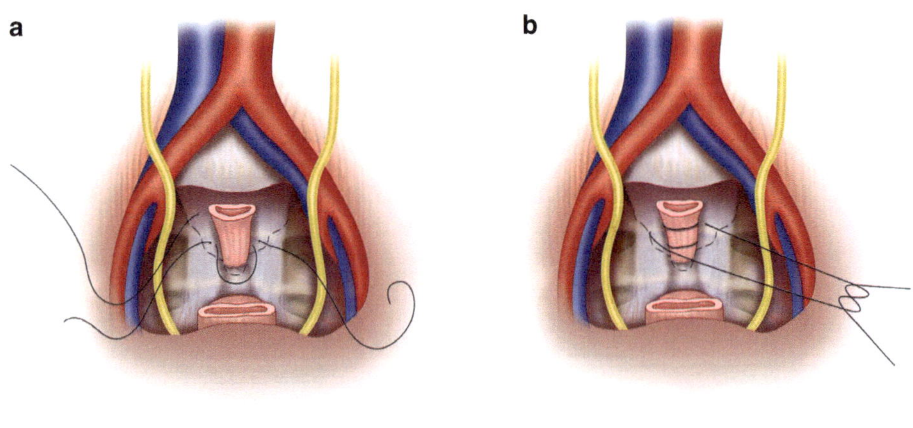

Fig. 36.12 Rectus abdominis muscle fragment sutured to presacral fascia to control bleeding

ity and decreased anal resting pressure. The incidence is significant with studies showing average rates of 44% [51].

Prevention

Unfortunately, there are no well-established strategies to prevent LARS. There is a relationship between anastomotic leakage and the development of LARS [25, 30]. Short-term improvements have been seen with colonic J pouch, side-to-end anastomosis and transverse coloplasty, but these benefits do not persist beyond 12–18 months [10, 27]. There is literature to suggest that a defunctioning stoma may contribute to impaired functional outcomes [33, 58], and that early closure may mitigate the severity of LARS [50]; however, the latter has not been replicated in subsequent studies. Trans-stomal irrigation, intraoperative nerve monitoring, pelvic floor physical therapy prior to stoma closure and transanal irrigation are techniques that may be helpful preventative measures and are currently under investigation [2].

Recognition

Patients will present with symptoms including frequency, urgency, fecal incontinence, clustering, and painful bowel movements. Their symptoms can be quantified using the LARS score (Fig. 36.13). Other etiologies including anastomotic stricture, tumor recurrence, radiation enteritis, bile salt, or pancreatic malabsorption and small bowel bacterial overgrowth should be ruled out prior to confirming the diagnosis of LARS.

Management

Initial management begins by increasing dietary fiber intake and adding fiber supplementation. For persistent symptoms, anti-motility agents including Imodium, loperamide, and tincture of opium should be prescribed.

Pelvic floor physical therapy and biofeedback should be recommended in conjunction with medical therapy. Retrograde colonic irrigation (RCI) helps to completely evacuate the neorectum and

Add the scores from each 5 answers to one final score.	
Do you ever have occasions when you cannot control your flatus (wind)?	
☐ No, never	0
☐ Yes, less than once per week	4
☐ Yes, at least once per week	7
Do you ever have any accidental leakage of liquid stool?	
☐ No, never	0
☐ Yes, less than once per week	3
☐ Yes, at least once per week	3
How often do you open your bowels?	
☐ More than 7 times per day (24 hours)	4
☐ 4–7 times per day (24 hours)	2
☐ 1–3 times per day (24 hours)	0
☐ Less than once per day (24 hours)	5
Do you ever have to open your bowels again within one hour of the last bowel opening?	
☐ No, never	0
☐ Yes, less than once per week	9
☐ Yes, at least once per week	11
Do you ever have such a strong urge to open your bowels that you have to rush to the toilet?	
☐ No, never	0
☐ Yes, less than once per week	11
☐ Yes, at least once per week	16
Total Score:	

Interpretation:	
0–20:	**No LARS**
21–29:	**Minor LARS**
30–42:	**Major LARS**

Fig. 36.13 LARS score (Emmertsen and Laurberg [19])

improve symptoms of fecal incontinence, frequency and clustering of bowel movements. RCI has also been shown to improve LARS scores [47]. Though not FDA-approved for LARS, there are several small series showing improvement of LARS and fecal incontinence with sacral nerve stimulation [26]. A systematic review assessing different interventions for LARS indicated that posterior tibial nerve stimulation was ineffective at improving LARS symptoms. Other interventions such as pelvic floor training, ramosetron and probiotics were effective in the short term, but their benefits could not be sustained in the long term. The best intervention to improve symptoms was RCI [18] . For those who continue to have debilitating symptoms despite these treatment strategies, fecal diversion is a surgical option that can afford these patients an improved quality of life.

Sexual and Urinary Dysfunction

Background

The cause of sexual dysfunction after rectal cancer treatment is multifactorial, due to a combination of autonomic pelvic nerve injury during surgery, chemoradiation-induced ovarian failure and radiation damage causing vaginal atrophy and fibrosis. Urinary incontinence is due to sympathetic nerve injury causing increased bladder tone, reduced bladder capacity, and urinary dysfunction.

Prevention

From a surgical perspective, an understanding of autonomic pelvic nerve anatomy is essential to prevent injury. The sympathetic autonomic plexus arises from T12-L2 and forms the superior hypogastric plexus (SHP) that emerges from the aorta at the level of the IMA (Fig. 36.14). High ligation of the IMA should be 1–2 cm from the origin of the aorta to avoid injury of this plexus. The SHP then splits into the right and left hypogastric nerves as they course over the sacral promontory (Figs. 36.14 and 36.15). As the operation commences into the pelvis, sharp dissection should be carried out in the avascular retrorectal space between the fascia propria anteriorly and the parietal fascia posteriorly to avoid injury of the hypogastric nerves (Fig. 36.16) Injury at this level may cause urinary urgency and incontinence [39].

The SHP then joins the pelvic splanchnic nerves (PSN) to form the inferior hypogastric plexus (IHP). The PSN enters at the level of S2-S4 and makes up the parasympathetic component. They lie in the lateral ligament joining the parietal fascia of the pelvic sidewall to the fascia propria medially. These nerves are responsible for detrusor contractility, vaginal lubrication, and genital swelling during sexual arousal. Damage at this level may cause decreased blood flow leading to reduced vaginal lubrication. The IHP continues anterolateral to the rectum, lateral

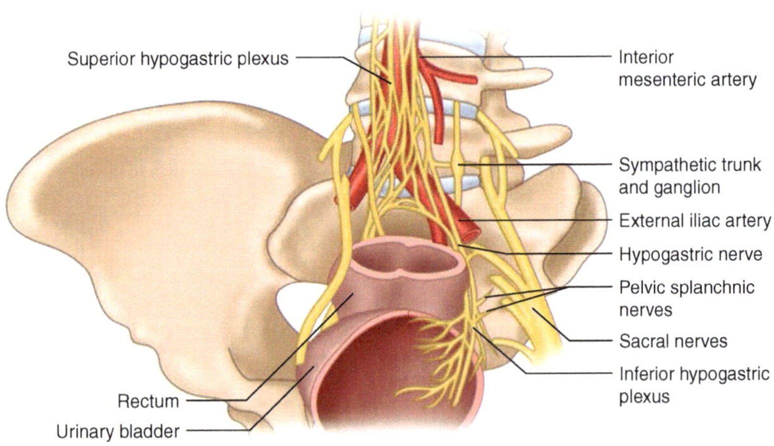

Fig. 36.14 Pelvic autonomic nerves

to the cervix, and extends to the lateral vaginal wall at the base of the bladder (Fig. 36.14). Injury to the PSN and IHP may occur if the TME dissection is taken too far laterally, or with excessive retraction of the rectum, displacing the IHP medially [39]. Because the IHP contains both sympathetic and parasympathetic nerve fibers, injury can result in both urogenital and sexual dysfunction.

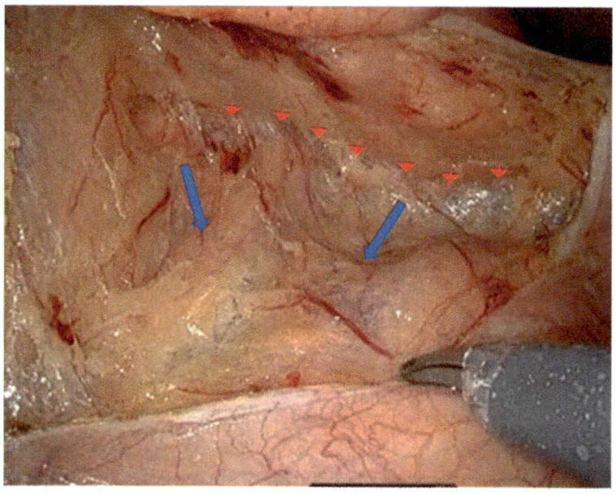

Fig. 36.15 Robotic view of hypogastric nerves over the sacral promontory during TME dissection. Blue arrows indicate hypogastric nerves over sacral promontory. Red arrows indicate plane of dissection between mesorectum and nerves

The anterior dissection around Denonvilliers fascia is less defined in women than in men. In women, the rectovaginal septum is described to have an anterior and posterior compartment. The posterior compartment is a continuation of the fascia propria of the rectum, and the anterior compartment is defined as Denonvilliers fascia, though this distinction is not always readily apparent [64]. Dissection in the plane to include Denonvilliers fascia is at high risk for autonomic nerve injury and is only required for anterior tumors, where a posterior vaginectomy may also be necessary. For posterolateral tumors, Denonvilliers fascia may be spared to avoid nerve injury.

Recognition

It is important for the provider to initiate conversations regarding sexual and urinary function once the patient has recovered from surgery, as

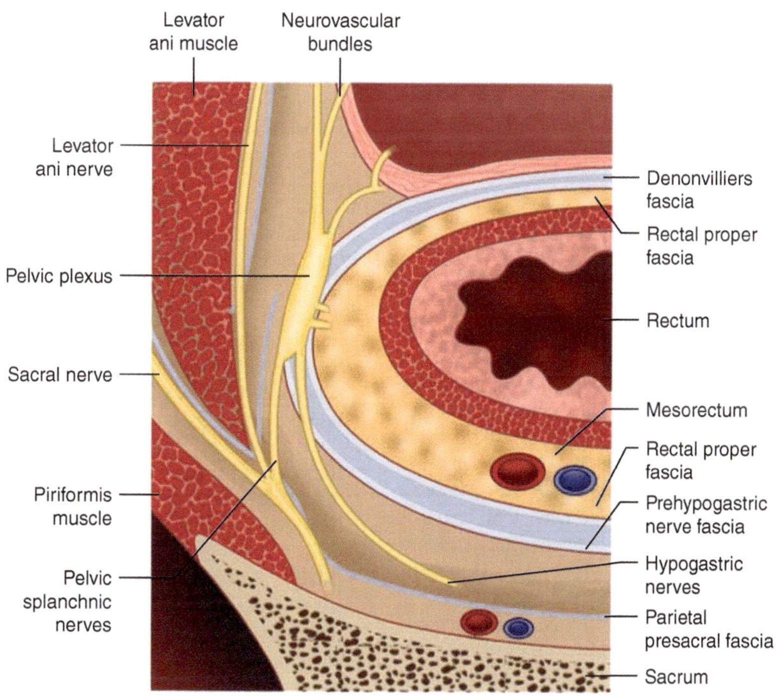

Fig. 36.16 Hypogastric nerves in relation to presacral fascia

many women may not be forthcoming with their concerns. Use of the Female Sexual Function Index-9 (FSFI-9) Questionnaire and the Pelvic Organ Prolapse/Incontinence Sexual International Urogynecological Association-Revised Questionnaire are useful tools for guiding diagnosis and management.

Treatment

A multidisciplinary approach between colorectal surgery, urogynecology and women's health is essential for optimal therapy. For patients suffering from sexual dysfunction, therapies including vaginal lubrication, topical and hormonal replacement therapy, pelvic floor physical therapy and psychological counseling are used depending on symptomatology. Patients with urinary incontinence, should have a referral to urology or urogynecology for medical management, pelvic floor physical therapy, and consideration of sacral nerve stimulation.

References

1. Alsanea N, Alabbad S. Use of the endostapler for the treatment of non-healing sinus secondary to a dehisced colorectal anastomosis. Tech Coloproctol. 2010;14:249–51. https://doi.org/10.1007/s10151-010-0600-5.
2. Annicchiarico A, Martellucci J, Solari S, et al. Low anterior resection syndrome: can it be prevented? Int J Color Dis. 2021;36:2535–52. https://doi.org/10.1007/s00384-021-04008-3.
3. Ballard DH, Gates MC, Hamidian Jahromi A, et al. Transrectal and transvaginal catheter drainages and aspirations for management of pelvic fluid collections: technique, technical success rates, and outcomes in 150 patients. Abdom Radiol (NY). 2019;44:2582–93. https://doi.org/10.1007/s00261-019-01974-9.
4. Blumetti J, Chaudhry V, Prasad L, Abcarian H. Delayed transanal repair of persistent coloanal anastomotic leak in diverted patients after resection for rectal cancer. Color Dis. 2012;14:1238–41. https://doi.org/10.1111/j.1463-1318.2012.02932.x.
5. Borstlap WAA, Musters GD, LPS S, et al. Vacuum-assisted early transanal closure of leaking low colorectal anastomoses: the CLEAN study. Surg Endosc. 2018;32:315–27. https://doi.org/10.1007/s00464-017-5679-6.
6. Borstlap WAA, Westerduin E, Aukema TS, et al. Anastomotic leakage and chronic presacral sinus formation after low anterior resection: results from a large cross-sectional study. Ann Surg. 2017;266:870–7. https://doi.org/10.1097/SLA.0000000000002429.
7. Braley SC, Schneider PD, Bold RJ, et al. Controlled tamponade of severe presacral venous hemorrhage: use of a breast implant sizer. Dis Colon Rectum. 2002;45:140–2. https://doi.org/10.1007/s10350-004-6130-3.
8. Braunschmid T, Hartig N, Baumann L, et al. Influence of multiple stapler firings used for rectal division on colorectal anastomotic leak rate. Surg Endosc. 2017;31:5318–26. https://doi.org/10.1007/s00464-017-5611-0.
9. Brehant O, Hanes A, Fuks D, et al. Stapled marsupialisation of chronic low rectal anastomotic sinuses. Int J Color Dis. 2009;24:1233–7. https://doi.org/10.1007/s00384-009-0780-5.
10. Brown CJ, Fenech D, McLeod RS. Reconstructive techniques after rectal resection for rectal cancer. Cochrane Database Syst Rev. 2008, 2008;(2):CD006040. https://doi.org/10.1002/14651858.CD006040.pub2.
11. Butch RJ, Mueller PR, Ferrucci JT, et al. Drainage of pelvic abscesses through the greater sciatic foramen. Radiology. 1986;158:487–91. https://doi.org/10.1148/radiology.158.2.3941878.
12. Cabellos Olivares M, Labalde Martínez M, Torralba M, et al. C-reactive protein as a marker of the surgical stress reduction within an ERAS protocol (Enhanced recovery after surgery) in colorectal surgery: a prospective cohort study. J Surg Oncol. 2018;117:717–24. https://doi.org/10.1002/jso.24909.
13. Calmels M, Collard MK, O'Connell L, et al. Redo-surgery after failed colorectal or coloanal anastomosis: morbidity, mortality and factors predictive of success. A retrospective study of 200 patients. Color Dis. 2022;24:511–9. https://doi.org/10.1111/codi.16025.
14. Casal Núñez JE, Vigorita V, Ruano Poblador A, et al. Presacral venous bleeding during mobilization in rectal cancer. World J Gastroenterol. 2017;23:1712–9. https://doi.org/10.3748/wjg.v23.i9.1712.
15. Chorti A, Stavrou G, Stelmach V, et al. Endoscopic repair of anastomotic leakage after low anterior resection for rectal cancer: a systematic review. Asian J Endosc Surg. 2020;13:141–6. https://doi.org/10.1111/ases.12733.
16. De Nardi P, Elmore U, Maggi G, et al. Intraoperative angiography with indocyanine green to assess anastomosis perfusion in patients undergoing laparoscopic colorectal resection: results of a multicenter randomized controlled trial. Surg Endosc. 2020;34:53–60. https://doi.org/10.1007/s00464-019-06730-0.
17. Dhindsa BS, Naga Y, Saghir SM, et al. Endo-sponge in management of anastomotic colorectal leaks: a systematic review and meta-analysis. Endosc Int Open. 2021;9:E1342–9. https://doi.org/10.1055/a-1490-8783.
18. Emile SH, Garoufalia Z, Barsom S, et al. Systematic review and meta-analysis of randomized clinical trials

on the treatment of low anterior resection syndrome. Surgery. 2023;173:1352–8. https://doi.org/10.1016/j.surg.2023.02.010.
19. Emmertsen KJ, Laurberg S. Low anterior resection syndrome score: development and validation of a symptom-based scoring system for bowel dysfunction after low anterior resection for rectal cancer. Ann Surg. 2012;255:922–8. https://doi.org/10.1097/SLA.0b013e31824f1c21.
20. Garcia-Granero A, Sánchez-Guillén L, Carreño O, et al. Importance of the Moskowitz artery in the laparoscopic medial approach to splenic flexure mobilization: a cadaveric study. Tech Coloproctol. 2017;21:567–72. https://doi.org/10.1007/s10151-017-1663-3.
21. Gee MS, Kim JY, Gervais DA, et al. Management of abdominal and pelvic abscesses that persist despite satisfactory percutaneous drainage catheter placement. AJR Am J Roentgenol. 2010;194:815–20. https://doi.org/10.2214/AJR.09.3282.
22. Ha GW, Kim JH, Lee MR. Oncologic impact of anastomotic leakage following colorectal cancer surgery: a systematic review and meta-analysis. Ann Surg Oncol. 2017;24:3289–99. https://doi.org/10.1245/s10434-017-5881-8.
23. Harisinghani MG, Gervais DA, Maher MM, et al. Transgluteal approach for percutaneous drainage of deep pelvic abscesses: 154 cases. Radiology. 2003;228:701–5. https://doi.org/10.1148/radiol.2283020924.
24. Harrison JL, Hooks VH, Pearl RK, et al. Muscle fragment welding for control of massive presacral bleeding during rectal mobilization: a review of eight cases. Dis Colon Rectum. 2003;46:1115–7. https://doi.org/10.1007/s10350-004-7289-3.
25. He S, Zhang J, Wang R, et al. Impact of long-course neoadjuvant radiation on postoperative low anterior resection syndrome and stoma status in rectal cancer: long-term functional follow-up of a randomized clinical trial. BJS Open. 2022;6:zrac127. https://doi.org/10.1093/bjsopen/zrac127.
26. Huang Y, Koh CE. Sacral nerve stimulation for bowel dysfunction following low anterior resection: a systematic review and meta-analysis. Color Dis. 2019;21:1240–8. https://doi.org/10.1111/codi.14690.
27. Hüttner FJ, Tenckhoff S, Jensen K, et al. Meta-analysis of reconstruction techniques after low anterior resection for rectal cancer. Br J Surg. 2015;102:735–45. https://doi.org/10.1002/bjs.9782.
28. Jafari MD, Pigazzi A, McLemore EC, et al. Perfusion Assessment in Left-Sided/Low Anterior Resection (PILLAR III): a randomized, controlled, parallel, multicenter study assessing perfusion outcomes with PINPOINT near-infrared fluorescence imaging in low anterior resection. Dis Colon Rectum. 2021;64:995–1002. https://doi.org/10.1097/DCR.0000000000002007.
29. Jain D, Sandhu N, Singhal S. Endoscopic electrocautery incision therapy for benign lower gastrointestinal tract anastomotic strictures. Ann Gastroenterol. 2017;30:473–85. https://doi.org/10.20524/aog.2017.0163.
30. Jutesten H, Buchwald PL, Angenete E, et al. High risk of low anterior resection syndrome in long-term follow-up after anastomotic leakage in anterior resection for rectal cancer. Dis Colon Rectum. 2022;65:1264–73. https://doi.org/10.1097/DCR.0000000000002334.
31. Kamal T, Pai A, Velchuru VR, et al. Should anastomotic assessment with flexible sigmoidoscopy be routine following laparoscopic restorative left colorectal resection? Color Dis. 2015;17:160–4. https://doi.org/10.1111/codi.12809.
32. Karatay E, Javadov M. The importance of the Moskowitz artery as a lesser-known collateral pathway in the medial laparoscopic approach to splenic flexure mobilisation and its evaluation with preoperative computed tomography. Wideochir Inne Tech Maloinwazyjne. 2021;16:305–11. https://doi.org/10.5114/wiitm.2020.100826.
33. Keane C, Sharma P, Yuan L, et al. Impact of temporary ileostomy on long-term quality of life and bowel function: a systematic review and meta-analysis. ANZ J Surg. 2020;90:687–92. https://doi.org/10.1111/ans.15552.
34. Kirat HT, Remzi FH, Shen B, Kiran RP. Pelvic abscess associated with anastomotic leak in patients with ileal pouch-anal anastomosis (IPAA): transanastomotic or CT-guided drainage? Int J Color Dis. 2011;26:1469–74. https://doi.org/10.1007/s00384-011-1272-y.
35. Lamazza A, Fiori E, Sterpetti AV, et al. Self-expandable metal stents in the treatment of benign anastomotic stricture after rectal resection for cancer. Color Dis. 2014;16:O150–3. https://doi.org/10.1111/codi.12488.
36. Lavryk OA, Bandi B, Shawki SF, et al. Turnbull-Cutait abdominoperineal pull-through operation: the Cleveland Clinic experience in the 21st century. Color Dis. 2022;24:1184–91. https://doi.org/10.1111/codi.16163.
37. Malik AH, East JE, Buchanan GN, Kennedy RH. Endoscopic haemostasis of staple-line haemorrhage following colorectal resection. Color Dis. 2008;10:616–8. https://doi.org/10.1111/j.1463-1318.2007.01459.x.
38. Meyer J, Naiken S, Christou N, et al. Reducing anastomotic leak in colorectal surgery: the old dogmas and the new challenges. World J Gastroenterol. 2019;25:5017–25. https://doi.org/10.3748/wjg.v25.i34.5017.
39. Moszkowicz D, Alsaid B, Bessede T, et al. Where does pelvic nerve injury occur during rectal surgery for cancer? Color Dis. 2011;13:1326–34. https://doi.org/10.1111/j.1463-1318.2010.02384.x.
40. Ng X, Chiou W, Chang S. Controlling a presacral hemorrhage by using a saline bag: report of a case. Dis Colon Rectum. 2008;51:972–4. https://doi.org/10.1007/s10350-007-9189-9.

41. Phitayakorn R, Delaney CP, Reynolds HL, et al. Standardized algorithms for management of anastomotic leaks and related abdominal and pelvic abscesses after colorectal surgery. World J Surg. 2008;32:1147–56. https://doi.org/10.1007/s00268-008-9468-1.
42. Picazo-Ferrera K, Jaurrieta-Rico C, Manzano-Robleda M, et al. Risk factors and endoscopic treatment for anastomotic stricture after resection in patients with colorectal cancer. Rev Gastroenterol Mex (Engl Ed). 2021;86:44–50. https://doi.org/10.1016/j.rgmx.2020.03.001.
43. Rahbari NN, Weitz J, Hohenberger W, et al. Definition and grading of anastomotic leakage following anterior resection of the rectum: a proposal by the International Study Group of Rectal Cancer. Surgery. 2010;147:339–51. https://doi.org/10.1016/j.surg.2009.10.012.
44. Remzi FH, Oncel M, Fazio VW. Muscle tamponade to control presacral venous bleeding: report of two cases. Dis Colon Rectum. 2002;45:1109–11. https://doi.org/10.1007/s10350-004-6369-8.
45. Ricciardi R, Roberts PL, Marcello PW, et al. Anastomotic leak testing after colorectal resection: what are the data? Arch Surg. 2009;144:407–11; discussion 411–412. https://doi.org/10.1001/archsurg.2009.43.
46. Rondelli F, Pasculli A, De Rosa M, et al. Is routine splenic flexure mobilization always necessary in laparotomic or laparoscopic anterior rectal resection? A systematic review and comprehensive meta-analysis. Updat Surg. 2021;73:1643–61. https://doi.org/10.1007/s13304-021-01135-y.
47. Rosen HR, Kneist W, Fürst A, et al. Randomized clinical trial of prophylactic transanal irrigation versus supportive therapy to prevent symptoms of low anterior resection syndrome after rectal resection. BJS Open. 2019;3:461–5. https://doi.org/10.1002/bjs5.50160.
48. Singh A, Kishore R, Saxena SS. Ligating internal iliac artery: success beyond hesitation. J Obstet Gynaecol India. 2016;66:235–41. https://doi.org/10.1007/s13224-016-0859-1.
49. Sirois-Giguère E, Boulanger-Gobeil C, Bouchard A, et al. Transanal drainage to treat anastomotic leaks after low anterior resection for rectal cancer: a valuable option. Dis Colon Rectum. 2013;56:586–92. https://doi.org/10.1097/DCR.0b013e31827687a4.
50. Sturiale A, Martellucci J, Zurli L, et al. Long-term functional follow-up after anterior rectal resection for cancer. Int J Color Dis. 2017;32:83–8. https://doi.org/10.1007/s00384-016-2659-6.
51. Sun R, Dai Z, Zhang Y, et al. The incidence and risk factors of low anterior resection syndrome (LARS) after sphincter-preserving surgery of rectal cancer: a systematic review and meta-analysis. Support Care Cancer. 2021;29:7249–58. https://doi.org/10.1007/s00520-021-06326-2.
52. Toh JWT, Matthews R, Kim S-H. Arc of Riolan-preserving splenic flexure takedown during anterior resection: potentially critical to prevent acute anastomotic ischemia. Dis Colon Rectum. 2018;61:411–4. https://doi.org/10.1097/DCR.0000000000000995.
53. van Doesburg IAJ, Boerma D, Bollen TL, et al. Large gluteal abscesses as a complication of transgluteal drainage of pelvic abscesses: analysis of three cases and a search of the literature. Dig Surg. 2009;26:329–32. https://doi.org/10.1159/000235821.
54. Vargas HD, Margolin DA . Anastomotic construction. ASCRS textbook of colon and rectal surgery, 2022. ASCRS U, www.ascrsu.com/ascrs/view/ASCRS-Textbook-of-Colon-and-Rectal-Surgery/2285072/all/Anastomotic_Construction.
55. Vignali A, Fazio VW, Lavery IC, et al. Factors associated with the occurrence of leaks in stapled rectal anastomoses: a review of 1,014 patients. J Am Coll Surg. 1997;185:105–13. https://doi.org/10.1016/s1072-7515(97)00018-5.
56. Wang QY, Shi WJ, Zhao YR, et al. New concepts in severe presacral hemorrhage during proctectomy. Arch Surg. 1985;120:1013–20. https://doi.org/10.1001/archsurg.1985.01390330025005.
57. Weidenhagen R, Gruetzner KU, Wiecken T, et al. Endoscopic vacuum-assisted closure of anastomotic leakage following anterior resection of the rectum: a new method. Surg Endosc. 2008;22:1818–25. https://doi.org/10.1007/s00464-007-9706-x.
58. Wells CI, Vather R, Chu MJJ, et al. Anterior resection syndrome—a risk factor analysis. J Gastrointest Surg. 2015;19:350–9. https://doi.org/10.1007/s11605-014-2679-x.
59. Westerduin E, Klaver CEL, van Geloven AAW, et al. Outcome after redo surgery for complicated colorectal and coloanal anastomosis: a systematic review. Dis Colon Rectum. 2018;61:988–98. https://doi.org/10.1097/DCR.0000000000001129.
60. Whitlow CB, Opelka FG, Gathright JB, Beck DE. Treatment of colorectal and ileoanal anastomotic sinuses. Dis Colon Rectum. 1997;40:760–3. https://doi.org/10.1007/BF02055427.
61. Wu Z, van de Haar RCJ, Sparreboom CL, et al. Is the intraoperative air leak test effective in the prevention of colorectal anastomotic leakage? A systematic review and meta-analysis. Int J Color Dis. 2016;31:1409–17. https://doi.org/10.1007/s00384-016-2616-4.
62. Yeung DE, Peterknecht E, Hajibandeh S, et al. C-reactive protein can predict anastomotic leak in colorectal surgery: a systematic review and meta-analysis. Int J Color Dis. 2021;36:1147–62. https://doi.org/10.1007/s00384-021-03854-5.
63. Zhou W, Xia L, Wang Z, et al. Transanal minimally invasive surgery for rectal anastomotic stenosis after colorectal cancer surgery. Dis Colon Rectum. 2022;65:1062–8. https://doi.org/10.1097/DCR.0000000000002361.
64. Zhu X-M, Yu G-Y, Zheng N-X, et al. Review of Denonvilliers' fascia: the controversies and consensuses. Gastroenterol Rep (Oxf). 2020;8:343–8. https://doi.org/10.1093/gastro/goaa053.

37 Pelvic Radiation Therapy

Sudha Amarnath

Introduction

Radiation therapy is used frequently in the treatment of female pelvic malignancies, including gynecologic, colorectal, and urologic cancers to help improve local control and/or survival. Radiation to the pelvis can be delivered using external beam or brachytherapy techniques and can be used in several different settings, often in combination with pelvic surgery. The most common uses of radiation include (1) Definitive treatment of cancer (e.g., locally advanced cervical cancer, medically inoperable endometrial cancer, rectal cancer in the era watch and wait), (2) Preoperative or neoadjuvant therapy for downstaging of a tumor to facilitate R0 resection and to sterilize microscopic disease (e.g., locally advanced rectal cancer, FIGO stage IIIB endometrial cancer), and (3) Postoperative or adjuvant therapy to sterilize microscopic or gross residual disease after surgery (e.g., FIGO stage III/IVA endometrial cancer, node-positive cervix cancer after radical hysterectomy). When radiotherapy is sequenced with surgery, the surgical team must be aware of the acute and late toxicities of radiation treatment and the implications these may have on their operation and the risk of peri-operative complications. This chapter describes the major potential toxicities of pelvic radiation therapy, acute and late, by organ site. Strong communication between the radiation oncology and surgical teams can help facilitate optimal timing of treatments and management of complications.

A Brief Primer on Radiation Therapy

External Beam Radiation Therapy

External beam radiation therapy (EBRT) most typically involves using a linear accelerator to deliver high-energy photons/x-rays to tissues in the body. The photons interact with electrons and water molecules to create free radicals that can directly or indirectly damage the DNA of cells. Biologically, cancer cells have less intact repair mechanisms to repair the DNA damage, and thus cancer cells die or become senescent, whereas surrounding normal tissue cells are better able to repair damage and can heal over time. Unfortunately, because the radiation beams must pass through normal tissues to get to the areas at risk (Fig. 37.1), inflammation and acute damage of surrounding normal tissues are common during and after treatment and are responsible for many of the acute side effects of radiation treatment. Weeks to months after completion of radiation, some patients may develop chronic late toxicities primarily related to scarring (e.g., fibro-

S. Amarnath (✉)
Department of Radiation Oncology, Cleveland Clinic Foundation, Cleveland, OH, USA

M. Hoffman et al. (eds.), *Major Complications of Female Pelvic Surgery*,
https://doi.org/10.1007/978-3-031-66772-5_37

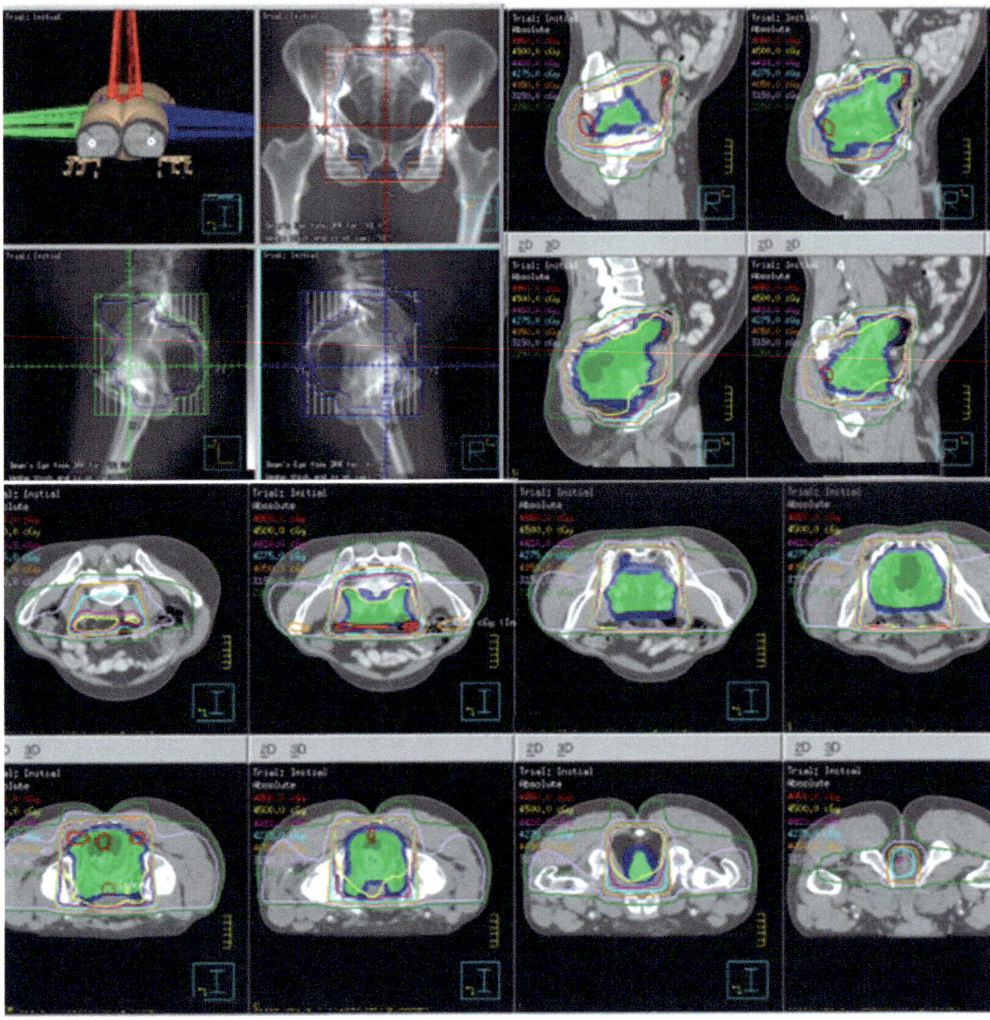

Fig. 37.1 An example pelvic radiotherapy plan using 3D-conformal radiation therapy to 45 Gy in 25 fractions

sis, stenosis), chronic inflammation (e.g., radiation proctitis/cystitis), or even tissue breakdown (e.g., ulceration, fistulae) [1]. Many of the side effects of external beam radiation therapy are dose-dependent and typically, the risk of toxicity increases with increasing doses of radiation. Modern radiation treatment planning techniques can help to reduce the risks of many toxicities but do not completely eliminate the risk of damage.

Brachytherapy

Brachytherapy is a specialized form of radiation where a radioactive source (typically Iridium-192 for gynecologic applications) is applied directly to a tumor or tissue at risk. An advantage of brachytherapy is that a smaller amount of normal tissue is exposed to radiation during the treatment, which allows for dose escalation to tumors for improved local control without as much toxicity risk to surrounding normal tissues. The disadvantage of brachytherapy is that it involves using applicators that are placed directly into tissues at risk (e.g., vagina, cervix/uterus, rectum), which requires a more invasive procedure for the patient. The side effects of brachytherapy can be similar to EBRT but are typically limited to smaller amounts of normal tissue.

Radiotherapy Toxicity

The side effects of radiation therapy are typically divided into three separate time points, acute, sub-acute, and late. Acute side effects occur during or within a few weeks of completing treatment and are typically caused by inflammation and the death of rapidly proliferating cells in normal tissue cells. Sub-acute side effects typically occur 4–12 weeks after treatment and represent prolonged recovery from acute effects. Late effects may occur months to years after treatment and can include fibrosis, vascular injury, and other gradual changes in more slowly dividing tissues. Late effects may be irreversible and may lead to end-organ damage. Any patient who receives radiation treatment is at risk for the development of a secondary malignancy due to residual DNA damage. This is a rare effect of treatment that, if it occurs, is most often seen approximately 10–20 years after treatment [2].

Several factors can influence the risk of radiation toxicity incidence and severity. These include radiation treatment factors such as the total dose of radiation prescribed, dose per fraction, treatment schedule, volume of normal tissue exposed, and number of years since prior radiation treatment (in the setting of re-irradiation). Patient factors can also influence the risk of toxicity such as smoking (a significant predictor for late bowel and bladder complications and can also decrease the efficacy of treatment) [3], and vascular disorders such as diabetes and hypertension (increases risk of effects from vascular injury and impacts wound healing) [4, 5]. Obesity, low body mass index, active collagen vascular disease, and inflammatory bowel disease may also increase the risk of acute and late toxicities [5–8].

Toxicities by System

Bladder/Ureters/Urethra

Background

Radiation-induced bladder and urinary acute effects are typically caused by inflammation and epithelial damage that leads to symptoms of dysuria, urgency, and increased frequency. Late toxicities are primarily due to epithelial and microvascular changes mediated by fibrosis that can lead to loss of compliance and capacity in the bladder and ureteral and/or urethral stenosis, as well as bleeding (radiation-induced hemorrhagic cystitis), and fistulae. Late effects typically arise 1–3 years after radiation treatment and are typically less common than late GI effects [9–12].

Possible Effects

- Acute: Urinary frequency, urgency, dysuria.
- Late: Radiation cystitis leading to bleeding, bladder dysfunction, ureteral/urethral stenosis/strictures, fistulae.

Prevention

Bladder toxicity can be minimized with proper radiation planning and delivery techniques to decrease the volume of GU structures that are irradiated, as well as decrease the volume of GU tissues that receive high doses (e.g., treating with full or empty bladder depending on clinical scenario, IMRT) [13].

Recognition

Patients typically present with signs/symptoms consistent with the toxicities listed above.

Management

Acute side effects from pelvic XRT can typically be managed with supportive care with medications as needed: dysuria (rule out urinary tract infection, then cranberry, pyridium) and urgency/frequency (e.g., oxybutynin, mirabegron). Late side effects should typically be managed conservatively with fluids, blood transfusions (as needed), and bladder irrigation to remove clots. Intravesical formalin and argon plasma coagulation can be tried at the time of cystoscopy. In more refractory cases, Botox injection and hyperbaric oxygen may be helpful [14, 15]. Surgical intervention is rarely indicated but may be helpful for urinary diversion in patients with vesicovaginal fistulae. Ureteral/urethral dilation, ureteral stent placement, urethrotomy, or open surgery may be necessary for ureteral and urethral stenosis and strictures [1].

Small Bowel

Background

The small bowel is the tissue most susceptible to damage within the pelvis during pelvic XRT. Although both the small and large bowel are at risk for toxicity, the small bowel is more vulnerable to damage due to its high epithelial mitotic rate, which leads to more acute side effects. The acute injury can progress to focal ischemia and fibrosis, which can lead to late effects of ulcers, strictures, obstruction, and bleeding [1]. The use of concurrent chemotherapy with radiation, such as 5-FU or capecitabine (frequently used in the treatment of GI cancers), can exacerbate these effects and cause enteritis of their own accord [16]. Patients over the age of 60 are at increased risk of small bowel obstruction or perforation [17]. Diabetes, atherosclerosis, IBD, and prior abdominal surgery can also increase the risk of toxicity.

Possible Effects

- Acute*:* diarrhea, bowel cramping, bloating, increased gas.
- Late*:* radiation enteritis, malabsorption, small bowel obstruction, bowel necrosis.

Prevention

Radiation effects on the small bowel can be decreased in some patients with appropriate treatment setup (full bladder, prone positioning with belly board). If postoperative pelvic XRT is planned or expected, mesh, omental, or other flaps can be used in the appropriate circumstance to help minimize the amount of small bowel in the pelvis [18, 19].

Recognition

Patients will typically present with signs or symptoms of the effects listed above. Bowel wall can be thickened and edematous on imaging.

Management

Patients are typically managed conservatively in the acute setting with fluids, anti-diarrheal agents (loperamide, diphenoxylate/atropine, tincture of opium), and other supportive medications (simethicone, dicyclomine). If the diarrhea is very severe, patients may require inpatient admission for supportive care and, in rare circumstances, may require the use of total parenteral nutrition (TPN). Late effects may also be managed conservatively with the supportive medications listed above but may require surgical intervention for small bowel obstructions and bowel necrosis. Patients with malabsorption may require vitamin replacement (esp. vitamin B12) or bile salt replacement [20].

Colon/Rectum

Background

Radiation toxicity in the large bowel/rectum is due to a similar mechanism of action as damage to the small bowel. Mucosal atrophy and loss of mucin-producing goblet cells contribute to possible late toxicities of treatment. Vascular sclerosis can lead to mucosal telangiectasias or ulceration more commonly in the colon and rectum than in the small bowel [5, 21].

Possible Effects

- Acute: Diarrhea, increased urgency/frequency, increased gas, mucositis → tenesmus and pain, cramping, hemorrhoidal irritation.
- Late*:* Radiation proctitis leading to changes in bowel habits, bleeding, ulceration, fistulae.

Prevention

Modern XRT treatment planning (intensity modulated radiation therapy-IMRT) can help avoid high doses to the rectum when it is not necessary for treatment (e.g., many gynecologic cancers, prostate cancers). Hydrogel spacers can help minimize rectal dose in the appropriate patient [13].

Recognition

Patients often present with diarrhea or bright red blood per rectum. Radiation proctitis can also be recognized on endoscopic exams (Fig. 37.2).

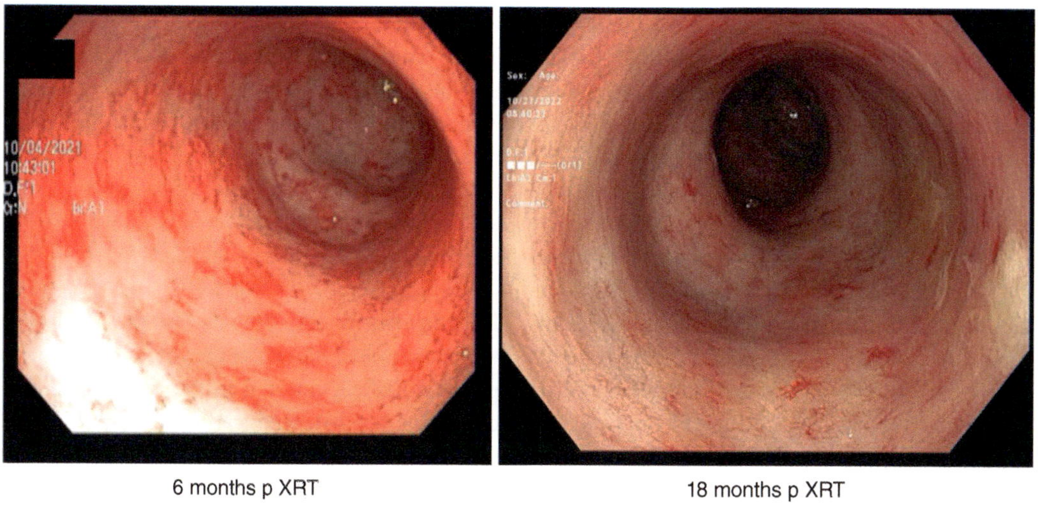

Fig. 37.2 Endoscopic images of radiation proctitis (6 months and 18 months after pelvic radiotherapy)

Management

Diarrhea is managed with fluids and anti-diarrheal agents as noted in small bowel section above. Hemorrhoids are managed conservatively with topical ointments. Symptomatic late radiation proctitis can be managed with enemas (sucralfate, hydrocortisone, and rebamipide can help protect injured mucosa) or with topical formalin or argon plasma coagulation (APC) at the time of colonoscopy [19]. Hyperbaric oxygen therapy may be helpful in more refractory cases [14, 22]. Diverting ostomy may be necessary in patients with recto-vaginal fistulas due to tumor or treatment.

Anus/Vulva/Skin

Background

The anus, anal margin, and vulvar are tissues that are susceptible to the acute and late effects of radiation primarily due to injury of the epithelial and deeper dermal layers of the skin and mucosa. Smoking, diabetes, and peripheral vascular disease can increase the risk of skin toxicity and impair long-term healing [1]. Scleroderma patients can also suffer from increased fibrosis and skin toxicity with radiation treatment. Obesity can increase the risk of toxicity due to higher doses of radiation delivered due to overlapping skin folds (i.e. pannus).

Possible Effects

- Acute*:* pain, itching, yeast infections. Radiation dermatitis (dryness, redness, desquamation).
- Late*:* Sphincter dysfunction, incontinence, stenosis, labial adhesions, dyspareunia, sexual dysfunction, scarring, fibrosis, hyperpigmentation, pain.

Prevention

Skin sparing can be achieved in most cases with modern radiation technology. When the anus, vulva, or groins must be targeted, using a frog leg setup can help minimize skin folds to decrease radiation dermatitis to the upper legs.

Recognition

Radiation dermatitis typically progresses from dry skin (often with associated itching) to redness/hyperpigmentation, and then peeling of the epithelial and dermal layers. This is often extremely painful.

Management

Skin toxicity is managed primarily with topical creams and ointments. Water/petroleum-based products can help provide a moisture barrier for healing and are safe for use during treatment. Aloe vera, witch hazel, topical anesthetics, and Sitz baths can also provide symptomatic relief. Zinc oxide and silver sulfadizene may be helpful after treatment [23]. Patients with non-healing ulcers should be referred to wound care specialists and may benefit from HBOT [22, 24]. Radiation fibrosis can be challenging to manage but can sometimes be treated with massage, oral pentoxifylline, and vitamin E [25, 26]. Patients with anal or vulvar adhesions or stenosis should be referred to colorectal surgery and urogynecology respectively.

Uterus

Background

Damage to the uterus from pelvic XRT is primarily due to late fibrosis causing decreased growth and compliance, as well as microvascular changes and arteriolar damage that leads to decreased fetoplacental blood flow [1]. These changes are dose-dependent—patients receiving lower doses of pelvic radiation may be able to carry a future pregnancy with increased risks; patients receiving more standard dosing of 45–50 Gy of XRT are unlikely to be able to carry a future pregnancy and typically will require a gestational carrier [27].

Possible Effects

- Acute*:* cramping with brachytherapy procedures.
- Late: altered blood flow and fibrosis → infertility/inability to carry a pregnancy, miscarriage, preterm labor, low birth weight, and placenta accreta.

Prevention

At this time, there are very few options to prevent radiation dosing to the uterus given its central pelvic location. Uterine transposition (moving the uterus with its associated blood supply out of the pelvis during radiation) is considered experimental [28].

Recognition

There are typically no symptoms associated with uterine late effects from radiation. If a patient has a history of prior pelvic XRT and is interested in pregnancy, they should be referred to reproductive endocrinology and infertility (REI) specialists and maternal-fetal medicine (MFM) specialists to help discuss options.

Management

Patients should be counselled on risks prior to pelvic XRT and referred to the appropriate specialists as needed. Referral to behavioral health specialists may also be beneficial for appropriate patients.

Ovaries

Background

The ovaries are exquisitely sensitive to radiation and loss of 50% of oocytes is seen at doses as low as 2–4 Gy. Long-term ovarian shutdown is both age and dose-dependent but is expected in women of all ages with more standard pelvic dosing used for pelvic malignancies (45–50 Gy) [29, 30].

Possible Effects

- Acute: none.
- Late*:* infertility, premature ovarian insufficiency (POI) → impact on cardiovascular, mental, neurologic, vaginal, and musculoskeletal health.

Prevention

Patients should be referred to REI prior to initiating pelvic XRT to discuss possible cryopreservation of embryos, oocytes, or ovarian tissue [29]. Laparoscopic ovarian transposition (moving the ovary (ies) with vascular pedicle outside the pelvis) is also a good option for well-selected patients under the age of 40 and may be performed at the time of other surgeries (i.e. nodal debulking/sampling). Ideally, ovaries should be transposed as high and lateral as possible in the abdomen and a minimum of 3 cm from the edge of the expected radiation treatment field [31].

Recognition

Patients will typically present with symptoms of menopause, including amenorrhea, hot flashes, mood changes, and fatigue. Hormone levels (FSH, E2) should be checked to assess for POI.

Management

Proper counselling and referrals prior to initiating pelvic XRT are of the utmost importance since none of the preventive measures outlined above can be performed after treatment has started. Women experiencing POI should be referred to a Women's Health and behavorial health specialist for discussion of possible hormone replacement therapy (HRT) if under age 40 and possible symptomatic treatment of hot flashes (e.g., venlafaxine, fezolinetant).

Vagina

Background

Vaginal effects from pelvic XRT are similarly due to epithelial and mucosal changes as described for other organs above [32]. These changes may lead to a diminishment of sexual function and quality of life [33].

Possible Effects

- Acute: increased vaginal discharge, mucositis, pain, itching, dryness, yeast infection.
- Late: fibrosis, ulceration, teleangiectasias, stenosis, dryness, discharge, adhesions, dyspareunia, sexual changes/dysfunction.

Prevention

Although prospective data is limited, national and international guidelines recommend the use of vaginal dilators to help mitigate the late adverse effects of radiation on the vaginal. Dilators help decrease adhesions and maintain the elasticity of the tissue. Lubrication with coconut oil or other vaginal moisturizers should be used to help with vaginal dryness [34].

Recognition

Patients may notice vaginal pain, dryness, dyspareunia, and/or vaginismus. Adhesions, loss of elasticity, vascular changes, and dryness after radiation may be appreciated on pelvic examination.

Management

Vaginal dilators per above. Appropriate patients may benefit from topical estrogen creams. Referral to urogynecology for dilation and surgical management of adhesions may be appropriate. Sexual health and behavioral health specialists may also be helpful [35]. Vitamin E, pentoxifylline, and hyperbaric oxygen may be appropriate for soft tissue necrosis of the vagina [22, 24–26]. Fistulas that develop between the vagina and bladder or vagina and rectum typically require surgical diversion and management.

Vascular/Lymphatics/Nerves

Background

Radiation may also have long-term effects on the vascularity of the pelvis (as noted in multiple organ systems above) that may also impair wound healing and lead to wound healing complications [1, 36]. Fibrosis of the lymphatic tissues (especially with groin irradiation) can lead to lymphedema of the legs. The nerves are quite resistant to radiation damage, but with higher doses of radiation (often seen with stereotactic body radiotherapy-SBRT, re-irradiation, or intraoperative radiotherapy-IORT), damage to the peripheral nerves is possible.

Possible Effects

- Acute: impaired blood flow → wound healing delays.
- Late: impaired blood flow → wound healing delays, lymphedema, peripheral neuropathy (numbness, tingling, pain).

Prevention

Accurate contouring and delineation of the nerves and the use of IMRT techniques may help reduce high-dose radiation to peripheral nerves.

Appropriate IORT dosing can also help reduce the risk of peripheral neuropathy.

Recognition

Patients may present with delayed wound healing or wound healing complications, leg swelling, numbness, tingling, or pain in a pelvic nerve distribution.

Management

Wound healing issues may need a referral for specialized wound care or plastic surgery. HBOT may also be helpful in appropriately selecting patients [37]. Patients at high risk for lymphedema should be referred to lymphedema physical therapy early for compression stocking fitting, massage, and other mitigation techniques [38]. Peripheral neuropathy may require management with medications that help with neuropathic pain.

References

1. Nicholas S, Chen L, Choflet A, Fader A, Guss Z, Hazell S, et al. Pelvic radiation and normal tissue toxicity. Semin Radiat Oncol. 2017;27(4):358–69.
2. Bentzen SM. Preventing or reducing late side effects of radiation therapy: radiobiology meets molecular pathology. Nat Rev Cancer. 2006;6(9):702–13.
3. Eifel PJ, Jhingran A, Bodurka DC, Levenback C, Thames H. Correlation of smoking history and other patient characteristics with major complications of pelvic radiation therapy for cervical cancer. J Clin Oncol. 2002;20(17):3651–7.
4. Maruyama Y, Van Nagell JR, Jr., Utley J, Vider ML, Parker JC. Radiation and small bowel complications in cervical carcinoma therapy. Radiology. 1974;112(3):699–703.
5. van Nagell JR Jr, Parker JC Jr, Maruyama Y, Utley J, Luckett P. Bladder or rectal injury following radiation therapy for cervical cancer. Am J Obstet Gynecol. 1974;119(6):727–32.
6. Mikkelsen TB, Sorensen B, Dieperink KB. Prediction of rehabilitation needs after treatment of cervical cancer: what do late adverse effects tell us? Support Care Cancer. 2017;25(3):823–31.
7. Wo J, Taghian A. Radiotherapy in setting of collagen vascular disease. Int J Radiat Oncol Biol Phys. 2007;69(5):1347–53.
8. Willett CG, Ooi CJ, Zietman AL, Menon V, Goldberg S, Sands BE, et al. Acute and late toxicity of patients with inflammatory bowel disease undergoing irradiation for abdominal and pelvic neoplasms. Int J Radiat Oncol Biol Phys. 2000;46(4):995–8.
9. Chorbinska J, Krajewski W, Zdrojowy R. Urological complications after radiation therapy-nothing ventured, nothing gained: a narrative review. Transl Cancer Res. 2021;10(2):1096–118.
10. Levenback C, Eifel PJ, Burke TW, Morris M, Gershenson DM. Hemorrhagic cystitis following radiotherapy for stage Ib cancer of the cervix. Gynecol Oncol. 1994;55(2):206–10.
11. Marks LB, Carroll PR, Dugan TC, Anscher MS. The response of the urinary bladder, urethra, and ureter to radiation and chemotherapy. Int J Radiat Oncol Biol Phys. 1995;31(5):1257–80.
12. Wit EM, Horenblas S. Urological complications after treatment of cervical cancer. Nat Rev Urol. 2014;11(2):110–7.
13. Zelefsky MJ, Levin EJ, Hunt M, Yamada Y, Shippy AM, Jackson A, et al. Incidence of late rectal and urinary toxicities after three-dimensional conformal radiotherapy and intensity-modulated radiotherapy for localized prostate cancer. Int J Radiat Oncol Biol Phys. 2008;70(4):1124–9.
14. Oscarsson N, Arnell P, Lodding P, Ricksten SE, Seeman-Lodding H. Hyperbaric oxygen treatment in radiation-induced cystitis and proctitis: a prospective cohort study on patient-perceived quality of recovery. Int J Radiat Oncol Biol Phys. 2013;87(4):670–5.
15. Chuang YC, Kim DK, Chiang PH, Chancellor MB. Bladder botulinum toxin A injection can benefit patients with radiation and chemical cystitis. BJU Int. 2008;102(6):704–6.
16. Cafiero F, Gipponi M, Peressini A, Bertoglio S, Lionetto R. Preliminary analysis of a randomized clinical trial of adjuvant postoperative RT vs. postoperative RT plus 5-FU and levamisole in patients with TNM stage II-III resectable rectal cancer. J Surg Oncol. 2000;75(2):80–8.
17. Yamada T, Ishihara S, Kawai M, Itoh Y, Naganawa S, Ikeda M. Analysis of late adverse events and their chronological changes after radiation therapy for cervical cancer. Nagoya J Med Sci. 2018;80(4):487–96.
18. Wang Y, Kong W, Lv N, Li F, Chen J, Jiao S, et al. Incidence of radiation enteritis in cervical cancer patients treated with definitive radiotherapy versus adjuvant radiotherapy. J Cancer Res Ther. 2018;14(Supplement):S120–S4.
19. Shadad AK, Sullivan FJ, Martin JD, Egan LJ. Gastrointestinal radiation injury: prevention and treatment. World J Gastroenterol. 2013;19(2):199–208.
20. Vistad I, Kristensen GB, Fossa SD, Dahl AA, Morkrid L. Intestinal malabsorption in long-term survivors of cervical cancer treated with radiotherapy. Int J Radiat Oncol Biol Phys. 2009;73(4):1141–7.
21. Shejul J, Chopra S, Ranjan N, Mahantshetty U, Mehta S, Patil P, et al. Temporal course of late rectal toxicity & impact of intervention in patients undergoing radiation for cervical cancer. Indian J Med Res. 2021;154(2):375–82.
22. Elad S, Cheng KKF, Lalla RV, Yarom N, Hong C, Logan RM, et al. MASCC/ISOO clinical practice

guidelines for the management of mucositis secondary to cancer therapy. Cancer. 2020;126(19):4423–31.
23. McQuestion M. Evidence-based skin care management in radiation therapy: clinical update. Semin Oncol Nurs. 2011;27(2):e1–17.
24. Williams JA Jr, Clarke D, Dennis WA, Dennis EJ 3rd, Smith ST. The treatment of pelvic soft tissue radiation necrosis with hyperbaric oxygen. Am J Obstet Gynecol. 1992;167(2):412–5; discussion 5–6.
25. Gothard L, Cornes P, Brooker S, Earl J, Glees J, Hall E, et al. Phase II study of vitamin E and pentoxifylline in patients with late side effects of pelvic radiotherapy. Radiother Oncol. 2005;75(3):334–41.
26. Dion MW, Hussey DH, Doornbos JF, Vigliotti AP, Wen BC, Anderson B. Preliminary results of a pilot study of pentoxifylline in the treatment of late radiation soft tissue necrosis. Int J Radiat Oncol Biol Phys. 1990;19(2):401–7.
27. Griffiths MJ, Winship AL, Hutt KJ. Do cancer therapies damage the uterus and compromise fertility? Hum Reprod Update. 2020;26(2):161–73.
28. Baiocchi G, Vieira M, Moretti-Marques R, Mantoan H, Faloppa C, Damasceno RCF, et al. Uterine transposition for gynecological cancers. Int J Gynecol Cancer. 2021;31(3):442–6.
29. Wallace WH, Anderson RA, Irvine DS. Fertility preservation for young patients with cancer: who is at risk and what can be offered? Lancet Oncol. 2005;6(4):209–18.
30. Wallace WH, Thomson AB, Saran F, Kelsey TW. Predicting age of ovarian failure after radiation to a field that includes the ovaries. Int J Radiat Oncol Biol Phys. 2005;62(3):738–44.
31. Morice P, Castaigne D, Haie-Meder C, Pautier P, El Hassan J, Duvillard P, et al. Laparoscopic ovarian transposition for pelvic malignancies: indications and functional outcomes. Fertil Steril. 1998;70(5):956–60.
32. Brand AH, Bull CA, Cakir B. Vaginal stenosis in patients treated with radiotherapy for carcinoma of the cervix. Int J Gynecol Cancer. 2006;16(1):288–93.
33. Flay LD, Matthews JH. The effects of radiotherapy and surgery on the sexual function of women treated for cervical cancer. Int J Radiat Oncol Biol Phys. 1995;31(2):399–404.
34. Damast S, Jeffery DD, Son CH, Hasan Y, Carter J, Lindau ST, et al. Literature review of vaginal stenosis and dilator use in radiation oncology. Pract Radiat Oncol. 2019;9(6):479–91.
35. Denton AS, Maher EJ. Interventions for the physical aspects of sexual dysfunction in women following pelvic radiotherapy. Cochrane Database Syst Rev. 2003;2003(1):CD003750.
36. Viswanathan AN, Lee LJ, Eswara JR, Horowitz NS, Konstantinopoulos PA, Mirabeau-Beale KL, et al. Complications of pelvic radiation in patients treated for gynecologic malignancies. Cancer. 2014;120(24):3870–83.
37. Moen I, Stuhr LE. Hyperbaric oxygen therapy and cancer—a review. Target Oncol. 2012;7(4):233–42.
38. Warren AG, Brorson H, Borud LJ, Slavin SA. Lymphedema: a comprehensive review. Ann Plast Surg. 2007;59(4):464–72.

38 Pelvic Exenteration for Central Pelvic Cancer

Desmond P. Barton, Owen M. Heath, Rasheed Shahnawaz, Qiu Sheng, Thompson Alan, and Kumar Pardeep

Introduction

Pelvic exenteration (PEx) was first described by Brunschwig in 1948 as a palliative procedure. He published on extended radical surgery for locally advanced gynaecological cancer (mainly primary and recurrent cervical cancer) where less radical surgery and/or radiation therapy had failed [1]. There was significant mortality and morbidity in his series, albeit 75 years ago. Most PEx are now performed with curative intent. To achieve cure there must be 1) no metastatic disease outside the operative field and 2) negative margins [2–4].

More extensive and longer operations are associated with increased morbidity [5]. Higher volume centres/surgical teams performing PEx have lower costs and intensive care usage [6]. During long-term follow-up, the postoperative complications and quality of life (QoL) can change. Obesity in the surgical population is an important confounding factor [7]. The impact of early postoperative complications include prolongation of hospital stay, delayed recovery, compromised QoL (which may not improve), increased costs and compromised survival [8].

Palliative exenteration is associated with increased morbidity and mortality, such that many question its role [9, 10]. As pelvic exenteration is associated with significant morbidity and mortality, case selection for such surgery with palliative intent is critical to avoid surgery-associated deterioration in QoL.

For gynaecological cancers, the most common indication for exenteration is recurrent cervical cancer following radiation therapy (RT) (Fig. 38.1). Most large surgical oncology centres perform these operations for a range of pelvic cancers. Traditionally pelvic exenteration was considered where there was no involvement of the pelvic sidewall, such as neuro-vascular structures and/or muscles/bone. Although these, so-called laterally extended or "out of the box" operations can be performed for pelvic sidewall recurrent pelvic cancers, their complications are beyond the scope of this article (see Chap. 39).

In colorectal practice, the main indications for PEx are locally advanced or recurrent rectal adenocarcinoma and anal squamous cell carcinoma. PEx is performed when these cancers directly invade adjacent structures or threaten the circumferential resection margin (CRM). PEx are performed where these cancers involve the urogenital organs anteriorly. En bloc sacrectomy can be performed when the cancer invades beyond the TME

D. P. Barton (✉) · O. M. Heath
Department of Gynaecological Oncology, The Royal Marsden Foundation Trust, London, UK
e-mail: desmond.barton@rmh.nhs.uk

R. Shahnawaz · Q. Sheng
Department of Colorectal Surgery, The Royal Marsden Foundation Trust, London, UK

T. Alan · K. Pardeep
Department of Uro-oncology, The Royal Marsden Foundation Trust, London, UK

M. Hoffman et al. (eds.), *Major Complications of Female Pelvic Surgery*,
https://doi.org/10.1007/978-3-031-66772-5_38

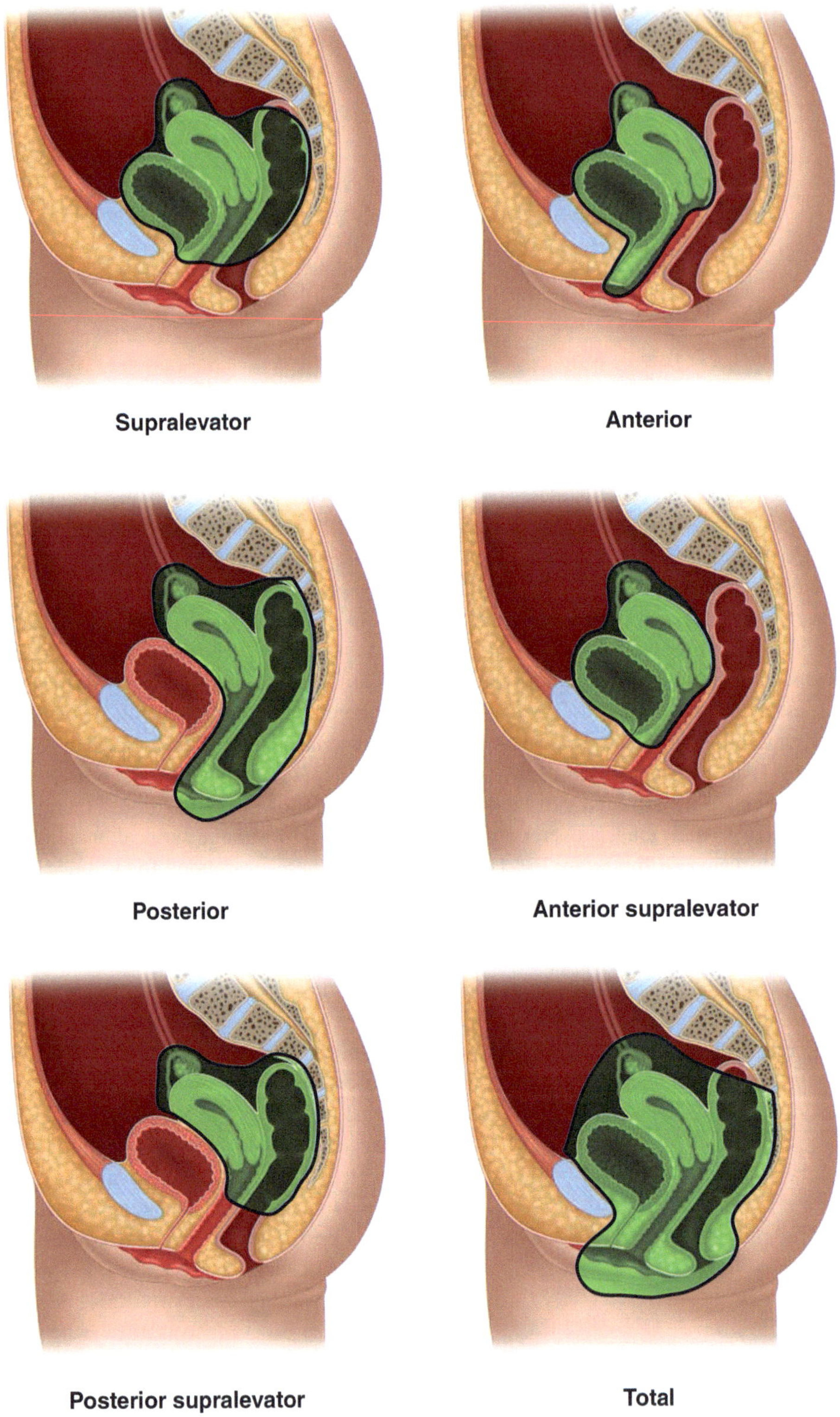

Fig. 38.1 The extent of pelvic exenteration may be individualized in selected cases depending on tumor location, organ function and prior treatment

plane posteriorly to involve the presacral fascia or the sacral cortex [11]. In one report on locally advanced rectal cancer, the perioperative mortality rate for PEx was 1.5%, and the 30-day postoperative major morbidity rate was 37.8%—with the most common being surgical site infection/collection. The 3-year survival rate was 56.4% with an R0 resection [12, 13].

In urological practice, the most common indications for anterior pelvic exenteration in female patients (anterior vagina and uterus in addition to urologic tract resection) are: muscle-invasive transitional cell carcinoma of the bladder (usually preceded by neo-adjuvant chemotherapy), high-grade non-invasive transitional carcinoma following failed intravesical BCG therapy, and as a salvage treatment following failed radiotherapy [14, 15]. It is also used in the treatment of adenocarcinoma or squamous cell carcinoma of the bladder, neither of which are radiosensitive. A less common indication is for selected cases of urethral cancer.

Assessment and Anticipation of Surgical Complications

Pre-Operative Considerations

Ideally, these multidisciplinary operations should be in a high-volume centre where there is co-location of services and the expertise of pathologists and radiologists is essential [12, 13, 17, 18]. The importance of the decision-making process (case selection) is emphasised in most reports on PEx.

Prevention, early recognition and comprehensive treatment of complications is an integral and necessary standard of care. As would be expected, patients with co-morbidities undergoing PEx have poorer outcomes [19–21]. More extensive operations (Fig. 38.1), particularly in the lateral and posterior compartments, are associated with an increased rate of complications (largely neurovascular) [22]. The Charlson comorbidity index, the POSSUM score (Physiological and Operative Severity Score for the enUmeration of Mortality and Morbidity) and other predictive models have been used to predict adverse outcomes, and an age-adjusted scoring system has been validated [23–27].

In anticipation of the consequences (complications) of PEx, the pre-operative period is when risk modification strategies should be implemented [16, 26]. These include:

- Revision of current medications.
- Correction of anaemia.
- Normalization of WBC and platelet counts.
- Pre-habilitation.
- Bowel preparation.
- Patients who have a pelvic fistula or have had urosepsis (with or without the presence of a nephrostomy tube or ureteric stent) are more predisposed to infection and a marked inflammatory response during and after surgery. It is unclear if "prophylactic" antibiotics before surgery reduce the risk or severity of such reactions.
- Consent: This must not be a rushed process. Setting realistic expectations from PEx—in terms of 5-year survival, complications and quality of life—is integral to the consent process.
- Psychological support may be necessary before and after surgery—in the short and the long term. It can be helpful to have other patients who have been through PEx surgery speak with those patients facing PEx [28]. It is also evident that patient expectations from surgery impact patient-reported outcomes [29].
- Multidisciplinary team (MDT) coordination: With comprehensive planning, there should be no surprises on the morning of surgery. There is evidence that patients undergoing PEx for gynecologic cancers are more obese obese and have more comorbidities [30].

Intra-Operative Complications

WHO Checklist

This is not a perfunctory exercise and will include patient identification, equipment checks, availability of blood and blood products and availability of surgeons from other disciplines. An important confirmation for some PEx is the availability of two "scrub teams" for the abdominal and perineal phases, and two sets of equipment including energy devices. There must also be a sufficient number of appropriately trained assistants with the surgical teams.

(a) Anaesthetic considerations
(b) Patient positioning

Most PEx are performed through an extended midline laparotomy and a fixed retraction system is used to keep the abdominal wall retracted. Prolonged retraction can traumatise the inferior epigastric pedicle, which is essential for the reconstruction of the pelvic floor/perineum using the rectus abdominis flap.

For laparoscopic and robotically assisted PEx the problems of prolonged "head-down" position and prolonged increased intraperitoneal pressure, include the compartment syndrome being more common [31]. During the procedure, the patient is periodically taken out of this position.

(c) Haemorrhage

In what is often a heavily pre-treated pelvis (and abdomen) with prior radiotherapy and surgery, the associated fibrosis, distorted anatomical planes and abnormal anatomy lead to an increased risk of intestinal injury and intra-operative bleeding.

Recognition of the cause, site, amount and rapidity of blood loss, and the stability of the patient—assessed from dialogue between senior members of the surgical and anaesthetic teams—is essential. In particular, communication must include notification of those steps of the operation where significant blood loss might be expected before that step is undertaken.

Pelvic packing/pressure, suturing of bleeding points, the use of haemostatic agents, and/or sacral tacks may be needed. Often it is necessary to change tact during the operation, apply pressure to control the bleeding area, proceed with another step when safe to do so, and then return to the site of bleeding. It is preferable to leave the most hazardous step to later in the operation when there has been more mobilisation of the specimen and greater access to the bleeding area. In those cases where pre-operative assessment indicates that vascular resection and reconstruction are thought possible, then the vascular surgeon should be involved in the pre-operative planning and readily available during surgery. When a translevator (sometimes referred to as an infralevator) PEx is being undertaken, dialogue and coordinated dissection between the abdominal and perineal teams are important. The abdominal phase should be completed with as full mobilisation as possible before the perineal phase is commenced.

Major haemorrhage is a risk of sacrectomy due to the proximity of major neurovascular structures to the resection margin, and confined physical space hindering access. Preoperative risk factors for major haemorrhage include large/difficult-to-access tumours, proximity to major vessels, previous surgery, and previous radiotherapy [32]. Blood products (pack red cells, fresh frozen plasma, platelets, and fibrinogen/thrombin agents) should be made available for use intraoperatively. Bleeding can occur as the result of vascular injury or generalised ooze from raw surfaces of bone or soft tissue.

Pre-emptive vascular mobilisation and control are essential prior to sacral resection. The presacral venous plexus and iliac vessels are the main sources of haemorrhage. Presacral haemostasis can usually be achieved by a combination of electrocautery, packing, and haemostatic dressings. The external iliac artery and vein are mobilised and controlled with vascular slings. The internal iliac artery and veins are identified and can be divided as required to achieve oncologic resection (see Chap. 39). In the case of urological cancers, major haemorrhage is unusual in female patients, even in those who have been irradiated previously, unless there is significant pelvic sidewall/vessel involvement. In such cases surgery is rarely performed, even for palliation, as the benefits are minimal.

The level of sacral transection is predetermined radiologically as part of the MDT approach to surgical planning. Sacrectomies are classified as high or low (below the level of the S2 nerve root foramen). High sacrectomy is associated with greater morbidity and poorer functional outcomes [34, 35]. L5, S1, and S2 nerve roots are identified in the posterior lateral compartments. Where 'high and wide' en bloc sacrectomies are performed, excision of the sacral nerve roots and sciatic nerve may be required to achieve an R0 margin. The resultant functional deficit (e.g. foot drop) requires intensive rehabilitation and orthotics. However, some have reported physical QoL can return to baseline 12 months after surgery [36]. Sacral osteotomy follows control and selective ligation of neurovascular structures. The height and angle of the sacral osteotomy in relation to the sacral cortex are determined on preoperative MRI. It is important to evaluate the level of thecal sac termination in relation to the osteotomy, as inadvertently opening the thecal sac can result in a CSF leak. Sacral division can be performed with an osteotome and mallet or other devices such as a pneumatic drill. The sacral division is usually started in the midline and extended laterally to divide the sacrospinous and sacrotuberous ligaments attaching the sacrum to the pelvis (see Chap. 40).

Whilst some surgeons prefer to start the operation with posterior dissection of the sacrum with the patient in the prone position, the authors' practice is to start in the Lloyd-Davies position to complete all abdomino-pelvic steps of the resection. Subsequently, the abdomen is closed and the patient is placed prone. The posterior aspects of the sacrectomy are completed to meet the anterior transection margin. This can be a hazardous phase of the operation due to the limited access to the pelvis for control of bleeding. Access can be improved by making a safe perineal entry point to the pelvis prior to prone positioning [33].

In addition to the higher risk of massive bleeding, sacrectomy is associate with a higher rate of wound dehiscence and perineal flap failure [37]. This procedure is also associated with significant long term postoperative pain [38]. Therefore, appropriate patient selection and counselling is paramount before embarking upon this procedure.

(d) Infection risk:

Not infrequently the tumour mass is partially necrotic/infected and during surgery there can be frequent fluid shifts and the development of a systemic inflammatory response (systemic inflammatory response syndrome—SIRS). Avoidance of peritoneal contamination with bowel contents and/or necrotic tumour is routine practice. With variably friable and fibrotic tissue, difficult access and altered anatomy, the manoeuvres of traction and counter-traction need to be controlled and not excessive to avoid tearing the specimen, or jeopardising surgical planes and margins. This is not always straightforward.

Specific Intra-Operative Considerations: Urology

Rectal injury is much less common in female urological exenterative surgery than in males because the vagina acts a barrier between the bladder and the rectum. For bladder cancers where a cystectomy with urinary diversion is indicated, consideration needs to be given to performing an en bloc hysterectomy (and in some cases partial vaginectomy).

The condition of the ureters (fibrosis) and ileum (for an ileal conduit) are assessed intra-operatively. The ileum, if fibrosed, may not be suitable as a conduit. Patients undergoing PEx and who have a ureteric stent(s) tend to have more fibrosed ureters, and post-PEx are more likely to develop urosepsis and a ureteral anastomotic stricture [39, 40]. The incidence and severity of complications of a urinary diversion are substantially higher in an irradiated than in a non-irradiated pelvis and it is unclear if the double-barrelled stoma, the continent or the incontinent urinary diversion confers long-term benefit with regards to lower risk of upper urinary tract infection and preservation of renal function [41–43]. (See Chaps. 15 and 16 for a more in-depth discussion regarding conduit complications and continent versus incontinent conduits.)

Specific Intra-Operative Considerations: Colorectal

In a supralevator exenterative procedure, there can be the option to perform a colorectal anastomosis. When an anastomosis has been made, the recommendation is to bring out a loop ileostomy, with the goal of reversing this some months later. Elderly patients often have significant diverticulosis or anal incontinence, and this may preclude a colorectal anastomosis. The stability of the patient, bowel preparation, and health of the proximal and distal (and length of) bowel are some of the factors that must be considered in deciding whether or not to do a colorectal anastomosis (see Chap. 36). A pelvic drain must be placed close to the anastomotic site. If possible, an omental transposition should be performed.

Specific Considerations: Plastic and Reconstructive (See Chap. 41)

(e) Intra-operative death: Whilst the 30-day mortality for PEx is often quoted as 1–2%, and the 90-day mortality slightly higher, the literature does not always clearly distinguish intra-operative from postoperative deaths [9, 12, 13, 20]. Obese patients and those with extended procedures for non-central relapse are at increased risk of serious complications and death within 90 days.

Post-Operative Complications

Immediate

Typically, the patient will be in intensive care and many will be intubated.

The specific problems

(a) Blood loss: Primary haemorrhage may be sudden or gradual and revealed or concealed. If sustained, substantial and associated with hypotension there is no recourse but to take the patient back to theatre. An experienced surgical and anaesthetic team should be involved in the decision making and the operation should ideally be by the team which performed the PEx. As with primary haemorrhage from other operations, often no source can be identified.

(b) Poor urine output: Where there has been a urinary diversion, a post-renal cause includes a blocked ureteric stent—these should be flushed regularly.

(c) Flap ischaemia and other flap problems—(see Chap. 41).

Early Complications—First 6 Weeks After Surgery

Within the first week, the problems typical of major abdominal and pelvic surgery can be seen, but with greater frequency and severity. Those more particularly associated with PEx include:

(a) Secondary haemorrhage: Unlike with significant primary haemorrhage, there is less need to take a patient with secondary haemorrhage back to theatre. With PEx and the prolonged catabolic phase, anaemia is not uncommon.

(b) Infection: This is the most common complication after major surgery. There are a number of guidelines on surgical site infection (SSI) [44, 45]. Although infection can be confirmed on bacteriology, and/or on imaging, in clinical practice the actual site and responsible organism(s) often remain elusive. The usual SSI are evident in PEx patients and more than one site can be a source. In particular these include urinary tract infection, donor and recipient sites of the reconstruction (including infected mesh), and as part of a cluster of problems referred to as the empty pelvis syndrome [46–48]. Patients undergoing PEx will be on peri-operative antibiotics, often for some days, and there is a risk of *C. difficile* "infection". With the often slow recovery and relative immobility, dependent wounds (donor and graft sites of the reconstruction) are prone to pressure and are often moist and oedematous—all of which contribute to wound breakdown. Given the anatomical location of these wounds, they cannot be self-cared for.

Abdominal wound infection is more likely if a mesh has been used in reconstruction of the anterior abdominal wall.

(c) Urological problems.

Urinary leak: Leakage from a urinary diversion will be identified with low urine output, high drain output and clinical suspicion. Urinary leakage is more common in the early postoperative period. The use of ureteric stents has been shown to reduce the rate of urinary leak. The serum urea and creatinine levels will rise and the patient's condition can vary. Pelvic or abdominal drain fluid biochemistry will confirm there is urine leakage. Occasionally this may manifest as leakage of fluid from the perineal wound. Nephrostomy tubes will be required in the short-term to manage the leak.

1. Breakdown of urinary diversion. This is a rare outcome where there is anastomotic failure, peritonitis, and an ill patient. Contrast studies will demonstrate the leak and its extent. Surgical intervention is considered, generally after a period of conservative management with a nephrostomy tube. It is more problematic to drain the urinoma/collection percutaneously as the anatomy is altered after PEx.
2. Infection—this may not be confirmed on urine culture as the patients are, or have very recently been, on antibiotics.
3. Stomal problems (see below).

(d) Intestinal tract problems:

1. The development of an enteric fistula, a potential consequence of the empty pelvis syndrome, has been offset to some extent by the use of a well-vascularised (bulky) flap that reconstitutes the pelvic floor and perineal/vaginal/perianal defect. Although such fistulae usually present in the perineum they can also present at the abdominal wound. This is a serious complication and can lead to chronic abscess formation, further fistulae and sepsis [46]. Conservative and subsequent surgical management are carefully considered [47, 48]. There is a substantial risk of prolonged hospitalisation, intestinal failure (that is, the patient is dependent on parenteral nutrition) and death. It may be necessary to call on the expertise of the "intestinal failure team".
2. Ileus: This is a common problem of major abdominal surgery and usually settles with conservative management. Some centres will routinely give parenteral nutrition after PEx. Delayed return of bowel function can sometimes take weeks to resolve and persistence with conservative management with parenteral nutrition usually results in resolution.
3. Bowel obstruction: This is rarely acute in nature. A prolonged period of conservative management including parenteral nutrition may be required. The decision to re-operate must not be premature, but must be considered if there are persistent signs of peritonitis.
4. Peritonitis—from an anastomotic leak. A leak may be contained in a walled off collection, which can be managed conservatively, or there may be a diffuse leak with generalised peritonitis. Omental transposition performed during PEx may contribute to containment of a leak. A localised collection can be managed conservatively with drainage, antibiotics and parenteral nutrition, whereas generalised peritoneal infection will usually require surgery. If a supralevator procedure has been performed with a colorectal anastomosis, there is an increased risk of anastomotic leak because of the prior pelvic radiotherapy. A proximal diversion, typically a loop ileostomy, is recommended. A loop ileostomy brings its own problems.
5. Stomal problems—see below.

(e) Stomal problems: Patients may struggle, mentally and physically, with the early adaptation to the stoma(s) and self-caring can take some weeks. The challenge can be greatest in those who have had a rectus abdominis flap reconstruction [49].

Stomal necrosis may develop—most often this is superficial, above the fascia. Endoscopic examination will reveal the level of demarcation. In some cases a laparotomy will be required for revision. Necrosis of a urinary conduit is very rare.

(f) Extensive subcutaneous oedema—rarely, a clinical picture similar to anasarca develops. Reduction of intravenous fluid, if possible, is important along with skilled nursing care to avoid pressure sores. This problem contributes to delay in mobilisation. There is debate about the use of salt-free albumen, parenteral nutrition and enteral nutrition in managing this problem. Extensive oedema of the vulva and perineum can be very upsetting to the patient and with the limited mobility and gravitational influences (dependent tissues), can be difficult to reverse.

(g) Pressure sores: The particular problems of malnourishment, immobilisation and subcutaneous oedema pre-dispose these patients to pressure sores. Skilled nursing care is essential.

(h) Thrombo-embolic problems: These have been reduced by the peri-operative use of stockings, sequential compression devices, prophylactic anticoagulation and early mobilisation—the last often not practical in a PEx patient. Central line infection/thrombosis is more common in PEx. A swollen lower limb post-PEx, whilst not unexpected, might also indicate an underlying thrombosis and a Doppler study is then indicated.

(i) Empty pelvis syndrome: A pelvic abscess is one consequence of the extensive dissection and resection, with a large residual "dead-space." The many potential sequelae of this are sometimes described as the "empty pelvis syndrome" [46, 47, 48]. A pelvic abscess can present insidiously with low grade fever or swinging pyrexia. There may be no other clinical signs or the patient may be septic. The usual investigations for source of infection will be needed. A CT of chest, abdomen and pelvis will be informative, and image-guided drainage may be required, but this can be technically difficult.

(j) High outputs from abdominal and pelvic drains: The cause may be a urinary tract leak and a check on drain biochemistry will confirm this. It is important to ensure there is not blockage of the ureteric stents or drains.

(k) Body image/psychological issues: With a midline scar(s), distorted anterior abdominal wall, stoma(s), and resected lower genital tract structures, body image issues are common and may become more significant in the long term. The features of PEx that can cause psychological problems include baseline or pre-operative psychological function, prolonged surgery, postoperative intubation, longer stay in intensive care, multiple medications and distorted body image. A patient with significant pre-morbid psychological problems may not be considered suitable for PEx. Psychological assessment and support should be available. Depression (reactive) and hallucinations are not uncommon. Patients who have been on HRT prior to surgery may have more challenges with vasomotor symptoms and mood swings after PEx.

Delayed Complications—In the First 12 Months

Within the first 6–12 months after PEx some of the problems mentioned above can manifest during this period and thereafter (50, 51). More specific problems include:

1. Stomal problems: These can relate to the patient's adjusting to stomas which in most cases are permanent. Aside from stomal retraction and stomal prolapse, PEx patients may have troublesome bowel activity as a result of prior radiotherapy. Abdominal wall weakness after surgery, especially when there has been reconstruction with a rectus abdominis flap, can compound the situation (see below). The presence of a stoma(s) has been reported to adversely affect the QoL [52].
2. Renal impairment: Associated with the risk of infection and anastomotic stricture, renal impairment can develop which is detectable only on biochemical profile (which should be checked regularly). Ureteral stenting and nephrostomy tube drainage may be required, followed by surgical revision- which is a major undertaking. In urological cancers, the rate of stricture formation is reported as being around 2%. In patients who have had

prior radiotherapy or long-term stenting, the rate is higher. To avoid anastamotic stricture, the anastomosis should be under low tension, the ureteric spatulation should be of adequate length with redundant ureteric tissue excised, and the length of the ileal segment should be adequate.

Ureteral stricture proximal to the anastomosis is more common on the left side. This is because the ureter is further mobilised (which can impair vascularity) and may be under more tension on the left to be able to join the conduit which usually is brought out on the right side. Such strictures are even more common in patients who have gynaecological cancers which have been previously treated with high-dose pelvic radiotherapy. They are much more common in such patients than those who have had radiotherapy for colorectal cancer. The majority of anastamotic ureteral stenoses are treated by nephrostomy insertion, balloon dilatation and stenting.

3. Lymphedema: This problem may affect one or both legs, the vulva, perineum, and/or reconstructive sites; for reasons that are not apparent lymphedema may not manifest until many months after PEx. It is often asymmetrical. As it may be a sign of recurrent disease, this should be excluded by clinical examination and imaging. Significant lymphedema distorts body image and reduces quality of life.
4. Abdominal wall problems: These can include reduced truncal mobility and flexibility. As the shape and configuration of the abdomen changes with increased laxity or herniation, the changing contours of the abdominal wall cause problems with application of stomal devices. In severe cases, stomal function can be compromised. Surgery to attempt to correct these problems is fraught with difficulty and is rarely considered.
5. Plastics reconstruction—discussed in Chap. 41.
6. Psychosexual: There is some evidence that patients who have had a vaginal reconstruction have improved psychosexual rehabilitation post-surgery. However, long-term data pre- and post-surgery are scant. Vaginal reconstruction does not necessarily achieve satisfactory functional results and realistic expectations should be set pre-operatively. Progressive vaginal stenosis or persistent discharge can develop.
7. Body image: Some or all of the changes noted in the early postoperative period can be improve or worsen with time.
8. Electrolyte/biochemical imbalances: These can be subtle and are more common in those who have had a urinary diversion. Some patients will develop ViB12 deficiency as a result of reduced function of the terminal ileum.
9. Quality of Life: There is evidence that QoL is lower after PEx but then improves by 12 months. Some suggest the baseline QoL is reached at 6 months [49], but other reports indicate a more prolonged time to improved quality of life and that older patients are less likely to regain this [50, 51]. Consideration should be given to starting or re-starting HRT.
10. Perianal pain: In women who have undergone a supralevator procedure (when the anal canal is preserved and where most often the patient has a permanent colostomy), tenesmoid pain may develop. When an anastomosis has been created, defecatory problems can persist.
11. Anorectal and urinary problems: When an anterior PEx has been performed, an unintended consequence is that anorectal dysfunction can develop; likewise, when a posterior PEx has been performed, the patient can develop bladder dysfunction. These problems can continue to worsen. Pelvic recurrence can also present in a similar manner. Worsening of these problems may require surgical intervention—a colostomy and urinary diversion, respectively.

Long-Term Beyond 12 Months

The problems and complications that can develop in the first year after a PEx may improve or worsen in the long-term. A dramatic or sudden development of a new symptom might indicate further recurrence. Often there is more than one problem that reduces the patient's QoL [9, 50, 51]. The fear of relapse remains.

1. Stomal problems: these can develop and worsen over time as abdominal wall weakness develops. Some patients develop a true parastomal hernia. This can worsen with time, contribute to stomal and body image problems and may not be improved by surgical appliances (abdominal wall supports). Surgery may be considered but is often unsuccessful.
2. Hernia: Abdominal wall weakness is more common than a true incisional hernia. Parastomal weakness develops and can lead to stomal prolapse, stomal retraction and stomal stenosis, all of which can impair stomal function. Prolapse of the pelvic floor reconstruction can develop (see Chap. 26). Mechanical support measures tend to be favoured over surgical intervention. Vaginal reconstruction can also herniate (see Chap. 41).
3. Lymphedema: Even in the absence of recurrent disease (which can present with lymphedema) this problem can develop many months after the PEx. It may be precipitated by a trivial injury to the lower limb, especially if cellulitis develops.
4. Renal impairment: This can be insidious in onset and regular biochemical profiles should be checked, which should include chloride and bicarbonate levels.
5. Plastics reconstruction—Chap. 41.
6. Psychosexual: See above. Progressive vaginal stenosis can develop despite vaginal dilatation.
7. Body image and QoL: Some or all of the changes noted in the early postoperative period may improve or worsen with time.
8. Electrolyte imbalances: These can be subtle and are more common in those who have had a urinary diversion.

Conclusion

PEx is a major surgical undertaking requiring the coordination of multiple teams in the decision making, surgery and aftercare. It is associated with significant complications during and after surgery, in the short and long-term, in at least 50% of patients. The pattern and severity of complications can change with time and affect quality of life. Complications can also be a sign of recurrence. Patients who have had PEx require regular and long-term surveillance and support from multiple health professionals. Arguably, patients do best in terms of oncologic outcome, QoL and complications when cared for by an experienced team.

References

1. Brunschwig A. Complete excision of pelvic viscera for advanced carcinoma: a one-stage abdominoperineal operation with end colostomy and bilateral ureteral implantation into the colon above the colostomy. Cancer. 1948;1:177–83. https://doi.org/10.1002/1097-0142(194807)1:2<177::aid-cncr2820010203>3.0.co;2-a.
2. The PelvEx Collaborative/a. Factors affecting outcomes following pelvic exenteration for locally recurrent rectal cancer. BJS. 2018;105:65–657. https://doi.org/10.1002/bjs.10734.
3. The PelvEx Collaborative/b. Pelvic Exenteration for advanced nonrectal pelvic malignancy. Ann Surg. 2019;270(5):899–905. https://doi.org/10.1097/SLA.0000000000003533.
4. Lampe B, Luengas-Wurzinger V, Weotz J, et al. Opportunities and limitations of pelvic exentera-tion surgery. Cancers. 2021;13:6162. https://doi.org/10.3390/cancers13246162.
5. Cheng H, Clymer JW, Chen BP-H, et al. Prolonger operative duration is associated with complications: a systematic review and meta-analysis. J Surg Res. 2018;229:134–44. https://doi.org/10.1016/j.jss.2018.03.022.
6. Althumairi AA, Canner JK, Gorin MA, et al. Reduction of costs for pelvic exenteration performed by high volume surgeons: analysis of the Maryland Health Service Cost Revies Commission database. Am Surg. 2016;82:46–52. https://doi.org/10.1177/000313481608200123.
7. Dencker EE, Bonde A, Troelsen A, Varadarajan KM, Silesen M. Postoperative complications: an observational study of trends in the United States from 2012 to 2018. BMC Surg. 2021;21:393. https://doi.org/10.1186/s12893-021-021-01392-z.
8. Fowler AJ, Yan YI, Prowle JR, et al. Long-term mortality following complications after elective surgery: a secondary analysis of pooled data from two prospective cohort studies. Br J Anaes. 2022;129:588–97. https://doi.org/10.1016/bja.2022.06.019.

9. The PelvEx Collaborative/c. Palliative pelvic exenteration: a systematic review of patient-centred outcomes. 2019. Eur J Surg Oncol. 2019;45:1787–95. https://doi.org/10.1016/j.ejso.2019.06.011.
10. Koh CE, Solomon MJ, Brown KG, Byrne CM, Lee P, Young JM. The evolution of pelvic exenteration practice at a single center: lessons learned from over 500 cases. Dis Colon Rectum. 2017;60:627–35. https://doi.org/10.1097/DCR0000000000000825.
11. Heald RJ. The 'Holy Plane' of rectal surgery. J R Soc Med. 1988;81(9):503–8. https://doi.org/10.1177/014107688808100904.
12. The PelvEx Collaborative/d. Changing outcomes following pelvic exenteration for locally advanced and recurrent rectal cancer. BJS Open. 2019;3:516–20. https://doi.org/10.1002/bjs5.50153.
13. The PelvEx Collaborative/e. Surgical and survival outcomes following pelvic exenteration for locally advanced primary rectal cancer: results from an international collaboration. Ann Surg. 2019;269(2) https://doi.org/10.1097/SLA.0000000000002528.
14. Cunneen C, Kelly M, Nason G, Ryan E, Creavin B, Winder D. The role of exenterative surgery in advanced urological neoplasms. Curr Urol. 2020;14:57–65. https://doi.org/10.1159/00499258.
15. Huang H, Yan B, Shang M, et al. Is hysterectomy beneficial in radical cystectomy for female patient with urothelial carcinoma of bladder? A retrospective analysis of consecutive 112 cases from a single institution. BMC Urol. 2019;19:28. https://doi.org/10.1186/s12894-019-0461-9.
16. The PelvEx Collaborative/f. Perioperative management and anaesthetic considerations in pelvic exenteration using Delphi methodology: results from PelvEx Collaborative. BJS Open. 2021; https://doi.org/10.1093/bjsopen/zraa055.
17. Carvalho F, Qiu S, Panagi V, et al. Total pelvic exenteration surgery- considerations for healthcare professionals. Eur J Surg Oncol. 2023;49:225–36. https://doi.org/10.1016/j.esjo.20222.08.011.
18. Modrall JG, Minter MA, et al. The surgeon volume-outcome relationship: not yet ready for policy. Ann Surg. 2018;267:863–7. https://doi.org/10.1097/SLA0000000000002334.
19. Climent M, Pera M. Preoperative optimization prior to exenteration. Chap 5. In: Winter DC, Kelly ME, editors. Surgical management of advanced pelvic cancer; 2021. p. 45–51. https://doi.org/10.1002/9781119518495.
20. Tortorella L, Casarin J, Mara KC, et al. Prediction of short-term surgical complications in women undergoing pelvic exenteration for gynecological malignancies. Gyn Oncologia. 2019;152:151–6. https://doi.org/10.1016/j.ygyno.2018.10.036.
21. CKP N, Sorensen CHK, Funder JA. Complications and survival after total pelvic exenteration. Eur J Surg Oncol. 2022;48:1362–7. https://doi.org/10.1016/j.ejso.2021.12.472.
22. Venchiarutti RL, Solomon MJ, Koh CE, Young JM, Steffens D. Pushing the boundaries of pelvic exenteration by maintaining survival at the cost of morbidity. Brit J Surg. 2019;106:1391–403. https://doi.org/10.1002/bjs.11203.
23. Charlson M, Szatrowski TP, Peterson J, Gold J. Validation of a combined comorbidity index. J Clin Epidemiol. 1994;47:1245–51. https://doi.org/10.1016/0895-4356(94)90129-5.
24. Copeland GP. The POSSUM system of surgical audit. Arch Surg. 2002;137:15–9. https://doi.org/10.1001/arch-surg.137.115.
25. Shim S-H, Lee SJ, Dong M, et al. Prediction model for 30-day morbidity after gynecological malignancy surgery. PLoS One. 2017;12(6):e0178610. https://doi.org/10.1371/journal.pone.0178610.
26. Van Kooten RT, Bahadoer RR, Peeters KCMJ, et al. Preoperative risk factors for major postoperative complications after complex gastrointestinal cancer surgery: a systematic review. Eur J Surg Oncol. 2021;47:3049–58. https://doi.org/10.1016/j.esgo.2021.07.021.
27. Dessai S, Fasal R, Dipon J, Adarsh D, Balasubramanian S. Age-adjusted Charlson comorbidity index and 30-day mortality in pelvic surgeries. South Asian J Cancer. 2018;7:240–3. https://doi.org/10.4103/sajc.sajc-241-17.
28. Harji DP, Williams A, McKigney N, Boissieras L, Denost Q, Fearnhead NS, Jenkins JT, Griffiths B. Utilising quality of life outcomes trajectories to aid patient decisions making in pelvic exenteration. Eur J Surg Oncol. 2022;48:2238–49. https://doi.org/10.1016/j.esjo.2022.08.011.
29. Waljee J, McGlinn EP, Davus Sear E, Chubg KC. Patient expectations and patient-reported outcomes in surgery: a systematic review. Surgery. 2014;155:799–808. https://doi.org/10.1016/j.surg.2013.12.015.
30. Matsuo K, Mandelbaum Adams CL, et al. Performance and outcome of pelvic exenteration for gynecologic malignancies: a population-based study. Gynecol Oncol. 2019;153:368–75. https://doi.org/10.1016/j.ygyno.2019.02.002.
31. Maerz DA, BecklN SAJ, Gainsburg. Complications of robotic-assisted laparoscopic surgery distant from the surgical site. Br J Anaes. 2017;118:492–503. https://doi.org/10.1093/bja.aex003.
32. Bonello VA, Bhangu A, Fitzgerald JEF, Rasheed S, Tekkis P. Intraoperative bleeding and haemostasis during pelvic surgery for locally advanced or recurrent rectal cancer: a prospective evaluation. Tech Coloproctol. 2014;18:887–93. https://doi.org/10.1007/s10151-014-1150-z.
33. Rogers AC, Jenkins JT, Rasheed S, et al. Towards standardisation of technique for en bloc sacrectomy for locally advanced and recurrent rectal cancer. J Clin Med. 2021;10(21) https://doi.org/10.3390/jcm10214921.
34. McCarthy ASE, Solomon MJ, Koh CE, Firouzbakht A, Jackson SA, Steffens D. Quality of life and functional outcomes following pelvic exenteration and

sacrectomy. Color Dis. 2020;22(5):521–8. https://doi.org/10.1111/codi.15044.
35. Sasikumar A, Bhan C, Jenkins JT, Antoniou A, Murphy J. Systematic review of pelvic exenteration with en bloc sacrectomy for recurrent rectal adenocarcinoma: R0 resection predicts disease-free survival. Dis Colon Rectum. 2017;60(3):346–52. https://doi.org/10.1097/DCR.0000000000000737.
36. Brown KGM, Solomon MJ, Lau YC, Steffens D, Austin KKS, Lee PJ. Sciatic and femoral nerve resection during extended radical surgery for advanced pelvic tumours: long-term survival, functional and quality-of-life outcomes. Ann Surg. 2021;273:982–8. https://doi.org/10.1097/SLA.0000000000003390.
37. Manrique OJ, Rajesh A, Asaad M, et al. Surgical outcomes after abdominoperineal resection with sacrectomy and soft tissue reconstruction: lessons learned. J Reconstr Microsurg. 2020;36(1):64–72. https://doi.org/10.1055/s-0039-1697629.
38. Lim JS, Koh CE, Liu H, Solomon MJ, Johnstone CSH. The price we pay for radical curative pelvic exenterations: prevalence and management of pain. Dis Colon Rectum. 2018;61(3):314–9. https://doi.org/10.1097/DCR.0000000000001013.
39. Davis NF, Burke JP, McDermott TED, Flynn R, Manecksha RP, Thornhill JA. Bricker versus Wallace anastomosis: a meta-analysis of ureteroenteric stricture rates after ileal conduit urinary diversion. Can Urol Assoc J. 2015;9(5–6):E284–90. https://doi.org/10.5489/cuaj.2692.
40. Mattei A, Birkhaeuser FD, Baermann C, Warncke SH, Studer UE. To stent or not to stent perioperatively the ureteroileal anastomosis of ileal orthotopic bladder substitutes and ileal conduits? Results of a prospective randomized trial. J Urol. 2008;179(2):582–6. https://doi.org/10.1016/j.juro.2007.09.066.
41. Hautmann R, Hautmann S, Hautmann O. Complications associated with urinary diversion. Nat Rev Urol. 2011;8:667–77. https://doi.org/10.1038/nrurol.2011.147.
42. Carter MF, Dalton DP, Garnett JE. Simultaneous diversion of the urinary and faecal streams utilizing a single abdominal stoma: the double-barrelled wet colostomy. J Urol. 1989;141:1189–91. https://doi.org/10.1016/s0022-5347(17)41210-9.
43. Urh A, Soliman PT, Schmeler KM, Westin S, Frumovitz M, Nick AM, Fellman B, Urbauer DL, Ramirez PT. Postoperative outcomes after continent versus incontinent urinary diversion at the time of pelvic exenteration for gynecologic malignancies. Gynecol Oncol. 2013;129:580–5. https://doi.org/10.1016/j.gyno.2013.02.024.
44. Ban KA, Minei JP, Laronmga C, et al. American College of Surgeons and surgical infection society: surgical site infection guidelines, 2016 update. J Am Coll Surg. 2017;224:59–74. https://doi.org/10.1016/j.jamcollsurg.2016.10.029.
45. https://www.nice.org.uk. Surgical site infections: prevention and treatment. 9NICE guideline [NG125].
46. Persson P, Ching P, Steele CW, Quinn M. Prevention and management of complications in pelvic exenteration. Eur J Surg Oncol. 2022;48:2277–83. https://doi.org/10.1016/j.ejso.2021.12.470.
47. Johnson YL, West MA, Gould L, et al. Empty pelvis syndrome: a systematic review of reconstruction techniques and their associated complications. Color Dis. 2022;24:16–26. https://doi.org/10.1111/codi.15956.
48. Sutton PA, Brown KGM, Ebrahimi N, et al. Long-term surgical complications following pelvic exenteration: operative management of the empty pelvis syndrome. Color Dis. 2022;24:1491. https://doi.org/10.1111/codi.16238.
49. Steffens D, Solomon MJ, Young JM, et al. Cohort study of long-term survival and quality of life following pelvic exenteration. BJS Open. 2018;2:328–35. https://doi.org/10.1002/bjs5.75.
50. Martinez A, Filleron T, Rouanet P, et al. Prospective assessment of first-year quality of life after pelvic exenteration for gynecologic malignancy: a French multicentric study. Ann Sur Oncologia. 2018;25:535–41. https://doi.org/10.1245/s10434-017-6120-z.
51. Armbruster SD, Sun AA, Westin SN, Bodurka DC, Ramondetta L, Meyer LA, Soliman PT. Prospective assessment of patient-reported outcomes in gynecologic cancer patients before and after pelvic exenteration. Gynecol Oncol. 2018;149:484–90. https://doi.org/10.1016/j.gyno.2018.03054.
52. Dessole M, Petrillo M, Lucidi A, et al. Quality of life after pelvic exenteration for gynecological malignancies. Int J Gyn Cancer. 2018;28:267–73. https://doi.org/10.1097/IGC.0000000000000612.

Resection of Recurrent Pelvic Sidewall Tumor

39

James D. McDonald and Ricardo J. Gonzalez

Introduction

Recurrent tumors of the pelvic sidewall are extremely difficult to manage as they commonly involve major nerves, vessels, and urinary tract structures including the ureters and bladder (Fig. 39.1 CT images). Often, these patients with pelvic recurrence have had prior pelvic surgery, systemic treatment, and radiation therapy. Unfortunately, when these tumors recur the treatment options available to maintain durable local control are limited as the disease has proven to be refractory to traditional or first-line therapies. Furthermore, depending on previous treatments, additional radiation may not be tolerable or effective. In these cases, extended surgical resection may be the only chance for disease control. The ability to achieve an R0 resection is the best predictor of survival in patients with pelvic sarcomas and tumors of gynecologic, urologic, and colorectal origin [1–4]. Unfortunately, however, traditional surgical approaches resulted in high complication rates and dismal outcomes in regard to the ability to achieve negative resection margins in patients with pelvic sidewall invasion. For these reasons, sidewall involvement was long considered an absolute contraindication to surgery [1, 5].

With the increased utility of pelvic exenteration as a method to obtain better local control, achieve negative resection margins, and improve survival with an acceptable morbidity and mortality rate there has been renewed interest in improving surgical approaches to address recurrent disease involving the pelvic sidewall in patients with gynecologic, urologic, and colorectal malignancies as well as soft tissue sarcomas. The utilization of extended pelvic resection for gynecologic malignancies was documented in the literature as early as the 1940s, but it did not gain traction until the late 1990s when Hockel first published his technique for resection in patients with pelvic wall recurrence [6, 7]. While the experience in extended sidewall resection for gynecologic malignancies grew, extending the indications for pelvic sidewall resection for colorectal malignancies also began to gain traction [8, 9]. As techniques for extended sidewall resection developed over time, there has been an improvement in R0 resection rates to as high as 66% with en bloc resection of vascular and other involved sidewall structures [10]. With increasing utilization of "ultra-radical" resection strategies to achieve R0 resection, there must be a clear understanding of the risks involved, with the overall complication

J. D. McDonald
Department of Surgery, University Surgixal Oncology, University of Tennessee Graduate School of Medicine, Knoxville, TN, USA
e-mail: James.McDonald@moffitt.org

R. J. Gonzalez (✉)
Sarcoma Department, Moffitt Cancer Center, Tampa, FL, USA
e-mail: Ricardo.Gonzalez@moffitt.org

M. Hoffman et al. (eds.), *Major Complications of Female Pelvic Surgery*,
https://doi.org/10.1007/978-3-031-66772-5_39

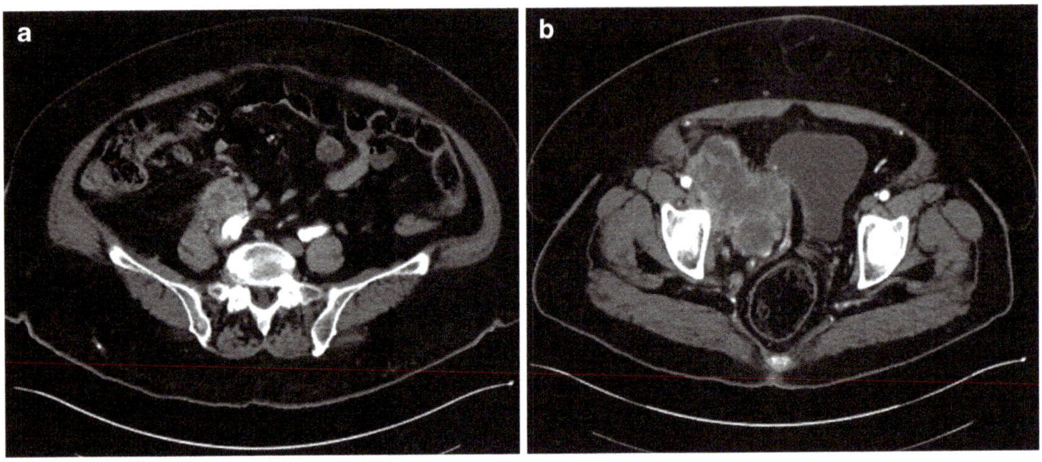

Fig. 39.1 Cross-sectional imaging showing pelvic sidewall disease involving the bifurcation of the CIA (**a**), as well as the acetabulum, bladder, and into the femoral canal (**b**)

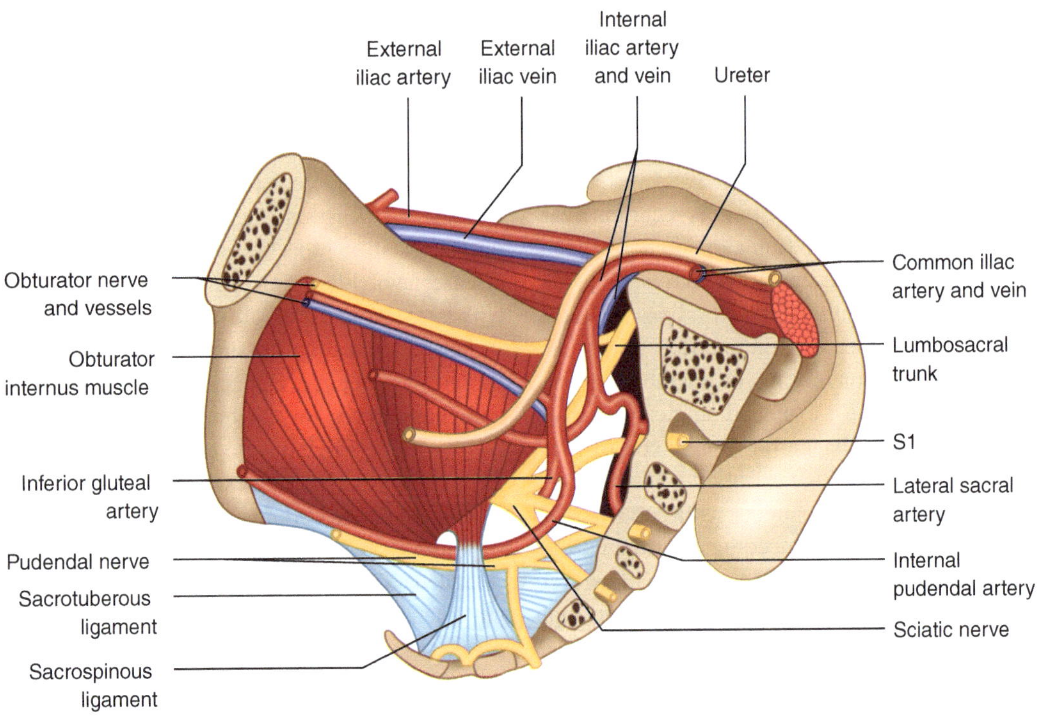

Fig. 39.2 Complex pelvic sidewall anatomy, with anatomic relationship of the boney pelvis, ureter, and major neurovascular structures

rate approaching 80%, and the major complication rate approaching 30% [10, 11].

At the fundamental level, the principal factor in the prevention of injury and complications during resection of recurrent pelvic sidewall tumors is to have a detailed and intimate knowledge of the relevant surgical anatomy of this area (Fig. 39.2 anatomy figures). A thorough description of the pelvic sidewall surgical anatomy and the lumbosacral triangle was first described and published by Maurice Marcille, a Parisian surgeon and anatomist, in his text "Lymphatiques et ganglions ilio-pelviens" in 1903 [12]. This area is considered the entryway to the pelvis and contains the ureter and the major neurovascular structures of the pelvis. More recently as surgeons have worked to improve the surgical approaches to the pelvic sidewall there has been a renewed interest in the surgical anatomy of this area [13]. While the focus of this chapter is the complications frequently encountered during the resection of recurrent pelvic sidewall tumors, the complication risk can be greatly reduced by thorough preoperative planning, appropriate knowledge of the relevant pelvic anatomy, and appropriate coordination with a multidisciplinary team that will frequently require Gynecologic Oncology, Surgical Oncology, Colorectal Surgery, Vascular Surgery, Urology, Neurosurgery and Plastics and Reconstructive Surgery.

Bowel Injury and Complications

Background

When attempting resection in patients with a recurrent pelvic sidewall tumor, it is important to understand and expect that these patients will have varying degrees of adhesions from prior surgery and/or radiation to the pelvis. Adhesions are often dense and frequently involve the large and small intestines we as the abdominopelvic sidewall and retroperitoneal structures. The initial step in any reoperative pelvic surgery is adhesiolysis to gain adequate exposure to the pelvis. During this lysis of adhesions both intentional and unintentional bowel injuries occur and the implications of this are typically determined by the timing with which these injuries are recognized. Additionally, when adhesions to the bowel mesentery are present, lysis of adhesions can result in segmental intestinal devascularization.

Prevention

In general, when performing enterolysis, the use of electrocautery should be minimized to prevent inadvertent thermal injury. Thermal injury, depending on the extent, may not be immediately evident. An unrecognized thermal bowel injury may present hours to days after the index operation. When it is determined that the adhesions between structures are too dense to safely attempt separation, segmental bowel resection is prudent. In these scenarios, our practice is to avoid any resection until the remainder of the involved bowel has been safely freed from surrounding structures. This approach minimizes the length of the bowel that requires resection and limits the number of anastomoses required for reconstruction.

Recognition

When dense adhesions are encountered during the initial stages of the operation, prompt recognition requires a high index of suspicion for potential bowel injury. Full-thickness injuries are easily identified immediately as there is stool or succus noted from the dissected area. Serosal injuries on the other hand are not as clear to the naked eye. When there is a concern for serosal injury, we will typically place a marking stitch in the area to re-evaluate the severity of the injury after a period of time. Another practice we employ to avoid any missed bowel injuries is to run the bowel and inspect it for any injured areas or devitalized segments. The bowel is run after completion of adhesiolysis and prior to placing retractors necessary to gain exposure to the pelvis, and then again at the end of the case. This duration of time allows for any suspicious area to declare or demarcate and to distinguish viable from non-viable bowel, especially in cases where blood flow is compromised. If the blood supply to a given segment of the bowel is in question, we will typically use a portable sterile Doppler or intraoperative indocyanine green fluorescence angiography to assess perfusion [14].

Management

The management of small and large bowel injuries identified at the index operation range from primary suture repair to segmental bowel resection with anastomosis. Partial thickness injuries are typically closed transversely using a Lembert suture technique to achieve the apposition of healthy bowel serosa [15]. A full-thickness small bowel injury involving less than 50% of the circumference is debrided back to healthy tissue and closed transversely to prevent narrowing of the lumen. Full-thickness bowel injuries are typically closed in two layers with the first layer performed in an interrupted or running fashion with care to take a healthy bite of serosa and a small bite of mucosa. A second layer of interrupted Lembert sutures is used to imbricate the first layer. While techniques vary, when a bowel resection is required, our practice is to perform a stapled side-to-side (functional end-to-end) anastomosis with sutured or stapled closure of the common enterotomy. A single or two-layer hand-sewn anastomosis is also an appropriate option. The choice between the different techniques is surgeon preference and there is no difference in complication rates between the two [16].

Urinary Tract Injury and Complications

Background

Injury and complications related to the urinary system during the resection of recurrent pelvic sidewall tumors are common. Up to 25% of patients experience a urinary-related complication that may include urinary retention, ureteral fistula, stricture, hydronephrosis, and/or bladder injury [10, 17]. When there is a planned ureteral resection and urinary diversion, the ureters are identified early but ligation and transection are reserved until the ureters have been dissected free to the level of tumor involvement. As the surgical plan moves urinary diversion to planned bladder preservation with the goal of maintaining bladder and ureteral continuity, the rate of ureteral injury increases. For this reason, preoperative ureteral stents are frequently employed to aid in early ureteral identification, and potentially identify injuries more readily.

Prevention

While there is conflicting data on the routine use of prophylactic ureteral stents in gynecologic and colorectal surgery to prevent injury, they are beneficial to assist in early ureteral identification when performing preoperative surgery, especially in the setting of previous radiation and bulky tumors [18–20]. With or without prophylactic stents, the safest way to identify the ureters early is to identify and isolate them in their normal anatomic position proximal to the previously operated field. Once identified, a vessel loop is placed around the ureter to assist in safe dissection and mobilization as it tracks down into the pelvis crossing the bifurcation of the common iliac artery, running medial to the internal iliac artery along the pelvic sidewall before entering the bladder posterlaterally. When mobilizing the ureter, it is important to remember that it has a segmental blood supply and in the pelvis, the blood supply for the ureter travels from the lateral vessels to the adventitial layer. Care should be taken to minimize dissection lateral to the ureter especially as it enters the bladder and to preserve the adventitia, in order to prevent ischemic injuries that may result in delayed urinary complications such as stricture or fistula [21].

Recognition

Intraoperatively, when ureteral stents are present, an injury is quickly and easily identified by visualizing the bright-colored stent through the ureteral defect. When stents are not placed, or when the injury is not immediately apparent then it may become evident by an accumulation of clear fluid in the surgical field. This can be confirmed by the administration of intravenous fluorescein which will turn urine green. When operating in the vicinity of the ureter within a difficult operative field, the surgeon must maintain a high level of vigilance. If a suspicious-looking tubular structure is transected or a lumen is identified in divided tissue, then further investigation to determine ureteral patency is required. If further dissection proves difficult or fruitless, then a cystoscopy should be performed to look for efflux of urine from the ureteral orifices. This is aided, if necessary, by the intravenous administration of 0.1 cc of fluorescein (followed by a 10 cc intravenous flush). Passage of a ureteral stent may also be attempted, with or without retrograde pyelography.

Delayed or missed ureteral injury can present as a urinoma, leakage of clear fluid from a wound (i.e. vagina) or drain, a prolonged ileus, flank pain, infection, hydronephrosis, or an unexplained rise in BUN and creatinine. When drains are in place, the fluid can be sent for a spot creatinine. Fluid creatinine at the level of 25–450 mg/dL is consistent with urine. If drain creatinine is equal to serum creatinine, then a ureteral injury is much less likely. CT-urogram is the imaging of choice to further evaluate the integrity of the ureters and to identify the location of injury.

Management

This subject is covered in more detail in Chap. 17.

Management of a ureteral injury is dependent on the mechanism, extent, and location of the injury, as well as the timing with which the injury is identified. In general, if identified within 72 hours of surgery, the recommendation is for re-exploration and repair of ureteral injury in the operating room. If the patient is unstable, infected, or has developed a urinoma, then temporary measures are taken. In these situations, if Urology is not already a member of the multidisciplinary team a consultation is warranted to provide their expertise in managing these difficult complications. Injury to the upper half of the ureter can typically be managed with direct uretero-ureterostomy, or by anastomosis to the contralateral ureter via transureteroureterostomy. Lower ureteral injuries are managed with ureteral reimplantation (which may include a psoas hitch) or bladder remodeling such as a Boari flap. The principles of ureteral repair are like other surgical anastomoses; adequate perfusion and minimal tension. Often this requires the injured ends to be debrided back to healthy bleeding edges along with adequate ureteral mobilization to ensure a tension-free repair and a gently approximated anastomosis with absorbable suture performed over a stent.

An injury that has a delay in diagnosis or is otherwise not amenable to repair in the operating room is managed with a percutaneous nephrostomy tube (PCN), percutaneous drainage of any urinoma, and subsequent ureteral stent placement if possible. In these cases, definitive repair is delayed until at least 6 weeks after the injury is stabilized.

Vascular Injury and Complications

Background

Vascular injury, in the context of extended lateral resection due to recurrent pelvic sidewall tumor, is a major intraoperative concern for surgeons. Depending on the extent of vascular involvement and resection necessary, there is an increase in operative time and intraoperative blood loss. When vascular reconstruction is required to achieve R0 resection margins, operative time, intraoperative blood loss, and vascular-related complication rates increase. These include post-operative graft complications such as acute thrombosis, distal limb ischemia leading to reperfusion injury and compartment syndrome, and graft infection [22].

Prevention

The key to the prevention of vascular injury and bleeding complications during reoperative pelvic surgery is to have a detailed knowledge of pelvic anatomy, understand the extent of disease as well as the necessary resection based on preoperative imaging, have a plan, and be prepared for a vascular repair, resection, and reconstruction. Finally, when need for vascular resection or isolation, the operating surgeon must adhere to the tenants of exposure and proximal and distal vascular control.

Experienced surgeons begin their approach to pelvic dissection by first gaining proximal control of the common iliac artery (CIA) with circumferential control using a vessel loop to allow for better retraction as your dissection proceeds distally. Next, due to its overlying orientation to the common iliac vein (CIV) circumferential dissection of the CIA is necessary to retract the artery laterally and expose the CIV. Once the CIA and CIV have been dissected out and controlled with vessel loops proximal and distal to the tumor, the dissection continues into the pelvis. As the pelvic dissection proceeds, care must be taken to control the branches of the ileopelvic arteriovenous system as these have the potential to become a significant source of bleeding. Next, the internal iliac artery (IIA) and vein (IIV) and external iliac artery (EIA) and vein (EIV) are encountered. These vessels are dissected out and circumferential control is once again obtained using vessel loops. Depending on the extent of resection it may be safe to proceed with ligation and transection of the IIA with a stapler or a suture ligature. Early division of the IIA allows for exposure to the IIV and its draining branches. These branches lie lateral to the IIA and can be accessed and easily ligated with the exposure created from the early division and retraction of the IIA. It is important to ligate the venous branches draining into the IIV prior to its ligation and division. If the IIV remains distended after the branches are ligated, you should be suspicious that there is a posterior branch that will need to be ligated prior to division. The inability to account for this may lead to unexpected bleeding that is often difficult to control. Ligation of the IIV will not typically result in any deficit. However, if ligation of both the EIV and IIV or the CIV is necessary due to tumor involvement, lower extremity edema may be significant postoperatively. However, this tends to be self-limited if collateral drainage is preserved during the dissection.

As the dissection is carried into the pelvis the surgeon must also be cognizant of the presacral venous plexus (PVP), which may be encountered if the dissection proceeds more medially. Failure to recognize that the dissection is encroaching on the PVP may result in difficult to control bleeding and can result in serious hemorrhage. Keeping the pelvic vascular dissection lateral and along the iliac artery and veins is the safest way to avoid bleeding from the PVP. When the resection requires more posterior dissection, bleeding from the PVP can be minimized by keeping the dissection anterior to the presacral fascia. In addition it is important to maintain awareness that the risk of inadvertent injury to the PVP is highest at the distal sacrum where Waldeyer's facia thickens and may become fused with the presacral fascia, especially if radiation has been previously delivered to this area [23].

In a patient with extensive vascular abutment or encasement who is otherwise an appropriate surgical candidate, the surgeon should anticipate that vascular reconstruction will be required. Attempts at resection without a plan for reconstruction should not be attempted as there is risk for life threatening bleeding. In these situations, the need for a multidisciplinary surgical team including the vascular surgeon is at a premium as there is growing data to support extended vascular resection as a single or two stage procedure. In highly selected patients with tumor involving the CIA or EIA, there are data to support pelvic exenteration with extended resection, including vascular resection and reconstruction [22, 24]. In instances where vascular reconstruction is required, it is recommended that this be performed during the initial stages of the operation to reestablish distal flow as soon as possible. Vascular reconstruction options include anatomical reconstruction with in-line interposition grafting of a resected segment or, in settings where in-line reconstruction is not feasible, extra-anatomical reconstruction with crossover femoral-to-femoral bypass grafting. The choice of conduit is driven by the degree of contamination expected or experienced, and the potential size mismatch. Our practice is to use either a cadaveric femoral vein graft or the contralateral greater saphenous vein as our vascular conduit as this minimizes risk of infectious or thrombotic complications [25]. As extended lateral pelvic resections become more commonly performed for gynecologic and colorectal malignancies involving major vessels of the pelvic sidewall, there has been increased interest in strategies to minimize complications. One such novel strategy is pre-emptive crossover femoral-to-femoral arterial bypass, performed as a separate procedure in advance of the planned surgical resection of the recurrent pelvic sidewall tumor [26–28]. This novel technique has been reported to reduce operative time, allow for appropriate amount of recovery time from the bypass procedure, and reduce the infectious complications related to the placement of a bypass graft at the time of a multivisceral resection.

Recognition

Vascular injury at the time of surgery is one of the most easily recognized complications in surgery. While easily recognized, gaining control of bleeding during reoperative pelvic surgery can be a challenge.

Management

Whether the bleeding is from an arterial or venous source, the best first step is to apply direct pressure to the area. This allows time to coordinate the resuscitative measures by the surgical team and anesthesia providers, as well as mobilize resources to the OR if necessary. Additionally, while bleeding is controlled with direct pressure, attempts should be made to ensure that there is adequate exposure and vascular control of the area of suspected bleeding. Depending on the source and the size of the vessel responsible, bleeding may be controlled with ligation or primary repair of the injured vessel. In some circumstances, such as bleeding from the internal iliac venous plexus, over-exuberant application of pressure may result in further tearing of delicate veins and exacerbation of bleeding.

Bleeding from the PVP poses a difficult challenge. The PVP is a valveless system that, when injured, can lead to significant blood loss [29]. In some cases when these vessels are inadvertently transected they can retract into the sacrum, making it nearly impossible to gain control with pressure alone. In any instance the initial step in control of presacral venous bleeding that does not resolve with electrocautery is pelvic packing with pressure. If bleeding is not controlled with packing, the addition of topical hemostatic agents, bone wax and cement, as well as sterile tacks or muscle patches to the area have been employed with success. Finally, spray electrocautery, argon beam coagulation, and circular suture ligation have been used as methods to obtain hemostasis [23].

Nerve Injury and Complication

Background

Major nerve (sciatic or femoral) resection is required in up to 30% of cases of laterally extended pelvic resection for recurrent pelvic sidewall tumors [6, 11, 22]. In settings where a nerve resection is planned, there should be a thorough preoperative physical assessment including evaluation of the contralateral side to ensure that the patient has the baseline functional capacity to compensate for anticipated motor deficits following nerve resection. Outcomes following major nerve resection can vary from minor sensory deficit to a significant motor deficit. While resection of a major nerve is not associated with worse survival, the negative impact that these motorsensory deficits may have on a patient's quality of life can be significant. Fortunately however, recent studies assessing quality of life after pelvic exenteration in patients who underwent femoral or sciatic nerve resection for lateral wall involvement for colorectal cancer found that there was a negative impact on quality of life at 6 months but that by 12 months most patients reported they were back to their preoperative functional baseline [30]. In patients who have required more extensive boney resection as in the case of hemipelvectomy for a pelvic sarcoma, the outcomes and impact on quality of life are more pronounced and are driven by the extent of resection and reconstruction required [31].

Prevention

After vascular control has been achieved and the internal iliac vessels have been ligated, extended lateral dissection takes place by gentle medial retraction of the specimen and vessels (Fig. 39.3c). The dissection proceeds lateral to the internal iliac vessels until the deep pelvic fascia is encountered. Once the deep pelvic fascia is incised then the lumbosacral trunk and sacral nerve roots on the piriformis muscle are exposed. The nerve roots are dissected away from the pelvic floor to the level of necessary resection, and beyond the tumor in cases where nerve preservation is planned.

Recognition

Unfortunately, unintended nerve injury is not always immediately evident during surgery. More frequently these are identified postoperatively when the patient has complaints of motor and/or sensory deficits that result from compression, traction, thermal spread, or a partial transection injury. When a nerve is transected, it can be more clearly identified intraoperatively. Depending on the nerve injured, the degree of injury, and how the injury occurred, attempts at repair may be considered.

Management

When neuropathy is identified with an unexpected motor and/or sensory deficit in the postoperative setting, the extent of injury may not be immediately evident. Traction or compression injury from a malpositioned retractor blade or stretch injury from dissection will typically improve with time [32]. Additionally, in setting of nerve resection, a multidisciplinary discussion with a neural reconstructive surgeon would be warranted to determine the benefit of nerve reconstruction on a case-by-case basis. As many of these patients undergoing laterally extended surgical resection have already received radiotherapy in or around the operative field, the deleterious effects of the radiation must be taken into account when dis-

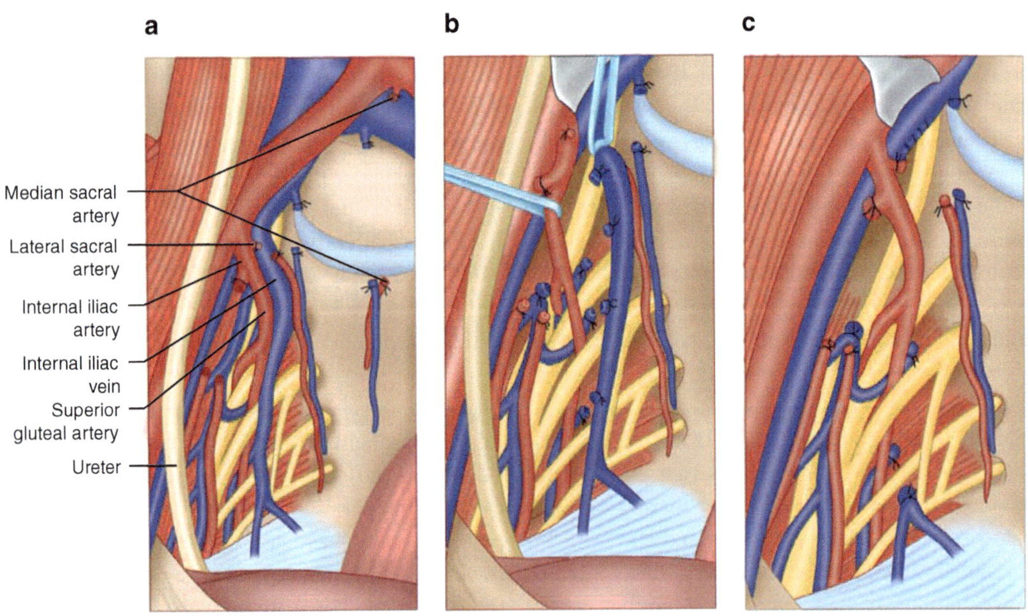

Fig. 39.3 Lateral pelvic sidewall neurovascular exposure. (**a**) In situ anatomic relationship of the ureter, major vessels, and nerves. (**b**) Sidewall vasculature controlled, and side-branches ligated. (**c**) Ligation and retraction of the major vessels exposing the lumbosacral plexus and pelvic nerves

cussing the role for reconstruction, and debridement of the grafting field must be performed to maximize chance of successful reconstruction [33].

As has been seen with the growing data and improved techniques for limb salvage and functional recovery after nerve resection for extremity soft tissues sarcomas, there appears to be benefit of nerve reconstruction after pelvic nerve resection as most patients report being at their preoperative functional baseline by 12 months post-surgery [30, 34, 35]. In those patients whose multidisciplinary team has determined that there would be benefit from nerve reconstruction, the primary modalities for reconstruction are primary repair, nerve grafting, and nerve transfer. Repair of femoral or obturator nerve injuries tend to have better results in regards to functional recovery and pain compared to those patients with attempted repair of sciatic or multilevel nerve injuries [36].

Summary

Pelvic sidewall tumor recurrence is a scenario that is common to Gynecologic and Surgical Oncologists, Colorectal Surgeons, and Urologists. As surgical techniques have improved, there has been a push to consider a patient's candidacy for surgery on a case-by-case basis and abandon the prior doctrine of sidewall involvement being an absolute contra-indication to surgery. In all scenarios where surgery is being considered there is definitive need for these cases to be presented in a multidisciplinary forum to determine if the patient is a suitable candidate for surgery, has reasonable chance to achieve a negative resection margin, and has the functional baseline necessary to achieve a desired functional recovery following surgery. Pre-requisites for any surgeon performing these complex operations include the need for a multispecialty surgical team, expert knowledge of the surgical anatomy, and an understanding of the major potential complications and management of such complications.

References

1. Moore HG, Shoup M, Riedel E, Minsky BD, Alektiar KM, Ercolani M, et al. Colorectal cancer pelvic recurrences: determinants of resectability. Dis Colon Rectum. 2004;47(10):1599–606.
2. Anthopoulos AP, Manetta A, Larson JE, Podczaski ES, Bartholomew MJ, Mortel R. Pelvic exenteration: a morbidity and mortality analysis of a seven-year experience. Gynecol Oncol. 1989;35(2):219–23.
3. Kraybill WG, Lopez MJ, Bricker EM. Total pelvic exenteration as a therapeutic option in advanced malignant disease of the pelvis. Surg Gynecol Obstet. 1988;166(3):259–63.
4. Mor E, Assaf D, Shemla S, Ben-Ami E, Mor-Hadar D, Halfon M, et al. Resection of recurrent pelvic soft tissue sarcoma: is the risk worth the reward? J Surg Res. 2023;283:914–22.
5. Pawlik TM, Skibber JM, Rodriguez-Bigas MA. Pelvic exenteration for advanced pelvic malignancies. Ann Surg Oncol. 2006;13(5):612–23.
6. Höckel M. Laterally extended endopelvic resection: surgical treatment of infrailiac pelvic wall recurrences of gynecologic malignancies. Am J Obstet Gynecol. 1999;180(2 Pt 1):306–12.
7. Mibayashi R. Mibayashi super-radical hysterectomy. Cervical cancer. Tokyo: Nakayama Shoten; 1970. p. 269–79.
8. Austin KKS, Solomon MJ. Pelvic exenteration with en bloc iliac vessel resection for lateral pelvic wall involvement. Dis Colon Rectum. 2009;52(7):1223–33.
9. Shaikh I, Aston W, Hellawell G, Ross D, Littler S, Burling D, et al. Extended lateral pelvic sidewall excision (ELSiE): an approach to optimize complete resection rates in locally advanced or recurrent anorectal cancer involving the pelvic sidewall. Tech Coloproctol. 2015;19(2):119–20.
10. Solomon MJ, Brown KG, Koh CE, Lee P, Austin KK, Masya L. Lateral pelvic compartment excision during pelvic exenteration. Br J Surg. 2015;102(13):1710–7.
11. Vizzielli G, Naik R, Dostalek L, Bizzarri N, Kucukmetin A, Tinelli G, et al. Laterally extended pelvic resection for gynaecological malignancies: a multicentric experience with out-of-the-box surgery. Ann Surg Oncol. 2019;26(2):523–30.
12. Marcille M. Lymphatiques et ganglions ilio-pelviens. Tribune Medicale. 1903:165–70.
13. Lee P, Francis KE, Solomon MJ, Ramsey-Stewart G, Austin KKS, Koh C. Triangle of Marcille: the anatomical gateway to lateral pelvic exenteration. ANZ J Surg. 2017;87(7–8):582–6.
14. Gurtner GC, Jones GE, Neligan PC, Newman MI, Phillips BT, Sacks JM, et al. Intraoperative laser angiography using the SPY system: review of the literature and recommendations for use. Ann Surg Innov Res. 2013;7(1):1.
15. Antoine Lembert 1802-1851. Study on intestinal suture with a description of a new procedure for

performing this surgical operation. 1826. Dis Colon Rectum. 1988;31(6):489–94.
16. Burch JM, Franciose RJ, Moore EE, Biffl WL, Offner PJ. Single-layer continuous versus two-layer interrupted intestinal anastomosis: a prospective randomized trial. Ann Surg. 2000;231(6):832–7.
17. Daix M, Martinez Gomez C, Angeles MA, Tock S, Gladieff L, Gabiache E, et al. Extended pelvic resection for gynecological malignancies: a review of out-of-the-box surgery. Gynecol Oncol. 2022;165(2):393–400.
18. Feng D, Tang Y, Yang Y, Wei X, Han P, Wei W. Does prophylactic ureteral catheter placement offer any advantage for laparoscopic gynecological surgery? A urologist' perspective from a systematic review and meta-analysis. Transl Androl Urol. 2020;9(5):2262–9.
19. Merola J, Arnold B, Luks V, Ibarra C, Resio B, Davis KA, et al. Prophylactic ureteral stent placement vs no ureteral stent placement during open colectomy. JAMA Surg. 2018;153(1):87–90.
20. da Silva G, Boutros M, Wexner SD. Role of prophylactic ureteric stents in colorectal surgery. Asian J Endosc Surg. 2012;5(3):105–10.
21. Sung VW, Wohlrab KJ. Chapter 26 – Urinary tract injury and genital tract fistulas. In: Sokol AI, Sokol ER, editors. General gynecology. Philadelphia: Mosby; 2007. p. 639–61.
22. Brown KG, Koh CE, Solomon MJ, Qasabian R, Robinson D, Dubenec S. Outcomes after en bloc iliac vessel excision and reconstruction during pelvic exenteration. Dis Colon Rectum. 2015;58(9):850–6.
23. Celentano V, Ausobsky JR, Vowden P. Surgical management of presacral bleeding. Ann R Coll Surg Engl. 2014;96(4):261–5.
24. Abdelsattar ZM, Mathis KL, Colibaseanu DT, Merchea A, Bower TC, Larson DW, et al. Surgery for locally advanced recurrent colorectal cancer involving the aortoiliac axis: can we achieve R0 resection and long-term survival? Dis Colon Rectum. 2013;56(6):711–6.
25. Chlupáč J, Filová E, Bačáková L. Blood vessel replacement: 50 years of development and tissue engineering paradigms in vascular surgery. Physiol Res. 2009;58(Suppl 2):S119–s40.
26. Martínez-Gómez C, Angeles MA, Saint-Lebes B, Migliorelli F, Martinez A, Ferron G. How to simplify out-of-the-box surgery in recurrent gynecologic malignancies compromising iliac vessels: preoperative femorofemoral crossover bypass. Int J Gynecol Cancer. 2019:ijgc-2019-000393.
27. Cibula D, Mitáš P. Laterally extended endopelvic resection with external iliac vessels resection and crossover ileofemoral bypass. Int J Gynecol Cancer. 2019;29(8):1338.
28. Peacock O, Smith N, Waters PS, Park-Yun Cheung F, McCormick JJ, Warrier SK, et al. Preemptive femoral-femoral crossover grafting of artery and vein before pelvic exenterative surgery for locally advanced and recurrent pelvic malignancy involving the Aortoiliac Axis. Dis Colon Rectum. 2021;64(1):e2–5.
29. Baqué P, Karimdjee B, Iannelli A, Benizri E, Rahili A, Benchimol D, et al. Anatomy of the presacral venous plexus: implications for rectal surgery. Surg Radiol Anat. 2004;26(5):355–8.
30. Brown KGM, Solomon MJ, Lau YC, Steffens D, Austin KKS, Lee PJ. Sciatic and femoral nerve resection during extended radical surgery for advanced pelvic tumours: long-term survival, functional, and quality-of-life outcomes. Ann Surg. 2021;273(5):982–8.
31. Beck LA, Einertson MJ, Winemiller MH, DePompolo RW, Hoppe KM, Sim FF. Functional outcomes and quality of life after tumor-related hemipelvectomy. Phys Ther. 2008;88(8):916–27.
32. Cardosi RJ, Cox CS, Hoffman MS. Postoperative neuropathies after major pelvic surgery. Obstet Gynecol. 2002;100(2):240–4.
33. Brandt K, Evans GR, Ang KK, Gürlek A, Peden E, Savel T, et al. Postoperative irradiation: are there long-term effects on nerve regeneration? J Reconstr Microsurg. 1999;15(6):421–5.
34. Martin E, Dullaart MJ, Verhoef C, Coert JH. A systematic review of functional outcomes after nerve reconstruction in extremity soft tissue sarcomas: a need for general implementation in the armamentarium. J Plast Reconstr Aesthet Surg. 2020;73(4):621–32.
35. O'Brien AL, West JM, Zewdu A, Grignol VP, Scharschmidt TJ, Moore AM. Nerve transfers to restore femoral nerve function following oncologic nerve resection. J Surg Oncol. 2021;124(1):33–40.
36. Nichols DS, Fenton J, Cox E, Dang J, Garbuzov A, McCall-Wright P, et al. Surgical interventions for lumbosacral plexus injuries: a systematic review. Plast Reconstr Surg Glob Open. 2022;10(8):e4436.

Resection of Tumors Involving the Pelvic Girdle

40

Alexander L. Lazarides, Shawna L. Watson, Guston G. Zervoudakis, Nora L. Watson, and David M. Joyce

Nerve Injury

Background

Tumors of the bony pelvis may affect nerves within the pelvis and peripherally once they have exited into the extremity. The rate of nerve injury for major pelvic tumor resection is quoted at 10–30%, though for sacrectomies, some degree of nerve involvement may be essentially guaranteed [1–4]. Large tumors arising from bone can distort local neurologic anatomy, or potentially involve important neurologic structures. Of particular risk are the sciatic nerve, the pudendal nerve, the femoral nerve and the obturator nerve.

Prevention

It is important to systematically identify and protect these critical neurologic structures. The authors advocate for early identification and, where necessary, mobilization of important neurologic structures early during a dissection. A fundamental understanding of the anatomic location of such nerves is critical when dealing with distorted anatomy, and ensuring sufficient exposure to identify nerves in their normal course may be necessary.

The femoral nerve arises from the lumbar plexus and then courses through the psoas muscle [5]. As such, tumors that involve the origin of the psoas may compromise the ability to salvage the femoral nerve. Once the nerve enters the abdomen, it can be reliably found within the interval between the iliacus and the psoas. In many bone tumors, the iliacus will serve as a suitable tumor margin; as such, the posas and the femoral nerve are often salvageable with careful dissection. The exit of the femoral nerve from the pelvis through the femoral triangle represents another predictable location to identify the nerve. The femoral nerve exits beneath the inguinal ligament and then travels between the sartorius laterally and adductor longus medially as it begins to divide to provide motor and sensory innervation [6].

The sciatic nerve is frequently at risk with tumors involving the sacrum and greater sciatic notch. The sciatic nerve arises from the lumbosacral plexus and courses out through the greater sciatic foramen [7]. The nerve may often be identified in relation to the piriformis, typically exiting below the piriformis; however, in approximately 13% of patients, the anatomic

A. L. Lazarides · G. G. Zervoudakis · N. L. Watson
D. M. Joyce (✉)
Department of Sarcoma, Moffitt Cancer Center, Tampa, FL, USA
e-mail: alexander.lazarides@moffitt.org; Guston.Zervoudakis@moffitt.org; David.joyce@moffitt.org

S. L. Watson
Department of Orthopaedic Surgery, University of South Florida, Tampa, FL, USA
e-mail: Shawna.Watson@moffitt.org

M. Hoffman et al. (eds.), *Major Complications of Female Pelvic Surgery*,
https://doi.org/10.1007/978-3-031-66772-5_40

location may be a variable [8]. The nerve then continues into the posterior compartment of the thigh. The nerve may predictably be found in the posterior thigh after its exit from the greater sciatic notch and often, dissection may be carried out from distal to proximal to ensure its protection throughout the case. Care should be taken as the vena commitantes that travel with the sciatic nerve can cause persistent bleeding. Frequently, the piriformis and the short external rotators may act as a barrier between the nerve and the tumor, allowing preservation.

Like the sciatic nerve, the pudendal nerve is commonly at risk with tumors involving the sacrum and the posterior column of the pelvis and acetabulum. The nerve arises from the S2-4 nerve roots [9]. The nerve exits the pelvis through the greater sciatic notch and then courses over the sacrospinous ligament before re-entering the pelvis through the lesser scatic notch. The nerve then passes through the pudendal canal along the medial wall of the obturator internus as it courses towards the pubic symphysis. The nerve may be predictably found proximal to the ischial spine and below the piriformis, coursing over the sacrospinous ligament as it exits the greater sciatic notch. This ligament is often frequently required to be released for pelvic or sacral resections; care must be taken to ensure protection of this nerve where able. In Type II (periacetabular) and Type III (ischium with superior and inferior rami) resection, the obturator and piriformis muscle bellies are frequently sufficient barriers to protect the pudendal nerve. Alternatively, in sacral resections, the nerve may be found shortly after the sacral nerve roots exit the sacrum.

The obturator nerve arises from the lumbar plexus and is frequently at risk in Type III pelvic resections where osteotomies or tumor involvement may place the nerve at risk. The nerve courses through the psoas major muscle before arising at the medial border of the psoas [10]. The nerve typically courses with the common and internal iliac vessels before coursing along the inner aspect of the pelvis along the obturator internus and exiting through the obturator canal. The obturator canal can predictably be found in the superior and lateral quadrant of the obturator ring and serves as a common anatomic landmark to identify this bundle.

Recognition

Intraoperatively, inadvertent nerve injury may be addressed with careful nerve repair, either direct end to end, or with interposition.

Postoperatively, the effects of nerve injury may not be immediately obvious. Femoral nerve injury will often manifest as weakness with ambulation, specifically loss of knee extensor function and weakness with hip flexion. Sensation may be affected, manifesting as loss of sensation of the anterior and medial thigh, as well as sensation in the saphenous distribution. The sciatic nerve will similarly present with a dramatic impact on functional and ambulatory capacity. Clinically, the manifestation of sciatic nerve injury will depend on the degree of impact. Often, the peroneal distribution is more easily impacted and will manifest as foot drop and sensory loss in the dorsal foot and first webspace. If more severe sciatic nerve injury occurs, there may be a complete loss of motor and sensory function below the level of the knee, save for the saphenous sensory distribution. Additionally, there may be weakness with knee flexion.

Damage to the pudendal nerve depends on the degree of impact. With a single-sided injury, bowel, bladder and sexual function may be variably impacted if the contralateral side is able to compensate. In the postoperative period, bowel and bladder function should be monitored closely and an injury suspected with persistent dysfunction and perineal pain.

Damage to the obturator nerve may not be as readily apparent and the clinical manifestations may not be as severe. Functionally, obturator nerve damage may manifest as weakness of the adductors and numbness in the obturator distribution to the medial thigh. Clinically, though, the manifestations of such an injury may not be as severe and may be readily compensated for by the remaining muscles.

Management

Management of neurologic injury depends on the nerve affected and the degree of impact [11]. Frequently, nerve injuries are neuropraxias, due to prolonged ischemia or stretch intraoperatively. While the time course is variable, supportive care is often all that is required with observation for the return of nerve function. For permanent injury, some instances may warrant nerve repair and grafting.

Whether a nerve recovers or not, bracing can be used to mitigate the effects of a nerve injury. From a motor functional perspective, the sciatic and femoral nerves hold particular importance. For femoral nerve injuries, a knee immobilizer or hinged knee brace locked in extension may be necessary to allow for optimal function with loss of knee extension to allow for safe ambulation. For sciatic nerve injuries, the extent of the injury may determine the type of brace that is required. For a drop foot, primarily affecting the peroneal distribution, an ankle-foot orthosis (AFO) may help manage the motor dysfunction. For more complete injuries, a more rigid orthosis may be required Regardless, for these injuries, fall precautions and gait aids are generally a necessity.

Management of a pudendal nerve injury depends on the degree of impact. In the postoperative period, bowel and bladder function should be monitored closely, and supportive measures provided until clinical resolution is seen. In cases of prolonged or permanent injury, it may be necessary to consider self-catheterization. In more severe cases, diversion may be necessary.

Frequently, obturator nerve injury requires no specific interventions. Physical therapy may be necessary to allow for appropriate compensation by the remaining muscles.

Vascular Injury

Background

Excessive blood loss is a common occurrence in hemipelvectomies and sacrectomies [1, 4]. There are several risk factors for bleeding including patient (obesity, age), tumor (size, location), and treatment (prior surgery, chemotherapy or radiotherapy) related factors. While the internal and external iliac vessels are of greatest concern for surgeons in pelvic and sacral bone resections, here we will also focus on the vessels external to the pelvis that are of equal import to consider in pelvic bone tumor resections.

Prevention

The best prevention is anticipation. Preoperatively, advanced imaging should be scrutinized and the relation of the major vessels to the tumor closely studied. Tumors that closely abut the major internal pelvic vessels should raise red flags and prompt the surgeon to anticipate the need for careful vascular dissection and the risk for potential vascular injury. Tumors that appear to impact the gluteal vessels may compromise important soft tissue flaps and prompt the surgeon to consider plastic surgery assistance for soft tissue coverage. In certain instances, limb salvage may be obviated if the external iliac vessels or femoral vessels are compromised and vascular reconstruction is not an option.

For major pelvic bone tumor resections, the authors advocate for a "high risk" anticipated blood loss protocol to be employed, which alerts all the members of the perioperative team as to the potential intraoperative needs related to major blood loss [12]. At the least, this should call for PRBCs, platelets and FFP to be available, as well as two large-bore peripheral IVs and an arterial line. For complex dissections, specialist vascular surgeons should be available to either assist directly with the dissection/ reconstruction or help manage an unanticipated injury.

Sacrectomy may have consideration for risk to vascular structures [13]. High sacrectomy, at the S1 or S2 levels places the common and internal iliac vessels are risk, particularly if more lateral osteotomies are required. Additionally, larger soft tissue tumors may displace vascular structures, such as the superior and inferior gluteal vessels, as they exit the pelvis. The sacrospinous ligament frequently must be released, and extreme care should be taken as injury to these structures may occur with aberrant dissection.

External to the pelvis, the superior gluteal vessels leave the greater sciatic notch above the piriformis muscle and provide blood supply to the superior portion of the gluteus maximus, the gluteus medius and minimus and the tensor fascia lata. The inferior gluteal vessels primarily supply the inferior portion of the gluteus maximus and the short external rotators (the piriformis and the quadratus femoris). These vessels are most at risk with Type IV and Type I pelvic resections.

The external iliac and femoral vessels are particularly at risk with Type III resections. These vessels are frequently protected within the pelvis by the iliacus and the psoas. As they exit the pelvis below the inguinal ligament, the muscles of the adductor compartment frequently serve as a barrier for tumor involvement as well. While it is uncommon for these vessels to be directly involved by pelvic tumor, large tumors may displace and distort the locally anatomy, predisposing them to injury. The bifurcation of the common femoral vessels often results in a tether point with the profunda femoris as it passes into the adductor compartment, and ligation of this branch may be necessary.

Recognition

Major vascular injury is readily identified with rapid and uncontrolled bleeding, though manifestation may be more subtle [14]. It is important to differentiate between venous and arterial bleeding. Full details of the management of intrapelvic major vascular injury are outlined elsewhere in this book.

Vascular injury external to the pelvis may be more challenging to identify. Of particular import is injury to the superior and inferior gluteal vessels. Injury may manifest by direct trauma or indirectly by thrombosis. Signs of these injuries may be subtle and may be recognized intraoperatively by loss of color, bleeding and contractility of the supplied musculature. The soft tissues should be scrutinized at the completion of every case. In cases of concern for flap perfusion, the use of intraoperative indocyanine green angiography may allow for intraoperative recognition of flap perfusion deficits and allow this to be addressed prior to leaving the operating room. Postoperatively, vascular injury commonly manifests with wound complications and flap breakdown.

Ligation of the profunda femoris is frequently required in pelvic tumor resections. Care should be taken as the medial femoral circumflex is an important supply for the femoral head and often branches from the common or deep femoral artery. Avascular necrosis, while rare, is a potential long-term sequelae of vascular injury and high ligation of the profunda femoris.

Loss of pulses to the distal extremity should prompt close evaluation of the external iliac artery as well as the common and superficial femoral vessels. While direct injury may not have occurred, thrombosis from manipulation is a possibility.

Management

The full details of the management of vascular injury to the internal and external iliac vessels are detailed elsewhere in this book.

Injury to the superior and inferior gluteal vessels is difficult to rectify. In some instances, thrombosis may resolve and the supplied musculature may remain viable. Nonetheless, wound complications and flap breakdown should be anticipated and careful wound monitoring should be employed. Early signs of soft tissue compromise should prompt the surgeon towards early debridement; plastic surgeons should be engaged early for assistance in these circumstances.

Injury to the common or superficial femoral artery may be devastating and may threaten the ability to salvage a limb. Early repair is recommended; in some instances, reconstruction may be necessitated, and a vascular surgeon should be called upon early. Prolonged ischemia should prompt consideration of compartment syndrome, and signs and symptoms of this should be carefully inspected for with a low threshold for prophylactic fasciotomy. In some instances, irreversible damage to the femoral vessels may require amputation.

Unique Considerations in Sacral Resections

Background

Sacrectomy may be necessary for surgical resection of bony metastases or, perhaps more often, as part of a combined surgical approach allowing greater visualization and access to—and/or composite resection of—the lower retroperitoneal pelvic contents such as the rectum. The sigmoid colon connects the descending colon to the rectum on the left side of the pelvis. At the approximate S3 level, the sigmoid colon becomes continuous with the rectum. The rectum lies just anterior to the S3/S4/S5 vertebral bodies until passing through the puborectalis and continuing as the anus.

Prevention

The most reliable way to preserve bladder, bowel and sexual dysfunction when performing a sacral resection is to preserve at least one of the two nerve roots present at each level [15]. Typically, this will be contralateral to the side that is most affected by the tumor.

Careful surgical planning is tantamount to executing a successful sacrectomy. Will the sacrectomy be performed en bloc with the intrapelvic resection, or will it be mobilized from the underlying structures prior to making the bony cuts? Radiated tissue may be adherent to the underlying bony structures and may place structures of the mesorectum (e.g., the blood supply and lymphatic drainage) at risk. The presacral/retrorectal space is a native plane between the mesorectal fascia and presacral (Waldeyer's) fascia, which may be developed during the surgical approach in order to protect the rectum from injury while performing bony cuts on the sacrum.

The sacrospinous and sacrotuberous ligaments are important for the stability of the pelvic ring and inhibitors of specimen removal if not properly divided [16]. Given their broad attachments on the sacrum, these are both most easily divided at their insertions on the ischial spine and ischial tuberosity, respectively. These ligaments may be elevated subperiosteally from their distal bony attachments to minimize the risk of injury to surrounding structures, such as the internal pudendal neurovasculature.

In some circumstances of anticipated dysfunction, or simply for wound protection, a prophylactic diverting colostomy may be performed prior to resection to potentially avoid or ameliorate serious complications associated with any subsequent bowel/bladder dysfunction [17, 18]. In some instances, this colostomy may be reversed once the final nerve function can be accurately assessed.

Recognition

In oncologic disease requiring high sacral resection, it may be necessary to sacrifice sacral nerve roots. The resulting sequelae can manifest variably along a spectrum of bowel and/or bladder dysfunctionality, depending on the bilaterality and number of levels sacrificed. Thus, diligence in monitoring for signs and symptoms of postoperative bowel or bladder dysfunction is pivotal. Alternatively, one may consider a reversable prophylactic diverting colostomy prior to resection as described above.

Management

Lumbopelvic stabilization and bony reconstruction may be required after any sacrectomy which destabilizes the lumbosacral articulation (L5-S1) or the sacroiliac articulation (S1/S2/S3-ilium) on either side [19]. Involvement of an orthopaedic oncology or spine surgeon may be required should lumbopelvic spinal instrumentation and/or custom endoprosthesic reconstruction be required. Often this will include contralateral posterior spinal instrumentation of the L2-S1/S2/ilium and spinal instrumentation cephalad to the defect ipsilaterally with a bar connection to the custom prosthesis on that side.

Fractures of the Pelvic Ring and Acetabulum

Background

In the setting of tumors involving the pelvic girdle, both the disease itself and the various modalities utilized throughout the treatment process are known risk factors for significant and generalized bone loss [20]. The structural integrity of the pelvic ring and acetabulum may be compromised via numerous venues including, but not limited to: direct bony involvement of tumor, metastases, local inflammatory milieu, chemotherapeutics, corticosteroids, malnutrition, or vascular compromise from required vessel sacrifice or periosteal stripping to obtain margins. As a result, pelvic fractures may occur during the treatment of female pelvic tumors.

Radiation can also weaken the bone to the point that the patient develops an insufficiency fracture. This occurs because the radiation both weakens the bone and ages it in a sense. Bone is constantly being stressed and remodels to strengthen the stressed area daily. The radiation degrades the ability of the bone to remodel thus degrading the ability of the osteoblasts to build bone. Small cracks eventually accumulate due to the delayed and limited ability of the bone to remodel after radiation and lead to enough accumulation of microfractures that a formal complete fracture develops which leads to pain.

Prevention

The first step in preventing fractures of the pelvic ring and acetabulum is awareness. By remaining cognizant of the detrimental effects that both the illness and treatment of pelvic girdle tumors can pose on the local bony infrastructure, there are preemptive steps that may be utilized to at least minimize the risk of fracture, if not prevent it completely. These include the utilization of antiresorptive medications such as bisphosphonates, appropriate nutritional management with Vitamin D and calcium monitoring, avoidance of high-impact activities, and physical therapy for core and peripelvic musculature strengthening. For instances involving significant concern for impending pathologic fracture, prophylactic fixation and operative stabilization may even be considered in the prevention of fracture.

When considering radiotherapy, novel techniques to spare and protect the bone may help mitigate the above developments.

Recognition

When treating patients presenting with tumors of the pelvic girdle, one must be wary of both occult and obvious fractures of the pelvic ring and acetabulum. Symptoms associated with stress and insufficiency fractures of the bony pelvis, including pain, difficulty with ambulation and ADLs and functional decline, may often be overlooked and attributed to the primary tumor/malignancy. Thus, one must be prudent in monitoring for any acute changes/increase in a patient's symptoms—particularly after a period of increased activity or an actual traumatic event. Imaging modalities for identifying potential pelvic fractures include those routinely used in examining the bony pelvis beginning with plain radiographs. It is important to maintain a low threshold for advanced imaging with CT or MRI imaging should there be concern for possible occult fractures not immediately identifiable on plain radiographs.

Management

Orthopaedic surgery consultation should be sought once a fracture has been identified. He or she will help to guide further workup and treatment recommendations including imaging studies, decision-making regarding surgical intervention versus close observation, and weightbearing/activity restrictions during the fracture healing period. Surgical treatment may include a combination of operative stabilization and/ or reconstruction.

The majority of these fractures are seen in the superior or inferior pubic rami and do not require surgical intervention. They are typically painful due to the fact that the origins of the adductors and sometimes hamstring muscles pull on these areas creating micromotion, which leads to pain with walking. The sacrum also will be in the radiation field and is a classic location for an insufficiency fracture. A radiograph can identify these insufficiency fractures but the majority require a combination of MRI and CT to identify. Treatment options are limited but can include a combination of cement and screw fixation. Nonoperative treatment is used for the majority of the cases.

Hardware Failure/Mechanical Complications

Background

Hardware failure in the setting of previous resection/reconstruction presents a very difficult problem [21, 22]. Outside of acute trauma, the breakdown of fixation may result from the failure of either hardware or bone. Thus, it is imperative to provide as robust a construct as possible at the initial procedure to account for the weakened state of the bony pelvis at the time of fixation as well as for potential disease progression.

Prevention

The best prevention is to consider not utilizing hardware or reconstruction at all. Patients can in fact do quite well with flail extremities, and in circumstances where the host wound is high risk, resection arthroplasty may be the more prudent choice [23].

If reconstruction is considered, then measures may be undertaken to minimize hardware failure risk. Infection is a major challenge with hardware reconstruction of pelvic defects; the use of extended antibiotic prophlyaxis protocols and bacteriostatic or resistant substances such as silver may help to minimize this risk. The use of plastic surgeons to optimize soft tissue coverage is also of utmost importance.

In resections involving the sacrum, consideration can be made for adding anterior spinal column fixation in conjunction with posterior instrumentation to minimize the risk of hardware failure. Finally, custom 3d printed reconstructions may optimize healing to host bone-to-implant interface.

Recognition

Recognition of hardware failure can fall anywhere on a wide spectrum from the complete breakdown of the construct to minor breakages such as a single screw, leaving the overall construct intact. Overt structure collapse will typically be easily appreciated on plain radiographs but, similar to the recognition of fractures as stated in the section above, advanced imaging should be obtained in the setting of acute trauma or change in symptoms absent obvious signs of hardware failure on basic imaging. However, as opposed to the previous section, the presence of existing hardware may obscure subsequent imaging and must be taken into account when choosing which advanced imaging modality to obtain.

Management

Management of hardware failure is often an extremely difficult task. Treatment will typically involve a thorough discussion with the patient and depend on factors including the full extent of fixation degradation, the patient's symptoms and goals of care, overall disease prognosis, and current stage of treatment.

Pelvic Cancer Complications Involving Bone

Osteomyelitis

Background

Patients having female pelvic cancers will often have radiation or compromise to the blood supply to the bones of the pelvis [24–26]. This places the area and its contents at high risk for development of infections and/ or fistulas. Additionally, compromised vascularity may predispose poor-quality bone to infection. Sequelae may include osteomyelitis of the pelvis or abscesses in the peripelvic region.

Prevention

Osteomyelitis is difficult to prevent, though radiation techniques that spare the bone and surgical techniques that preserve the periosteum and blood supply to the bone while limiting soft tissue stripping may help mitigate these problems from arising in the future. Osteomyelitis typically occurs via hematogenous spread, direct contiguous spread from nearby wounds or structures, or direct inoculation. It is a risk in patients with recurrent bacteremia or sepsis, including patients with chronic wounds near the bone, chronic indwelling lines or immunocompromised or diabetic patients.

Recognition

Typically, when osteomyelitis is suspected or identified it may or may not be associated with an abscess. Signs and symptoms of osteomyelitis may include systemic symptoms such as fever, hypotension, and tachycardia. Additionally, manifestations may include pain, redness and warmth, open wounds or sinuses that probe directly to the bone. Close evaluation is necessary to ensure patients are not manifesting signs of sepsis, as this may be an urgency or an emergency.

Management

It is important to recognize osteomyelitis early, as the first line of treatment for osteomyelitis without abscess is antibiotics alone. In early osteomyelitis, this is frequently sufficient. Often times the osteomyelitis returns because the source of the infection was not addressed. In cases of recurrent osteomyelitis, a fistula from the urogenital or intestinal tract must be considered as this often results in a persistent fluid collection bathing the area [27]. Patients can develop abscess through the obturator foramen or under the pubic symphysis that can eventually track into the thigh (Fig. 40.1).

The infection will not be eradicated unless the source is removed and in chronic infection, bony changes occur that will not resolve without surgical management [26, 28]. With pubic symphysis osteomyelitis or septic arthritis of the pubic symphysis, a simple debridement at that location is unlikely to resolve the issue in a previously radiated field. Source control with debridement is the solution that will eradicate the infection. A simple washout or mechanical debridement with limited resection of the pubic symphysis may not be enough. If the patient has had radiation or has had long-standing osteomyelitis a radical debridement may be necessary, which means removing the unhealthy or dead tissue in the radiated field and can require cutting back to the pubic root and ischial tuberosity to find healthier bleeding bone. This resection often requires a plastics surgery team to place a flap and possible mesh to limit the hernia likely created. Sometimes the anterior, inner(medial), and posterior thighs require debridement because an infection can track along the adductor or hamstring muscles into the distal thigh (Fig. 40.1). Often times after osteomyelitis resection a wound vac can be placed in the front of the pelvis to temporize and allow the remaining tissue to declare itself healthy enough to remain. At the initial presentation of pubic symphysis osteomyelitis, an aspiration for cultures or even a bone culture with a biopsy can help direct appropriate antibiotics. As long as the patient is stable a drain can be placed in the abscess or fluid collection as a temporizing method, which allows the appropriate surgical services to formulate a plan to treat the infection. Operating immediately in a stable patient can lead to nonhealing draining wounds that complicate closure at a later time. The key to treating these infections is to remove the source, and some fistula tracts may not be elongated pathways that track to the bone at all but rather are plastered to the side of the bone. If the anterior pelvic bone is resected patients can usually stand immediately, although ambulation can be difficult due to the detachment of the adductors (Fig. 40.2). Depending on age and deconditioning, the patient will require a walker for about 3 to 4 months and typically will not gain a lot of function or strength back till about 6–8 months. However, patients can expect to get back to work and limited athletic activities such as golf. Typically, patients with long standing osteomyelitis develop pubic symphysis instability which causes pain due to the infection degrading the ligaments ventrally. Patients typically look bet-

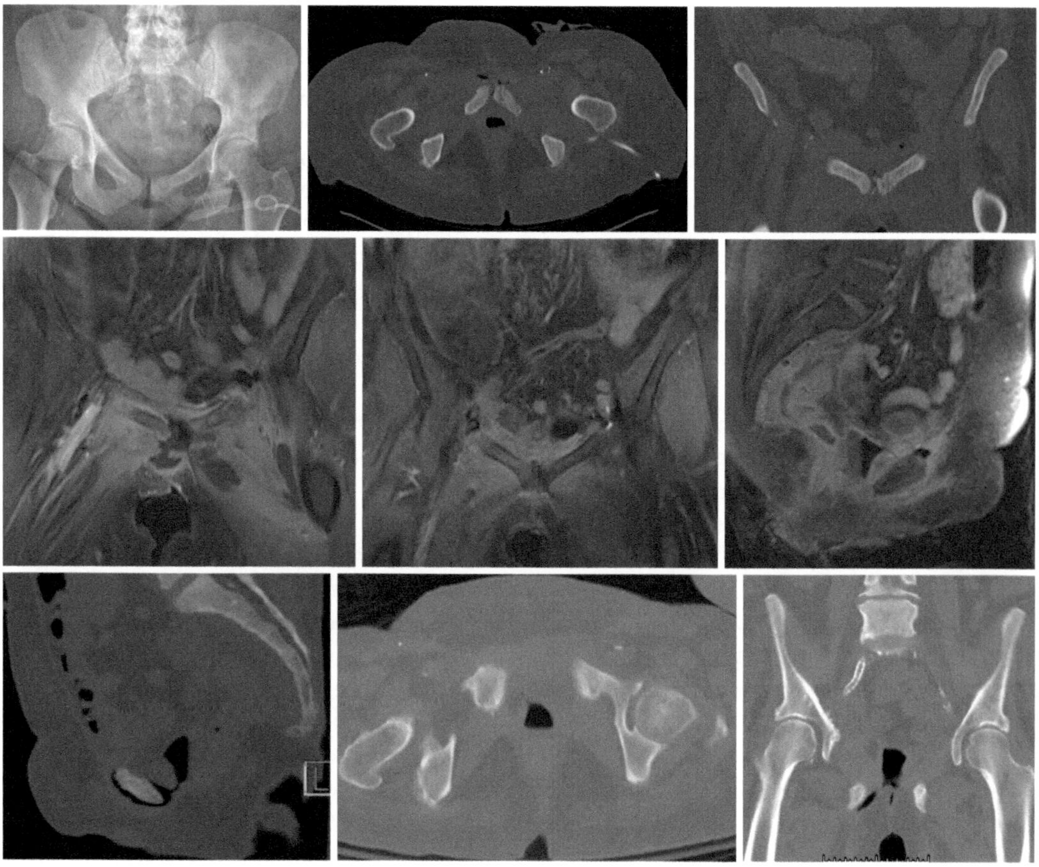

Fig. 40.1 A 51-year-old female who was diagnosed with stage IIb squamous carcinoma of the cervix in 2006 and treated with chemotherapy and radiation with recurrence in 2007 and had anterior pelvic exenteration and ileal colic continent urinary diversion, plastic flap neovagina, en bloc hysterectomy and flaps, and 4 months later a modified radical vulvectomy with lymphadenectomy and flaps with evidence of colonic vaginal fistula with subsequent wound issues with 50.4 Gy of postoperative radiation. Fistula identified in 2020 later developing osteomyelitis and discharge in 2021 that progressed to bilateral leg abscess seen on MRI with associated gas seen on CT and fistula seen on both sagittal CT and MRI

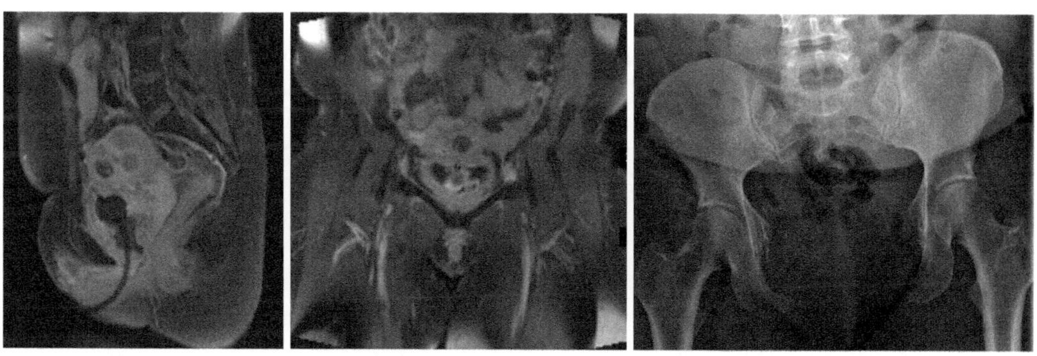

Fig. 40.2 A 50-year-old female with recurrent squamous cell carcinoma of vagina previously treated with chemotherapy and radiation that involved the need for anterior bone resection (radical) and flap

ter 1–2 days after surgery because the infection has been removed.

Radiation Complications of Pelvic Bone

Radiation Osteitis

Radiation osteitis is a complication encountered in female pelvic cancer patients who have required radiation during part of their treatment. The bone can become inflamed and develop a reaction that mimics osteomyelitis. If the periosteum is irritated enough it can be significantly painful. This is generally benign and a self-limiting condition.

Recurrent and Metastatic Lesions

Background

Women with soft tissue pelvic cancer can develop local metastasis to the pelvis through either hematogenous or lymphatic spread.

Prevention

Appropriate treatment.

Recognition

Patients will typically present with pain, neurologic changes or diminished functional capacity/activity. Systemically they may manifest symptoms of increased bone resorption and turnover including hypercalcemia, GI discomfort, kidney stones, and mental status changes.

Appropriate cancer specific staging and surveillance will typically be sufficient. Evaluation should begin with radiographs of the area of concern. In circumstances of uncertainty, advanced imaging, including an MRI with and without contrast, may help to clarify bony involvement by metastatic disease.

Management

Single or multiple lesions in the pelvis can be treated with radiation and/or surgery.

There are some locations of the pelvis that can be affected by metastases and not affect the load-bearing aspect of the bony pelvis. These lesions typically will be treated with radiation.

The portions of the pelvis that are required to be structurally sound in order to walk are the pelvic ring and acetabulum. These portions of the bone include S1, S2, the posterior column and superior dome of the acetabulum and the sciatic buttress from the acetabulum into the bone of the sacroiliac joints. These sections if affected by disease often require some form of surgical treatment in combination with radiation. If a single lesion (either metastasis or local recurrence) is identified and it has been some time since the index treatment with no other metastasis then surgical resection can be considered(Figs. 40.3 and 40.4). If there is early local recurrence or metastasis to the bone with or without distant metastasis, removal down to residual micro-

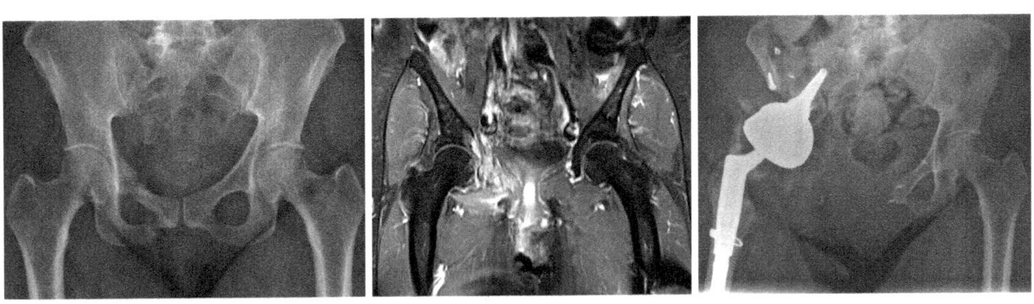

Fig. 40.3 A 60-year-old female with a history of vulvar cancer resected in 2016 with recurrence involving inferior and superior rami and adjacent soft tissue requiring hemipelvectomy and compassionate reconstruction in 2020 that allows her to walk

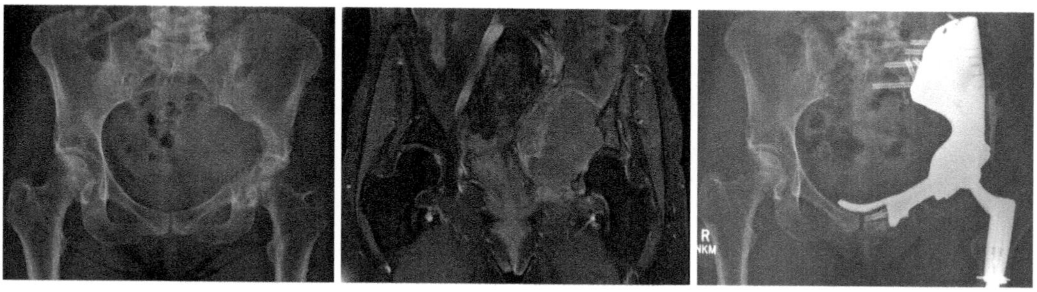

Fig. 40.4 A 59-year-old female with uterine/endometrial cancer who had a resection and vaginal radiation in 2012 who developed a local recurrence with no other metastases and underwent resection and custom reconstruction in 2020 who walks with a cane and is disease free 3 years from surgery

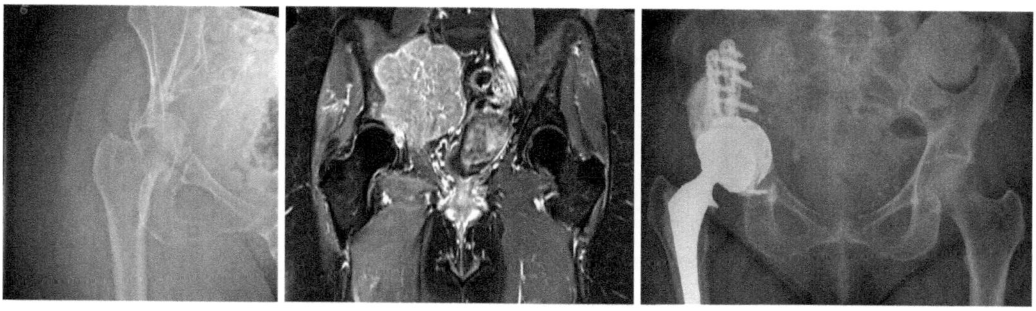

Fig. 40.5 60-year-old female with a history of well-differentiated endometrial adenocarcinoma resected in 2016 with pathologic fracture due to high-grade recurrence with large soft tissue component involving the iliac vessels

scopic disease and stabilization of the weight-bearing bone is undertaken (Fig. 40.5).

Radiation Associated Sarcomas

Background

The female pelvic cancer patient often has had a combination of surgery, radiation and chemotherapy to address the primary site of cancer. Having radiation can, for a small subset of patients, lead to the development of a radiation-associated sarcoma in the pelvis. This typically occurs around 7–10 years out and can be seen as early as 3–4 years out from radiation [29].

Prevention

Preventing radiation-associated sarcomas can be difficult if treatment of the initial cancer necessitates radiotherapy as part of the treatment regimen. Techniques to spare surrounding tissues may help to mitigate some of this risk. In younger patients, the long-term morbidity of radiotherapy should be weighed carefully against the need for local control and overall survival from the primary cancer.

Recognition

It is important to understand this phenomenon because surgeons may think a recurrence has happened and not recognize that an entirely different cancer has formed that requires a different approach for treatment. An open biopsy would be inappropriate in this scenario with a sarcoma as it could significantly affect the morbidity of the resection due to contamination and if a radiation-associated sarcoma is being considered, appropriate and early referral to a specialist should be made by sending it to the appropriate orthopaedic oncologist or sarcoma surgeon.

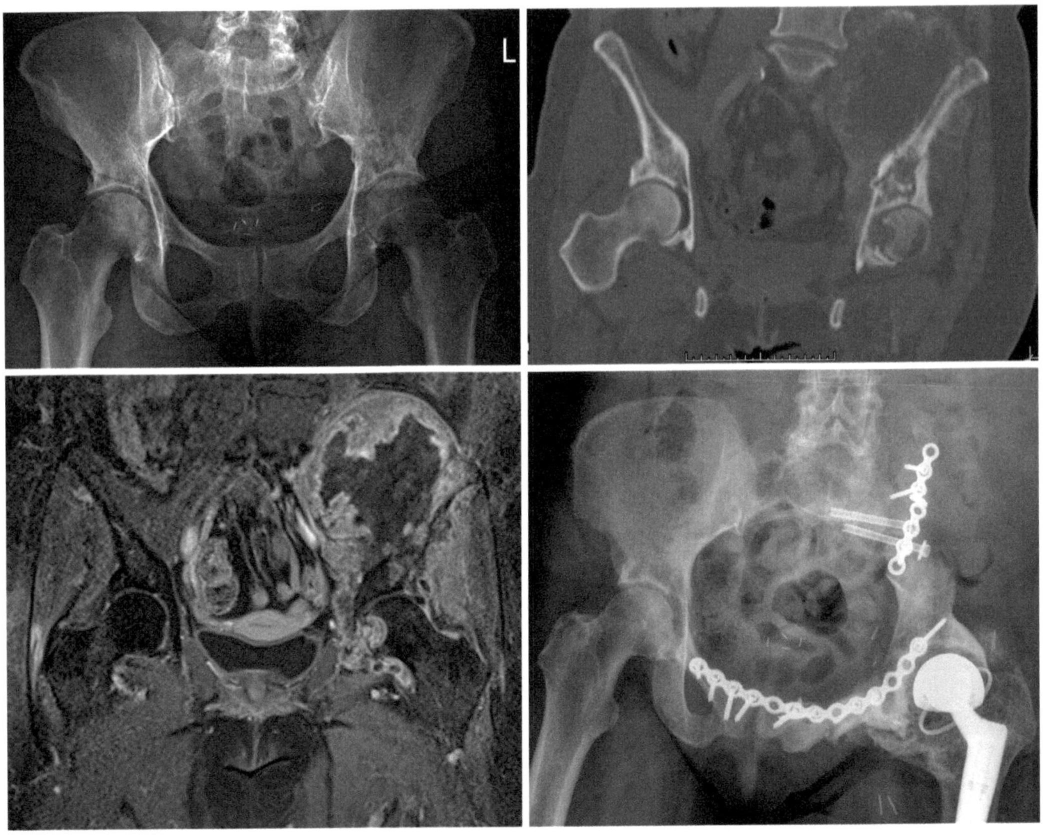

Fig. 40.6 A 49-year-old female with cervical cancer treated in 2004 with radiation and developed a mass in 2017 thought to be recurrence but was found to be consistent with radiation-associated sarcoma that underwent resection and reconstruction with allograft and hip reconstruction

Management

These are treated with some form of adjuvant treatment and surgery with the majority undergoing resection alone. If the tumor involves bone the orthopaedic oncologist can resect the affected parts of the pelvis (i.e., a hemipelvectomy) and reconstruct parts of the pelvis that are needed to ambulate (Fig. 40.6). Parts of the pelvis can be resected that do not need to be reconstructed. The bony pelvis itself serves as a way to contain the viscera and serves as a foundation for weight bearing and muscle origins to ambulate. If the front of the pelvis, not involving the joint, is affected and resected and not replaced the plastic surgery team can place a flap and mesh with the aid of suture anchors to limit the development of a hernia. If the hip joint is involved and is resected it can be reconstructed with both custom and compassionate use devices.

Wound Healing Considerations

Background

Surgical wound complications are a common outcome of oncologic surgery [1–4]. Multiple factors may contribute to this such as a patient's nutritional/medical status, previous surgeries in the same location, radiation, prolonged surgical time, and type and timing (staged vs. primary closure) of plastic surgery intervention.

Prevention

Prevention of wound dehiscence and superficial infection is the first and foremost important part of care. It is important to consider all aspects, such as discussing with patients their perioperative nutrition. One purpose of ERAS (enhanced recovery after surgery) is to increase the perioperative nutritional intake. Proper wound care education also needs to be discussed with the patient prior to surgery and postoperatively.

Previous surgeries and radiation to the surgical site prior to a hemipelvectomy do increase the risk of wound breakdown [30, 31]. Typically, these surgeries and treatments were done in the past with no thought of the patient possibly needing a large pelvic reconstruction in the future. Carefully planning surgical incision and reconstruction with the team is imperative to optimize soft tissue closure over the reconstruction, to decrease tension on the soft tissues.

Attention to the manor of closure also needs to be addressed to decrease adverse outcomes. Patients can be primarily closed without plastic reconstruction versus complex closure with large flaps to ensure plenty of muscular and soft tissue coverage between the implant and subcutaneous tissue. Again, decreasing tension at surgical incisions and soft tissue coverage are key. At times an incisional wound vac can be used to protect the area from drainage that may help decrease maceration of the incision edges during the healing process. The use of creams or ointments on the surgical areas are not recommended as the edges of skin become swollen. The powder is not recommended as it often becomes a paste.

Recognition

As with most complications related to surgery, early recognition is important. Frequent wound checks while the patient is recovering in the hospital and checks during the first 6–8 weeks are important. Most commonly skin healing fails between weeks 6–8 regardless of how the skin looks at week 4. Patient's incisions can be followed in person and via serial photographs.

Recommendations for follow-up will depend on the type of closure. The common areas for breakdown are at the apexes of the incision and incisions that are in soft tissue creases and under skin folds due to skin tension and increased moisture, respectively.

Educating the patient on signs and symptoms of early breakdown when they are a recovering outpatient is also key, and patients should be instructed to contact the surgical team at first sight of concern. An enlarging fluid collection (seroma/hematoma), redness, warmth, or new/increased active drainage, a large area of eschar sloughing off the incision, and darkening of the skin (necrosis) should be addressed or watched closely for changes. Early use of antibiotics is warranted especially in patients that have had radiation in the past.

Management

Depending on how the wound is breaking down, different methods can be used to address the problem. All patients who have had a history of radiation should be on prophylactic oral antibiotics until their wound is healed.

Simple and small areas of wound dehiscence can usually be addressed with a drying agent such as Betadine wash BID, leave dry to air, then cover with light nonstick dressing and paper tape. Larger and deeper areas can be cared for with wet-to-dry dressings.

Areas of soft tissue necrosis are often watched, and the large eschar is not removed until it declares itself. Evaluation by the surgeon is needed to determine if bedside debridement followed by wound care or surgical intervention is needed.

Large wound dehiscence with metal prostheses exposed requires immediate attention via the oncologic orthopaedic surgeon and plastic surgery. Cultures should also be done intraoperatively with ID consult and IV antibiotics.

References

1. Schwab JH, Healey JH, Rose P, Casas-Ganem J, Boland PJ. The surgical management of sacral chordomas. Spine (Phila Pa 1976). 2009;34(24):2700–4.
2. Zeifang F, Buchner M, Zahlten-Hinguranage A, Bernd L, Sabo D. Complications following operative treatment of primary malignant bone tumours in the pelvis. Eur J Surg Oncol. 2004;30(8):893–9.
3. Tunn PU, Fehlberg S, Andreou D, Kettelhack C. Endoprosthesis in the operative treatment of bone tumours of the pelvis. Z Orthop Unfall. 2007;145(6):753–9.
4. Capanna R, van Horn JR, Guernelli N, Briccoli A, Ruggieri P, Biagini R, et al. Complications of pel-

vic resections. Arch Orthop Trauma Surg (1978). 1987;106(2):71–7.
5. Jakubowicz M. Topography of the femoral nerve in relation to components of the iliopsoas muscle in human fetuses. Folia Morphol (Warsz). 1991;50(1–2):91–101.
6. Kalinin RE, Suchkov IA, Klimentova EA, Shanaev IN. Clinical anatomy of deep femoral vessels in the area of femoral triangle. Angiol Sosud Khir. 2021;27(1):17–23.
7. Ribeiro FS, Bettencourt Pires MA, Silva Junior EX, Casal D, Casanova-Martinez D, Pais D, et al. Rethinking sciatica in view of a bilateral anatomical variation of the sciatic nerve, with low origin and high division: historical, anatomical and clinical approach. Acta Medica Port. 2018;31(10):568–75. Epub 20181031
8. Eastlack J, Tenorio L, Wadhwa V, Scott K, Starr A, Chhabra A. Sciatic neuromuscular variants on MR neurography: frequency study and interobserver performance. Br J Radiol. 2017;90(1079):20170116. Epub 20170822.
9. Schraffordt SE, Tjandra JJ, Eizenberg N, Dwyer PL. Anatomy of the pudendal nerve and its terminal branches: a cadaver study. ANZ J Surg. 2004;74(1–2):23–6.
10. Yoshida T, Nakamoto T, Kamibayashi T. Ultrasound-guided obturator nerve block: a focused review on anatomy and updated techniques. Biomed Res Int. 2017;2017:7023750. Epub 20170209.
11. Hasija R, Kelly JJ, Shah NV, Newman JM, Chan JJ, Robinson J, et al. Nerve injuries associated with total hip arthroplasty. J Clin Orthop Trauma. 2018;9(1):81–6. Epub 20171028.
12. Malone DL, Hess JR, Fingerhut A. Massive transfusion practices around the globe and a suggestion for a common massive transfusion protocol. J Trauma. 2006;60(6 Suppl):S91–6.
13. Tang X, Guo W, Yang R, Tang S, Ji T. Risk factors for blood loss during sacral tumor resection. Clin Orthop Relat Res. 2009;467(6):1599–604. Epub 20080910.
14. Yoo TK, Min SK, Ahn S, Kim SY, Min SI, Park YJ, et al. Major vascular injury during nonvascular surgeries. Ann Vasc Surg. 2012;26(6):825–32. Epub 20120622.
15. Moran D, Zadnik PL, Taylor T, Groves ML, Yurter A, Wolinsky JP, et al. Maintenance of bowel, bladder, and motor functions after sacrectomy. Spine J. 2015;15(2):222–9. Epub 20140906.
16. Hammer N, Hoch A, Klima S, Le Joncour JB, Rouquette C, Ramezani M. Effects of cutting the sacrospinous and sacrotuberous ligaments. Clin Anat. 2019;32(2):231–7. Epub 20181121.
17. Guo Y, Palmer JL, Shen L, Kaur G, Willey J, Zhang T, et al. Bowel and bladder continence, wound healing, and functional outcomes in patients who underwent sacrectomy. J Neurosurg Spine. 2005;3(2):106–10.
18. Rose PS, Sciubba DM. Technique of oncologic sacrectomy. In: Sciubba DM, editor. Spinal tumor surgery: a case-based approach. Springer; 2019.
19. Wellings EP, Houdek MT, Owen AR, Bakri K, Yaszemski MJ, Sim FH, et al. Comparison of free vascularized fibular flaps and allograft fibular strut grafts to supplement spinopelvic reconstruction for sacral malignancies. Bone Joint J. 2021;103-B(8):1414–20.
20. Chung YK, Lee YK, Yoon BH, Suh DH, Koo KH. Pelvic insufficiency fractures in cervical cancer after radiation therapy: a meta-analysis and review. In Vivo. 2021;35(2):1109–15.
21. Fisher NE, Patton JT, Grimer RJ, Porter D, Jeys L, Tillman RM, et al. Ice-cream cone reconstruction of the pelvis: a new type of pelvic replacement: early results. J Bone Joint Surg Br. 2011;93(5):684–8.
22. Fujiwara T, Medellin Rincon MR, Sambri A, Tsuda Y, Clark R, Stevenson J, et al. Limb-salvage reconstruction following resection of pelvic bone sarcomas involving the acetabulum. Bone Joint J. 2021;103-B(4):795–803.
23. Beadel GP, McLaughlin CE, Aljassir F, Turcotte RE, Isler MH, Ferguson P, et al. Iliosacral resection for primary bone tumors: is pelvic reconstruction necessary? Clin Orthop Relat Res. 2005;438:22–9.
24. Micha JP, Goldstein BH, Rettenmaier MA, Caillouette JT, Fee MJ, Brown JV 3rd. Pelvic radiation necrosis and osteomyelitis following chemoradiation for advanced stage vulvar and cervical carcinoma. Gynecol Oncol. 2006;101(2):349–52. Epub 20060126.
25. Ambrosini F, Zegna L, Testino N, Vecchio E, Mantica G, Suardi N, et al. Management of osteomyelitis of the pubic symphysis following urinary fistula in patients with radiation-induced urethral strictures after prostate cancer treatment. Cent European J Urol. 2022;75(3):284–9. Epub 20220916.
26. Dudareva M, Ferguson J, Riley N, Stubbs D, Atkins B, McNally M. Osteomyelitis of the pelvic bones: a multidisciplinary approach to treatment. J Bone Jt Infect. 2017;2(4):184–93. Epub 20171009.
27. Mandava A, Koppula V, Sharma G, Kandati M, Raju K, Subramanyeshwar RT. Evaluation of genitourinary fistulas in pelvic malignancies with etiopathologic correlation: role of cross sectional imaging in detection and management. Br J Radiol. 2020;93(1111):20200049. Epub 20200615.
28. Gupta S, Zura RD, Hendershot EF, Peterson AC. Pubic symphysis osteomyelitis in the prostate cancer survivor: clinical presentation, evaluation, and management. Urology. 2015;85(3):684–90.
29. Lazarides AL, Burke ZDC, Gundavda MK, Novak R, Ghert M, Wilson DA, et al. How do the outcomes of radiation-associated pelvic and sacral bone sarcomas compare to primary osteosarcomas following surgical resection? Cancers (Basel). 2022;14(9). Epub 20220427.
30. Gu Q, Wang D, Cui C, Gao Y, Xia G, Cui X. Effects of radiation on wound healing. J Environ Pathol Toxicol Oncol. 1998;17(2):117–23.
31. Ogura K, Boland PJ, Fabbri N, Healey JH. Rate and risk factors for wound complications after internal hemipelvectomy. Bone Joint J. 2020;102-B(3):280–4.

Pelvic Reconstructive Procedures

41

Julian Pribaz and Kristen Whalen

Background

Trauma and extensive extirpative gynecologic, urologic and/or colorectal surgery for malignancy can result in large pelvic defects that require complex soft tissue reconstruction by plastic surgeons.

It should be remembered that this is a team surgery and attention to detail during the extirpative and reconstructive phases are equally important to maximize patient outcomes and prevent complications. The extirpative surgeon must strive for complete tumor excision with clear margins, have minimal blood loss, and avoid fecal and urinary contamination. This chapter will focus on optimizing the reconstructive aspects of this team surgical event.

The goals of female pelvic reconstructive surgery are to provide durable external soft tissue coverage, obliterate internal dead space, and restore aesthetics and sexual function when possible.

Options for pelvic reconstruction are numerous and include primary closure, skin grafts, and flaps. Local and regional pedicled flaps such as the vertical rectus abdominis myocutaneous flap, omental flap, gracilis flap, Singapore flap, other thigh flaps, and gluteal flaps are the mainstay of pelvic reconstruction. Distant free tissue transfer can be considered when locoregional donor sites are not available, although this is exceedingly rare [1, 2].

Flap reconstruction helps decrease complications compared to primary closure and skin grafting because it provides healthy, well-vascularized tissue (which enables delivery of antibiotics to this unfavorable milieu), obliterates dead space and decreases tension on the skin closure [3, 4]. Primary closure following abdominoperineal resection or pelvic exenteration is more likely to have delayed wound healing which prolongs patients' recovery, negatively affects quality of life, and delays adjuvant therapy [4].

The choice of flap reconstruction is determined by the location, size and depth of the defect, the availability of donor tissues, and the goal of reconstruction [5–7]. Multiple flaps may be necessary for composite reconstruction of extremely large defects or for vaginal reconstruction [7–9].

There are several inherent challenges in reconstructing pelvic defects. This unique anatomic area is dependent, exposed to external pressure and shear forces, and is difficult to keep clean due to moisture, high bacterial counts, and contamination from feces and/or urine [6, 9, 10]. Many of these patients have a history of radiation which results in decreased vascularity and

J. Pribaz (✉) · K. Whalen
Department of Plastic Surgery, University of South Florida Morsani College of Medicine, Tampa, FL, USA
e-mail: jpribaz@usf.edu; kswhalen@usf.edu

M. Hoffman et al. (eds.), *Major Complications of Female Pelvic Surgery*,
https://doi.org/10.1007/978-3-031-66772-5_41

pliability of local tissues. Additionally, patients may be elderly and debilitated, with poor nutritional status and other co-morbidities. These factors all contribute to a poor wound-healing environment [6].

Complications after pelvic reconstructive surgery are common and include:

- Wound dehiscence and delayed wound healing.
- Fluid collection (hematoma, seroma).
- Infection.
- Partial or total flap loss.
- Fistula.

Donor site morbidity can occur as well, specifically abdominal bulge or hernia formation following rectus abdominis flaps and cellulitis and fluid collections following thigh flaps [1, 11]. In general, the vertical rectus abdominis myocutaneous flap has a lower complication rate over thigh and gluteal based flaps [4, 11]. However, certain clinical situations including patients with prior abdominal surgeries, morbid obesity, hernias, or ostomy placement through both rectus muscles may preclude the use of abdominal-based flaps.

The use of perforator flaps such as deep inferior epigastric perforator flap, anterolateral thigh flap, gluteal perforator flap, or perineal perforator-based island flaps that spare muscle have reduced donor site morbidity [4, 12]. In general, donor sites should be carefully chosen keeping complication profile and possible future surgical needs in mind [7].

Overall complication rates after pelvic defect reconstruction with flaps are high, nearing 40% [13]. This is somewhat attributable to the increased co-morbidities of patients requiring extensive pelvic resections and reconstruction. Preparedness on behalf of the reconstructive surgeon is essential in anticipating and managing complications in this high-risk patient population. One must recognize settings that predispose patients to potential complications such as previous failed procedures, trauma, and extensive radiation damage and adjust the reconstructive plan accordingly.

While the first reconstructive option should have the most reliable and predictable outcome, some flaps will invariably fall short. The surgeon must critically analyze why a complication occurred and optimize contributing risk factors. Lastly, one must have several backup plans, or lifeboats, and consider these during the initial operation so as not to burn bridges that may be needed in the future. This is where surgeon experience and judgment are invaluable.

Prevention

Prevention and mitigation of complications in this difficult group of patients should be considered during ALL phases of treatment, namely pre-, intra- and postoperatively.

Preoperative

Thorough preoperative evaluation of patients is critical in planning the optimal reconstructive surgery to minimize complications from the outset. A detailed history is performed to ascertain the patient's medical and surgical history, as well as treatment goals including the desire for sexual function. Modifiable patient risk factors, such as obesity, tobacco use, anemia, diabetes, clotting disorders, and malnutrition, should be identified and optimized prior to surgery [2, 8, 11, 14]. When treating high-risk patients, it is important to counsel them appropriately about outcome expectations [11].

Patient examination should focus on anatomic features involved, evidence of radiation damage, and availability of donor sites including areas of excess soft tissue, preexisting scars, undermining, ostomies, and hernias. If the vascular integrity of potential donor sites is in question, a handheld Doppler exam or computed tomography angiography can be performed preoperatively.

Close communication with the extirpative surgeons regarding the expected extent of resection and diversion of the urogenital or anorectal system is helpful in developing a reconstructive plan. Finally, one must review all previous operative procedures and available imaging to prevent errors from poor flap selection.

Intraoperative

Wide surgical preparation and draping of the pelvis and donor sites is essential for exposure. A position change may be required to appropriately access and mobilize donor tissue, such as switching to prone positioning to elevate gluteal flaps for posterior perineal defects.

In addition to antiseptic skin preparation, prophylactic intravenous antibiotics should be administered within 60 minutes of the start of surgery and re-dosed as indicated to prevent infection. Every effort should be made to optimize surgical efficiency to decrease operative time as lengthy surgeries have increased risks of complications [5].

The reconstructive surgeon must first critically evaluate the extent of the anatomic defect including deep space and skin involvement (Fig. 41.1). Any heavily radiated, devitalized, or traumatized tissue that remains should be debrided back to healthy, vascularized tissue to facilitate healing. It is important to wait until the final debridement before finalizing your flap design.

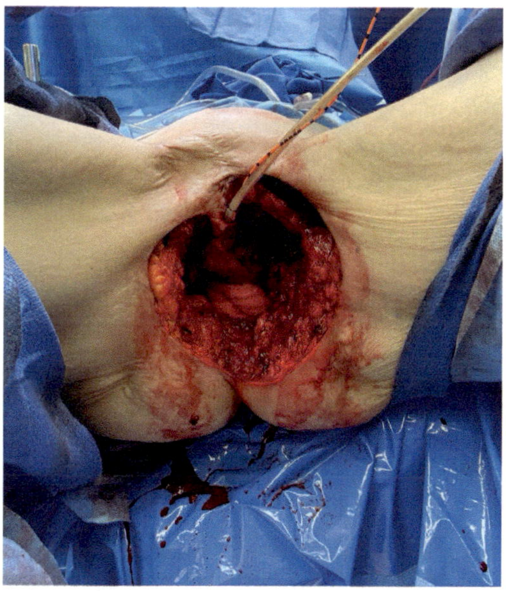

Fig. 41.1 Large pelvic defect with internal dead space and external skin defect

Thoughtful and meticulous flap design, dissection, and inset are imperative in achieving a successful reconstruction.

In cases of a large pelvic defect with a deep space component, the surgical plan should include obliteration of the dead space with bulky muscle, omental or de-epithelized flaps. The extra tissue helps cover exposed pelvic structures and mechanically supports the internal organs. This can effectively prevent internal herniation, prolapse and fluid collection which all predispose the patient to infection, incisional dehiscence, and fistulae [3, 4, 8, 15].

In cases of a large skin defect, the flap should incorporate a skin paddle to replace the resected perineal skin. Otherwise, there would be undue tension on primary skin closure and an increased risk of incisional dehiscence [3]. A skin paddle can also be utilized to resurface vaginal defects. Intraoperative templates are useful in designing the flap dimensions. However, the skin paddle should be slightly oversized to account for tissue thickness, edema, and rotation, and to avoid a tight closure which could compress the vascular pedicle [16] (Fig. 41.2).

When designing and elevating flaps, the reconstructive surgeon must have a thorough understanding of the vascularity of the various flaps including pedicle location, arc of rotation,

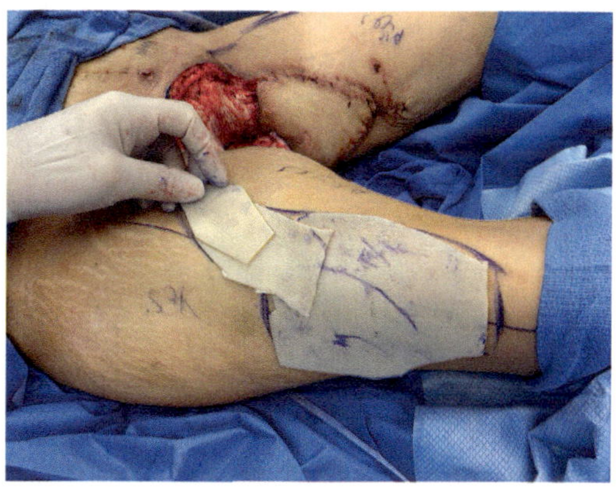

Fig. 41.2 Flap design based on an intraoperative template of a perineal defect made with hydrocolloid dressing

and location and reliability of cutaneous perforators. With this knowledge, surgeons can make modifications to flap design to meet the unique requirements of the defect [17]. Dominant perforators should be incorporated into the flap design when feasible to improve vascularity. A handheld doppler is helpful in identifying perforators for this purpose.

In the case of rectus abdominis flaps, designing the skin paddle over the robust periumbilical perforators improves perfusion. The skin paddle can also be oriented obliquely and extend beyond the costal margin to increase the length of the flap for use in large or posteriorly oriented defects [18, 19]. Any part of the flap that cannot reach the perineum should be de-epithelialized rather than de-skinned because maintenance of the dermal plexus improves vascularity to the distally oriented skin paddle. Leaving the inferior attachment of the rectus muscle is advised to prevent stretching, twisting, kinking, or avulsion of the vascular pedicle once it is transposed into the pelvis (Fig. 41.3).

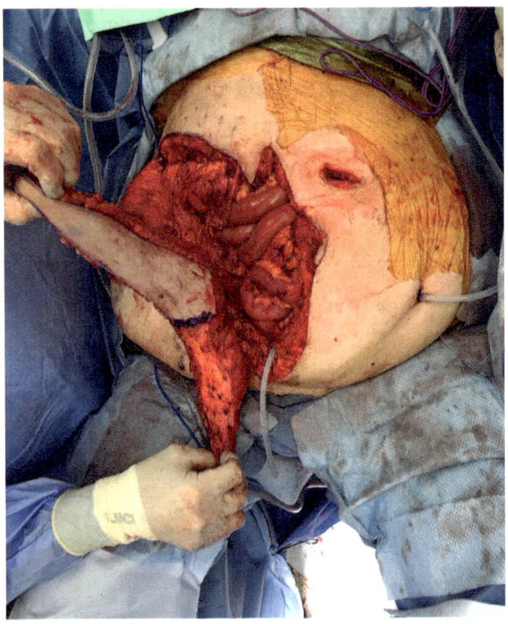

Fig. 41.3 Design of an extended oblique vertical rectus abdominus myocutaneous (VRAM) flap. Note the intrapelvic portion is de-epithelialized to preserve the subdermal plexus and the inferior muscular attachment to the pubis is maintained to prevent pedicle kinking, twisting, and avulsion when transferring the flap into the pelvis

For advancement flaps from the thigh or buttocks, the flap should be designed large enough to include reliable perforators, provide sufficient skin coverage, and allow for flap re-advancement if needed [19]. The leading edges can also be de-epithelialized to fill internal dead space (Fig. 41.4).

It is important to discuss preserving the omentum with the extirpative surgeons if you are planning to incorporate it into the reconstruction. The omentum should be adequately dissected based on the right or left gastroepiploic pedicle to avoid tension on the blood supply and prevent a tight intrabdominal band that may lead to internal hernia [7].

Once the flap has been elevated, it can be transferred to the recipient site. One must release all scar contractures and radiated tissue to avoid constriction and pressure on the flap, which can develop once postoperative edema has set in. If there is any concern about the vascularity of the flap, the subcutaneous tunnel should be released to accommodate the transferred tissue. The skin paddle can be extended to include a wide skin bridge to cover the tracks of the pedicled flap and eliminate the need for a tunnel (Fig. 41.5).

When performing free tissue transfer (which is uncommon, due to the large number of regional flap options), recipient vessels must be inspected

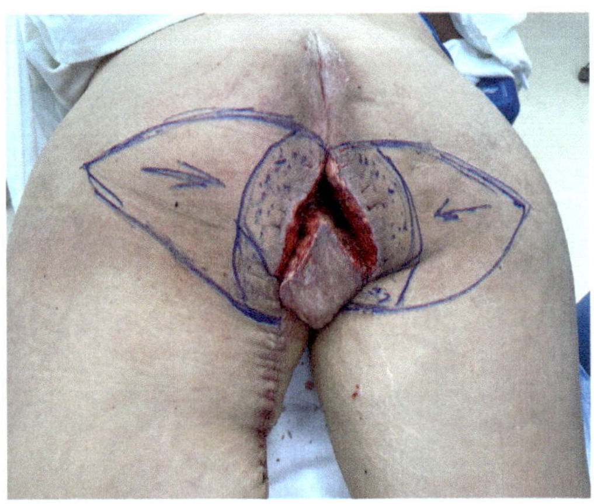

Fig. 41.4 Design of bilateral V-Y gluteal fasciocutaneous flaps for secondary reconstruction after dehiscence and distal flap necrosis of a VRAM flap. Note the leading edges are marked for de-epithelialization to fill internal dead space

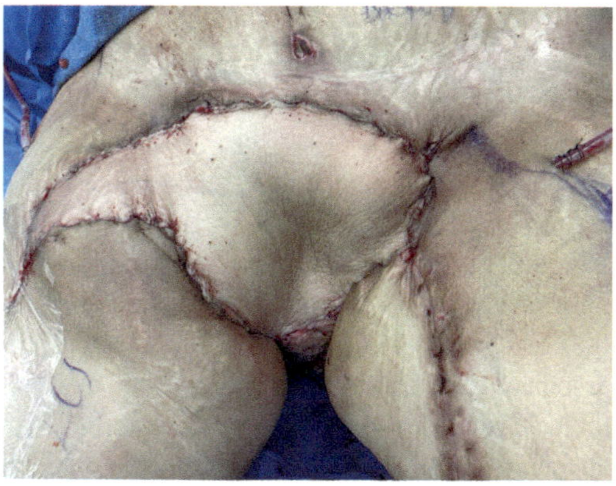

Fig. 41.5 Right pedicled anterolateral thigh with an extended skin paddle to cover the pedicle's course and prevent the need for a constrictive subcutaneous tunnel

intraoperatively to ensure they are intact and outside of the zone of radiation. If local vessels are unavailable, an arteriovenous vascular loop from regional vessels can be created with a vein graft [20].

Intraoperative flap perfusion can be assessed by observing clinical bleeding patterns or by the use of SPY angiography technology. Tissue with evidence of poor blood flow should be excised prior to flap inset.

In addition to the recipient site, one must also consider the donor site's morbidity. To reduce the risk of bulge or herniation formation after transfer of rectus abdominis muscles, it is critical to restore the abdominal wall. The fascia can be closed primarily when harvesting a muscle-only rectus abdominis flap. In cases that require a myocutaneous flap, the anterior rectus sheath and overlying soft tissue are harvested with the muscle resulting in a fascial defect. Adjunctive techniques to reduce abdominal wall morbidity in this setting include fascia-sparing rectus muscle harvest with primary fascial closure, component separation with primary fascial closure, or placement of an inlay mesh that is inset on proper anatomic tension [15, 18]. Biologic mesh should be considered in contaminated or infected wound beds.

In patients where the abdominal donor site is not available due to previous surgeries or multiple ostomies, the thigh or gluteal tissue can be used. These flaps are ideally harvested as fasciocutaneous flaps in ambulatory patients to preserve mobility [8, 14]. A pinch test verifies that the donor site can be closed primarily without excessive tension. Incisions should be oriented along resting skin tension lines to allow for larger flap harvest and inconspicuous donor site closure. Skin grafting of the donor site may be required if it cannot be closed primarily.

Measures should be taken to prevent fluid collection which can later become a source of infection. Careful hemostasis is essential during all stages of the operation. Multiple drains should be placed including at least one large caliber drain in the pelvis and a drain beneath the flap. Progressive tension sutures can also be considered to minimize dead space at the donor site.

The flap should be inset loosely to prevent kinking of the pedicle or perforators [7]. A meticulous multilayer, water-tight cutaneous closure should be performed while avoiding overly tightened sutures that can result in tissue necrosis.

There are several options for dressings and the choice is often surgeon dependent. The ideal dressing absorbs drainage, protects the incision from shear forces, minimizes trauma to surrounding skin, and allows regular monitoring of the incision and flaps by the surgical team. Absorbent abdominal gauze pads and mesh panties are simple, cheap and achieve the above goals. Dressings should be changed at least daily and as needed for saturation or contamination.

Postoperative

Protocols vary based on surgeon and institutional preference, but postoperative activity modification and positioning is critical in preventing pressure induced necrosis and dehiscence in the early postoperative period. Optimal positioning depends on the exact location of the flap but ranges from prone to supine and lateral decubitus. Air-fluidized mattresses are a useful adjunct for pressure offloading. Some surgeons opt for bed rest for the first 1–3 days, while others encourage early ambulation to prevent venous thromboembolism. Sitting or waist flexion greater than 30 degrees is generally prohibited for 3–6 weeks to avoid direct pressure on the flap and tension on the skin closure. Once patients start ambulating, they should be instructed to log-roll to stand with the guidance of a physical therapist [2, 4, 9].

Due to the dependent nature of these surgical sites, the incisions are prone to fluid egression and maceration. It is important to keep the incisions dry with frequent dry dressing changes. Closed suction drains should be maintained for several weeks until output is less than approximately 30 cc per day to prevent fluid collections in gravity-dependent zones [2, 4]. It is also advisable to leave perineal drains in place until the intrabdominal drains have been removed by the extirpative surgeons. Sutures are removed once incisions are fully healed.

Postoperative antibiotics, especially in patients with foreign materials such as mesh, should be considered to prevent infection. Patients are closely monitored for derangements such as anemia, hyperglycemia, hypothermia, hypovolemia, and malnutrition and optimized accordingly.

Recognition

Early identification of complications is best achieved with close postoperative monitoring. Patients are typically hospitalized for 7 to 14 days and seen in the clinic weekly or biweekly until drains are removed and complete healing is observed.

Wound Dehiscence and Delayed Wound Healing

Delayed wound healing is the most common complication after female pelvic reconstructive surgery and requires timely diagnosis and treatment. Wound dehiscence or delayed healing is recognized on exam as lack of completely opposed skin edges greater than two weeks after surgery.

Fluid Collection

Superficial fluid collections can be palpated on exam and may be associated with incisional drainage. Clear drainage is most consistent with a seroma but can also indicate a urine leak. Sanguineous drainage suggests a hematoma and purulence is concerning for an abscess. Laboratory studies are useful to evaluate for associated anemia or leukocytosis. Fluid analysis including culture, cytology, and creatinine can also help determine the etiology of the collection and guide treatment.

Infection

Superficial infection can be diagnosed on exam with findings of warmth, erythema, edema, and tenderness. Deeper organ space infections are best identified with imaging such as ultrasound or computed tomography. Significant pain, necrotic tissue with malodorous drainage, and rapidly progressive sepsis are signs of a serious necrotizing soft tissue infection. This clinical diagnosis requires a high index of suspicion and warrants prompt surgical exploration.

Partial or Total Flap Loss

Pedicled and free flaps are susceptible to vascular compromise by pedicle compression, clotting, or kinking which necessitate timely intervention in the operating room to prevent flap loss [2]. These patients should be closely monitored postoperatively by experienced clinicians with serial flap checks which include flap color, turgor, capillary refill, temperature, and doppler when applicable. Flaps that are pale, cool and have weak or absent arterial doppler signals and slow capillary refill likely have arterial insufficiency. Flaps with dark, purplish discoloration, edema, and brisk capillary refill are suffering from venous insufficiency. Early recognition of a perfusion problem is essential in salvaging flaps.

Fistula

Fistulae can be identified on exam by abnormal connections between anatomic structures such as the skin, bladder, vagina, and rectum. Patients may note abnormal drainage as well. Static and dynamic imaging can be helpful in further characterization of the fistula.

Donor Site Complications

Donor site hernia can be diagnosed as a palpable bulge on physical exam or with computed tomographic scans. As with flap recipient sites, donor sites are also subject to wound dehiscence, fluid collections, and infection and are recognized as above. In the case of abdominal incisional dehiscence, the wound should be gently probed or imaged to assess for fascial integrity.

Management

Wound Dehiscence and Delayed Wound Healing

Small wounds that are superficial and involve less than one-third of the incision can be managed conservatively with local wound care such as saline moist-to-dry gauze packing. These wounds typically completely heal by secondary intention. Larger wounds can be treated with negative-pressure wound therapy or operative debridement and secondary closure to accelerate healing. Expedited healing is especially important when the patient requires adjuvant therapy [2, 11].

Fluid Collection

Fluid collections including hematoma, seroma, and abscesses should be treated with percutaneous or open drainage. A simple seroma can be treated with serial aspiration or drain placement. A larger, persistent collection or abscess may necessitate extensive incision and drainage. In the case of an abscess, patients should be placed on culture-directed antibiotic therapy. A patient with a suspected urine leak should be evaluated and treated by the appropriate surgical team.

Infection

Cellulitis and local wound infection defined as localized erythema without fluid collection or dehiscence can be treated with antibiotic therapy.

Open, infected wounds are best treated with frequent dressing changes that promote mechanical debridement and drainage of purulent and necrotic tissue. Loosely packed moist-to-dry dressings with saline or Dakin's solution can be utilized for this purpose.

Deep organ space infections are diagnosed on imaging or re-exploration and are often dealt with by the ablative surgeon with serial debridement, removal of infected prosthetics, drain placement, and infectious disease consultation for antibiotic management.

Partial or Total Flap Loss

If a flap shows acute signs of arterial or venous insufficiency, it should be explored in the operating room emergently. One must investigate the pedicle for compression or kinking. In the case of a free flap, the arterial or venous anastomosis needs to be revised if there is a clot present.

Flaps that have early signs of venous congestion can be treated conservatively with leech therapy to improve flap circulation [21]. Progressive venous insufficiency warrants operative exploration as above.

Partial flap loss, defined as necrosis involving less than one-third of the flap volume, should be treated with bedside or formal operative debridement once the necrotic tissue has fully demarcated. This can be followed by local wound care, negative-pressure wound therapy, delayed primary closure, or flap re-advancement.

When larger or total flap loss occurs, the nonviable flap should be excised in the operating

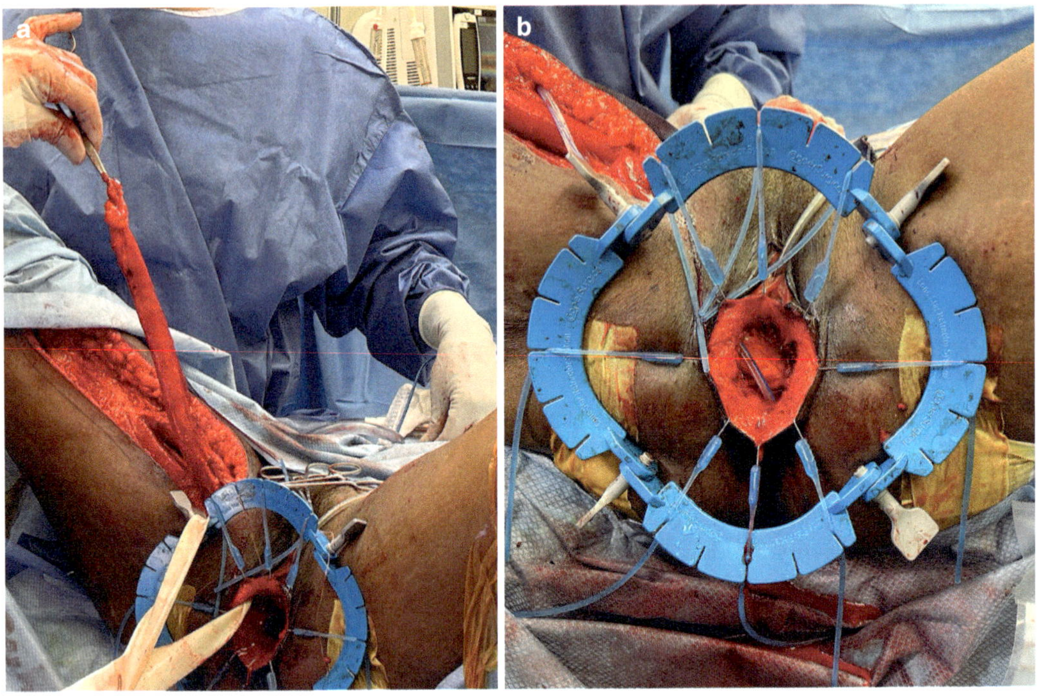

Fig. 41.6 (**a**) Right pedicled gracilis muscle flap isolated on its vascular pedicle. (**b**) Gracilis muscle flap inset for repair of rectovaginal fistula

room. The resulting defect can be temporized with negative-pressure wound therapy until definitive reconstruction with a lifeboat flap is performed. One should already have a secondary and tertiary reconstructive option in mind in the event of flap loss (Fig. 41.5a–b).

Fistula

Extensive fistulae can be addressed with a muscle or musculocutaneous flap to obliterate dead space and separate the involved anatomic organs. The gracilis flap is an ideal choice as it is located outside of the field of radiation and is typically spared in abdominal-based extirpative surgeries (Fig. 41.6a–b) [22, 23].

Donor Site Complications

A clinically significant donor site hernia or bulge can be addressed with exploration and repair with inlay or only mesh for abdominal wall support. Donor site dehiscence, fluid collections, and infection are treated as above.

Conclusion

Reconstruction plays an important role in facilitating extensive pelvic resections in the setting of malignancy. Complications are unfortunately a reality of reconstructive surgery and commonly occur in the pelvis due to its poor wound-healing environment. It is imperative to minimize risks at every stage of patient care, carefully analyze complications when they do occur, be prepared with a lifeboat for salvage reconstruction, and learn from mistakes to prevent them in the future.

References

1. Witte DYS, van Ramshorst GH, Lapid O, Bouman M-B, Tuynman JB. Flap reconstruction of perineal defects after pelvic exenteration: a systematic description of four choices of surgical reconstruction

methods. Plast Reconstr Surg. 2021;147(6):1420–35. https://doi.org/10.1097/prs.0000000000007976.
2. Hollenbeck ST, Toranto JD, Taylor BJ, et al. Perineal and lower extremity reconstruction. Plast Reconstr Surg. 2011;128(5):551e–63e. https://doi.org/10.1097/PRS.0b013e31822b6b87.
3. Devulapalli C, Jia Wei AT, DiBiagio JR, et al. Primary versus flap closure of perineal defects following oncologic resection: a systematic review and meta-analysis. Plast Reconstr Surg. 2016;137(5):1602–13. https://doi.org/10.1097/prs.0000000000002107.
4. Wang ED, Conkling N, Xu X, et al. Perineal flap reconstruction following oncologic anorectal extirpation: an outcomes assessment. Plast Reconstr Surg. 2015;135(1):176e–84e. https://doi.org/10.1097/prs.0000000000000837.
5. Jones HW, Rock JA. Te Linde's operative gynecology. In: Jones HW, Rock JA, editors. Books@Ovid. 11th ed. Wolters Kluwer; 2015.
6. Weichman KE, Matros E, Disa JJ. Reconstruction of peripelvic oncologic defects. Plast Reconstr Surg. 2017;140(4):601e–12e. https://doi.org/10.1097/prs.0000000000003703.
7. Westbom C, Talbot S. An Algorithmic Approach to Perineal Reconstruction. Plast Reconstr Surg Glob Open. 2019;7(12):e2572. https://doi.org/10.1097/GOX.0000000000002572.
8. Bialowas C, Nguyen B, Patel A. Best solutions for perineal and pressure sore reconstruction. Plast Reconstr Surg. 2021;148(6):1026e–39e. https://doi.org/10.1097/prs.0000000000008509.
9. Mericli AF, Martin JP, Campbell CA. An algorithmic anatomical subunit approach to pelvic wound reconstruction. Plast Reconstr Surg. 2016;137(3):1004–17. https://doi.org/10.1097/01.prs.0000479973.45051.b6.
10. Larson EL, McGinley KJ, Foglia AR, Talbot GH, Leyden JJ. Composition and antimicrobic resistance of skin flora in hospitalized and healthy adults. J Clin Microbiol. 1986;23(3):604–8. https://doi.org/10.1128/jcm.23.3.604-608.1986.
11. Nelson RA, Butler CE. Surgical outcomes of VRAM versus thigh flaps for immediate reconstruction of pelvic and perineal cancer resection defects. Plast Reconstr Surg. 2009;123(1):175–83. https://doi.org/10.1097/PRS.0b013e3181904df7.
12. Kim JT, Yew Ming Ho S, Hwang JH, Lee JH. Perineal perforator-based island flaps: the next frontier in perineal reconstruction. Plast Reconstr Surg. 2014;133(5):683e–7e. https://doi.org/10.1097/prs.0000000000000146.
13. Zeiderman MR, Nuño M, Sahar DE, Farkas LM. Trends in flap reconstruction of pelvic oncologic defects: analysis of the national inpatient sample. J Plast Reconstr Aesthet Surg. 2021;74(9):2085–94. https://doi.org/10.1016/j.bjps.2020.12.067.
14. Althumairi AA, Canner JK, Gearhart SL, Safar B, Sacks J, Efron JE. Predictors of perineal wound complications and prolonged time to perineal wound healing after abdominoperineal resection. World J Surg. 2016;40(7):1755–62. https://doi.org/10.1007/s00268-016-3450-0.
15. Campbell CA, Butler CE. Use of adjuvant techniques improves surgical outcomes of complex vertical rectus abdominis myocutaneous flap reconstructions of pelvic cancer defects. Plast Reconstr Surg. 2011;128(2):447–58. https://doi.org/10.1097/PRS.0b013e31821e6fd2.
16. Driessen C, van Hout N, van Kuppenveld P, et al. Usefulness of a template-based anterolateral thigh flap for reconstruction of head and neck defects. Microsurgery. 2020;40(7):776–82. https://doi.org/10.1002/micr.30637.
17. Weinstein B, King KS, Triggs W, Harrington MA, Pribaz J. Bilobed gracilis flap: a novel alternative for pelvic and perineal reconstruction. Plast Reconstr Surg. 2020;145(1):231.
18. Baumann DP, Butler CE. Component separation improves outcomes in VRAM flap donor sites with excessive fascial tension. Plast Reconstr Surg. 2010;126(5):1573–80. https://doi.org/10.1097/PRS.0b013e3181ef8d00.
19. Mougalian SS, Soulos PR, Killelea BK, et al. Use of neoadjuvant chemotherapy for patients with stage I to III breast cancer in the United States. Cancer. 2015;121(15):2544–52. https://doi.org/10.1002/cncr.29348.
20. Wong S, Garvey P, Skibber J, Yu P. Reconstruction of pelvic exenteration defects with anterolateral thigh–vastus lateralis muscle flaps. Plast Reconstr Surg. 2009;124(4):1177–85. https://doi.org/10.1097/PRS.0b013e3181b5a40f.
21. Hackenberger PN, Janis JE. A comprehensive review of medicinal leeches in plastic and reconstructive surgery. Plast Reconstr Surg Glob Open. 2019;7(12):e2555. https://doi.org/10.1097/gox.0000000000002555.
22. Hotouras A, Ribas Y, Zakeri S, Murphy J, Bhan C, Chan CL. Gracilis muscle interposition for rectovaginal and anovaginal fistula repair: a systematic literature review. Color Dis. 2015;17(2):104–10. https://doi.org/10.1111/codi.12791.
23. Zhang C, Yang X, Bi H. Application of depithelized gracilis adipofascial flap for pelvic floor reconstruction after pelvic exenteration. BMC Surg. 2022;22(1):304. https://doi.org/10.1186/s12893-022-01755-0.

Index

A
Abdominal perineal resection (APR), 389
Abdominal wall problems, 435
Abdominal wound infection, 432
Ablative procedures, 338
Abnormal placentation, 51, 52, 312
Activated partial thromboplastin time (aPTT), 7
Active voiding trial, 369
Acute coagulopathy, 313
Acute enteritis, 396, 397
Adhesiolysis, 441
Adjunctive techniques, 467
Aging-related impairments, 24, 26, 27
Alvimopan, 15, 16
Anal cancer, 394
Anal sphincteroplasty, 342
Anal squamous cell carcinoma, 388, 395
Anastomotic bleeding, 408
Anastomotic leak, 161
Anastomotic strictures, 406, 408
Angular pregnancies, 306
Anorectal and urinary problems, 435
Anorectal fistula, 215, 216
Anorectal manometry, 223
Antegrade colonic irrigation, 344
Anticoagulation, 7
Anus, anal margin, and vulvar, 421
Apical tenderness, 373
APR/ELAPE for rectal cancer, 391
Arterial embolization, 360
Asherman's syndrome, 47

B
Bilateral uterine artery ligation, 294
Bilateral V-Y gluteal fasciocutaneous flaps, 466
Bipolar thermal energy, 283
Bladder cancer (BCa), 117
Bladder defects, 328
Bladder dysfunction, 368, 369
Bladder injury, 297, 298, 327, 366, 367
  during pelvic dissection, 281
  management, 65, 66, 281, 282
  prevention, 64
  recognition, 64, 65
  risk factors, 64
Bladder toxicity, 419
Body image/psychological issues, 434
Bowel injury, 67, 68, 247, 248, 298
  and complications, 441, 442
  genital tract prolapse, 76
Bowel obstruction, 433
Brachytherapy, 417, 418

C
Carbohydrate loading, 14
Carbon dioxide embolism, 247
CAUTI, 371
Cellulitis and local wound infection, 469
Cervical and cesarean scar ectopic pregnancy, 306, 307
Cervical injury, 313, 314
Cesarean birth, 291
Cesarean delivery, 294
Cesarean hysterectomy, 293
  incidence, 319
  PAS, 321, 322, 324, 325
Charles procedure, 338
Charlson comorbidity index, 429
Chemoprophylaxis, 4–6
Chemoradiotherapy (CRT), 387
Chylous ascites, 361
Clinical coagulopathy, 327
Clitoral-sparing surgery, 345
Colonic reservoir, 148, 149
Colo-rectal anastomosis, 432
Colorectal anastomotic leak (AL), 401–403
Colorectal dysfunction, 369, 370
Colorectal malignancies, 439
Colorectal surgery, 441
Complex advanced fistula therapy, 216, 217
Complex pelvic sidewall anatomy, 440

M. Hoffman et al. (eds.), *Major Complications of Female Pelvic Surgery*,
https://doi.org/10.1007/978-3-031-66772-5

Composite pelvic resection, ovarian cancer
anastomotic bleeding, 384
anastomotic leak, 381–383
anastomotic stricture, 384, 385
bowel injury, 383, 384
post-operative hemorrhage, 378, 379
ureteral injury, 379, 380
vascular injury, 377, 378
Computed tomography pulmonary angiography (CT-PE), 7
Conduit necrosis, 161
Contemporary cesarean delivery of a term infant, 294
Continent cutaneous urinary diversion (CCUD)
afferent segment, 152
colonic reservoir, 148, 149
efferent segment, 150, 152
ileal reservoir, 149
ileocaecal reservoir, 146–148
incidence, 145
outcome, complications, and gender, 149, 150
Continuous bladder irrigation (CBI), 119
Cornuostomy, 306
Crohn's disease, 215, 216
Cryptoglandular abscess, 207–209
Cystitis, 120

D
D-dimer, 6
Deep infiltrating endometriosis (DIE)
bladder endometriosis, 257
diagnosis, 255
gastro-intestinal endometriosis, 260, 262
nerve-sparing surgery, 256
pathophysiology, 255
surgical approach, 256
treatment, 256
ureteral complications, 258–260
ureteral endometriosis, 257, 258
ureteral injury, 258–260
Deep organ space infections, 469
Delayed/missed ureteral injury, 443
Delayed wound healing, 468
Delorme's procedure, 238
Delphi technique, 404
Denonvilliers fascia, 413
Direct oral anticoagulants (DOACs), 7
Discitis, 236, 237
Disruption of the mesentery, 358–359
Disseminated intravascular coagulation (DIC), 313, 325, 327
Donor site complications, 470
Donor site hernia, 469
Donor site morbidity, 464
Duodenum, 359
Dysuria, 120, 121

E
Early pregnancy loss, 313
Ectopic pregnancy
complications, 301
diagnosis, 301
medical and surgical management, 301
Electrolyte/biochemical imbalances, 435
Empty pelvis syndrome, 434
Endoluminal approaches, *see* Transanal local excision (TAE)
Endometritis, 299
Endopelvic fascia, 89
Endorectal advancement flap (ERAF), 213, 214
Endoscopic mucosal resection (EMR), 190
Endoscopic submucosal dissection (ESD), 190
Endosponge, 404
Enhanced recovery after surgery (ERAS)
history, 13
immunonutrition, 17
intraoperative considerations, 15
postoperative considerations, 15, 16
prehabilitation, 17
preoperative considerations, 14, 15
RC/PLND/UD, 13
thromboembolic events, 17
USC protocol, 14
Enteric fistula, 433
Enterocutaneous fistula, 160, 161
Entrapped ovary, 273
Estrogen-based contraception, 4
Extensive fistulae, 470
Extensive subcutaneous edema, 434
External beam radiation therapy (EBRT), 417
External iliac vein, 353
Extra-levator abdominal perineal resection (ELAPE), 389

F
Fecal diversion, 344, 383, 403
Fecal incontinence (FI), 200
after radical vulvectomy, 344
anal insertion devices, 225
bowel function, 221
bulking agents, 226
complications, 395
definition, 221
diagnosis and evaluation, 222, 223
gynecologic malignancy, 222
OASIS, 221
prevention, 200
PTNS, 227
radiation therapy, 222
radiofrequency tissue remodeling, 226
recognition, 201
risk factors, 200
SNM, 227, 228
treatment, 201, 224, 225, 228
vaginal bowel control systems, 225, 226
VMR, 228
Female pelvic surgery
healing problems, 389

locally progressive/recurrent disease, 389
pelvic exenteration (*see* Pelvic exenteration (PEx))
positive resection margins, 389
salvage surgeries, 389
Female pelvis, 286, 287
Female urethra, 280
Female urethrectomy
advancement meatoplasty, 106, 107
distal urethrectomy, 103, 106, 107
higher-stage urethral cancers, 104
meatal stenosis and distal urethral stricture, 105, 106
meatotomy, 106
noncancerous diseases, 105
pubovaginal slings, 112, 113
PUC, 103
radical urethrectomy, 104, 105
SUI, 107–112
surgical intervention, 105
vulvar and vaginal cancers, 105
Femoral nerve injuries, 451
Femoral triangle, 335
Fistulae, 469
Fistula-in-ano
anatomy, 210
ERAF, 213, 214
etiology, 209
fistula plug/fibrin glue, 212
fistulotomy, 211
history, 209
imaging, 211
LIFT, 212, 213
location, 210
minimally invasive techniques, 214, 215
seton placement, 211, 212
subcutaneous/submucosal fistulas, 209
treatment, 211
Fistula laser tract closure (FiLaC), 214
Flap design, 465
Flap reconstruction, 463
Floating villi technique, 304
Fluid collections, 469
Fractures of pelvic ring and acetabulum, 454, 455
Frailty
aging, 23, 24
assessment, 24, 25
benefits, 25, 26
definition, 23
geriatricians and geriatric care providers, 27, 28
health-related outcomes, 25
interventions, 26, 27
Fried Frailty Index, 24
Future pregnancy outcome, 305

G
Gastrointestinal (GI) complications, 15
Gastro-intestinal endometriosis, 260, 262
General emotional support in preoperative and postoperative phases, 344
Generous meatotomy, 95
Genital tract prolapse
bowel injury, 76
intraoperative injuries
management, 75
prevention, 73, 74
recognition, 74
sacrospinous ligament fixation and sacral colpopexy, 73
nerve injury, 76–78
post operative complications, 78
urinary tract injury, 75, 76
Genitourinary complications, 277–280
Geriatric comanagement, 27
Giant liposarcoma, 284
Gonadotropin releasing hormone (GnRH), 43
Gracilis myocutaneous flap, 342
Gracilis neosphincter/artificial sphincter, 344
Groin dissection, 339
Groin pain, 85
GROINSS-V-1 prospective trial, 333
GROINSS-V-I study, 339
Gut microbiome, 35
Gynecologic cancers, 340
Gynecologic oncology, 441

H
Hardware failure, 455
Hematuria, 177
Hemipelvectomies, 451
Hemoperitoneum, 303
Hemorrhage, 320
after dilation and curettage/dilation and evacuation, 309
management, 63, 64
prevention, 62
recognition, 62, 63
risk factors, 61
Hernia, 436
Horseshoe abscess, 208
Human chorionic gonadotropin (hGC), 301
Hypogastric (internal iliac) arteries and veins, 283
Hysterectomy, 307
bladder injury, 64–66
bowel injury, 67, 68
hemorrhage
management, 63, 64
recognition, 62, 63
risk factors, 61
indications, 61
prevention, 62
ureteral injury, 66, 67
vaginal cuff dehiscence, 68, 69

I
Ileal conduit urinary diversion
anastomotic leak, 161
conduit necrosis, 161
enterocutaneous fistula, 160, 161

Ileal conduit urinary diversion (*cont.*)
  ileus and bowel obstruction, 160
  infection, 159, 160
  metabolic disturbances, 161, 162
  parastomal hernias, 157, 158
  sexual side effects and quality of life impact, 162
  stomal stenosis, 158, 159
  stoma-related complications, 157
  ureterointestinal strictures, 159
Ileal reservoir, 149
Ileocaecal reservoir, 146–148
Ileus/bowel obstruction, 138, 433
Impaired perineal wound healing, 389–391
Infertility
  bleeding and hysterectomy
    blood loss, 43
    management, 46–47
    prevention, 43, 45
    recognition, 45
  IUA, 47, 48
  ovarian reserve and loss of ovary, 55, 56
  uterine perforation, 49, 50
  uterine rupture and abnormal placentation, 51, 52
  volume overload, hysteroscopic procedures, 52–55
Inflammatory bowel disease (IBD)
  early postoperative complications
    anastomotic/pouch leaks and pelvic abscesses, 267–269
    SSIs, 267
  intraoperative complications
    reproductive organs, 265, 266
    ureter and bladder injury, 265
    vessels, 266, 267
  late postoperative complications
    anastomotic/pouch fistulas, 269–271
    entrapped ovary, 273
    infertility, 271, 272
    sexual dysfunction, 272
    unhealed perineal wound, 272, 273
Inguinal lymphadenectomy, 340
Inguinofemoral lymphadenectomy (IFL)
  early and aggressive surgical resection, 340
  infection, 340
  management of lymphedema, 338
  physiologic surgical options, 338
  prevention of lymphedema, 334, 335
  surgical management of lymphedema, 338
  surgical site complications, 340
  vascularized lymph nodes, 338
Intermittent self-catheterization (ISC), 369
Internal iliac venous plexus, 352
International Study Group of Rectal Cancer, 401
Interstitial pregnancy, 306
Intestinal anastomosis, 138
Intraoperative flap perfusion, 467
Intrauterine adhesive disease (IUA)
  management, 48
  prevalence, 47
  prevention, 47
  recognition, 48
Intrauterine pregnancy (IUP), 301, 305
Introital stenosis, 345
Intussusception, 176, 177
Inversion of the uterine corpus, 296, 297

L
Laceration of the vaginal wall, 277
Laparoendoscopic single-site surgery (LESS), 337
Laparoscopic entry and complications, 304
Laparoscopy, 303
Large bowel obstruction (LBO), 394
Large infected presacral fluid collection, 391
Lateral pelvic sidewall neurovascular exposure, 446
Lateral venorrhaphy, 354
LigaSure technology, 339
Ligation of intersphincteric fistula tract (LIFT), 212, 213, 216
Local excision for anal squamous cell cancer, 387
Low anterior resection syndrome (LARS), 410–412
Lower extremity lymphedema (LEL), 333
Lumbopelvic stabilization, 453
Lumbosacral plexus, 286
Lundiana pouch, 146
Lymphadenectomy, 351, 353
Lymphaticovenular anastomosis, 338
Lymphatic system, 352
Lymphedema, 356, 435, 436
Lymphocyst, 360
Lymphovenous anastomosis (LVA), 337
Lymphovenous bypass, 338

M
Major hemorrhage, 430
Major nerve (sciatic or femoral) resection, 445
Major pelvic bone tumor resections, 451
Malabsorption, 143
Malnutrition
  clinical assessments, 31–33
  consequences, 33, 34
  definition, 31
  gastrointestinal anatomic and functional alterations, 34
  neoadjuvant therapy, 34, 35
  preoperative malnutrition
    gut microbiome, 35
    mitigation, 35, 36
    prevalence, 33
Marshall-Marchetti-Krantz (MMK) procedure, 90
Massive hemorrhage, hemodynamic instability, 303–304
Massive obstetric hemorrhage, 321–325
Meatal stenosis, 105, 106
Mechanical bowel preparation (MBP), 14
Mechanical complications, 455
Mechanical tamponade, 293
Mechanism of venous injury, 283
Mechanism of venous laceration, 285
Mesenchymal stem cells (MSCs), 216
Mesentery of the sigmoid colon, 358, 359
Metabolic disturbances, 161, 162

Metabolic imbalance, 143
Methotrexate, 302, 305
Microsurgical anastomosis, 337
Microsurgical lymphatic bypass, 356
Midurethral slings (MUS), 84–88
  bladder injury, 85
  De Novo Irritative Voiding Symptoms, 88
  mesh erosion, 85
  pain, 85, 88
  recurrent incontinence, 88
  SIS, 85
  TOT, 84, 85
  TVT, 84
  voiding dysfunction, 88
Mild lymphedema, 356
Minimally invasive surgery
  incision site hernia, 250, 251
  obesity, 251
  surgical energy and thermal injury, 248–250
  Trendelenburg complications, 252
  trocar injury, 245–248
Mitrofanoff procedure, 150
Mixed augmentation ileum and caecum (MAINZ) pouch I, 146
Modified radical vulvectomy
  IFL, 339
  and inguinal lymphadenectomy, 333
Muscle flap transposition, 391
Muscle transfer techniques, 344

N
Narcotic pain, 15
Nasogastric (NG) tubes, 15
Necrotizing infection, 299, 339
Negative-pressure wound therapy (NPWT), 340
Neobladders
  early postoperative complications
    ileus/bowel obstruction, 138
    intestinal anastomosis, 138
    perioperative bleeding, 137
    urological anastomosis and suture lines, 138, 139
    UTI, 140
    vesicovaginal fistula, 139
  indication, 137
  long-term complications
    malabsorption, 143
    metabolic imbalance, 143
    pelvic organ prolapse, 142, 143
    psychological effects, 143
    sexual dysfunctions, 142
    short bowel syndrome, 143, 144
    urinary incontinence, 140, 141
    urinary retention, 141, 142
    urinary strictures, 141, 142
    urinary tract infections, 143
  urinary diversions, 137
Neostigmine, 16
Nephrostomy tubes, 433
Nerve injury, 356, 357, 449, 450
  and complication, 445–447
  genital tract prolapse, 76–78
Neurologic injury, 285, 286, 451
Neurosurgery, 441
Non-diagnostic laparoscopy, 304
Non-gynecologic tumors in the female pelvis, 276–277
Non-muscle invasive BCa (NMIBC), 117
Non-tubal ectopic pregnancy, 305–307
Non-urogynecological pelvic masse, 276

O
Obesity, 251
Obstetric anal sphincter injury (OASIS), 221
Obstetric hemorrhage, 320
Obturator nerve, 450, 451
Obturator neuropathy, 357
Open/laparoscopic surgery, 351
Orthopaedic surgery consultation, 454
Orthotopic neobladder, 140, 141, 143
Osteomyelitis, 455, 456
Ovarian cancer, composite pelvic resection
  anastomotic bleeding, 384
  anastomotic leak, 381–383
  anastomotic stricture, 384, 385
  bowel injury, 383, 384
  post-operative hemorrhage/hematomas, 378, 379
  ureteral injury, 379, 380
  vascular injury, 377
Ovarian sparing surgery for ovarian ectopic pregnancies, 307
Ovaries, 422

P
Palliative exenteration, 427
Parastomal hernias, 157, 158
Partial cystectomy (PC)
  advantages, 123
  complications, 125, 126
  contraindications, 123
  indications, 123
  oncological outcomes, 126, 127
  preoperative work-up, 124
  surgical technique, 124, 125
Partial/total flap loss, 469–470
Pedicled and free flaps, 468
Pedicled omentoplasty, 335
Pelvic abscess, 372, 401, 434
Pelvic and paraaortic lymphadenectomy (PPLND)
  arterial embolization, 360
  chylous ascites, 361
  complications, 351
  duodenum, 359, 360
  lymphedema, 356
  lymphocyst, 360
  mesentery of the sigmoid colon, 358, 359
  nerve injury, 356, 358
  ureteral injuries, 358
  vascular injury, 352, 353, 356

Pelvic and paraaortic lymph node removal, 351
Pelvic cancer, 455–458
Pelvic defect reconstruction with flaps, 464
Pelvic exclusion techniques, 393
Pelvic exenteration (PEx)
  circumferential resection margin, 427
  decision-making process, 429, 436
  delayed complications, 434, 435
  description, 427
  early complications, 432–434
  indications, 427
  infection risk, 431
  intra-operative complications, 429–432
  morbidity, 427
  multidisciplinary team (MDT) coordination, 429
  parastomal hernia, 436
  post-operative complications, 427, 432
  pre-operative considerations, 429
  prevention, early recognition and comprehensive treatment of complications, 429
  psychological support, 429
  radiation therapy, 427
  risk modification strategies, 429
  scrub teams, 429
  surgical site infection/collection, 429
Pelvic floor physical therapy and biofeedback, 411
Pelvic fluid collections/abscess/organ space infection, 387, 391, 392
Pelvic girdle tumors, 454
Pelvic lymphadenectomy, 351, 356
Pelvic lymph node dissection (PLND), 13
Pelvic organ prolapse, 142, 143
Pelvic Organ Prolapse Quantification system (POP-Q), 341
Pelvic radiotherapy, 417–424
Pelvic reconstructive procedures
  anatomic area, 463
  bulge/herniation formation, 467
  complication rate, 464
  early identification, 468
  extirpative and reconstructive phases, 463
  free tissue transfer, 466
  operative procedures, 465
  patient examination, 464
  perforator flaps, 464
  periumbilical perforators, 466
  postoperative activity modification and positioning, 467
  post-operative antibiotics, 468
  pre-operative evaluation, 464
  prevention and mitigation of, 464
  primary closure, 463
  prophylactic intravenous antibiotics, 465
  risk factors, 464
  skin grafts, and flaps, 463
  wide surgical preparation and draping of the pelvis and donor sites, 465
Pelvic resection for gynecologic malignancies, 439
Pelvic ring and acetabulum, fractures, 454, 455
Pelvic sidewall disease, 440
Pelvic sidewall tumor, 447
Percutaneous tibial nerve stimulation (PTNS), 227
Perianal abscess, 207–209
Perianal cancer without sphincter involvement, 389
Perianal pain, 435
Perineal dehiscence, abdominal perineal resection for anal cancer, 278
Perineal hernia, 278, 387, 392, 393
Perineal wound
  complications, 387
  dehiscence, 390
Peritonitis, 433
Persistent ectopic pregnancy (PEP), 305
Placenta accreta, 312
Placenta accreta spectrum (PAS), 319, 321–324, 327, 328
Plastics reconstruction, 432, 435, 436, 441
Positive pregnancy test, 303
POSSUM score, 429
Postabortal infection, 315
Post-abortion hemorrhage, 309
Post-cesarean infections, 298, 299
Posterior tibial nerve modulation, 344
Postoperative groin cellulitis, 339
Postoperative sexual function, extensive perineal excision, 343
Postpartum hemorrhage, 292, 293
Post-polypectomy syndrome, 191, 194
Preoperative relational dissatisfaction, 345
Presacral sinuses, 273
Presacral venous bleeding, 409, 410
Presacral venous plexus (PVP), 444
Pressure sores, 434
Primary anal reconstruction, 342
Primary haemorrhage, 432
Primary urethral cancers (PUC), 103
Procidentia, *see* Rectal prolapse
Progressive obstructive symptoms complications, 394
Progressive vaginal stenosis, 436
Propensity score matched analysis, 339
Prophylactic antibiotics, 197
Prophylactic use of endovascular interventions, 322
Psychosexual, 435
Pubovaginal slings (PVS), 110, 111
  bladder perforation, 89
  De Novo Irritative Voiding Symptoms, 89
  fascia lata, 112
  overview, 88, 89
  rectus sheath, 112, 113
  recurrent incontinence, 90
  sling erosion, 113
  urinary retention, 89
Pudendal nerve, 450
  damage, 450
  injury, 451
  terminal motor latencies, 344
Pudendal neuropathy, 344

Q

Quality of life, 435

R

Radiation associated sarcomas, 459–460
Radiation-induced bladder and urinary acute effects, 419
Radiation osteitis, 458
Radiation proctitis, 421
Radiation therapy, female pelvic malignancies, 417
Radiation toxicity, 420
  incidence and severity, 419
  in the large bowel/rectum, 420
Radiation treatment
  acute toxicities, 417, 419
  late toxicities, 417, 419, 420
Radical cystectomy
  bladder cancer, 129
  complications, 130
    bleeding/thromboembolic, 131, 132
    cardiopulmonary, 131
    gastrointestinal, 131
    genitourinary, 130
    infection, 130
    lymphocele, 132
    neurologic, 132
    organ-sparing cystectomy, 133
    ovary removal risks, 133
    vaginal, 133
  surgical approach, 129, 130
Radical hysterectomy, 365
  blood supply of ureter, 366
  complications, 363
    bladder dysfunction, 366–369
    colorectal dysfunction, 369, 370
    rectal injury, 367
    sexual dysfunction, 372, 373
    surgical site infection, 370–372
    urinary tract injury, 364, 365
    vaginal dehiscence, 370
  neuroanatomy, 368
  oncologic resection of a pelvic malignancy, 363
  ureter through the parametrium, 364
Radical lymphadenectomy, 340
Radical vulvar surgery, 341
Radical vulvectomy, 342
  functional impairments, 341, 342
  IFL, 339
  infection, 340
  loco-regional recurrence after wide local excision, 345
  and lymphadenectomy, 339
  NPWT, 340
  surgical debridement, 340
  vacuum-assisted closure in complex wound failures, 340
Radiofrequency tissue remodeling, 226
Radionuclide lymphoscintigraphy, 333
Reconstructive surgery, 342
Rectal carcinoma, 401–403, 405, 406, 408–410, 412, 414
Rectal hyposensitivity, 223
Rectal injury, 367, 431
Rectal prolapse
  abdominal procedures, 232–233
  abdominal surgery complications, 233, 234
  anastomotic leaks, 237
  definition, 231
  diagnosis, 231
  discitis, 236, 237
  hemorrhagic complications, 234, 235
  intraabdominal collections/ seromas/ abscess, 237
  mesh complications, 235, 236
  multicompartment prolapse repairs, 239
  perineal surgery, 238, 239
  postoperative constipation/fecal impaction, 239
  postoperative pain, 238
  preoperative procedures, 232
  risk factors, 231
  SBO, 237
  surgical repair, 231
  ureteral injury, 237
Rectopexy, 234, 235
Rectosigmoid anastomosis, 381
Rectosigmoid carcinoma, 401–404, 406, 408–410, 412, 413
Rectosigmoid junction, 397, 398
Rectovaginal fistulas (RVFs), 395, 396
Rectus muscle flap, 390
Recurrent and metastatic lesions, 458–459
Recurrent ectopic pregnancy (REP), 305
Recurrent pelvic sidewall tumor resection
  extended surgical resection, 439
  management, 439
  recurrence, 439
  recurrent pelvic sidewall tumors, 440
  surgical approaches, 439
Regional anesthesia, 15
Renal impairment, 434, 436
Residual pregnancy tissue/blood products, 315
Retropubic suspensions, 90
Right pedicled anterolateral thigh with an extended skin paddle, 467
Right pedicled gracilis muscle flap, 470
Robot-assisted RC (RARC), 15
Robotic-assisted video-endoscopic inguinal lymphadenectomy (RAVEIL), 337
Ruptured ectopic pregnancy, 303, 304

S

Sacral nerve neuromodulation (SNM), 227
Sacral nerve stimulation, 344, 414
Sacral resection, 453
Sacral transection, 430
Sacrectomy, 431, 451, 453, 454
Salpingectomy, 305

Salpingostomy, 305
Saphenous vein preservation, 335
Sarcoma, 275
Sciatic nerve, 449
Secondary lymphedema after lymphadenectomy, 333
Sentinel lymph node (SLN) dissection, 333
  mapping, 338
  sampling, 339
Sexual dysfunction, 142, 272, 341, 372, 373
  physiological changes, 345
  rectal cancer treatment, 412, 413
  vulvar cancer, 345
Sexual intercourse, 277
Short bowel syndrome, 143, 144
Simple cesarean hysterectomy, 319, 320
Single incision laparoscopic surgery (SILS), 250
Single incision slings (SIS), 85
Sinus tract marsupialization, 405
Skin toxicity, 421
Small bowel, 420
Small bowel obstruction (SBO), 237, 387, 393, 394
SolestaR injection, 226
Sphincteroplasty, 344
Staccato tapping, 118
Stomal problems, 433
Stomal stenosis, 158, 159
Stress urinary incontinence (SUI), 368
  definition, 83
  female urethrectomy, 107–112
  injectable therapy, 83, 84
  MUS, 84–88
    bladder injury, 85
    De Novo Irritative Voiding Symptoms, 88
    mesh erosion, 85
    pain, 85, 88
    recurrent incontinence, 88
    SIS, 85
    TOT, 84, 85
    TVT, 84
    voiding dysfunction, 88
  PVS
    bladder perforation, 89
    De Novo Irritative Voiding Symptoms, 89
    overview, 88, 89
    recurrent incontinence, 90
    urinary retention, 89
  retropubic suspensions
    Burch procedure, 90
    overview, 90
    recurrent incontinence, 90
    voiding dysfunction, 90
  urethral diverticulectomy, 97, 98
Subclinical AL, 405
Subjective Global Assessment (SGA), 31
Suction-assisted lipectomy, 338
Suction thrombectomy, 8
Superficial fluid collections, 468
Superficial infection, 468
Supralevator abscesses, 207
Supralevator exenterative procedure, 432
Suprasphincteric fistulas, 210
Surgical abortion, 309, 310, 312–316
Surgical oncology, 441
Surgical site infection (SSI), 267, 298, 320, 321, 370–372
Surgical wound complications, 460
Sustained thermal injury, 281
Suture rectopexy (SR), 237
Sympathetic and parasympathetic nerve injuries, 286
Symptomatic strictures, 397, 398

T

Tamoxifen, 4
Tension-free vaginal tape (TVT), 84
Thermal damage, 364
Thermal injury, 365
Thrombo-embolic problems, 434
Thrombolysis, 8
Traction/compression injury, 286
Transanal local excision (TAE)
  abscess
    management, 198
    prevention, 197
    recognition, 197
    surgical site infections, 197
  bleeding
    management, 196
    prevention, 195, 196
    recognition, 196
    risk factors, 195
  conventional retractors and sutures, 189
  EMR and ESD, 190
  fecal incontinence, 200
    management, 201
    prevention, 200
    recognition, 201
    risk factors, 200
  perforation
    delayed perforations, 191
    ESD, 191
    intra-procedural perforations, 190
    management, 194, 195
    post-polypectomy syndrome, 191
    prevention, 191–194
    recognition, 194
  polyps, 189
  screening, 189
  strictures, 198–200
  TAMIS, 189, 190
  urinary retention, 201, 202
Transanal minimally invasive surgery (TAMIS), 189, 190, 192, 193, 195, 200
Transobturator tape (TOT), 84, 85
Transsphincteric fistulas, 209, 210
Transurethral macroplastique injection, 110, 111
Transurethral resection of a bladder tumor (TURBT)
  bleeding and reoperation/transfusion, 119, 120
  non-infective cystitis and voiding discomfort, 120, 121

perforation, 117, 118
risk factors, 117
symptom, 117
UTIs, 120
Transvaginal marsupialization, 95
Trauma and extensive extirpative gynecologic, urologic and/or colorectal surgery for malignancy, 463
Trendelenburg complications, 252
Trocar injury, 245–248
Trocar site hernia, 250, 251
Tubal ectopic pregnancy, 301–305
Tubal rupture and hemoperitoneum, 304
Tumor of female pelvis, 275, 276
Tumors of bony pelvis, 449
Turnbull-Cutait technique, 217

U
Uncontrolled obstetric hemorrhage, 320
Underwater EMR (UEMR), 192
Unfractionated heparin, 7
Unhealed perineal wound, 272, 273
Unilateral/bilateral lower extremity edema, 356
Unilateral/bilateral rhomboid flaps/local advancement flaps, 342
Unintended hysterotomy extension, 294–296
Unintended nerve injury, 446
Ureteral avulsion, 176, 177
Ureteral endometriosis (UE), 257, 258
Ureteral injury, 66, 67, 358, 363, 365, 366
anatomy, 167
DIE, 255, 256, 258, 259
management
bladder flap, 171
delayed recognition, 169
methylene blue, 168
mucosal apposition, 169
non-refluxing anastomosis, 171, 172
perforation, 168
psoas hitch, 169
reconstruction, 169
penetrating trauma, 167
prevention and evaluation, 168
Ureteral stents, 442
Ureteral stricture, 435
Ureteral wall injury, 176
Ureterointestinal strictures, 159
Ureteroscopy
early postoperative complication
intravascular stent misplacement, 180
pain and ureteral obstruction, 179
post obstructive diuresis, 180
premature labor, 179
ureteral stent discomfort, 179
ureteral stent migration, 180
urinoma, perirenal abscess and hematomas, 178
UTI and sepsis, 178, 179
vascular anomalies, 178
intraoperative complication
access, 177
bleeding, 177
ureteral avulsion and intussusception, 176, 177
ureteral wall injury, 176
late postoperative complication
neglected stents, 181, 182
ureteral stricture, 181
upper urinary tract, 175
Ureters (fibrosis), 431
Urethral bulking agent (UBA), 83, 84
Urethral diverticulectomy (UD)
complications, 97
diagnosis, 94, 95
differential diagnosis, 95
excision and reconstruction, 96, 97
indications, 95
pathophysiology, 93
prevalence and presentation, 94
recurrences, 99, 100
stress urinary incontinence, 97, 98
stricture, 99
surgical management, 95
urethrovaginal fistula, 98, 99
Urethral eversion, 344, 345
Urethrovaginal fistula, 98, 99
Urinary diversion (UD), 13, 16, 431, 433
Urinary dysfunction, 412, 413
Urinary incontinence, 140, 141, 341
anatomical distortions, 344
sympathetic nerve injury, 412
Urinary injury, 280, 281
Urinary leak, 433
Urinary retention, 141, 142, 201, 202
Urinary strictures, 141, 142
Urinary tract infections (UTIs), 16, 372
neobladders, 140, 143
ureteroscopy, 178, 179
Urinary tract injury
complications, 442, 443
genital tract prolapse, 75, 76
Urine/bowel contents, 298
Urinomas, 380
Urologic Injury, 327
Urological practice, 429
Urology, 441
Uterine artery embolization (UAE), 293, 307
Uterine atony, 309, 310
Uterine injury, 314
Uterine perforation, 49, 50, 314
Uterine rupture, 51, 52, 296
Uterine scar dehiscence, 296
Uterine scar rupture, 319
Uterus damage, 422
"Utra-radical" resection strategies, 439

V
Vacuum assisted closure (VAC) dressings, 391
Vaginal bowel control systems, 225, 226
Vaginal cuff dehiscence, 68, 69
Vaginal dehiscence and evisceration, 370

Vaginal effects, pelvic XRT, 423
Vaginal lubrication, 412
Vaginal preparation, hysterectomy, 339
Vascular injury, 282, 352–355, 451–453
  and complications, 443–445
  during resection of pelvic tumors, 282, 285
Vascular ligation techniques, 293
Vascular/lymphatics/nerves, radiation, 423, 424
Vascular sclerosis, 420
Vascular surgery, 441
Venous injury, 283
Venous thromboembolism (VTE)
  diagnosis, 6, 7
  epidemiology, 3
  prevention, 4–6
  risk factors, 3, 4
  treatment, 7–9
Ventral mesh rectopexy (VMR), 228, 235
Vertical rectus abdominus myocutaneous (VRAM) flap, 389, 390, 466
Vesicovaginal fistula, 139
Video-assisted anal fistula treatment (VAAFT), 214
Video-endoscopic inguinal lymphadenectomy (VEIL), 337
Vitamin B12 deficiency, 143
Vitamin K antagonists, 7
Vulvar reconstruction, 342
Vulvectomy, 333, 338, 340, 341
Vulvovaginal carcinoma surgery, 342
Vulvovaginal oncologic surgery, 343
Vulvovaginal reconstruction, 342
V-Y advancement gluteal fold flap, 342

W

Wexner fecal incontinence scale, 342
WHO checklist, 429–432
Wound breakdown, 339
Wound dehiscence
  and delayed wound healing, 468, 469
  and superficial infection, 460, 461
Wound infection, 299, 339

GPSR Compliance

The European Union's (EU) General Product Safety Regulation (GPSR) is a set of rules that requires consumer products to be safe and our obligations to ensure this.

If you have any concerns about our products, you can contact us on ProductSafety@springernature.com

In case Publisher is established outside the EU, the EU authorized representative is:

Springer Nature Customer Service Center GmbH
Europaplatz 3
69115 Heidelberg, Germany

Batch number: 10044841

Printed by Printforce, the Netherlands